Nanotherapeutics for the Treatment of Hepatocellular Carcinoma

Edited by

Biswajit Mukherjee

Department of Pharmaceutical Technology,
Jadavpur University,
Kolkata 700032,
India

&

Former Guest Scientist, German Cancer Research Center (DKFZ),
Heidelberg, Germany

Nanotherapeutics for the Treatment of Hepatocellular Carcinoma

Editor: Biswajit Mukherjee

ISBN (Online): 978-981-5039-74-0

ISBN (Print): 978-981-5039-75-7

ISBN (Paperback): 978-981-5039-76-4

Bentham Science Publishers Pte. Ltd.
80 Robinson Road #02-00
Singapore 068898
Singapore
Email: subscriptions@benthamscience.net

CONTENTS

PREFACE

Cancer is a fatal disease, and hepatocellular carcinoma (HCC) has become a predominant cause of cancer-related deaths. Existing therapy against the HCC is inadequate for several reasons, such as late diagnosis, HCC being asymptomatic at the initial stage, liver resection or transplantation as an advisable treatment option, non-availability of the liver for transplantation, rejection of the transplanted liver by the body, nonspecific chemotherapy that causes damages to cancerous as well as normal hepatic cells, fast rejection of free drug/small molecules from hepatic tumors, the formation of resistance against chemotherapy by cancer cells, and the dearth of the non-targeted drug system.

Hence, it is essential to deliver the drug/formulation specifically to the cancer cells to induce apoptosis and reduction or cessation of proliferation, keeping normal healthy cells unaffected. Nanoscale drug delivery systems show such capabilities for targeted drug delivery to the HCC specific cells, avoiding the normal cells. Several investigations showed how productive and beneficial nanotherapy is in successfully delivering a drug in HCC cells by specifically targeting cancer cells. Commercial availability of the new formulations has been explored and is already in the pipeline of commercialization. Hence, it is important to understand nanotherapy and its correlation to HCC patients to control HCC in a better and satisfactory way. However, technology still needs to be improved for ease of manufacturing and cost-effective production of nanotherapy against HCC. More efforts are required to concentrate on the targeting aspects of the formulation of HCC cells.

The content of this book would be suitable for medical students, medical faculties, researchers of medicines, biomedical scientists, and researchers studying and working in hepatocellular carcinoma and nanotherapy. In this book, several chapters by the authoritative experts of the field have explored all the areas of nanotherapeutics against HCC. The readers will benefit from the knowledge shared by the experts. Thus, nanotherapeutics have shown considerable potential and tremendous impetus for rapid translation from the pre-clinical to the clinical domain to significantly prolong the survival in HCC. Based on the recent investigations, the book is intended to highlight the impact of nanotherapeutics in HCC treatment and its future direction.

Biswajit Mukherjee
Department of Pharmaceutical Technology,
Jadavpur University,
Kolkata 700032,
India,

List of Contributors

Akhil Suresh	Department of Pharmaceutics, Manipal College of Pharmaceutical Sciences, Manipal Academy of Higher Education, Manipal, Karnataka, India
Apala Chakraborty	Department of Pharmaceutical Technology, Jadavpur University, Kolkata 700032, WB, India
Ashique Al Hoque	Department of Pharmaceutical Technology, Jadavpur University, Kolkata 700032, WB, India
Asma Aktar	Department of Pharmacy, Jashore University of Science and Technology, Jashore-7408, Bangladesh
Ben J. Slotman	Amsterdam UMC, Vrije Universiteit Amsterdam, Department of Radiation Oncology, Cancer Center Amsterdam,
Biswadip Sinha	Institute of Pharmacy, Dept. of Pharmaceutics, Biopharmaceutics & Nutricosmetics, Freie University of Berlin, Berlin, Germany
Biswajit Mukherjee	Department of Pharmaceutical Technology, Jadavpur University, Kolkata 700032, India
Bivek Chaulagain	Department of Pharmaceutical Sciences, North Dakota State University, Fargo, North Dakota 58105, USA
Buddhadev Layek	Department of Pharmaceutical Sciences, North Dakota State University, Fargo, North Dakota 58105, USA
Chamalki Madhusha	Department of Chemistry, Faculty of Applied Sciences, University of Sri Jayewardenepura, Gangodawila, Nugegoda, Sri Lanka
Chetan H Metha	Department of Pharmaceutics, Manipal College of Pharmaceutical Sciences, Manipal Academy of Higher Education, Manipal, Karnataka, India
D. Nedra Karunaratne	Department of Chemistry, University of Peradeniya, Peradeniya, Sri Lanka
Debasmita Dutta	Department of Molecular and Human Genetics, Baylor College of Medicine, Houston, Texas 77030, United States Department of Pharmaceutical Technology, Jadavpur University, Kolkata-700032, West Bengal, India
Disni Dedunupitiya	Department of Chemistry, Faculty of Science, University of Peradeniya, Peradeniya, Sri Lanka
Elisa Giovannetti	Amsterdam UMC, Vrije Universiteit Amsterdam, Department of Medical Oncology, Cancer Center Amsterdam, The Netherlands, Fondazione Pisana per la Scienza, Pisa, Italy
Geethi K. Pamunuwa	Department of Horticulture and Landscape Gardening, Faculty of Agriculture and Plantation Management, Wayamba University of Sri Lanka, Makandura, Gonawila, Sri Lanka
Imalka Munaweera	Department of Chemistry, Faculty of Applied Sciences, University of Sri Jayewardenepura, Gangodawila, Nugegoda, Sri Lanka Instrument Center, Faculty of Applied Sciences, University of Sri Jayewardenepura, Gangodawila, Nugegoda, Sri Lanka

Iman Ehsan	Department of Pharmaceutical Technology, Jadavpur University, Kolkata 700032, India
Jagdish Singh	Department of Pharmaceutical Sciences, North Dakota State University, Fargo, North Dakota 58105, USA
Kishor Mazumder	School of Optometry and Vision Science, UNSW Medicine, University of New South Wales (UNSW), Sydney, NSW, Australia School of Biomedical Sciences, Charles Sturt University, Wagga Wagga, NSW 2650, Australia Department of Pharmacy, Jashore University of Science and Technology, Jashore-7408, Bangladesh
Laboni Das	School of Pharmacy, Techno India University, EM-4, Sector-V, Salt Lake, Kolkata, WB, India
Md. Emran Hossain	Department of Pharmacy, Jashore University of Science and Technology, Jashore-7408, Bangladesh
Manasadeepa Rajagopalan	East West College of Pharmacy, Bangalore, Karnataka, 560091, India
Manisheeta Ray	Department of Pharmaceutical Technology, Jadavpur University, Kolkata 700032, India
Maria Lucia A.D Lestari	Faculty of Pharmacy Universitas Airlangga Surabaya, Department of Pharmaceutical Science, Surabaya, Indonesia
Moumita Dhara	Department of Pharmaceutical Technology, Jadavpur University, Kolkata-700032, West Bengal, India
N Udupa	Department of Pharmaceutics, Manipal College of Pharmaceutical Sciences, Manipal Academy of Higher Education, Manipal, Karnataka, India
Nilwala Kottegoda	Department of Chemistry, Faculty of Applied Sciences, University of Sri Jayewardenepura, Gangodawila, Nugegoda, Sri Lanka Center for Advanced Materials Research (CAMR), Faculty of Applied Sciences, University of Sri Jayewardenepura, Gangodawila, Nugegoda, Sri Lanka
Nuwanthi P. Katuwavila	Faculty of Engineering and Science, National School of Business Management, Mahenwatte, Pitipana, Homagama, Sri Lanka
Pei Pei Che	Amsterdam UMC, Vrije Universiteit Amsterdam, Department of Radiation Oncology, Cancer Center Amsterdam, Amsterdam UMC, Vrije Universiteit Amsterdam, Department of Medical Oncology, Cancer Center Amsterdam, The Netherlands,
Peter Sminia	Amsterdam UMC, Vrije Universiteit Amsterdam, Department of Radiation Oncology, Cancer Center Amsterdam,
Prasanta Ghosh	Department of Pharmaceutical Technology, Jadavpur University, Kolkata 700032, India
Ramkrishna Sen	Department of Pharmaceutical Technology, Jadavpur University, Kolkata 700032, India
Richard N. L. Lamptey	Department of Pharmaceutical Sciences, North Dakota State University, Fargo, North Dakota 58105, USA

Riddhi Trivedi	Department of Pharmaceutical Sciences, North Dakota State University, Fargo, North Dakota 58105, USA
Samrat Chakraborty	Department of Pharmaceutical Technology, Jadavpur University, Kolkata 700032, India
Sanchari Bhattacharya	Guru Nanak Institute of Pharmaceutical Science and Technology, 157 f, Nilgunj Rd, Sahid Colony, Panihati, Kolkata, West Bengal, India
Sanjay Arora	Department of Pharmaceutical Sciences, North Dakota State University, Fargo, North Dakota 58105, USA
Shreyasi Chakraborty	Department of Pharmaceutical Technology, Jadavpur University, Kolkata 700032, WB, India
Somenath Datta	Duke Molecular Physiology Institute (DMPI), Duke University School of Medicine, Durham, North Carolina, USA
Suresh Ajmeera	School of Biological Sciences, National Institute of Science Education and Research, HBNI, Khordha, Jatni, Odisha, 752050, India
Srinivas Mutalik	Department of Pharmaceutics, Manipal College of Pharmaceutical Sciences, Manipal Academy of Higher Education, Manipal, Karnataka, India
Susanthi Jayasinghe	Department of Chemistry, Faculty of Science, University of Peradeniya, Peradeniya, Sri Lanka
Thusini D. Wijerathne	Department of Chemistry, University of Peradeniya, Peradeniya, Sri Lanka
Usha Y Nayak	Department of Pharmaceutics, Manipal College of Pharmaceutical Sciences, Manipal Academy of Higher Education, Manipal, Karnataka, India
V Badireenath Konkimalla	School of Biological Sciences, National Institute of Science Education and Research, HBNI, Khordha, Jatni, Odisha, 752050, India
Varalakshmi Velagacherla	Department of Pharmaceutics, Manipal College of Pharmaceutical Sciences, Manipal Academy of Higher Education, Manipal, Karnataka, India
Veranja Karunaratne	Department of Chemistry, Faculty of Science, University of Peradeniya, Peradeniya, Sri Lanka

CHAPTER 1

Hepatocellular Carcinoma: Diagnosis, Molecular Pathogenesis, Biomarkers, and Conventional Therapy

Biswajit Mukherjee[*, 1], Manasadeepa Rajagopalan[2], Samrat Chakraborty[1], Prasanta Ghosh[1], Manisheeta Ray[1], Ramkrishna Sen[1] and Iman Ehsan[1]

[1] *Department of Pharmaceutical Technology, Jadavpur University, Kolkata 700032, India*

[2] *East West College of Pharmacy, Bangalore, Karnataka 560091, India*

Abstract: Hepatocellular carcinoma (HCC), the most common liver malignancy, has been a significant cause of cancer-related deaths worldwide. Cirrhosis, hepatic viral infections, fatty liver, and alcohol consumption are notable risk factors associated with HCC. Furthermore, a crucial challenge in the therapeutic management of HCC patients is the late-stage diagnosis, primarily due to the asymptomatic early stage. Despite the availability of various preventive techniques, diagnoses, and several treatment options, the mortality rate persists. Ongoing investigation on exploring molecular pathogenesis of HCC and identifying different prognostic and diagnostic markers may intervene in the conventional mode of treatment option for better therapeutic management of the disease. Subsequently, tumor site and its size, extrahepatic spread, and liver function are the underlying fundamental factors in treating treatment modality. The development in both surgical and non-surgical methods has resulted in admirable benefits in the survival rates. Understanding the mechanism(s) of tumor progression and the ability of the tumor cells to develop resistance against drugs is extremely important for designing future therapy concerning HCC. This chapter has accumulated the current literature and provided a vivid description of HCC based on its classification, risk factors, stage-based diagnosis systems, molecular pathogenesis, prognostic/diagnostic markers, and the existing conventional treatment approaches.

Keywords: Cellular signaling pathway, Cirrhosis, HCC molecular pathogenesis, HCC- prognostic/diagnostic markers, HCC risk factors, Hepatocellular carcinoma (HCC), cell signaling during HCC development, Ongoing therapy against HCC, Stage-based diagnosis, Tumor microenvironment.

* **Corresponding author Biswajit Mukherjee:** Department of Pharmaceutical Technology, Jadavpur University, Kolkata 700032, India; Tel/Fax: +913324146677; Emails: biswajit55@yahoo.com, biswajit.mukherjee@jadavpuruniversity.in

INTRODUCTION

Hepatocellular carcinoma (HCC) is a malignant form of highly progressive primary liver cancer. It originates from hepatocytes. Around 0.9 million new cases and 0.8 million deaths of liver cancer patients globally have been reported in 2020 by the International Agency for Research on Cancer. Increasing mortality rates and late-stage diagnosis often make HCC a tremendous challenge for its better therapeutic management. Hence patients detected with early-stage HCC possess a greater chance of getting a positive response with different treatment protocols. HCC may not show any symptoms at an early stage of cancer. Still, with the disease's progress, the symptoms such as pain at the right side of the upper abdominal part, fatigue, bloating, loss of appetite, nausea, vomiting, fever, pale bowels, and dark urine may appear. Several risk factors are associated with infected livers, fatty liver, and chronic alcohol consumption in a high amount. In the case of cirrhotic liver, the treatment decisions become limited except the finding of liver transplantation. Due to cirrhosis, any planned liver resection gets limited since the remaining liver may not tolerate volume loss and regenerate. However, an effective treatment method for HCC and cirrhosis of the liver is orthotopic liver transplantation (OLT), but early-stage HCC detection is required for such cases. HCC and cirrhosis are more significant in patients with hepatitis C virus (HCV) infection.

Several upstream or downstream regulators in various signaling cascades activate/ inactivate to continue uncontrolled proliferation in the cancerous processes (Mello and Attardi 2018, Nam and van Deursen 2014, Dolgin 2017). Epigenetic alterations may cause DNA methylation and other histone modifications that confer significant alteration to the genome. The epigenetic modification may inactivate tumor suppressor genes or cause the sudden activation of oncogenes. These may ultimately cause cancer (Kanwal and Gupta, 2012). Thus, a vivid understanding of the tumor microenvironment only can lead to exploring molecular pathogenesis more accurately and minutely to access the more appropriate and convincing therapeutic management of HCC. Suitable diagnostic and prognostic biomarkers are still essential to identify the disease early as the treatment decisions strictly depend on the tumor stage.

Hence, in this chapter, we want to introduce HCC with its classification, risk factors, and various diagnostic staging based on current literature. Tumor microenvironment and molecular pathogenesis during HCC development and progression, along with prognostic/diagnostic HCC markers, have been explored here. The existing conventional treatment approaches give a better understanding of the current way of therapeutic management of HCC.

CANCER AND ITS TYPES

The liver is the largest organ that primarily undergoes detoxification, metabolism, break-down of blood cells, protein synthesis, and bile synthesis. The liver predominantly contains hepatocytes. However, other cell types such as perisinusoidal fat-storing cells or ito cells, hepatic stellate cells, Kupffer cells, and hepatic sinusoidal endothelial cells are also available in the liver (Guyton and Hall 2006, Fox 2011). Neoplasm that grows in epithelial cells is carcinoma, whereas mesenchymal (connective tissue) origin is a sarcoma. Both types appear in the liver.

Primary liver cancer begins in the liver and secondary liver cancer cells where neoplastic cells develop in a different organ and migrate to the liver.

Primary Liver Cancer

Hepatocellular Carcinoma (HCC)

The most common primary liver cancer that accounts for nearly 75 percent of all liver cancers in adults is HCC. It originates from hepatocytes. HCC usually metastasizes to the lungs, bone marrow, and other digestive organs, including the stomach, pancreas, and small and large intestines, including the colon.

Intrahepatic Cholangiocarcinoma (Bile Duct Cancer)

Intrahepatic cholangiocarcinomas originate from epithelial cells of the cell-lining present in small bile ducts. The type accounts for 10-20% of hepatic cancers (Gupta and Dixon 2017).

Angiosarcoma and Hemangiosarcoma

They are primarily rare forms of primary hepatic cancer. Their origin is the endothelial cells of hepatic blood vessels. The reports suggest that these forms of cancer are familiar to people who had prolonged exposure to chemicals such as thorium dioxide and vinyl chloride (Molina and Hernandez 2003, Bolt 2005).

Hepatoblastoma

Unifocal immature fetal precursor liver cells seem to be the origin of this scarce hepatoblastoma. Although rare, hepatoblastoma is only seen in infants and children, usually up to three years of age. Hepatoblastoma can metastasize. (Hoshida *et al.*, 2012, Meyers *et al.*, 2012, Wang *et al.*, 2013).

Secondary Liver Cancer

Secondary cancer is advanced liver cancer. The aptest cancer to spread is bowel cancer, as blood supply from the small bowel is well-connected to the liver by the hepato-portal vein. Melanoma, breast cancer, stomach, esophagus, pancreas, kidney, ovary, and lung usually spread to the liver. Secondary liver cancer is more prevalent in Australia (Cancer Council 2020).

Occasionally, secondary liver cancer appears before the diagnosis of primary cancer, and thus, primary cancer remains undiagnosed in patients who have been diagnosed with secondary liver cancer. It is also popular as a cancer of unknown primary (Hoshida *et al.*, 2012).

DETAIL DESCRIPTION OF HCC

Hepatocellular carcinoma (HCC) is recognized as the most prevalent form of primary liver cancer as its occurrence ranges between 80-90%, among all types of primary liver cancer (Chen *et al.*, 2019; Galun *et al.*, 2017; Ladju *et al.*, 2017; Li *et al.*, 2016; Mohamed *et al.*, 2017; Zhang *et al.*, 2016). The majority of HCC cases in Asia and sub-Saharan Africa are due to predominantly elevated incidences of hepatitis B (HBV) virus-induced hepatic infection. Globally, the incidences of HCC show a steep rise accompanied by a high mortality rate, making HCC one of the most devastating neoplasias (Galun *et al.*, 2017; Li *et al.*, 2016; Zhang *et al.*, 2016). Chronic inflammatory hepatocellular damage from various etiologies may be a risk factor for HCC (Aravalli *et al.*, 2013; Yang *et al.*, 2019; Yapali and Tozun, 2018). More risk factors of HCC include chronic hepatitis for hepatitis B (HBV) and C viruses (HCV) infections, vinyl chloride, tobacco, foodstuffs contaminated with aflatoxin B1 (AFB_1), excessive consumption of alcohol, non-alcoholic fatty liver disease (NAFLD), obesity, diet, excessive drinking of coffee, oral contraceptives, hemochromatosis, genetic and congenital abnormalities (Balogh *et al.*, 2016; Marrero *et al.*, 2018). The impact of these risk factors for the development of HCC varies depending on the geographical regions, lending diagnosis, prognosis, and treatment recommendation (Marrero *et al.*, 2010). HCC shows an extreme preference for males as compared to females. The occurrence of HCC in males is four times and eight times higher than in females in the low-incidence and high-incidence regions, respectively (Balogh *et al.*, 2016; Marrero *et al.*, 2018; Yapali and Tozun, 2018). The findings of the HCC BRIDGE study conducted on 18,031 patients enrolled from 42 sites in 14 different countries have revealed that the mean age for the diagnosis of HCC was 69, 65, and 62 years in Japan, Europe, and North America, respectively (Park *et al.*, 2015). In Africa, a population-based study did not provide convincing high-quality data. The outcomes of a tertiary-referra-

-center-based cohort study on 1,552 patients enrolled from 14 centers in seven African countries showed that the onset of HCC diagnosis was 45 years, as found in the literature published in 2015 (Yang *et al.*, 2015). Like diagnosis and onset, wide variations in the overall survival of HCC-patients globally occurred. The median survival of HCC-patients was drastically low in sub-Saharan Africa (2.5 months) (Yang *et al.* 2015; Yang *et al.*, 2017a), indicating severe lacuna in a surveillance program and availability of productive treatment strategies. Taiwan and Japan have experienced the highest clinical outcomes in HCC-patients for the regular, extensive surveillance program. The plan consisted of an assessment of multiple tumor biomarkers, namely, alpha-fetoprotein (AFP), the *Lens culinaris* agglutinin reactive glycoform (AFP-L3), des-gama-carboxyprothrombin (DCP), and also imaging in the high-risk individuals by liver ultrasonography to detect unknown or suspicious liver nodules. Thus, they were capable of detecting the adults with a risk of HCC (Kudo 2018a). The clinical outcomes in China, Korea, North America, and Europe are significantly poor compared to Japan and Taiwan. It is because more than 60% of patients develop intermediate or advanced stage HCC. Egypt provided the best clinical outcome among the different African countries as patients' overall survival was significantly higher than the other sub-Saharan and East African countries. The reason could be a lesser proportion (69%) of HCC-patients transformed into an intermediate or advanced stage as compared to a higher proportion (76%) of medium and advanced-stage HCC-patients in other African countries (95%). Further, effective treatment options are accessible to a more significant proportion (76%) of HCC-patients in Egypt as compared to a low ratio (3%) of treated patients who had access to the treatment against HCC in other African countries (Yang *et al.*, 2015; Yang *et al.*, 2017a; Kudo 2018a; Yang and Roberts 2010).

India has also experienced a steep rise in the primary liver cancer from the last decade. Nowadays, HCC has become one of the leading gastrointestinal (GI) cancers in India (Acharya *et al.*, 2014; Kumar *et al.*, 2014). The consensus guidelines for tackling HCC in the USA, Europe, and North America are inadequate to address the issues related to the management of HCC in India. The most important limitation is the socio-economic condition of India. Thus the majority of Indians cannot afford the costly treatments suggested by these guidelines.

Further, the different surveillance strategies such as awareness for the interception of HCC, screening to identify high-risk groups, inability to diagnose HCC at the early stages, and inadequate availability of palliative and curative treatments lead to a diagnosis of HCC at the intermediate and the advanced forms. In 2011, the Indian National Association for Study of the Liver (INASL) had developed a Task-Force on HCC to design consensus guidelines based on clinical features of

HCC, especially the disease pattern and clinical practices in India. Importantly, nationalized representative data depicting the epidemiology of HCC is not available. Cancer is not a reportable disease in India, and registries mostly have an urban focus (Kumar *et al.*, 2014; Acharya, 2014).

The information obtained cancer registry website (www.ncrpindia.org, accessed on 11.01.21) has depicted that the last registry published by the Indian Council of Medical Research (ICMR) in 2008 provided information on all the types of cancer for a period of two years (2006-2008) (http://www.ncrpindia.org/Reports/PBCR_2006_2008.aspx, accessed 11.01.21; https://www.ncdirindia.org/ncrp/ca/about.aspx, accessed on 11.01.21). Besides, World Health Organization (WHO) also provided clues regarding the epidemiology of HCC in India. Based on the information supplied by the ICMR and WHO (http://www.ncrpindia.org/Reports/PBCR_2006_2008.aspx, accessed 11.01.21; https://www.ncdirindia.org/ncrp/ca/about.aspx; accessed on 11.01.21; http://ci5.iarc.fr/, accessed 11.01.21), the following consensus statements have been finalized by the Task-Force as described below:

(a) In India, age-adjusted incidence rates of HCC in men and women range between 0.7 to 7.5 and 0.2 to 2.2, respectively, per 100,000 populations, per year.

(b) HCC has shown a strong preference for male and male: female ratio was 4:1.

(c) The age of HCC patients showed broad variation that ranged between 40-70 years.

(d) The transformation of cirrhosis into HCC is 1.6% per year in India.

(e) 6.8/100,000 and 5.1/100,000 are the age-standardized mortality rate in men and women, respectively, in India.

(f) Most hepatic neoplasia in India is derived from cirrhosis, chronic viral hepatitis such as HBV and HCV infections, alcohol consumption, and aflatoxin exposure.

(g) Diabetes mellitus, non-alcoholic fatty liver disease (NAFLD), smoking, and tobacco have contributed significantly to HCC development and are also considered risk factors.

(h) Data implicating the impact of the genetic predisposition for HCC are inadequate to consider it a risk factor.

Staging System in HCC

Cancer staging is a crucial aspect to provide necessary information that helps decide the best possible therapeutic management (Aravalli *et al.,* 2013; Yang *et al.,* 2019; Balogh *et al.,* 2016; Marrero *et al.,* 2018). Further, the staging system provides various valuable information such as the proper selection of primary and adjuvant therapy, helping to assess prognosis, to assist in analyzing outcomes of the therapeutic regimen/treatment strategies, and for appropriate channeling of information to avoid any uncertainty (Pons *et al.,* 2005; Karademir 2018; Subramaniam *et al.,* 2013). In oncology, the tumor stage has a sole impact on the prognosis of patients having a solid tumor. Thus other co-factors such as age or histologic grade are rarely considered for staging. HCC is an exceptional neoplasm as it originates primarily from underlying cirrhotic condition and, thus tumor staging and histologic grade have an impact on suitability and applicability of treatment strategies (Pons *et al.,* 2005; Marrero *et al.,* 2010; Marrero *et al.,* 2018, Yang *et al.,* 2019). The various metabolic alterations at the origin of neoplasia and the degree of hepatic impairment due to neoplastic transformation make HCC highly heterogeneous, as reported in the literature (Aravalli *et al.,* 2013; Yang *et al.,* 2019). Thus, the staging system's efficiency depends on its capability to address the issues such as tumor stage, liver function, and physical status on the disease's prognosis (Pons *et al.,* 2005; Marrero *et al.,* 2018, Yang *et al.,* 2019). Eight different stagings belong to HCC, but no one has universal acceptance (Pons *et al.,* 2005, Subramaniam *et al.,* 2013; Marrero *et al.,* 2018). Europe frequently employed the Barcelona-clinic liver cancers (BCLC) system and the Italian liver Program (CLIP), whereas Japan integrated staging (JIS) has owned in recognition as a standard system in Japan for directing liver cancer (Pons *et al.,* 2005; Marrero *et al.,* 2018; Yang *et al.,* 2019).

In TNM staging, the number and size of the original tumor are denoted by T (tumor). Nodes (N) signify the presence of cancer in regional (nearby) lymph nodes. M (metastases) indicates the spreading of HCC from the primary site to a distant body part. Lungs and bones are the most preferred sites for the metastasis of HCC (Pons *et al.,* 2005; Subramaniam *et al.,* 2013; Karademir, 2018). The American Joint Committee on Cancer (AJCC) has approved the staging. Each stage has a characteristic number (0-4) and a letter “X”. The intensity of severity is denoted by a number. The higher number indicates more rigor than the lower number (Llovet *et al.,* 1998; Marsh *et al.,* 2000; Vauthey *et al.,* 2002). For example, the score T2 indicates a giant tumor as compared to the score T1. The letter “X” marks the unavailability of clear-cut information regarding cancer. The TNM staging has exhibited significantly superior performance as a prognostic predictor for the patients undergoing surgery than those undergoing resection or transplantation. An improved TNM staging version has appeared by incorporating tumor stage and fibrosis (Szklaruk *et al.,* 2003; Pons *et al.,* 2005; Karademir, 2018).

Among the myriads of staging systems, the BCLC system has been maximally explored to properly assess prognosis in HCC patients (Balogh *et al.,* 2016; Marrero *et al.,* 2018; Liu *et al.,* 2016). The findings obtained from a plethora of cohort studies and randomized clinical trials (RCTs) led to the development BCLC staging system (Llovet *et al.,* 1999; Former *et al.,* 2018). Ideally, it is a single unified proposal to establish a liaison between evaluating prognosis and selecting the most suitable treatment strategies, including their advancement to make them highly potent (Balogh *et al.,* 2016; Marrero *et al.,* 2018; Giannini *et al.,* 2016). Thus, it is more likely a classification system than a scoring system (Llovet *et al.,* 1999; Balogh *et al.,* 2016; Former *et al.,* 2018; Yang *et al.,* 2019). The plan had several variables such as tumor stage, liver functional status, overall physical status, and cancer-related symptoms. BCLC acts as a bridge between these variables and various treatment option systems (Marrero *et al.,* 2005; Cillo *et al.,* 2006; Chen *et al.,* 2009). Further, the global acceptability of BCLC staging as a guide for HCC treatment is maximum (Marrero *et al.,* 2018, Yang *et al.,* 2019). Minor tuning requires depending on some specialized individual cases, especially in patients with impaired liver function. Based on the variables mentioned above, BCLC staging assigned HCC patients into five categories, namely, 0, A, B, C, D (Cillo *et al.,* 2006; Chen *et al.,* 2009).

The classification of HCC-patients under various categories, namely, stage 0 (very early stage), if they have no abnormalities in liver function (Child-Pugh A), one asymptomatic tumor < 2cm without vascular invasion or satellites. The therapy recommended for stage A is resection.

Patients with Child-Pugh score A or B, a single tumor of any size or 2-3 tumors of size < 3cm, are assigned into stage A (early stage). The radical approach comprising resection, transplantation, adjuvant resection, or percutaneous treatment is recognized as optimal therapy as reported in the literature (Cillo *et al.,* 2006; Chen *et al.,* 2009).

Patients with Child-Pugh score A or B, multiple tumors, and without extrahepatic metastases belong to stage B (intermediate stage). Chemoembolization may be beneficial for these patients.

The stage C (advanced stage) patients have Child-Pugh score A or B accompanied with multiple tumors and extrahepatic metastases and relatively good performance status (PS) (1-2). Patients may receive newer agents derived from potential findings of RCTs.

The HCC patients with Child-Pugh C status at any tumor stage and below-par PS (>2) belong to stage D (terminal phase). The patients with an end-stage disease condition receive a recommendation for symptomatic treatment (Cillo *et al.*, 2006; Chen *et al.*, 2009).

Kudo *et al.* (2003) proposed the Japan Integrated Staging System (JIS). This system's basis was a cohort study employing 722 patients who had undergone treatments at two Japanese institutions. JIS score is a compiled system of Child-Pugh grade and Japanese TNM developed by the Liver Cancer Study Group of Japan (LCSGJ) (Makuuchi *et al.*, 2003). The three parameters, such as vascular invasion, single and multiple nodules, and their diameter, either ≤ or > 20 cm, are backbones of the JIS scoring system. In JIS staging, the patients receive a scoring of 0, 1, and 2 based on Child-Pugh status A, B, C, D, respectively. Subsequently, the scores such as 0, 1, 2, and 3 have become with Japanese TNM staging I, II, III, and IV, respectively. The summation of these scores finally divides patients into six groups (0-5) (Kudo *et al.*, 2004; Toyoda *et al.*, 2005). The cumulative 10-year survival rates of patients with the JIS system and with the Italian program (CLIP) were 65% and 23%, respectively, indicating the significantly superior ability of the JIS system in stratifying of early diagnosed HCC patients (Kudo *et al.*, 2004; Toyoda *et al.*, 2005). In the exiting JIS staging system, replacing the encephalopathy component with indocyanine green clearance (ICG-R15) achieves more effective and timely HCC-screening. Further refinement has made prognosis prediction highly accurate by the JIS system, leading to biomarker combined JIS (bm-JIS). The biomarkers included in bm-JIS are α-fetoprotein (AFP), AFP-Lens culinaris agglutinin-reactive (AFP-L3), and des-gamma-carboxy prothrombin (DCP) (Ikai *et al.*, 2006; Kitai *et al.*, 2008). This staging system's performance remained unassessed in HCC-patients of Western countries, where HCC has been detected at the early stage (Karademir 2018).

The retrospective analysis of 435 patients undergoing treatment at 16 Italian institutions led to CLIP development in 1998 (the cancer of the Liver Italian Program (CLIP) investigators. 1998). The fundamental focus behind the development of CLIP was to overcome the shortcomings associated with the TNM staging. Child-Pugh status of the patients, tumor morphology and extension, portal vein thrombosis, and AFP levels are the fundamental components of CLIP score (Farinati *et al.*, 2000; Llovet and Bruix, 2000; Ueno *et al.*, 2001). Each of the sub-component under these variables receives a Scoring system. For example, Child-Pugh status, A, B, and C are similar to scores 0, 1, 2. Based on the variable tumor morphology and extension, the characteristics, namely, uninodular and extension ≤50 percent, multinodular and extension ≤50 percent, and massive or extension >50 percent, depict scores 0, 1, 2, respectively. The levels of AFP <400 and ≥ 400 have been assigned with scores 0 and 1, respectively. The presence and the absence of portal vein thrombosis have scores of 0 and 1, respectively. The final CLIP score is the summation of all the subscores, and depending on the final score, patients have been stratified into six groups (0-6). The CLIP calculation is very facile and well-coordinated with survival (Liu *et al.,* 2016). The lower number signifies a superior prognosis as compared to a higher number. CLIP score fails to provide conclusive information regarding the impact of underlying liver diseases, performance status, and extrahepatic metastasis on the outcomes. Notably, the CLIP score is incapable of predicting the appropriate therapy for the HCC-patients. The prospective CLIP validation findings in 196 patients revealed that the CLIP score's predictive potency was significantly superior to the Okuda staging system (Liu *et al.*, 2016). Even though several cohort studies (Canadian, Italian and Japanese) had externally validated the CLIP score, the main disadvantage is that it fails to predict early-stage HCC patients who could benefit from radical treatment (Pons *et al.*, 2005).

A study consisting of 850 patients first proposed the Okuda system in 1985 (Okuda *et al.,* 1985). The factors of the Okuda staging include the size of the tumor ($\leq$ or $>$ 50% of the entire liver), the presence of ascites, levels of serum albumin ($\leq$ or $>$ 3.0 g/dL), and bilirubin levels ($\leq$ or $>$ 3.0 mg/dL). The variables assessment has resulted in a classification of HCC-patients into three stages. They are, namely, I (not advanced), II (moderately advanced), and III (very advanced) (Shouval, 2002). The Okuda system is the most widely explored classification system in Western countries (Cillo *et al.,* 2006; Liu *et al.,* 2016). Briefly, the Okuda system is an integrated system capable of addressing the extent of underlying cirrhosis and tumor features from a single platform (Pons *et al.,* 2005). In the past, normally, HCC cases were diagnosed at the advanced stage, making a huge impact on the popularity and acceptability of the Okuda system. The advancement in surveillance and imaging techniques makes a remarkable impact on HCC diagnosis, and nowadays, patients are diagnosed efficiently at an early asymptomatic stage of disease (Karademir 2018). Further, the probability of the tumor occupying half of the liver space nowadays is a remote possibility leading to the loss of glory of the Okuda system. Importantly, Okuda is incapable of differentiating moderately advanced HCC patients; thus, the Okuda system's major focus is identifying patients with the end-stage disease to exclude from therapeutic trials due to their inferior prognosis (Rabe *et al.,* 2003; Giannini *et al.,* 2004). The Okuda system is a crude classification system where tumor size is designated arbitrarily (Shouval 2002). The potential shortcomings associated with Okuda staging include the inability to provide information regarding various crucial aspects of the tumor, which greatly impact the prognosis of early phase HCC patients. These include nature of tumour (unifocal/multifocal/diffuse), existence of vascular invasion and size (< 2cm). Moreover, the Okuda system's predictive potential is significantly lower than the modern staging system available for HCC classification (Subramaniam *et al.*, 2013; Karademir, 2018). Despite several disadvantages, till now Okuda system has a global acceptance and is considered as standard. The new scoring system's performance has been analyzed compared to the Okuda stage (Levy *et al.*, 2002; Liu *et al.*, 2016).

The Hong Kong Liver Cancer (HKLC) classification developed by Yau *et al.* (2014) was on the cohort study employing 3856 HCC patients who were predominantly infected with HBV virus and had undergone treatment at a single institution. Similar to BCLC, HKLC also bridges stages of HCC with the treatment recommendations. The pillars of HKLC are the five established prognostic factors: Eastern Cooperative Oncology Group (ECOG) PS, Child-Pugh grade, condition of the tumor, and presence of extrahepatic vascular invasion metastasis. Based on these prognostic factors, patients had five principal groups and nine subgroups with distinct survival outcomes (Sohn *et al.*, 2017). Compared to BCLC, HKLC has a significantly superior discriminatory potential between patients with moderate tumor-related symptoms and more severe symptoms (Adhoute *et al.*, 2015).

Further, HKLC can recognize patients at intermediate or advanced HCC, probably requiring highly aggressive treatments. Therefore, the patients' survival outcomes are significantly higher in HKLC staging than BCLC due to the potent stratification of patients into distinct groups and intrusive treatment recommendations (Yau *et al.*, 2014; Adhoute *et al.*, 2015; Sohn *et al.*, 2017). Despite its high potential prognostic ability, several issues associated with HKLC have highlighted some critical drawbacks. Firstly, overlapping as observed between nine subgroups of HKLC diminished its clinical applicability. Although reports revealing the decrement of subgroups from 9 to 5 are available, their external validations are still warranted (Adhoute *et al.*, 2015; Sohn *et al.*, 2017). Secondly, the performance of HKLC in non-HBV-related cases is yet to validate. Thus its ability to link the treatment recommendations is specific and may not be generalizable. The pooled data obtained from a prospective European cohort with 1693 patients have revealed that the predictive power of BCLC classification on overall survival was significantly superior to the HKLC counterpart (Kolly *et al.*, 2016). Finally, evidence-based criteria developed for the prognosis assessment revealed that BCLC is the sole classification system that can meet all cancer staging standards (Forner *et al.*, 2018; Yang *et al.*, 2019).

Risk Factors for HCC

Pre-existing cirrhosis links to nearly 70-90% of HCC-patients (Singh *et al.*, 2018; Yang *et al.*, 2019; Balogh *et al.*, 2016; Marrero *et al.*, 2018). Thus, the etiological agents responsible for chronic liver injury lead to cirrhosis and are risk factors for

HCC. The prime causes of cirrhosis and HCC include HBV, HCV, alcohol intake, and NAFLD. Other factors contributing to HCC development include hereditary hemochromatosis, primary biliary cholangitis (PBC), and Wilson's disease (Yang *et al.*, 2019; Balogh *et al.*, 2016; Marrero *et al.*, 2018).

Viral hepatitis due to chronic HBV infection and HCV infection makes remarkably significant contributions to HCC development as it accounts for nearly 80% of HCC cases globally (El-Serag, 2012; Yang JD and Roberts, 2010). Chronic HBV infection plays a pivotal role in developing HCC in East African and most African countries, excluding northern Africa, where HCV exhibits its prevalence (Park *et al.*, 2015; Yang *et al.*, 2015). The statistics have revealed that globally, 257 million individuals will develop chronic HBV infection and HBV–associated acute hepatitis, chronic hepatitis, cirrhosis, and HCC, resulting in 20 million deaths between 2015 and 2030 (Yang *et al.*, 2019). Among them, HCC will solely contribute to 5 million deaths. HBV contains a double-stranded circular DNA molecule having eight different genotypes (A-H) in further geographic distribution. For example, the most prevalent genotypes in Europe and the Middle East are A and D. In contrast, the predominant genotypes are C and B in Asia. The development of HCC is significantly higher with genotype C than A, B, and D (Balogh *et al.*, 2016; Marrero *et al.*, 2018). The HBV genome contains four overlapping transcription units which encode nucleocapsid or core protein comprising of hepatitis B core antigen (HBcAg), envelope protein containing hepatitis B surface antigen (HBsAg), polymerase, and the X protein (HBx), having a pivotal role for the development of HCC (Yoon, 2018). Several reports in the literature have revealed that integrating the viral genome with the host genome leads to an oncogenic transformation in hepatic cells upon chronic HBV infection (Sung *et al.*, 2012). The findings of the next-generation sequencing (NGS) study revealed that the integration of the HBV genome occurred in 80% of HBV-positive HCC cases. Further, a more extensive association was with tumor tissues than non-tumor tissues (Nault *et al.*, 2013). Three cancer-associated genes, namely, telomerase reverse transcriptase (TERT), mixed-lineage leukemia 4 (MLL4), and cyclin E1 ($CCNE_1$), were frequently observed at the integration sites in HBV positive tumors, signifying considerably good association between integration sites and hepatic neoplasia. The published literature highlighted that more than 50% of HCC tissues had exhibited mutation in TERT promoter (Sung *et al.*, 2012; Nault *et al.*, 2013). Plenty of pieces of evidence have suggested that HBx performs crucial roles in the development of HCC *via* a plethora of mechanisms at the cellular and molecular level (Sung *et al.*, 2012; Nault *et al.*, 2013; Bell *et al.*, 2015; Zhang *et al.*, 2012). They include: (a) transactivation of various oncogenes such as Yes-associated protein (YAP), (b) changes in DNA specificity of cyclic AMP (cAMP) -response element-binding protein (CREB) along with the activation of transcription factor 2 (ATF-2) that lead to binding and stimulation of HBV enhancer, (c) modification of DNA binding specificity of p53 suppressor leading to altered expression of its target genes, and (d) regulation of an array of cellular signaling pathways such as Src-dependent pathway, PI3K-Akt pathway, inflammation-associated NF-κβ/STAT-3 and wnt/β-catenin pathway (Sung *et al.*, 2012; Nault *et al.*, 2013; Bell *et al.*, 2015; Zhang *et al.*, 2012; Chan *et al.*, 2013; Cha *et al.*, 2004; Tian *et al.*, 2013). Moreover, HBx has the potential to influence the epigenetic alteration by hypermethylation or hypomethylation of oncogenes and tumor suppressor genes, thus boosting the histone acetylation and deacetylation of tumor-associated genes with the alteration of several microRNAs (miRNAs) (Zhu *et al.*, 2010; Kong *et al.*, 2011; Chen *et al.*, 2013c). The modes of transmission of HBV include contaminated blood transfusions, intravenous injections, and sexual contact. The transmission of infection from mother to fetus through vertical transmission is the predominant cause of HBV infection worldwide. Interestingly, chronic HBV infection has the unique ability to transform normal hepatocytes into neoplastic hepatocytes (Yang *et al.*, 2019; Balogh *et al.*, 2016; Marrero *et al.*, 2018). The hepatocarcinogenesis induced by HBV can be reduced remarkably upon using antiviral agents capable of treating hepatitis B. For example, a significantly superior reduction in 5-year incidence of HCC (13.7% in control *vs.* 3.7% upon treatment) was available in the literature upon therapy with antiviral agents, especially in cirrhotic patients (Hosaka *et al.*, 2013).

HCV-induced HCC is prevalent in North America, Europe, Japan, parts of central Asia, including Mongolia, northern Africa, and in the Middle East, especially in Egypt (Yoon, 2018; Singh *et al.*, 2018; Yang *et al.*, 2019; Balogh *et al.*, 2016; Marrero *et al.*, 2018). The small single-stranded RNA virus HCV possesses significantly high genetic variability. Western countries and the Far East observe genotypes I, II, and III, while the Middle East follows type IV genotypes (Choo *et al.*, 1991). The genome of HCV is 9.6-kb long, encoding a large polyprotein (Rusyn and Lemon 2014). The cleavage of this protein at the multiple sites leads to the creation of a minimum of 10 proteins along with the structural proteins [core, envelope (E1 and E2)], and non-structural (NS) proteins (p7, NS_2, NS_3, NS_4A, NS_4B, NS_5A, and NS_5B). Outcomes of various epidemiologic studies revealed that globally HCV is recognized as one of the prime risk factors, leading to the development of HCC (Lerat *et al.*, 2011; Lindenbach *et al.*, 2005). Plenty of studies has revealed the direct influence of HCV to induce malignant transformation, especially the potential of HCV core protein to activate STAT3 *via* IL-6 autocrine pathway, leading to enhancement in the activity of telomerase (Tacke *et al.*, 2011; Zhu *et al.*, 2010; He *et al.*, 2007). Further, NS_4A elevates cells' proliferation by upregulating phosphorylation of extracellular signal-related kinases (ERKs) and inhibiting p53-mediated apoptosis and p21 promoter activity (Kwun *et al.*, 2001, Yu *et al.*, 2012). Apart from the above mechanisms, plenty of evidence in the literature (Korenaga *et al.*, 2005; Munakata *et al.*, 2005; Choi *et al.*, 2006; Tsai *et al.*, 2012) has suggested several mechanisms through which HCV induces oncogenic transformation. They include as follows: (a) oxidative stress resulting in DNA mutagenesis, (b) intense and stable inflammation promoted by NF-κβ, (c) transformation of tumor suppressor genes, (d) direct modulation of the wnt/β-catenin pathway by NS_5A, and (e) interaction between TGF-β receptor and NS_5A leading to blockade of TGF-β signaling. The presence of pre-existing cirrhosis is the most familiar feature of HCV-induced HCC.

Non-alcoholic steatohepatitis (NASH), a type of NAFLD accompanied by advanced fibrosis, has been observed in patients more than 50 years and who had diabetes or obesity. Annually, NASH's progress to HCC occurs at a rate of 0.5% (Younossi *et al.*, 2016a). Chronic metabolic disorders such as diabetes and obesity significantly increase the chances of HCC. The liver plays a crucial role in glucose metabolism, highlighting the direct impact of diabetes mellitus on the liver resulting in chronic hepatitis, fatty liver, liver failure, and cirrhosis (White *et al.*, 2012; Yang *et al.*, 2017a; Younossi 2016b). The evidence in the literature has recognized diabetes as an independent risk factor of HCC, and the risk of HCC is increased by 2 to 3 folds (Welzel *et al.*, 2013; El-Serag *et al.*, 2006). Plenty of reports in the literature (Mittal *et al.*, 2016; Huang *et al.*, 2018; West *et al.*, 2017) have suggested that failure in the regulation anti-inflammatory pathway cascade loses control of cellular proliferation by the pleiotropic effect of insulin resulting in induction of carcinogenesis. Further, insulin-like growth factor and insulin receptor substrate I can boost cellular proliferation and downregulation of apoptosis, respectively (Park *et al.*, 2010; Balkau *et al.*, 2001; Yoshimoto *et al.*, 2013). Obesity and various hepatobiliary diseases, namely, NAFLD, steatosis, and cryptogenic cirrhosis, may lead to hepatocytes' malignant transformation and induction of HCC (Callee *et al.*, 2003; Reddy and Rao, 2006). Obesity alone boosts the risk of HCC by 1.5 to 4-folds. In overweight subjects and obese patients, the relative risks of HCC were 117% and 189%, respectively (Larson and Wolk 2007). The occurrence of HCC-NAFLD has been observed predominantly in men. The HCC developed in men exhibits significantly reduced fibrosis and cirrhosis, and half of the HCC-NAFLD patients revealed the absence of cirrhosis (Monsour *et al.*, 2013; Turati *et al.*, 2014). Tumors showed a significantly reduced AFP level and elevated des-γ-carboxy prothrombin level than HCV-related HCC (Wakai *et al.*, 2011; Tokushige *et al.*, 2010).

The attributable population fraction (PAF) determines the quantitative assessment of disease risk factors. Evaluation of a population-based study comprising 6,991 HCC- patients more aged than 68 years resulted in the PAF (Welzel *et al.*, 2013). The study's findings revealed that the elimination of diabetes and obesity resulted in a 40% reduction in HCC events. The percentage of decline was much superior upon the elimination of other factors, including HCV. There is a lack of high-quality population-based studies to analyze the association between NAFLD and HCC. However, the preliminary investigations' outcome has suggested that proper assessment of characteristic metabolic syndromes would be the thrust area for effective management and prevention for HCC (Marrero *et al.,* 2018).

Overconsumption of alcohol is a primary global concern as it leads to fatty liver, alcoholic steatohepatitis (ASH), cirrhosis, and finally, resulting in the development of HCC (Schwartz and Reinus 2012). Chronic alcohol consumption activates cytochrome P450 2E1(CYP2E1), a component of cytochrome P450 mixed-function oxidase system, that functions on diverse biological activities such as enhancement of alcohol metabolism, elevation in oxidative stress, hepatotoxicity, and cooperation between several drugs, xenobiotics, and carcinogens (Neuman *et al.,* 2015). Aldehyde produced by alcohol metabolism is crucial for oxidative stress and subsequent liver damage (Yoon 2018). Alcoholic liver disease (ALD) and alcoholic cirrhosis contribute 20-25% and 1.3 -3% of HCC cases annually. The PAF of ALD as a risk factor of HCC ranges between 13-23%, and race and sex play a significant role in the risk factor (Welzel *et al.,* 2013; Massarweh and El-Serag 2017). The function of alcohol as an independent risk factor for HCC potentiates explicitly by the presence of viral hepatitis (Marrero *et al.,* 2018).

Aflatoxin, potent mycotoxins, has strong hepatocarcinogenic effects and can contaminate wide varieties of staple cereals and oilseeds (Yang *et al.,* 2019; Gouas *et al.,* 2009). An area with widespread contamination with aflatoxins exhibits elevated incidences of HCC (Gouas *et al.,* 2009). For example, a faulty post-harvesting process results in exposure of West African countries' general population to aflatoxins. In contrast, there has been a minimum exposure to people of Western countries. The probability of HCC development upon aflatoxin exposure directly depends on the dose and duration. The active form of aflatoxin responsible for hepatocarcinogenesis is aflatoxin B1(AFB1), produced by *Aspergillus sp*. The principal mechanism of AFB1 includes mutation at codon 249 of tumor suppressor gene *TP53* due to the substitution of arginine by serine (*R249S*), specifically in HCC. The substitution, which accounts for 50-90% of *TP53* mutation, is highly predominant in the HCC-patients having high aflatoxin exposure (Weng *et al.,* 2017). The synergy between HBV infection and aflatoxin exposure lends to a remarkable intensification of risk factors of HCC (Yang *et al.,* 2019). Induction of cytochrome P450s by chronic HBV infection boosts inactive AFB1 into an active mutagenic metabolite, AFB1-8, 9-epoxide. The probability of mutation of TP53 by AFB1 has been increased significantly due to hepatocyte necrosis and regeneration induced by chronic HBV infection. Further, HBV oncogenic protein inhibits the nucleotide excision repair mechanism to remove AFB1-DNA adducts (Yang *et al.*, 2019).

Aristolochic acid (AA), a highly mutagenic compound, is obtained from plants such as *Aristolicia* and *Asarum,* which grow worldwide (Arlt *et al.*, 2002). The outcome of the next-generation sequencing (NGS) study revealed that the fraction of HCC patients of Asian origin, especially from China, Taiwan, Vietnam, and South East Asia, showed high mutation rates with similar patterns mutational characteristics that occurred upon exposure to AA. The findings of a large study encompassing 1400 patients revealed that 78%, 47%, 29%, 13%, 2.7%, 4.8%, and 1.7% of HCC patients from Taiwan, China, Southeast Asia, Korea, Japan, North America, and Europe exhibited the signature mutational characters of AA (Rosenquist and Grollman 2016; Ng *et al.*, 2017; Hsieh *et al.*, 2008; Chen *et al.*, 2018). A randomly sampled cohort study comprising of 200,000 patients registered under National Health Insurance in 1997 and 2003 confirmed exposure of one-third of the Taiwanese population to AA (Hsieh *et al.*, 2008).

An estimate that reveals the risk of hereditary hemochromatosis in HCC ranges between 100- 200-folds. Thalassemia (an iron overload state) has no direct correlation with HCC. However, a high prevalence of HCV has been observed in Thalassemic individuals and eventually may increase the risk of HCC in them. Consumption of beer in non-galvanized steel drums increases the risk of HCC than the storage of it in iron resulting in an elevated risk of HCC at least ten times than that of regular iron drums. A population-based cohort study with patients with hereditary hemochromatosis and 5973 members of their first-degree relatives (Elmberg *et al.*, 2003) revealed that HCC was developed in 62 patients having a standardized incidence ratio of 21 (95% confidence interval (CI), 16-22). The risk of developing HCC was more in men than in women, and the incidence risk of developing nonhepatic malignant transformation is nil. Cirrhosis developed from primary biliary cholangitis (PBC) is also recognized as one of the viable risk factors of HCC. A study conducted for three years, with 273 patients with cirrhosis developed from PBC, showed the incidence of HCC was 5.9%. (Marrero *et al.*, 2018) A systemic review comprising 6528 patients with autoimmune hepatitis (AIH) with a median follow-up of 8 years for HCC incidence showed that the pooled incidence rate was 3.1 per person-years, defining AIH as one of the risk factors of HCC (Tansel *et al.*, 2017).

A prospective study employing cirrhosis patients due to alpha-1 antitrypsin deficiency and a median follow-up time of 5.2 years revealed that the annual incidence of HCC was 0.9% (Antoury *et al.*, 2015).

Pathophysiology of HCC

Characteristic well-defined confirmed features of initiation and developmental process of HCC are not yet figured out distinctively with the defined molecular and histopathological markers (Aravalli *et al.*, 2013; Sia *et al.*, 2017). Plenty of evidence in the literature suggests that continuous build-up of mutation and genetic changes in preneoplastic hepatocytes leads to hepatic neoplastic transformation and, eventually, the development of HCC (El-Serag and Rudolph 2007; Farazi and DePinho 2006; Chakraborty *et al.*, 2020). The tumor rarely accompanies the single lesion and, more commonly, with multiple lesions. The neoplastic cells of well-differentiated tumors depict normal hepatocytes' characteristics, whereas cells of poorly differentiated tumors are big and hardly distinguishable from metastatic tumors of other origins (Aravalli *et al.*, 2013; Sia *et al.*, 2017). The building blocks for the basic hepatic structure include parenchymal (hepatocytes and cholangiocytes) and nonparenchymal cells (fibroblasts, stellate cells, Kupffer cells, and endothelial cells) (Stranger 2015; Knouse *et al.*, 2014). The differences in opinion exist over the existence of stem cells in the adult liver. The sinusoidal lumen and perisinusoidal space of Disse contain intrahepatic lymphocytes and liver-specific natural killer cells (NK cells). Hepatocytes contribute a principal share (60-80%) of the hepatic mass. Architectural organization of the liver reveals that coordinated assembling of cells results in the formation of the lobules. Lobules are further differentiated into functional regions or zones. Liver zones are important parts, especially for hepatocytes, as the zones strongly influence the action of hepatocytes without hampering their phenotype. Hepatocytes are predominantly polyploid (4N, 8N, *etc.*). Polyploid cells constitute 50% of the human liver and 90% of the mouse liver (Stranger 2015; Knouse *et al.*, 2014). The insult by toxic substances followed by the immune response triggers inflammation in the liver *via* activation of Kupffer cells and hepatic stellate cells (HSCs), leading to necrosis. Liver fibrosis and cirrhosis may happen during this process (Severi *et al.*, 2010). Cirrhosis, the leading stage of fibrosis, has some signature characteristics such as deformation of liver parenchyma, septae, and nodule formation, a shift in the blood flow, and a high possibility of liver failure. Cirrhosis results in considerably high mortality and morbidity and gains the status of a single largest risk factor for the development of HCC (Friedman *et al.*, 2008; Roskams and Kojiro, 2010). Information regarding the molecular mechanisms responsible for the transition of cirrhosis into hepatic malignancy is unspecified. Further, the periodic necrosis in hepatocytes accompanied by regeneration due to an elevation in cell turnover leads to liver sensitization towards different mutagenic agents' adverse effects. Finally, genetic and epigenetic alteration may occur, resulting in dysplastic foci, nodules, and eventually HCC (Severi *et al.*, 2010; Friedman *et al.*, 2008; Roskams and Kojiro, 2010). The three commonest cellular patterns which constitute the growth pattern of HCC are trabecular, pseudo glandular (or pseudoscalar), and solid (or compact). The coexistence of these patterns can be observed in the same lesion. Further, the cells can abruptly undergo transition from one pattern to another (Quaglian 2018). Several variations have been observed in tumor cells as follow: (a) accumulation of fat, (b) disseminated differentiation of cytoplasm (clear cell change), ground glass appearance, (c) incorporation of Mallory–Denk bodies, and oncogenesis (Ziol *et al.*, 2018; Okamura 2005; Salomao *et al.*, 2010; Si *et al.*, 2004). HCC tumor possesses intra- and/ inter morphological heterogeneity as well as stem cell-like properties that have been observed in some subtypes of hepatic neoplasia and intrahepatic cholangiocarcinoma (iCCAs) such as HCC with CK19-positive cells (Roskams *et al.*, 2003; Lee *et al.*, 2006; Wang *et al.*, 2011; Singh *et al.*, 2013). Numerous hypotheses have been developed based on the above observations. They include: (a) both hepatocytes and cholangiocytes have evolved from a common progenitor cells (hepatoblasts) and eventually lead to the formation of primary liver tumours, (b) mature hepatocytes and cholangiocytes give rise to birth of two distinct tumour, namely HCC and iCCA, respectively, (c) sequential alterations of genome result in dedifferentiation of mature hepatocytes into precursor cells which might finally convert into HCC cells equipped with the markers of progenitor cells, (d) potential of adult hepatocytes to trans-differentiate into biliary-like cells ultimately leads to the formation of iCCA, (e) progenitor cells that arise from mature hepatocytes have the ability to transform to HCCs and iCCAs possessing progenitor-like features, (f) unlike hepatocytes, plasticity and transformation potential are absent in mature cholangiocytes resulting in their transformation specifically into iCCA (Tanimizu *et al.*, 2013; Chen *et al.*, 2012; Tarlow *et al.*, 2014; Guest *et al.*, 2014).

Molecular and Cellular Features of the Tumor Microenvironment

The tissue environment performs a pivotal role in malignant hepatic tumor formation and development (Leonardi *et al.*, 2012; Yang *et al.*, 2011; Qin *et al.*, 2020). The process of carcinogenesis includes transforming healthy hepatocytes into preneoplastic lesions, which finally transform into a malignant tumor. The direct or indirect interplay between several different types of cells with extracellular matrix (ECM) components such as collagen, fibronectin, laminin, glycosaminoglycans, hyaluronan, and proteoglycan leads to malignant transformation through the acquisition of abnormal phenotype. The elements of tumor stroma are known as cancer-associated fibroblast (CAFs), macrophages (liver resident Kupffer cells, and other tumor-infiltrating cells), leukocytes, HSCs, endothelial cells, pericytes, neutrophils, and dendritic cells (Wu *et al.*, 2012; Schrader and Iredale 2011, Severi *et al.*, 2010). In HCC, CAFs play a crucial role in the initiation and progression of the tumor by producing several components such as epidermal growth factor (EGF), hepatocyte growth factor (HGF), fibroblast growth factor (FGF), interleukin-6 (IL-6), chemokine (C-X-C motif) ligand 12 (CXCL12), matrix metalloproteinase (MMP)-3, and 9 (MMP-3 and MMP-9). IL-8, cyclooxygenase-2 (COX-2), and secreted acidic protein rich in cysteine (SPARC) have also been synthesized by CAFs to boost the macrophage production and recruitment, which significantly elevate the triggering of CAFs through the production of tumor necrosis factor-α (TNF-α) and platelet-derived growth factor (PDGF) (Mueller *et al.* 2007; Zhang *et al.,* 2007; Aravalli *et al.,* 2013; Yang *et al.*, 2017b). Several cytokines such as IL-4, IL-6, and transforming growth factor-β (TGF-β) lead to polarization of tumor-associated macrophages (TAMs) into M2-mononuclear phagocyte-like cells, which further express cytokines such as IL-10 and TGF-β, chemokines, namely, CCL17, CCL22, and CCL24, vascular endothelial growth factor (VEGF) and EGF resulting in recruitment of regulatory T-cells (Tregs) to boost the angiogenesis (Mantovani *et al.,* 2011; Movahedi *et al.,* 2010). The tumor microenvironment contains liver-specific TAMs, namely, Kupffer cells and resident macrophages. Liver-specific TAMs have the potential to spoil the $CD8^+$ cytotoxic T-lymphocyte (CTL)-mediated immune response through ligand-receptor interaction between programmed death-ligand 1 (PD-L1) and the cell surface protein program death 1 (PD-1) at the surface of $CD8^+$ cells. Further, Kupffer cells and HSCs upon stimulation by pro-inflammatory cytokines such as IL-1β, TNF-α, and PDGF produce osteopontin, one of the key players in various cell signaling pathways involved in inflammation, tumor progression, and metastasis (Ramaiah and Rittling 2008; Leonardi *et al.,* 2012). The role of dendritic cells (DCs) is to process antigen and present the antigen properly to the infiltrating CTLs through their expression at the surface of dendritic cells. The endocytic activity of DCs is significantly high. Accumulating evidence in the literature has highlighted that high endocytic exercise helps the tumor breach immune surveillance (Lin *et al.,* 2010). Glycipan 3 (GPC3) is specifically overexpressed in HCC, signifying poor prognosis. The published literature findings revealed that expression of GPC3 epitope on the surface of human monocyte-derived DCs *in vitro* resulted in induction of functional T-cells to produce interferon-γ (O'Beirne *et al.,* 2010). Thus, the GPC3 epitope needs to assess CTL response in patients receiving immunotherapy. Another study's outcome revealed that the suppression of the immune response of DCs in the tumor microenvironment by infiltrating $CD4^+$/$CD25^+$ Tregs increased tumor size (Lee *et al.,* 2012).

During liver injury, the transdifferentiation of collagen-producing cells, HSCs, leads to the formation of myofibroblast-like cells that produce cytokines, chemokines, growth factors, and ECM. Further, the phenotypic transformation of HSCs is crucial for the development of hepatic fibrosis. The inducers of HSC activation and proliferation include HBV-encoded X protein, HCV-nonstructural protein, MMP-9, PDGF, TGF-β, Janus kinase (JNK), insulin-like growth factor

(IGF)-binding protein, and cathepsin B and D and HSCs activation leads to liver fibrosis and subsequently HCC development (Friedman *et al.*, 2008; Leonardi *et al.*, 2012).

The endothelial cells express several angiogenic receptors, namely, VEFGR, EGFR, EGF homology domains-2(Tie-2), PDGFR, and C-X-C chemokine receptors (CXCRs). The ligand-receptor interactions regulate several signaling pathways involved in survival, proliferation, mobilization, and endothelial cell invasion (Leonardi *et al.*, 2012). HCC shows the significant overexpression of TGF-β, which performs the chemoattractant role for CD105, boosting angiogenesis in the tumor. The angiogenesis activity was significantly elevated in CD105-positive endothelial cells (Aravalli *et al.*, 2013). Further, they exhibit considerably high resistance to chemotherapeutic drugs and inhibitors of angiogenesis. The one crucial aspect for cancer cells' progression includes infiltration of T cells into the tumor microenvironment. The number of $CD4^+/CD25^+$ is remarkably high in malignant hepatic tissues as compared to the adjacent benign tissues. $CD4^+/CD25^+$ Tregs reduced the proliferation, activation, and degranulation of $CD8^+$ T cells and the production of granzymes (A and B) and perforin (Aravalli *et al.*, 2013). This observation of several studies showed that a significant reduction in CD8+ T cells and elevated Treg numbers indicated inferior prognosis, specifically after resection (Chen *et al.*, 2012; Mathai *et al.*, 2012; Wang *et al.*, 2012). Researchers have identified an immune-gene signature comprising 14 genes that encode pro-inflammatory cytokines such as TNF-α and IFN-γ and chemokines such as CXCL10, CCL5, and CCL2. The infiltration of lymphocytes is guided by the immune-gene signature, resulting in precise predictions of patients' survival at early stages. Further, pronounced neutrophil activity has resulted in malfunctioning of immune regulation, signifying poor prognosis, especially after resectioning HCC (Chew *et al.*, 2012; Li *et al.*, 2011).

The structural support and anchorage to parenchymal cells have been provided by ECM and maintain the intracellular communication through the different types of proteoglycans such as heparan sulfate, chondroitin sulfate, and keratin sulfate. One of these proteoglycans' crucial functions is to ease the storage of various growth factors such as HGF, FGF, PDGF, and VEGF within the ECM. Among the different proteoglycans, heparan sulfate proteoglycans have a strong impact on the pathogenesis of HCC (Leorandi *et al.*, 2012; Wu *et al.*, 2012).

The most abundant protein in ECM is collagen, which assists the migration and proliferation of cells in tumor stroma. The heterotrimeric component protein of tumor stroma, laminin, is involved in various biological activities such as angiogenesis, aggregation of the basement membrane and cellular attachment, migration, growth, proliferation, and differentiation. Among the different subtypes, laminin-5 (Ln-5) expression has been observed in HCC nodules, and the expression is associated with the acquisition of metastatic phenotype. The combined action of Ln-5 and TGF-β boosts the epithelial-to-mesenchymal transition (Aravalli *et al.,* 2013).

The surface protein integrin plays a crucial role in cell-matrix and cell-cell adhesion. The various members of integrin have a positive and negative impact on the development of carcinogenesis. For example, β1 integrin caused significant depletion in cell adhesion. It elicited the potential to inhibit the S-phase kinase-associated protein2 (Skp2)-dependent degeneration of p27 through the participation of phosphoinositide 3-kinase (PI3K) pathway leading to a substantial reduction in proliferation of malignant hepatocytes, SMMC-7721. On the contrary, α6β4 and α3β1 integrins showed their potential for considerable increment in Ln-5-dependent migration and invasion of malignant hepatic cells. Therefore, depending on the subtypes, integrins either cause enhancement or inhibit cell growth in HCC (Bergamini *et al.,* 2007; Kikkawa *et al.,* 2008; Mizuno *et al.,* 2008).

Importance of Cancer Stem Cells in HCC

At the initial phase of tumor development, the transformation and the continuous growth of a single or few cells begin as a subpopulation of mutated cells, which guide tumor growth and progression (Merlo *et al.,* 2006). This hypothesis, known as the "stochastic or clonal evolution model," highlights that single mutated cell has the uncontrolled proliferative potential to form tumors and helps acquire resistance (Aravalli *et al.,* 2013). A more recent theory highlighting the "stem cell characteristics" of a small quiescent cell population, which guides tumor growth, recurrence, and resistance against chemotherapeutics, has challenged the clonal evolution theory concept. This model's fundamental concept states that multipotency allows few cells within a tumor to acquire characteristics such as self-renewal and heterogeneity within a tumor to reiterate the original tumor (Ma *et al.,* 2007; Visvader and Lindeman 2008). Neoplastic hepatocytes such as Huh-7 and PLC-5 have a side population (SP) of cells having stem cell-like characteristics, thus providing enough impetus in support of the concept highlighting the role of cancer stem cells (CSCs) to develop HCC (Chiba *et al.,* 2006). The findings of several experimental studies have supported the fact that the origin of HCC might be from progenitor cells (Sia *et al.,* 2017). For example, genetic alterations in mice produce an impact on the Hippo pathway in the liver, resulting in an expansion of progenitor-like cells and, finally, developing HCC, iCCA, and mixed hepatocellular cholangiocarcinoma (HCC-CCA)(Lee *et al.,* 2010). The activated oncogenes (H-RAS and SV40LT)-expressing different mouse hepatic cells such as hepatic progenitors, hepatoblasts and hepatocytes can undergo transformation leading to the development of iCCA or HCC (Holczbauer *et al.*, 2013). The subpopulation of stem cells or progenitor cells may exist in peribiliary glands present on the entire biliary tree, resulting in iCCA and fibrolamellar HCC (FLC) (Cardinale *et al.*, 2012; Cardinale *et al.*, 2011; Torbenson 2012).

Further, the Notch signaling pathway's activation results in the development of HCC and iCCA (Villanueva *et al.*, 2012; Zender *et al.*, 2013). Significantly higher abundance of mutated genes encoding isocitrate dehydrogenase has been observed in iCCA as compared to HCC and are associated with decreased hepatocyte differentiation and foster cellular proliferation of oval cells and biliary transformation after liver injury in collaboration with KRAS (Kirsten rat sarcoma viral oncogene homolog) mutation (Saha *et al.*, 2014; Ikenoue *et al.*, 2017). In brief, the above experimental evidence provides the necessary impetus regarding progenitor cells' potential in developing the two most frequent primary liver cancers, such as HCC and iCCA.

Further, several experimental pieces of evidence highlighted the potential of adult hepatocytes as a cell of origin for liver cancer development (Mu *et al.*, 2015; Shin *et al.*, 2016; Jörs *et al.*, 2015; He *et al.*, 2013; Marquardt 2016). The outcome of the studies employing fate-tracing system has highlighted the role of adult hepatocytes rather than progenitor cells for the origination of liver cancer as observed in hepatoxin-induced and carcinogen-free (Mdr2 knockout) model (Mu *et al.*, 2015; Shin *et al.*, 2016; Jörs *et al.*, 2015). Interestingly, data pointed out progenitor markers such as EPCAM (epithelial cell adhesion molecule), SOX9 (SRY-Box Transcription Factor 9), PROM1 (Prominin 1)-expressing cancer cells, $Foxl1^{+}$ that have no notable contribution for the development of HCC tumor (Shin *et al.* 2016). Further, in consensus with another study (Mu *et al.*, 2015), this study highlighted that HCC did not arise from biliary cells. The study also highlighted that the expression of hepatocyte-specific p62 resulted in induction of c-MYC, activation of mTORC1, and ultimately initiation of HCC (Umemura *et al.*, 2016). The superior plasticity property of adult hepatocytes allows them to maintain uniformity with cells acting as the origin of cancer.

Moreover, plasticity assists in dedifferentiation into progenitor state as well as restoration of hepatocyte pool. The loss of tumor suppressor TP53 drives mature hepatocytes' dedifferentiation into Nestin-positive progenitor-like cells, which subsequently expand and acquire lineage-specific oncogenic lesions such as a mutation in WNT and NOTCH leading to the development of HCC and iCCA, respectively. Regardless of origin (whether progenitor cells or adult hepatocytes), HCC with stem cell properties exhibit highly aggressive clinical behavior and inferior prognosis than HCC cells without stem cell features. The discrepancies between HCC cells that originate from mice and humans impair the study. Thus, more concrete studies are required to assess the situation responsible for transforming adult hepatocytes leading to tumor formation. Finally, the study will bridge the gap between pre-clinical and clinical stages involving patients with extensive liver damage. The investigation should identify cells that become exceedingly susceptible to the HCC associated oncogenic mutations, such as in TERT promoter or CTNNB1 (Sia *et al.*, 2017).

Inflammation and HCC

The causative agents for liver inflammation include viruses, bacteria, metabolites of alcohol, drugs, and chemicals. The liver's inability to convert medicines and chemicals to non-reactive or non-immunogenic substances due to impaired hepatic metabolism usually accumulates toxic substances that lead to liver damage (Fallot *et al.*, 2012; Severi *et al.*, 2010). In response to liver damage, chemokines and cytokines are released by Kupffer cells and other different cells, leading to inflammation development (Aravalli *et al.*, 2013; Singh *et al.*, 2018). Further, uncontrolled cellular proliferation accompanied by liver inflammation can significantly impact the pathogenesis of liver cancer. Plenty of studies (Aravalli *et al.*, 2013; Singh *et al.*, 2018; Naugler and Karin 2008a) have suggested that primarily liver injury due to viral hepatitis results from host immune response triggered by viral antigen. The coordinated action of humoral and cellular immunity results in clearance of viral pathogen principally through three mechanisms as follows: (a) direct destruction of infected hepatocytes through the participation of virus-specific T-cell, (b) antibody-mediated humoral response resulting in the elimination of free viral particles, (c) the release of specific inflammatory cytokines by activated mononuclear cells and inactivation of virus non-cytopathically in infected hepatocytes. Cytokines and chemokines produced by several different cells are present in the liver. The cell surface receptors of several cytokines such as IL-1β, IL-6, and TNF-α are present in hepatocytes. Liver sinusoidal endothelial cells function both as a source and target of cytokines. Kupffer cells produce the majority of them (Leonardi *et al.*, 2012). Several reports (Nakagawa *et al.*, 2009; Wong *et al.*, 2009; Naugler and Karin 2008b) revealed that IL-6 is of prime importance among the various cytokines due to its direct HCC-correlation, especially in the presence of cirrhosis. Chronic hepatitis leads to elevated production of IL-6 by activated Kupffer cells. Several investigations revealed a significantly elevated serum IL-6 level in viral hepatitis induced by chronic HCV/HBV infection, alcoholic hepatitis, and non-alcoholic steatohepatitis. IL-6 knockout mice showed a massive reduction in diethylnitrosamine (DENA)-induced HCC development, signifying the direct implication of IL-6 signaling in experimental carcinogenesis (Aravalli *et al.*, 2013; Singh *et al.*, 2018). Accumulating evidence suggested that IL-6 substantially uplifts the proliferation of hepatic tumor cells by diminishing the apoptosis process *via* activation of signal transducer and activator of transcription 3 (STAT3) (Yu *et al.*, 2009). Further, IL-6 establishes an essential liaison between HCC and obesity. The production of IL-6 in Kupffer cells is significantly inhibited by estrogen, signifying gender biases in HCC development (Aravalli *et al.*, 2013).

TNF-α is the pro-inflammatory immune mediator produced by Kupffer cells and other immune cells. Chronic tissue injury affects NF-κB and Akt pathways and may participate in tumor development and progression. Further, it can induce oxidative stress in primary murine hepatocytes by forming metabolite 8-ox--deoxyguanosine (8-oxodG), resulting in extensive DNA damage (Leonardi *et al.*, 2012). Interestingly, the role of TNF-α is still questionable as the findings in published literature highlight the elevated as well as reduced expression of TNF-α in HCC (Leonardi *et al.*, 2012; Aravalli *et al.*, 2007).

IL-1β induces activation, proliferation, and transdifferentiation into the myofibroblastic phenotype of HSCs. Further, it triggers HSC for the production and activation of MMP, especially MMP-9. IL-1β in neoplastic hepatocytes such as HepG2, Hep3B, and Huh-7 induced the expression of TNF-based apoptosis-inducing ligand (Han *et al.*, 2004; Leonardi *et al.*, 2012).

The transcription factor NF-κB plays a crucial role in innate immunity and inflammatory signaling pathways in the liver. Upon activation, Dimeric NF-κB undergoes nuclear translocation followed by its attachment with a particular nuclear factor resulting in stimulation in the transcription of genes involved in immune response, inflammation, survival, and cell proliferation. NF-κB activates in all forms of chronic liver diseases such as viral hepatitis, alcoholic or non-alcoholic, and biliary liver diseases. The inflammatory HCC model (hepatocyte-specific lymphotoxin αβ transgenic mouse model) highlighted the positive impetus of NF-κβ in a transgenic mouse model. The hepatocyte-specific deletion Inhibitor of nuclear factor kappa-B kinase (IKK-β) resulted in inhibition of NF-κβ, leading to a significant reduction in progression of HCC (Singh *et al.*, 2018).

Globally, HBV-positive patients with metastatic HCC show a Th1/Th2-like cytokine shift. The change results in a significant elevation in expressions of Th2-like cytokine profile (IL-4, IL-8, IL-10, and IL-5) and subsequently reduced expressions of Th1-like cytokines (IL-1α, IL-1β, IL-2, IL-12p35, IL-12p40, IL-15, TNF-α, and interferon–γ (IFN-γ)). The literature findings highlighted the direct correlation between cytokine shift and metastatic phenotype, indicating anti-inflammatory/immune-suppressive responses that may help induce HCC (Budhu *et al.*, 2006; Aravalli *et al.*, 2013).

IL-12 functions as a tumor suppressor by promoting the production of IFN-γ in natural killer (NK) cells and naïve T cells. The principal role of IL-12 is to induce differentiation of T-cells resulting in the enhancement of cell-mediated immune response. Further, it serves as a vital link between innate and adaptive immune systems. The serum of patients suffering from chronic hepatitis, cirrhosis, and HCC exhibited significantly elevated expression of IL-12. The rat liver revealing expression of IL-12 from adenoviral vector showed a 60% reduction in tumor growth upon treatment with DENA. The reason could be IL-12 mediated activation of NK cells and downregulation of angiogenesis. Further, intratumoral injection of IL-12 in HCC-induced rats resulted in infiltration of lymphocytes into tumor promoted by NK cells, $CD3^+$ cells, and Mac-1 positive cells resulting in significant inhibition of angiogenesis and subsequently the tumor growth (Leonardi *et al.,* 2012; Aravalli *et al.,* 2013). An attempt has explored the potential of IL-12 anti-tumor therapeutics against HCC. However, the clinical applicability of IL-12 is questionable due to high systemic toxicity associated with an elevated level of IFN-γ due to high-dose therapy required to exhibit therapeutic efficacy. The growing number of findings in the literature highlighted single-nucleotide polymorphisms (SNPs) in various cytokines—for example, the use of C31T polymorphism in IL-1β as a genetic marker for hepatitis-related HCC. Similarly, C626G and A628C polymorphisms of TRAIL 1 receptor indicated an increased possibility of developing HCC (Bochud *et al.,* 2012; Joshita *et al.,* 2012, Marabita *et al.,* 2011).

Oxidative Stress in HCC

All living systems maintain a reducing cellular redox environment within their cells by managing a constant metabolic energy input controlled by enzymes having a wide variation in cellular functions. An impairment in normal redox state leads to elevated reactive oxygen species (ROS) and reactive nitrogen species (RNS), leading to oxidative stress. Persistent oxidative stress in chronic hepatic inflammation irrespective of etiology and liver cirrhosis, as reported in the literature, generates high amounts of reactive oxygen species (ROS). The principal resource of free radicals include mitochondrial and cytochrome P450 enzymes of hepatocytes (Das *et al.,* 2010), endotoxin-activated Kupffer cells, and neutrophils. ROS and RNS play an essential role in the transcription and activation of cytokines and growth factors, leading to the pathogenesis and progression of HCC. ROS level under the physiological level plays a pivotal role in several cellular processes such as oxidative phosphorylation, cellular proliferation, apoptosis, and senescence. Different antioxidant enzymes such as superoxide dismutase (SOD), catalase (CAT), thioredoxin (TRX), glutathione peroxidase (Gpx) are the key players to maintain the ROS levels within the physiological level (Ghosh *et al.,* 2014). Persistent oxidative stress due to chronic inflammation results in the generation of high levels of ROS and antioxidant enzymes that are incapable of neutralizing them, leading to their attack on mitochondria. Mitochondrial DNA (mtDNA) is prone to attack due to the lack of protective histone, limited genetic repair system, and the proximity to the high level of ROS (Trachootham *et al.*, 2009). Mutation in mtDNA alters various metabolic activities dependent on mitochondria, such as calcium ion homeostasis, oxidative phosphorylation, *etc.*

Further, ROS that leak from mitochondria results in mutation of DNA leading to physiological and biochemical alterations in the cells resulting in the sequential conversion of normal hepatocytes into malignant hepatocytes through the acquisition of several neoplastic characteristics such as uncontrolled cellular proliferation, activation of mitogenic signaling, and disruption of the cellular death signaling pathway, promotion of epithelial-mesenchymal transition, metastasis, angiogenesis and chemoresistance (Wang *et al.*, 2018). The compelling number of reports has revealed that malignant cells are adapted to function at a higher level of endogenous stress as compared to normal cells both *in vitro* and *in vivo* (Trachootham *et al.*, 2009; Wang *et al.*, 2018; Ma *et al.*, 2016; Dong *et al.*, 2016). Multiple pathways in cancer cells are involved for the activation of redox-sensitive transcription factors such as nuclear factor-κB (NF-κB), nuclear erythroid 2-related factor 2 (Nrf2), c-jun, and hypoxia-inducible factor-1 (HIF-1), leading to upregulation of antioxidant molecules such as SOD, catalase, thioredoxin, and GSH antioxidant system. Expressions of cell-survival molecules such as Bcl-2 family proteins and the Akt survival pathway by redox-sensitive transcription factors may be other mechanisms that confer drug-resistant capacity. Further, an alteration in the function of cell death factors (such as caspases) also contributes to redox adaptation. These adaptive redox mechanisms help the cancer cells to escape from severe oxidative damage and survive under stress and ROS-mediated mutation.

Further, ROS activate many signaling cascades such as Ras/Raf *via* oxidative modification and MAPK. Reports in the literature have revealed ROS-induced activation of p38 MAPK as one of the key players responsible for HCC progression (Aravalli *et al.*, 2013). Oxidative stress in the liver activates hepatic stellate cells, resulting in extracellular matrix deposition leading to liver fibrogenesis. Lipid peroxidation resulted in the accumulation of malonaldehyde (MDA) in the serum of chronic hepatitis patients. The levels of superoxide radicals, MDA, GSH/glutathione disulfide (GSSG), and redox enzymes' activities were significantly higher in HBV-associated HCC patients than healthy individuals (Andrea *et al.*, 2015; Marra *et al.*, 2011). Thus, HCC presents two relevant concerns: (i) occurrence of cirrhotic background resulting in a profound decrease in quality of life and survival of patients and (ii) oxidative stress and chronic inflammation responsible for pleiotropic pathogenesis of HCC.

Epithelial-Mesenchymal Transition (EMT)

EMT plays a prime role in embryogenesis as it is involved in the generation of mesoderm, which organizes into multiple layers. Cancer progression and metastasis frequently undergo activation of EMT. Further, chemoresistance and recurrence developed in cancer directly correlate with the acquisition of the EMT features. EMT can generate cells possessing the characteristics of stem cells and the invasive metastasis characteristics observed frequently in cancer (Iwatsuki *et al.*, 2010; Thiery *et al.*, 2009). An array of transcription factors, namely Twist, Snail, and Slug, activated during embryogenesis also played an essential role in tumor progression (Sanker *et al.*, 2019). TGF-β secreted by stromal liver parenchyma cells and enhancement in PDGF signaling in ras-transformed malignant hepatocytes stimulate EMT and tumor progression. Downregulation of E-cadherin (CDH1) and hepatocyte nuclear factor (HNF)-4α and upregulation of Twist, Snail, Slug, and Vimentin are often observed in liver cancer, signifying poor prognosis (Aravalli *et al.*, 2013). A mouse model of HCC both *in vitro* and *in vivo* exhibited destabilization of adherent junctions along with the acquisition of invasion and metastatic ability due to EMT. Outcomes of the study showed that overexpression of four genes such as CDH1, an inhibitor of DNA binding 2 (ID2), MMP 9, and transcription factor 3 (TCF3) in HCV-infected HCC patients indicated poor prognosis, highlighting the importance of this four-gene signature in molecular classification of HCC (Kim *et al.*, 2010; Ding *et al.*, 2010).

Hypoxia and HCC

Hypoxia boosts the entire key process of HCC development, and they include proliferation, angiogenesis, metastasis, and radio and chemoresistance of cells belonging to HCC. Hypoxia-inducible factor -1 (HIF-1), an important oxygen-dependent DNA regulatory element, acts as a master regulator to promote the plethora of signature characteristics of malignancy such as epithelial-mesenchymal transitions (EMT), intravasation, oxidative defense, extravasation, invasion of the extracellular matrix, and secondary growth of metastases, *i.e.*, overall development of malignant transformation at a low partial pressure of oxygen (Li *et al.*, 2018). Accumulating evidence in published literature has revealed that HIF-1α exerts multiple effects resulting in aggravation and poor prognosis in HCC (Luo *et al.*, 2014; Bowyer *et al.*, 2017; Wilson *et al.*, 2014; Thambi *et al.*, 2014; Yu *et al.*, 2017). They include: (a) upregulation of genes involved in glycolytic pathway cascade such as phosphoglycerate kinase 1 (PGK1), hexokinase-2 (HK2), glyceraldehyde-3-phosphate dehydrogenase

(GAPDH) and phosphofructokinase (PFK), glucose transporters (*e.g. GLUT1*) and *LDH* leading to enhancement of ATP production anaerobically by converting glucose to lactate, (b) function as a transcriptional activator of vascular endothelial growth factor (VEGF), transforming growth factor alpha (TGF- α) and insulin-like growth factor (IGF)-2 leading to cellular proliferation and survival, (c) promotion of angiogenesis to support oxygen and nutrient delivery, (d) promotion of EMT transition for the acquisition of metastatic phenotype, (e) imparting resistance against chemo and radio therapeutics resulting poor prognosis, (f) elevated the synthesis of monocarboxylate transporters (responsible for expulsion of lactate into the extracellular space) and carbonic anhydrase (CA) -9 and 12 (responsible for generation of HCO_3 by using CO_2), thus reduces the chance of death due to hypoxic acidosis due to lactate generation leading to elongation of cellular survival of malignant population.

A report in published literature has highlighted that CA9 mediated cytokines' expression in Hep3B cells in the presence of the hypoxic condition, indicating its role as one of the vital tumor markers of HCC. Comparative microarray to analyze the gene expressions of HepG2 cells in a chronic hypoxic condition and that in HCC patients (van Malenstein *et al.*, 2010) revealed that chronic hypoxia resulted in the expression of 7 sets of various genres, including FGF21 and cyclin D1. Hypoxia resulted in the downregulation of endogenous degradation machinery in neoplastic hepatocytes leading to enhanced production and intracellular accumulation of β-catenin. The embryogenic hepatic development is regulated by bone morphogenic proteins (BMPs) (Maegdefrau *et al.*, 2009). Among the BMP family, the elevated expression of BMP-4 is promoted by hypoxia in HCC, resulting in vasculogenesis and tumor progression. Further, the high-mobility group box 1 (HMGB1) upregulates the expressions of caspase-1 and inflammatory cytokines in hypoxic HCC cells, leading to the tumor's extensive invasiveness and metastasis. Hypoxia-induced autophagy induced chemoresistance in HCC cells (Du *et al.*, 2012; Yan *et al.*, 2012; Song *et al.*, 2009).

Impairment of Cell Cycle in HCC

Malfunctioning of the cell cycle regulators is the common feature in malignant cells resulting in angiogenesis, uncontrolled proliferation, hyperplasia, and, finally, tumor formation. The healthy liver usually remains at a quiescent state, and gradual renewal of cells takes place. They possess the powerful regenerative ability, and they enter into the cell cycle in response to the mitogenic signal and subsequently advance for cell division (Michalopoulos 2010). Cyclin and cyclin-dependent kinases (Cdk) and de-novo expression of the *CYCLIN D1* gene are induced by cytokines and growth factors. The checkpoint regulators strictly control cellular proliferation and prevent the entry of quiescent hepatocytes into the cell cycle (Sharma *et al.*, 2014). The retinoblastoma (pRb) and other proteins downregulate the expression of the E2F transcription factor, leading to a significant decrement in its activity (Henley and Dick 2012). The binding of Cdk4/6 with the members (p15/16/17/18/19) of the Ink4 family of Cdk inhibitors leads to a significant decrease in the formation of cyclin D-Cdk4/6 complex (Singh *et al.*, 2018). The gene expression profiling of HCC samples resulted in identifying a "proliferation cluster" that depicts enhanced expression of proliferation-associated genes. The downregulated expression of p16/pRb genes or impairment in the function of proteins encoded by these genes may result in tumorigenesis as the proper functioning of p16/pRb restricts the entry of quiescent cells into the cell cycle. The changes in the expression of pRb are less frequent in HCC. The expression levels members of the CDK interacting protein (Cip)/ kinase inhibitory protein (Kip) family, namely, p21/27 that have been decreased persistently in HCC samples resulting in the promotion of cellular movement through various phases of the cell cycle (Singh *et al.*, 2018).

Loss of Senescence Control

Senescence has distinct morphological features of irreversible growth inhibition of cells. The exact mechanism responsible for hepatocytes' senescence is not known (Singh *et al.*, 2018). The one mechanism could be a continuous decrease in the telomeric segment through the hepatocytes' partial proliferative ability. The telomere-independent tools, including free radical and oncogene-dependent senescence, have been predicted as probable mechanisms for monitoring senescence in hepatocytes in chronic liver diseases. The DNA damage initiated by free radical and oncogene-mediated senescence stimulates ATM/Chk/p53 pathway leading to cell arrest at the G1 phase. A similar mechanism has been followed by p16/pRb pathway also. The malfunctioning of DNA damage checkpoints and regulators of the cell cycle produces a conducive environment for uncontrolled proliferation of mutated hepatocytes at the senescence phase leading to malignant transformation. Different types of human HCC have shown variations in the extent of mutation in the p53 pathway as depicted below (a) p53 mutation has been observed approximately 50% and 20-30% of aflatoxin-mediated and non–aflatoxin-mediated HCC, respectively, (b) HCC with a mutation in p53 pathway seldom report $p14^{ARF}$, (c) overexpression of Mdm2 has been observed in HCC, (d) human HCC has shown overexpression of oncoprotein gankyrin that restricts overexpression of pRb and p53 (Singh *et al.*, 2018).

Alterations of genes such as p16, p15, and RB1 of the pRb pathway were in above 80% of HCC cases. Methylation of promoter of the gene (p15/p16) and deletion or mutation of RB1 gene generally occurs. Among them, methylation of the promoter of p16 leads to downregulation of the gene. The transformation of the precancerous lesion into neoplasia requires activation of telomerase. Cirrhosis reveals telomerase-dependent senescence arrest. Reactivation of TERT acts as a circumvention to vigorously promote HCC to progress aggressively. Activation of telomerase is a rate-limiting step for the initiation of cellular immortality.

Interestingly, activation has been observed in most HCC cases, whereas it is absent in normal hepatocytes. The surface proteins (viral X and PreS2) and HCV core protein may enhance telomerase activity. Thus, activation of telomerase activity and changes in senescence controlling genes are the substantial predisposing factors for the hepatic neoplastic transformation (Singh *et al.*, 2018).

Apoptosis and HCC

Inflammatory liver disease, development of fibrosis, and HCC cause different types of liver injury and related chronic cell death. The principal cell death processes with HCC follow apoptosis (programmed) and necrosis (accidental). The other modes of cell death, such as autophagy, necroptosis, pyroptosis, ferroptosis alone or in combination, also contribute to the development and progression of HCC (Eguchi *et al.*, 2014). Several molecular anomalies resulting in impairment in the regulation of apoptotic process lead to malignant transformation and development of HCC. Among them, the most frequent alteration found in HCC is the mutation of the *TP53 gene.* Resistance to apoptosis conferred by death receptor ligands, such as FasL or TNF-related apoptosis-inducing ligand (TRAIL), has also been reported in HCC (Ranjan and Pathak 2016). Overactivation of anti-apoptotic pathways makes a significant contribution to disrupting the balance between death and survival in HCC. Overexpression of apoptosis counteracting molecules such as Bcl-XL, Mcl-1, cellular inhibitor of apoptosis protein-1 (c-IAP1), X-linked inhibitor-of-apoptosis protein (XIAP), cause cellular survival in HCC cells. The upregulation of expressions of growth factors and the molecules associated with machinery are responsible for cleavage of their proforms to active peptides in HCC. The resistance to apoptosis occurs in HCC, induced by the activation of the JAK/STAT, PI3K/AKT, and RAS/ERKs pathways. Finally, the published investigations have suggested that inflammatory processes and EMT have also contributed to cell survival in HCC (Singh *et al.*, 2018).

Cellular Signalling Pathways in HCC

Hepatocarcinogenesis is a complex multi-stage process that requires the participation of several signaling pathways. This signaling cascade promotes the growth, proliferation, and survival of neoplastic hepatocytes. Briefly, we have discussed the signaling pathways involved in hepatocarcinogenesis below.

EGF/TGF-α pathway

Overexpression of EGF has been reported in chronic hepatitis, cirrhosis, and HCC. Further, EGFR is recognized as a poor prognostic factor of HCC and is associated with rapid tumor growth and intrahepatic metastases. Overexpression of TGF-α has been found in the pre-neoplastic lesion, indicating its role in early HCC (Buckley *et al.*, 2008; Scaggiante *et al.*, 2016; Komposch and Sibilia 2016). Epidermal growth factor (EGF) and its close associate transforming growth factor α (TGF-α) bind to epidermal growth factor receptor (EGFR), and activation of this pathway results in tumor growth and progression.

Insulin Growth Factor (IGF) Pathway

The circulating ligands such as IGF-I, IGF-II, and their receptor IGF-IR constitute this pathway (Mekuria and Abdhi 2017; Pollak 2012). Progressive upregulation of IGF-II and IGF substrates at mRNA and protein levels has been observed during hepatocarcinogenesis, as evidenced in neoplastic hepatocytes. They are involved in cellular proliferation and inhibition of apoptosis (Breuhahn and Schirmacher 2008).

HGF/c-Met Pathway

Mesenchymal cells secrete cytokines and hepatocyte growth factor (HGF) that bind with the c-Met receptor (Alessandro *et al.*, 2015). The pivotal roles of the HGF/c-Met pathway to promote cellular proliferation, survival, and cellular motility have been implicated in various cancers, including HCC (Ang *et al.*, 2013). Further, the overexpressed c-Met has increased metastatic potential and poor prognosis in HCC (Giordano and Columbano 2014).

Signaling Pathways Involved in Neovascularization in HCC

Angiogenesis plays a crucial role in HCC due to its highly vascular nature (Elsamanoudy *et al.*, 2016). This process requires paracrine and autocrine interactions between tumor cells and vascular endothelial cells. The released pro-angiogenic factors from tumor cells in response to the hypoxic condition and nutrient deprivation activate endothelial cells, which disrupt the extracellular matrix leading to the release of angiogenic factors such as vascular endothelial growth factor (VEGF), fibroblast growth factor (FGF), platelet-derived growth factor (PDGF), and transforming growth factor β (TGF-β). These angiogenic factors initiate activation of endothelial cells through tyrosine kinase receptors (TKR) and intracellular mediators such as mitogen-activated protein kinase (MAPK), phosphoinositide 3-kinase (PI3K)/Akt/mammalian target of rapamycin (mTOR) pathways resulting in proliferation and migration of endothelial cells.

The proliferated endothelial cells form a new tubular structure and lumen for new blood vessels. Finally, activation and recruitment of pericytes stabilize the new blood vessels. Plenty of literature has revealed the role of VEGF and FGF as the most vital stimuli for tumor angiogenesis in HCC. VEGF is considered the most potent angiogenic factor in HCC (Tumanova and Shchegolev 2015; Nana *et al.*, 2016).

MAPK Pathways

The aberrant upstream signals such as EGFR signaling, IGF signaling, together with the inactivation of tumor suppressor genes by aberrant methylation, probably result in activation of intracellular signaling pathway, MAP kinase kinase (MEK 1/2) through Ras leading to activation of extracellular signal-regulated kinase (ERK1/2) by phosphorylation (Min *et al.*, 2011; Schmitz *et al.*, 2008). Stimulation of ERK further activates numerous nuclear and cytosolic proteins involved in cellular proliferation, inhibition of apoptosis, angiogenesis, and metastasis. Reports in the literature revealed that overexpression of MEK 1/2, ERK 1/2, and phosphorylation of ERK1/2 was observed in HCC patients, indicating its critical role in HCC tumorigenesis (Yu *et al.*, 2015; Roskoski 2010).

PI3K/Akt/mTOR Pathway

PI3K/Akt/mTOR pathway plays a pivotal role in carcinogenesis, including HCC (Bunney and Katan 2010). Numerous factors contribute to activation of Akt, such as tyrosine kinase receptor (EGF or IGF signaling), constitutive activation of PI3K, and loss of function of tumor suppressor gene, PTEN, by epigenetic silencing or somatic mutations (Llovet and Bruix, 2008; Villanueva *et al.*, 2008). A growing number of reports in the literature has suggested a positive correlation between activated Akt and poor prognosis in HCC (Llovet and Bruix, 2008; Menon *et al.*, 2012)

mTOR, an essential mediator of the PI3K-Akt pathway, acts as a central regulator of cell growth and proliferation. It allows cells' progress from the G1 phase to the S phase of the cell cycle by sensing the nutritional status. An activated mTOR pathway was observed in HCC, as reported in the literature (Sabatini 2006).

Signaling Pathways Related to Cell Differentiation and Development

Wnt-β Catenin Pathway

Wnt-β catenin plays a crucial role in regulating the developmental process, namely differentiation, cellular migration, and hepatocytes' survival (Saito-Diaz *et al.*, 2013). Wnt canonical pathway describes a cascade that translocates β catenin from cell membrane to nucleus upon activation. It acts as a coactivator of the T-cell factor/lymphoid enhancer factor (TCF/LEF) family of transcription factors and regulators of specific activity of oncogenes such as *c-myc, cyclin D,* and *survivin*. Wnt ligands' stimulation of Frizzled receptor produces a signal for uncoupling of β catenin from E-cadherin at the plasma membrane (Saito-Diaz *et al.,* 2013).

Evidence in the literature reported Wnt cascade activation in HCC, especially in HCV-induced HCC (Wasiberg and Saba 2015). Further, the accumulation of β-catenin protein has been observed in the nuclei of neoplastic hepatocytes around 40-70% of patients with HCC. Aberrant methylation of tumor suppressors such adenomatous polyposis coli (APC) and E-cadherin and autocrine/paracrine secretion of Wnt ligands activate Wnt canonical ligands (Waisberg and Saba 2015).

Hedgehog (Hh) Signaling

In cellular differentiation and regeneration, and stem cell biology, Hh signaling regulates cellular proliferation, apoptosis, and migration (Lee *et al.,* 2016). Three related Hh ligands are sonic hedgehog (SHh), Indian hedgehog (iHh), and desert hedgehog. Among the different hedgehog ligands, the association of SHh with HCC has been reported in the literature (Mohammed *et al.,* 2016; Lian-Yi *et al.,* 2014). Chen *et al.* (2013a) revealed that SHh induced cell migration and invasion in HCC *via* focal adhesion kinase/Akt signaling-mediated production of matrix-metalloproteinase-2 and -9.

Notch Pathway

It regulates the cellular differentiation pathway during embryonic development and adulthood and is highly conserved (Yamamoto *et al.,* 2014). In the liver, it controls biliary fate and morphogenesis. Many types of cancer, including HCC, can be developed due to the notch pathway's deregulation (Kevin *et al.,* 2015). Distinct roles of this pathway in HCC have been reported in the literature (Kevin *et al.,* 2015; Villanueva *et al.,* 2012; Yamamoto *et al.,* 2014). For example, some studies have revealed that overexpression of notch 1 inhibited HCC by promoting cell cycle arrest and apoptosis. Contrary to this, some studies have reported the positive role of notch 1 in the pathogenesis of HCC as it enabled the formation of hepatic tumors in mice (Gramantieri *et al.,* 2007).

Hippo Pathway

This evolutionarily conserved pathway regulates apoptosis, cellular differentiation, and proliferation and controls organ size (Hong *et al.,* 2015). The failure in regulation of this pathway has been associated with cancer development. Evidence in literature has suggested that Yes-associated protein 1 (YAP 1), a critical hippo pathway component, might act as an independent prognostic indicator of HCC patients (Kang *et al.,* 2016; Li *et al.,* 2012a). Further, plenty of reports in the literature (Vicente *et al.,* 2015; Li *et al.,* 2012a; Su-Xia *et al.,* 2014) has highlighted the role of activated YAP1 in HCC and correlates YAP1 expression to the stages, serum AFP level, and prognosis of HCC. An alteration in the hippo pathway might result in activation of YAP1 (Kang *et al.,* 2016; Li *et al.,* 2012a).

Target Receptor(s) and Biomarker Proteins in HCC

Asialoglycoprotein Receptor

Asialoglycoprotein receptor (ASGP-R) is mainly present on the surface of hepatic cells. It is made up of a single subunit having an average molecular weight of 41,000 (Weigel 1981). It has the galactose terminal and galactosamine residues (Elanggar *et al.,* 2019; Weigel 1982). It plays a significant role in the clearance of the desialylated protein from serum through endocytosis and lysosomal degradation. The majority of well-differentiated HCC expresses asialoglycoprotein receptors, and expression of asialoglycoprotein has been reported in four out of six well-differentiated HCC (Hyodo *et al.,* 1993). This interpretation was further supported by Trere *et al.* (1999) as they reported the expression of ASGP-R in 80% of well-differentiated and 20% of poorly-differentiated HCC. Additionally, they said that ASGP-R was present in the plasma membrane of DNA-synthesizing cells. Finally, several studies have concluded that the potential of ASGP-R as a surface biomarker to recognize HCC and could be explored for neoplastic hepatocyte-specific targeted drug delivery (Quan *et al.,* 2015; Thapa *et al.,* 2015; D'Souza and Devarajan 2015).

Glypican-3 (GPC3)

Glypican 3, most commonly known as GPC3, a member of heparan sulfate proteoglycans, contains three segments: core protein, heparan sulfate chain glycosyl-phosphatidyl inositol (GPI). The covalent GPI anchor mediates the attachment of GPC3 protein to the hepatocyte membrane. The N-terminal secretory signal peptide and hydrophobic domain must add GPI anchor to the C-terminus (Filmus and Selleck 2001; Zhang *et al.,* 2016). Several studies have reported that a predominantly high expression of GPC3 occurs in HCC tumor tissue, and minimal expression of it is observed in non-tumor liver tissues (Mu *et al.,* 2014). Further, several studies concluded that the canonical Wnt model positively modulates the expression of GPC3, and its upregulation leads to neoplastic transformation (Capurro *et al.,* 2005). Two heparan sulfate side chains and the core protein of GPC3 probably form a complex with Wnt at the cell surface (Baumhoer *et al.,* 2008). Evidence in literature has suggested that GPC3 may promote the translocation of transcription factor β-catenin by stimulating the Wnt pathway (Polakis 2012). Further, the literature has also reported the role of transcription factor c-Myc as a regulator of GPC3 expression through the Wnt pathway (Li *et al.,* 2012b). Thus, targeted drug delivery to target GPC3 is being explored by researchers to achieve better therapeutic outcomes (Feng *et al.,* 2013; Hanaoka *et al.,* 2015; Wang *et al.,* 2016).

Transferrin Receptor (TfR)

TfR is a transmembrane glycoprotein and is also known as CD71. It is composed of two homodimers joined by intermolecular disulfide bonds. Each subunit is made of 760 amino acids and has three domains such as the extracellular domain of 671 amino acids with a large extracellular C-terminal domain, transmembrane domain composed of 28 amino acids and short single-pass domain, the intracellular domain of 61 amino acids, and N-terminal domain (Tros de Ilarduya and Duzgunes 2013). TfR overexpression as compared to normal cells has been found in different types of malignant cells, including HCC. Further, researchers reported that TfR-2, homologous to TfR1, was predominantly expressed in hepatocytes and erythrocytes of the small intestine. Thus, it can be explored to develop targeted drug delivery in HCC (Tortorella and Karagiannis 2014).

Heat Shock Protein 70 (HSP70)

It is a molecular chaperone that is activated in response to stress and protection for cell survival. HSP70 is under the strict control of upstream transcription factor heat shock factor-1 (HSF-1). Upregulation of HSF-1 helps HSP70 promote tumor invasion and metastasis in HCC (Jin *et al.,* 2011; Fang *et al.,* 2012; Liu *et al.,* 2014). Further, the study conducted by Liu *et al.* (2014) reported the abundant expression of 14-3-3σ in HCC tumors, and upregulation of 14-3-3σ positively modulates the expression of HSP70, which in turn induces cellular proliferation *via* β-catenin/HSF-1 dependent pathway. Thus, HSP70 and its downstream regulator, 14-3-3σ, and upstream regulator modulate the HCC development as HSP70 overexpression results in microvascular thrombi formation in HCC patients as a potential prognostic biomarker of HCC. HSP70 can be explored to develop targeted therapy in HCC due to its predominant upregulation that has been observed exclusively in neoplastic hepatocytes (Jin *et al.,* 2011; Fang *et al.,* 2012).

Tumor-Associated Glycoprotein-72 (TAG-72)

TAG-72 is a mucin-1 (MUC-1) like macromolecular glycoprotein. Overexpression of TAG-72 has been observed in most adenocarcinomas such as gastric, colon, and pancreatic cancer (Chauhan *et al.,* 2007; Zhang *et al.,* 2012). The relationship between TAG-72 and HCC was established by Zhang *et al.* (2012). They performed analysis on sixty pairs of HCC and paracarcinomatous (PCLT) tissues and 10 normal liver (NL) tissues; for Western blot and immunohistochemistry analysis. They found a significantly high TAG-72 protein expression in HCC tissues compared to PCLT and NL tissues. They concluded that elevated TAG 72 correlated with TNM stage, Edmondson-Steiner grade, vein invasion, and multiple tumor nodes. Further, they highlighted that overexpression of TAG-72 resulted in shorter overall survival. Thus, TAG-72 can be considered a potential prognostic marker for HCC and may be explored for vital clinical implications such as developing neoplastic hepatocyte-specific targeted drug delivery (Chauhan *et al.,* 2007; Chauhan and Lahiri 2016).

Golgi Protein73 (GP73)

GP73 is a type-II Golgi-specific membrane protein that is encoded by the *GOLMI* gene on chromosome 9q21.33. The elevated level of GP73 in several types of malignancy, such as lung adenocarcinoma, seminomas, and renal cell cancer, has more pronounced activity in liver diseases, especially in HCC (Norton *et al.,* 2008). Several studies have reported an elevated level of serum GP73 in primary hepatic carcinoma (PHC). Further, reports are available on fucosylated GP73 (FC-GP73), and these findings suggested that FC-GP73 was more sensitive and specific for the diagnosis of HCC as compared to GP73. However, the definitive role of GP73 on tumor size, stage, recurrence, and prognosis needs to investigate extensively to explore GP73 for clinical application (Block *et al.,* 2010; Kladney *et al.,* 2000).

Ki-67 Antigen

Ki-67 is a nuclear protein that is involved in cellular proliferation. The elevated level of Ki-67 has been observed in grade 1 to grade IV HCC tumors. Thus, expression of this proliferative biomarker has a direct correlation with the severity of the disease (Scholzen and Gerdes 2000; Mohamed *et al.,* 2008)

Somatostatin Receptor (SSTR)

SSTR, a superfamily of transmembrane G-protein coupled receptors, has varied expression densities in the brain, gut, endocrine, exocrine pancreas, adrenals, thyroid, kidneys, and immune cells (Patel 1999). The expression of SSTR has been reported in various liver diseases such as acute hepatitis, chronic hepatitis, cirrhosis, and HCC (Kouroumalis *et al.,* 1998). SSTR was found to express in 41% of HCC patients (24/59), whereas expression of SSTR was absent in normal liver cells such as hepatocytes and hepatic stellate cells, as evidenced from the study (Reynaert *et al.,* 2004). The expression levels of different subtypes such as SSTR1, SSTR2, SSTR3, SSTR4, and SSTR5 of SSTR receptor in HCC were found to be 46, 41, 64, 0, and 75%, respectively (Reynaert *et al.,* 2004). These findings were further supported by several other studies (Notas 2004; Blaker 2004). Thus, the antibodies capable of binding to SSTR3 and SSTR4 can develop targeted therapy against HCC.

Homodimeric Glycoprotein (AF-20)

The presence of AF-20 specifically in HCC tissue was reported in various studies (Wilson *et al.,* 1988). It is a dimer where a disulfide bond joins an individual subunit of molecular weight of 90 kDa. It is initially synthesized as a precursor core protein of 82 kDa with two added mannose units. One of the mannose units is modified to a complex polysaccharide, leading to a mature 90 kDa monomer (Moradpour *et al.,* 1995). Studies have shown the high expression of AF-20 in Huh-7 cells and on the surface of Friendship of China and United States-FOCUS human HCC cells where FOCUS was considered a model for studying hepatitis B virus-associated HCC (Wilson *et al.,* 1988). The predominantly specific expression of AF-20 on FOCUS human cells can be explored as a possible delivery approach in HCC (Zhang *et al.,* 2016).

Osteopontin (OPN)

OPN is a multi-functional protein of the extracellular matrix and participates in several biological processes (Qin 2014). Researchers demonstrated that OPN might promote cancer-stem-like phenotype *via* the αvB3-NF-κB-HIF-α pathway. They stated that OPN binds to integrin αvB3 leading to activation of the transcription factor, NF-κB resulting in upregulation of HIF-α and its downstream gene BMI1 to exert steaminess-like properties (Wang *et al.,* 2014). Further, they found that depletion in OPN resulted in a series of incidences such as a reduction in the stem cell-associated gene(s), side population cell fraction, formation of hepato-spheroids, and tumorigenicity in immune-deficient mice. These outcomes were supported by another study where they found that reduction of OPN resulted in attenuation of hepatocarcinogenesis (Shang *et al.,* 2012; Liu *et al.,* 2015). The association between pre-diagnostic OPN level and HCC incidence was established by Duarte-Salles *et al.* (2016) by a cohort study. They found that the addition of α-fetoprotein (AFP) to the OPN levels increased the sensitivity of this cohort. Several other studies also reported that OPN and AFP increased the sensitivity and specificity of diagnosis of HCC (Fouad *et al.*, 2015; Weber 2011; De Stefano *et al.*, 2018). Thus, OPN can function as a diagnostic and prognostic marker in HCC as it imparts stem cell-like properties, which are essential for HCC development.

Des-γ-Carboxyprothrombin

Des-γ-carboxyprothrombin (DCP) is also known as prothrombin-induced vitamin K absence-II (PIVKA II). Impairment in vitamin K-dependent post-translational γ-carboxylation of glutamic acid residues results in the formation of DCP, a non-functional precursor of prothrombin (Koike *et al.*, 2001). As per the published literature, an excessive synthesis of prothrombin precursors by HCC cells directly correlates with cancer progression, tumor diameter, and portal vein thrombosis (Matsubara 2012). The structural resemblance between DCP and hepatocyte growth factor renders dual functionality on DCP (Gao *et al.*, 2012). It functions as an autologous growth factor to stimulate the proliferation of HCC and paracrine factor to integrate HCC with vascular endothelial cells resulting in the promotion of angiogenesis *via* activation of VEGF and EGF (Zhu *et al.*, 2014). Further, the overall sensitivity and specificity of DCP for HCC diagnosis have ranged between 67-71% and 84-92% (Gao *et al.*, 2012; Zhu *et al.*, 2014; Yu *et al.*, 2016).

α-Fetoprotein (AFP)

AFP is produced in the liver during fetal development. Thus it is considered a fetal analog of serum albumin. Three different isoforms (AFP-L1, AFP-L2, AFP-L3) of AFP have been reported so far. They differ from each other in their binding affinity to Lens cularis agglutinin (LCA). The portion that comprises AFP-L3 shows an influential association with LCA compared to the parts that include AFP-L1 and AFPL-2 (Sterling *et al.*, 2009). Evidence in the literature revealed a close association of AFP-L3 with HCC (Lai *et al.*, 2017; Abdel-Aziz *et al.*, 2016). The simultaneous determination of AFP-L3, AFP with p-53 or with DCP revealed that the simultaneous determination provided better sensitivity and specificity than their counterpart (Lai *et al.*, 2017; Abdel-Aziz *et al.*, 2016). AFP does not assist in therapeutic decisions as a prognostic marker, especially in patients pre-treated with normal AFP levels. Differences in opinion have been observed regarding the determination of AFP level after post-treatment (Best 2016; Hadziyannis *et al.*, 2013).

Squamous Cell Carcinoma Antigen (SCCA)

SCCA, a serine protease inhibitor, is present in the squamous epithelium. It has established its clinical potential to identify patients with progressive liver diseases as a risk for HCC (Biasiolo *et al.*, 2016). Several clinical data have suggested that the overall diagnostic sensitivity of SCCA or SCCA-IgM immune complex (IC) was lower than that of AFP. However, a combination of AFP and SCCA-IgM was found to provide much better sensitivity despite a modest decrease in specificity than their counterparts (Pozzan *et al.*, 2014). Interesting pieces of evidence claiming the potential of SCCA-IgM as an independent predictor towards the progression of HCC in patients with cirrhosis are also available in the literature (Biasiolo *et al.*, 2016; Pozzan *et al.*, 2014). This fact was further supported by a retrospective study conducted on 57 cirrhotic patients. Additionally, abundant production of isoform SCCA2 by HCC, especially in those belonging to aggressive liver tumors, has also been reported in the literature (Pozzan *et al.*, 2014; Lou *et al.*, 2017). An extensive investigation can assess its diagnostic performance compared to AFP or SCCA-IgM to explore a possible therapeutic target (Biasiolo *et al.*, 2016).

Hepatocyte Paraffin 1 (HepPar1)

HepPar1 is a monoclonal antibody that is produced from failed liver xenografts. The antigen detected by HepPar1 is localized in fetal and adult livers (Villari *et al.*, 2002). It recognizes an epitope, which is most likely a component of mitochondria of neoplastic hepatocytes (Zimmerman *et al.*, 2001). It has the potential to distinguish between HCC and secondary or metastatic neoplasms. Researchers have reported that strong expression of HepPar1 was seen in the majority of HCC tumors (35/48), but the minimal expression was seen in nonhepatic tumors such as lung, gallbladder, stomach, pancreas, colon, and malignant melanoma (Xue *et al.*, 2015).

APO-J

APO-J is also known as clusterin. It is a glycoprotein containing seven glycosylated sites (Comunale *et al.*, 2011). The literature reports have highlighted its superior sensitivity compared to AFP (Nafee *et al.*, 2012; Zheng *et al.*, 2015). The level of APO-J was found to decrease significantly. Thus researchers concluded that it could be used as an independent marker of HCC (Nafee *et al.*, 2012; Zheng *et al.*, 2015). The outcomes of other studies supported the previous finding and highlighted that it could monitor HCC progression and metastasis (Nafee *et al.*, 2012; Zheng *et al.*, 2015).

DKK-1 (Dickkopf-p1)

DKK-1 can diagnose HCC at the very early stages. Further, it can detect HCC in patients where AFP fails to detect (Shen *et al.*, 2016; Tsai *et al.*, 2012). The study conducted by Zhu *et al.* (2013) highlighted its ability to act as a biomarker in patients undergoing liver transplantation, resulting in the prediction of prognosis of such patients. However, more studies are required to establish its potential as a biomarker.

Human Carbonyl Reductase 2 (HCR2)

HCR2 expresses in the liver and kidneys. It detoxifies the ROS and alpha carbonyl. The liver's tumor part shows significantly less carbonyl reductase 2 than the standard counterpart (Wang *et al.,* 2009). The downregulation of HCR2 promotes cancer growth by triggering the damage caused by ROS and other carcinogens (Liu *et al.,* 2006).

Midkine

The heparin-binding growth factor, midkine, is expressed at the time of early embryogenesis. Midkine overexpresses during wound healing, tumorigenesis, and inflammation (Zhu *et al.,* 2013). It cannot be used as a biomarker in advanced stages of HCC due to the marginal elevation in the level as compared to AFP. The expression of midkine increased at the early stages of HCC (Nault 2014).

Nerve Growth Factor (NGF)

NGF, a neurotrophin member, is involved in various physiological processes such as differentiation, survival, and preservation of the peripheral and central nervous systems. The level of NGF is correlated with tumor growth, invasion, and metastasis (Levi-Montalcini 1987). NGF normally binds with high-affinity and low-affinity receptors, namely, trkANGF and $p75^{NTR}$, respectively. The significant overexpression of $trkA^{NGF}$ has been observed in HCC. It has the potential to distinguish between cirrhosis that leads to HCC and cirrhosis that does not result in HCC development (Rasi G *et al.,* 2007).

Vascular Endothelial Growth Factor (VEGF)

VEGF is a glycosylated cytokine that acts as a mitogen and is a mediator of various cellular processes such as vascular permeability, angiogenesis, vasculogenesis, and endothelial cell growth-reduced survival (Treiber *et al.,* 2006; Zhu *et al.,* 2013). The characteristics of tumor and environment promote VEGF expression, leading to VEGF signaling and downstream MAPK cascade initiation. The level of VEGF predicts the HCC recurrence. Thus, it is an essential biomarker, indicating HCC patients' survival (Poon *et al.,* 2004; Llovet *et al.,* 2012).

Transforming Growth Factor-β (TGF-β)

TGF-β plays a pivotal role in regulating cellular proliferation and differentiation in HCC cells (Bedossa *et al.,* 1995). Elevation of TGF level has been observed in HCC patients (Liu *et al.,* 2015). Plenty of reports in the literature has highlighted the dual role of TGF-β as a biomarker and prognostic marker. Further, the close associate of TGF-β, mucin1, activates JNK/AP1 leading to regulation of TGF- β signaling (Li *et al.,* 2015; Lou *et al.,* 2017; De Stefano *et al.,* 2018). Thus, mucin1 has also been explored as a therapeutic target.

Epidermal Growth Factor (EGFR)

EGFR acts as an essential player in all phases of hepatic injury, starting from the very early stages of inflammation to HCC development, including fibrogenesis and neoplastic transformation (Berasain and Avila 2014). Among the different EGFR proteins, researchers reported detecting ErbB3 in the serum of the early stage of HCC and have also been associated with portal vein invasion and metastasis (Hsieh *et al.,* 2011; Chen *et al.,* 2013 a/b). Reports are available stating induction of miRNA-7 in HCC cells by HBV, and HBx protein was found to downregulate the EGFR expression (Berasain and Avila 2014; Lanaya *et al.,* 2014; Hu *et al.,* 2015). Several studies also evaluated the potential role of soluble EGFR in the HCC metastasis *in vivo* model (Lanaya *et al.,* 2014; Hu *et al.,* 2015).

Hepatocyte Growth Factor (HGF)

HGF is a cytokine that is released by nonparenchymal *Ito* cells in the liver (Nakamura *et al.,* 1997). The information on prognosis provided by tissue HGF is either little or insignificant. Consistently, a high level of plasma HGF was observed in patients with HCC compared to normal subjects, as reported in the literature (Mizuguchi *et al.,* 2004; Yamagamim *et al.,* 2002). Further, circulating HGF level has been directly correlated with a downward shifting of overall survival and upward shifting of tumor size, grade, recurrence, metastasis, and postoperative complications after partial hepatectomy (Mizuguchi *et al.,* 2004; Yamagamim *et al.,* 2002). Researchers have highlighted that an increase in circulating HGF has also been observed in many pathological liver conditions such as hepatitis and a more severe stage of liver cirrhosis (Mizuguchi *et al.,* 2004). However, it is not a specific biomarker of HCC.

α-1-Fucosidase

This lysosomal enzyme cleaves the fucose glycosidic bond present in glycolipids and glycoproteins. The liver's various pathological conditions, such as cirrhosis, hepatitis, and HCC, result in elevated expression of α-1-fucosidase, which is recognized as one of the early HCC biomarkers having a cut-off value of 870 nm/mL/h (Tangkijvanich *et al.,* 1999). The level of α-1-fucosidase is elevated at least six months before the HCC development, and in 85% of HCC patients, the value that has been observed is 700 nm/mL/h (Wang *et al.,* 2014).

Annexin A2

Annexin A2, a calcium-ion-dependent phospholipid-binding protein, is present at the cell surface. It is involved in cell mobility, protein interaction with the actin cytoskeleton, and endocytosis (Lokman *et al.,* 2014). Overexpression of annexin A2 was observed in HCC, and it showed an inverse relationship with the survival rates. It exhibited higher sensitivity and specificity as compared to AFP to detect early-stage HCC (Sun *et al.,* 2013; Zhang *et al.,* 2015).

Micro RNA

Micro RNAs (miRNA) are short single-stranded endogenous non-coding RNA molecules that act by an RNA silencing mechanism. The initiation of transcription of miRNA from an intronic region of the host gene results in pri-miRNA transcription, which is further processed. It is then transported to the cytoplasm by Exportin. In the cytoplasm, the enzyme dicer also processes, resulting in an entirely mature miRNA molecule. It regulates the gene expression by targeting the messenger RNA (mRNA) molecules through multiple mechanisms, namely, binding within the complementary sequence within mRNA molecule, splitting of mRNA molecule, the axing of poly(A) tail, and default translation of mRNA into protein by ribosomes (Lou *et al.,* 2017; De Stefano *et al.,* 2018). Plenty of reports in the literature has revealed that miRNAs are involved in various physiological processes such as cellular proliferation, differentiation, metabolism, and apoptosis (Macfarlane *et al.,* 2010; Shen *et al.,* 2016). Several studies have highlighted the dysregulation of miRNA at various stages of HCC (Bertoli *et al.,* 2015; Casanova-Salas, 2014). Attempts have explored miRNA as a potential biomarker for diagnosis, prognosis, staging, and prediction of therapeutic responses in HCC (Li *et al.,* 2016; Jin *et al.,* 2017; Jin *et al.,* 2019). For example, there was an overexpression of miR-122 in serum in HCC patients compared to healthy individuals, and therapy provided a decline in its level (Mohamed *et al.,* 2017). A study conducted by Li *et al.* (2010) in 500 serum samples showed that the changes in the expression level of three mRNAs, such as miR-25, miR-375, and let-7f, resulted in a distinguished difference between HCC and healthy controls. Further, the level of miR-16, miR-195, and miR-199a in serum individually or in combination might have the ability to distinguish between HCC and chronic hepatitis (Jiang *et al.,* 2015). A cluster of seven miRNAs (miR-29a, miR-29c, miR-133a, miR-143, miR-145, miR-192, and miR-505) was able to detect HCC with higher sensitivity as compared to AFP (Lin *et al.,* 2015). The literature has reported that four panels of miRNA comprising miT-20a-5p, miR-320a, miR-32--3p, and miR-375 have the potential to differentiate HCC from benign liver lesions. Thus the role of circulating miRNA has been highlighted as a potential diagnostic marker in HCC (Huang *et al.,* 2009). Literature has also depicted miRNA's role as a prognostic tool due to its ability to determine tumor size, nodal, and metastasis stage of HCC, invasion, recurrence, and overall survival (Liang *et al.,* 2013;Yang *et al.,* 2010). Su *et al.* (2014) reported the predominant role of miR-25 on tumor size and metastasis. Large tumors and a high risk of metastasis in primary HCC samples after surgery have been associated with the overexpression of miR-183 and miR-17-5p. A study that dealt with overall profiling of miRNAs has revealed that upregulation of multiple miRNAs such as miR-25, miR-372, miR-155, and miR-182 indicated shorter survival time, whereas downregulation of miR-29a-5p, miR-100, miR-29, miR-101, and miR-148a signified cure of HCC and increased survival (Xiong *et al.,* 2018; Zhu *et al.,* 2014; Zhang *et al.,* 2013). Locked nucleic acids known as antagomirs have been developed as therapeutics to suppress oncogenic miRNA expression (Janssen *et al.,* 2013). Further, upregulation and downregulation of specific miRNA result in drug resistance in neoplastic cells. Thus, attempts have been made to develop antagomirs to target these miRNAs to improve the drug's sensitivity. In conclusion, miRNAs' profiling and expression provide significance to developing targeted therapeutics in the future (Chauhan and Lahiri 2016).

Circular RNAs

Circular RNAs derived from precursor messenger RNAs (Pre-mRNA) are members of small non-coding RNAs. Advancement in bioinformatics and high-throughput sequencing helps identify several circular RNAs in different tissues and explore their role in human pathological and physiological processes (Han *et al.,* 2017; Han *et al.,* 2018; De Stefano *et al.,* 2018). They are involved in various critical biological functions, including autophagy, cell cycle, apoptosis, and proliferation. Specific characteristics such as stability, abundance, a high proportion of conservation among different species, cell type, and stage-specificity offer significant promise for their application as new biomarkers (Han *et al.,* 2017; Han *et al.,* 2018; De Stefano *et al.,* 2018). A study conducted by Yao *et al.* (2017) assessed the expression of circZKSCAN1 (has_circ_0001727) in HCC samples and tissues. Downregulation of circZKSCAN1 was statistically significant in HCC tissues compared to the adjacent non-tumor tissue areas. Thus, this study's outcome has lent enough impetus to the role of circZKSCAN1 as a potential biomarker of HCC diagnosis and prognosis.

Cancer Stem Markers

HCC has a heterogeneous cell population of cells like most other types of cancer. Many studies have revealed that a small subpopulation of HCC tumor cells can be self-renewal and can differentiate, known as stemness. The resemblance between these cells and stems cells, these cells are coined as cancer stem cells (CSCs). They show specific properties such as excellent efflux potential, dysregulating signaling pathways, slow growth, and small colonies. Even though most research has focused on targeting bulk tumor cells, targeting CSCs is the new arena requiring extensive investigations (Reya *et al.*, 2001; Chen *et al.*, 2013b; Chen *et al.*, 2016). Thus, exploring CSC in cancer stem markers in primary HCC tumors may help develop several effective cancer therapeutics in the future. Some of the CSCs have been described below

CD44

It is a cell adhesion molecule that is a multi-functional and multi-structural transmembrane protein. It contains three domains: N-terminal extracellular binding region, variant exons inserting membrane-proximal part (v1-10), a transmembrane domain, ankyrin and ezrin, radixin, moesin (ERM) protein binding cytoplasmic domain. Special attention has been provided towards different isoforms of CD44, which are generated due to variant exons (Yan *et al.*, 2015; Goodison *et al.*, 1999). These isoforms are expressed in cancerous tissue but restricted in normal tissues. The immunohistochemical method showed that isoforms of CD44 were in 22% of HCC tumor cells but did not express in normal liver cells (Mathew *et al.*, 1996). Further, the study reported that the presence of CD44 increased sensitivity to the AFP level. The hallmark characters of tumors, such as metastasis and growth, may be promoted by CD44 overexpression. Thus, the development of anti-CD44 therapy could be a promising option for HCC (Endo and Terada, 2000; Xie *et al.*, 2008; Sano *et al.*, 2003).

CD133

CD133, known as human prominin-1, is primarily involved in the plasma membrane protrusion in embryonic epithelia. CD-133 positive cells exhibited significant overexpression of Wnt/β-catenin, Notch, Hedgehog/Bmi, and Oct3/4 expression compared to negative counterpart (De Stefano *et al.*, 2018). Further, an experiment in the mouse model showed the more aggressive tumor initiated by $CD133^{+}$ cells than CD133 cells. Even $CD133^{+}$ resulted in an elevated level of serum AFP in HCC patients who had undergone liver transplantation. CD133 was also associated with poor overall survival and high recurrence risk after transplantation (Yin *et al.*, 2007).

CD90

CD90, which is known as Thy-1, is glycosylated phosphatidylinositol (GPI)-anchored protein. The expression of CD90 in diverse types of cells serves as one of the key players in regulating various biological processes such as apoptosis, cell adhesion, fibrosis, cell-cell, and cell-matrix adhesion (Sukowati *et al.*, 2013). All these processes play a crucial role in cancer development. The relationship between $CD90^+$ and organ metastasis in HCC was reported in a clinic-based pathological study. Different types of experiments conducted by the researchers have highlighted the potential role of CD90 in HCC development, drug resistance, and progression. Therefore, targeting CD90 populations may result in effective therapeutics against HCC (Yang *et al.*, 2008; Yamashita *et al.*, 2013).

Epithelial Cell Adhesion Molecule (EpCAM)

EpCAM is a type 1 transmembrane glycoprotein that is involved in cell-cell homophilic interactions in the mucosal epithelium. Stem cell traits such as self-renewal and differentiation features were observed in EpCAM positive HCC tumor specimens (Yamashita *et al.*, 2013; Terris *et al.*, 2010). The blocking of expression of EpCAM by RNA interferences showed inhibition of spheroid formation reduced cellular invasion and tumorigenesis in HCC cells. These outcomes provided enough positive impetus to explore EpCAM as a molecular target in HCC (Matsumoto *et al.*, 2017).

SURVEILLANCE AND HCC

The objective of the surveillance program in HCC is to decrease patients' mortality substantially and improve clinical outcomes. The intensity of risk factors guides the decision dealing with the entry of a patient into the surveillance program. Several factors, such as the patients' age, overall health, functional status, competence, and preparedness, adhere to the surveillance (Balogh *et al.*, 2016). The study correlating the incidence threshold of HCC and initiation of the surveillance program is not available. Therefore, decision analysis has been performed to lay out the instructions relating to the incidence of HCC, which may lead to a successful surveillance program. Principally, surveillance is treated as potent if it escalates the survival at least 100 days. In terms of cost-effectivity, a surveillance program that costs less than 50,000 USD/year of life gained is recognized as standard. Plenty of published study on the decision analysis and cost-effective models for HCC is available. For example, a theoretical cohort study conducted by Sarasin *et al.* on patients having Child-Pugh A cirrhosis revealed that the percentage (1.5%) HCC incidence/per year increased the survival by at least three months (Balogh *et al.*, 2016; Marrero *et al.*, 2018; Yang *et al.*, 2019). The percentage of HCC incidence below this threshold did not have any notable impact on survival. Unlike the observation reported by Sarasin *et al.* (1996), Lin *et al.* (2004) pointed out that irrespective of HCC incidence, the surveillance encompassing AFP and ultrasound were effective. Despite a wide variation in observation obtained from different published models of HCC, preferably surveillance should be performed when the annual incidence of HCC is 1.5% /year provided irrespective of etiology of cirrhosis pre-disposing factor. In non-cirrhotic hepatitis B patients, the surveillance using AFP and ultrasound was cost-effective at the annual threshold incidence of HCC, which was 0.2% /year. Thus, the criteria for screening cirrhotic patients should be given as a preference for the screening of HCC. As per the norms, the screening might have little value for patients with autoimmune hepatitis cirrhosis and primary biliary cirrhosis. Further, advanced/decompensated cirrhotic patients who are excluded from transplantation procedures are considered ineligible for the screening procedure. These patients' very short lifespan prevents them from the survival benefit obtained from the surveillance program (Balogh *et al.*, 2016; Marrero *et al.*, 2018; Yang *et al.*, 2019).

Radiographic tests and serological markers have been utilized for effective screening. Radiological investigations that have been utilized in the screening process are ultrasound, multiphase computerized tomography (CT), and magnetic resonance imaging (MRI) with contrast. Since the early 1980s, the identification of intrahepatic lesions has been performed *via* ultrasound. The sensitivity of ultrasound shows a strong dependence on the equipment and operator. Thus a wide variation (35-84%) has been observed (Chevret *et al.* 199; Balogh *et al.*, 2016). The guidelines framed by the American Association for the Study of Liver Diseases (AASLD) have suggested applying liver ultrasound with or without AFP determination every six months to perform the surveillance in HCC. AFP and ultrasound together increase the overall survival (OS). AASLD has framed the guidelines for execution, interpretation, and reporting of US examinations in HCC surveillance. Based on these guidelines, the ultrasound examination results depicted negative, provided no focal abnormalities or benign lesions such as cysts. The work becomes the nondiagnosed provided size of the lesion is <10 mm and is not precisely benign. A positive impact in ultrasound examination is characterized by lesions having a size $\geq$ 10 mm. The size of malignant nodules < 10 mm is rare. It gives the rationality to fix the 10-mm size as a threshold. Further, guidelines highlight that if a lesion <10 mm have been shown malignant transformation at all, the smaller-sized nodules arising from malignancy are troublesome for definitive diagnosis. Thus, close monitoring of patients is warranted in the regularized HCC screening (Marrero *et al.*, 2018).

The prime function of AFP is to regulate fatty acids in fetal and proliferating adult liver cells. AFP has been the most widely explored serum biomarker for the diagnosis of HCC since the 1980s. Plenty of studies has assessed that sensitivity and specificity of AFP determination ranged between 21-64% and 82-93%, respectively. The positive result in AFP determination was denoted by the value >20ng/ml. The major drawback associated with AFP determination is that the AFP level has been elevated in acute hepatitis without any sign of HCC development. The racial differences were also observed (42.9% and 60% among blacks and nonblacks, respectively) in the responsiveness of AFP (>20ng/ml). Further, decreased sensitivity of AFP has been observed in the case of tiny HCC lesions. The report in the literature (Balogh *et al.*, 2016; Marrero *et al.*, 2018; Yang *et al.*, 2019) suggested the level of AFP >400ng/ml could be recognized as conclusive in diagnosing the HCC despite the reduced sensitivity at the elevated cut-off value. Besides AFP, several other biomarkers such as Lens-culinaris agglutinin-reactive fraction of AFP (known as AFP-L3) and DCP have been approved by the US Food and Drug Administration (FDA) for the screening of HCC cases. The specificity of AFP-L3 is distinctively superior as compared to AFP. However, its sensitivity is lower than that of AFP. Interestingly, AFP-L3 characterizes tumors with high aggressiveness, reduced doubling time, substantially good vascular invasiveness, and intrahepatic metastatic quality. The measurement of AFP-L3 has been expressed as a percentage of AFP, and literature (Marrero *et al.*, 2018; Yang *et al.*, 2019) has stated that strong specificity of AFP-L3 for HCC when AFP-L3 value reaches >20ng/ml. Patients having a high risk of developing HCC are denoted by the level of AFP-L3 >10%. The post-translational impairment in the vitamin K-dependent carboxylase system leads to the formation of DCP. The specificity of DCP (91%) is significantly higher than AFP (70%). The fruitful tumor resection results in the normalization of DCP. The good sensitivity and specificity of DCP in differentiating HCC from chronic hepatitis and cirrhosis has been observed at a level above 123 mAU/ml (Marrero *et al.*, 2018; Yang *et al.*, 2019). The integration of these three markers with a threshold value (DCP >40 mU/ml + AFP >20ng/ml and AFP-L3 >10%) leads to the diagnosis of HCC with the highest accuracy. The reported sensitivity and specificity were 82.2% and 82.4%, respectively (Marrero *et al.*, 2018; Yang *et al.*, 2019). A diagnostic model to incorporate all the three biomarkers together with the patients' age and sex has been proposed, which finally has given the birth of the gender, Age, AFP-L3, AFP, and DCP (GALAD) model. The phase II study of the GALAD model has shown highly promising findings. It necessitates exploring its potential in phase III and phase IV stages to assess a large cohort study (Marrero *et al.*, 2018).

Efforts have been made to design studies to assess novel cancer biomarkers and evaluate methylated regions of DNA, DNA mutation resulting in cancer development, miRNA, long noncoding RNAs, native and posttranslational modified protein, and biochemical metabolites. Findings reveal differential expression of various biomolecules released from the exosomes of neoplastic cells and normal cells. The Early Detection Research Network (EDRN) is an initiative of the National Cancer Institute (NCI) to bring together several institutions for rapid translation of the information on biomarkers into clinical applications and their exploration for up-gradation of surveillance program resulting in successful identification of risk factors and diagnosis at the early stages. The diagnostic potency of cross-sectional and contrast-enhanced CT or MRI is significantly superior as compared to ultrasound. However, their surveillance usage has not been recommended due to insufficient data and high cost (Balogh *et al.,* 2016; Marrero *et al.,* 2018; Yang *et al.,* 2019).

A cohort study comprising 407 cirrhotic patients analyzed the potential of MRI (liver-specific contrast) with ultrasound to perform surveillance in HCC (Balogh *et al.,* 2016). Findings revealed that out of 407 patients, 43 patients resulted in malignant transformation and, finally, the formation of HCC. Among the 43 patients, 26 patients by MRI, one patient by ultrasound, and 11 patients by both modalities had been detected. Both the modalities failed to identify five patients. Further studies are needed to explore the superior utility of MRI over ultrasound to perform effective surveillance, especially in cases where the suboptimal performance of ultrasound occurs due to body habitant and other criteria. Abbreviated MRI examination protocol has been developed to potentiate the activity of cross-sectional MRI and reduce contrast exposure and duration of scanning. The abbreviated protocol characteristically reveals a T-weighted image obtained during the hepatobiliary phase of post-gadoxetate disodium injection followed by T2-weighted imaging and diffusion-weighted imaging (Balogh *et al.,* 2016; Marrero *et al.,* 2018). The sensitivities and specificities of the protocol ranged between 80-90% and 91-98%, respectively. The studies which are still at the pipeline may clarify the suitability of CT, MRI including abbreviated one over ultrasound, along with safety and cost-effectiveness under some specified cases such as patients with truncal obesity or with distinct parenchymal heterogeneity that arises clearly from cirrhosis (Balogh *et al.,* 2016; Marrero *et al.,* 2018; Yang *et al.,* 2019).

TREATMENT STRATEGIES

The long latent period associated with HCC leads to disease diagnosis at the advanced stages where patients are symptomatic and possess some extent of liver impairment. No treatment strategies at this stage offer survival. Further, substantially high morbidity has been associated with all the available therapy. A study assessing the Marketscan database of 700,000 patients who had to apply at least once for NAFLD/NASH/HCV revealed that one-fourth of the patients diagnosed with HCC had no idea of HCC before detection. The study pointed to routine conductance of HCC screening in 21.1% and 22.3% of HCV-infected patients. Interestingly, one-third of the patients under the continuous supervision of expert hepatologists revealed inconsistent HCC screening. Appropriate screening and *vigilance* may result in diagnosis at the early stages with liver function restoration (Yang *et al.*, 2019).

Generally, the stage and magnitude of liver damage guide the selection of optimal treatment strategies for HCC. In HCC, treatment strategies are primarily of two types: palliative and curative (Fig. **1**). The curative treatments such as surgical resection, liver transplantation, percutaneous ablation, palliative treatments, namely transarterial chemoembolization (TACE), radioembolization, and systemic therapy, are followed in intermediate and advanced stages of HCC (Kumari *et al.,* 2018; Gomma and Waked 2015). Irrespective of treatment approaches, achieving the optimal therapeutic outcome in HCC requires multidisciplinary approaches. It requires various experts, such as hepatologists, radiologists, pathologists, medical oncologists, interventional radiologists, transplant surgeons, and hepatobiliary surgeons.

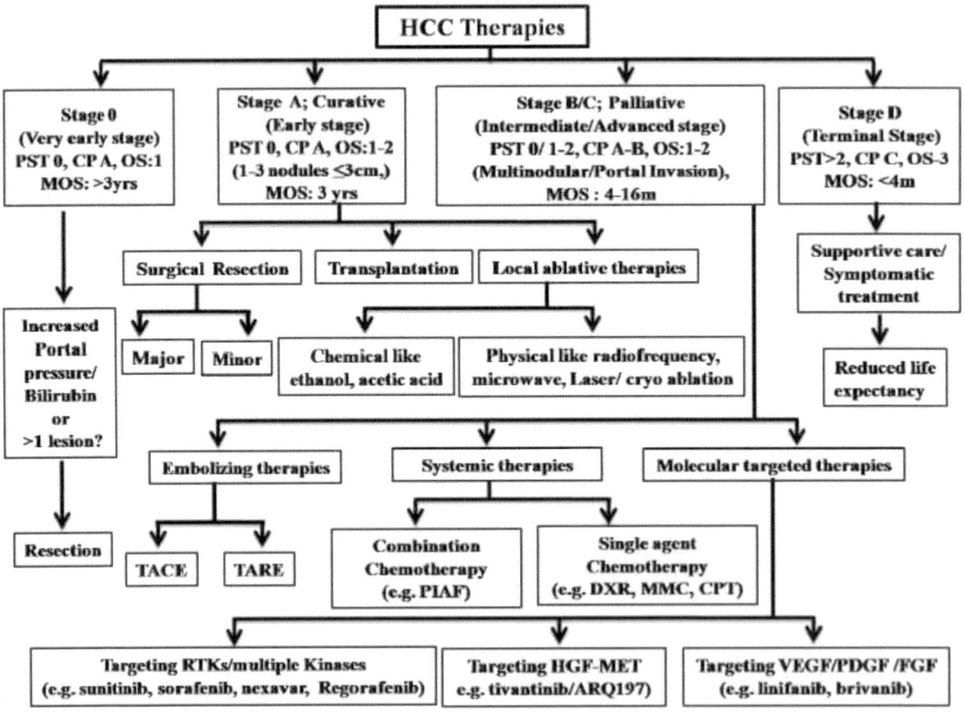

Fig. (1). Schematic representation of Barcelona Liver Cancer (BCLC) classification and recommended treatment modalities based on the category. (In figure; PST: Performance status test CP: Child-Pugh OS: Okuda stage MOS: Median overall survival).

Curative Treatments

Surgical Resection

Surgical resection has the highest potential among the various treatment strategies for noncirrhotic patients and provides an excellent curative rate with a 5-year survival that ranges between 41%-74%. Several factors, such as size and location of the tumor, basal liver function, the status of the remaining (non-tumor) liver volume, and a tumor-free portion of liver suitable for post-resection mortality and morbidity, govern the faith of the resection. The typical resection candidates have a single primary tumor located in the liver without a radiologic sign of vascular invasion. The rest of the liver can adequately maintain liver function. The optimal candidate selection is of prime importance to restrict the mortality and morbidity associated with surgery. The technical aspect of surgery is maintained with candidates having a normal synthetic function and adequate residual volume (volume of the liver without tumor). The removal of giant tumors requires major hepatectomy, whereas partial hepatectomy is preferred in the cirrhotic liver or in benign liver tumors. Further, surgical resection is not performed in cirrhotic patients with multiple tumors and extra-hepatic masses, involving the central bile duct, and presence of portal hypertension (Balogh *et al.,* 2016; Marrero *et al.*, 2018; Yang *et al.*, 2019; Yang *et al.*, 2012).

There are great techniques for assessing liver function. The most practical and common is the Child-Pugh grading system, which is mainly considered for partial hepatectomy patients. This technique is prevalently used for evaluating the functional status of the liver. The patients considered for liver transplantation are assessed through the Model for End-stage Liver Disease (MELD) scoring system. The patients with Child-Pugh class B or C liver function and elevated MELD scores should opt for liver transplantation.

Surgical Resection in Advanced HCC

Patients with an advanced stage of HCC, namely, large tumors that measure more than 10cm diameter and extrahepatic metastases or macroscopic vascular invasion, are recommended for surgery since no other treatment option such as chemotherapy, liver transplantation, or systemic ablation works.

In large HCC, with more than 10 cm in diameter, about 40 to 166 patients were evaluated, and extensive hepatic resection was done. The postoperative mortality and morbidity and increasing blood loss were compared with those of patients with smaller HCC. Mortality and survival rates of 5 years were 2-3.3% and 28-33%, respectively (Kishi *et al.*, 2011).

The presence of macroscopic vascular invasion is an essential criterion for the prognosis of HCC patients. Since HCC occupies adjacent venous tributaries, it provides a very high risk of extra or intra-hepatic metastases. Surgical resection of HCC patients with macroscopic vascular invasion is challenging and risky because of poor survival benefits. However, a better survival possibility can be expected from surgical resection than non-surgical treatment protocols.

From some study reports, it can be seen that surgical resection for patients with HCC and with the portal venous invasion of the main trunk (Vp4) or right or left main trunk (Vp3) cannot be recommended due to poor survival benefits when compared to HCC patients with portal venous invasion of secondary tributaries (Vp2) or peripheral tributaries (Vp1) (Kishi *et al.*, 2011). However, reports for aggressive resection for HCC patients with Vp3 or Vp4 show 10 to 42% survival rates of 5 years. Portal vein tumor resection involves two processes- one is the resection of a specific segment of the portal vein, and the other one involves peeling-off technique by placing a portal venotomy followed by a detachment of tumor bulk and removal from the inner portion of the portal vein (Wu *et al.*, 2000). Invasion of HCC in the bile duct or inferior vena cava is pretty infrequent as compared to foray in the portal vein. Generally, there is no such difference in the postoperative prognosis of patients with or without bile duct tumor thrombi.

In the case of extrahepatic metastases, aggressive resection shows limited benefits. The survival rate of 5 years of 20 patients after hepatic resection having extrahepatic recurrence was limited to 30 percent only (Yang *et al.*, 2007). In the case of extrahepatic metastases from HCC, the most affected organ is the lungs. Pulmonary metastases accounted for 50-60% of patients with HCC associated with extrahepatic metastases. Studies show patients' 5-year survival rate following pulmonary resection in the range of 27-33%. Although the research has been conducted with a limited number of patients, as in most cases of pulmonary metastases, multiple lesions can be observed, for which it is not recommended to go for pulmonary resection with more than three lesions.

Anatomical Resection

As mentioned earlier, HCC tends to invade the adjacent portal vein resulting in intrahepatic metastases. Simultaneously, extensive hepatic resection cannot be performed in cases where the liver's condition is severely damaged. To control this problem, Makuuchi *et al.*, 2008 proposed a type of hepatectomy called anatomic subsegmentectomy. Here, intraoperative ultrasonography is done by injecting indigo carmine dye to the portal venous tributaries to identify hepatic tumors' specific locations. Positive staining areas are then marked with electrocautery. By determining the size and location of tumors, resection of one or more than one segment is done. The report showed postoperative prognosis after anatomic resection with an overall recurrence-free survival of patients with solitary or small HCC (Mazzaferro V *et al.,* 1996, H. Imamura *et al.,* 1999, M. Yamamoto *et al.,* 2001, K. Hasegawa *et al.,* 2005, S. Eguchi *et al.,* 2008, T. Kamiyama *et al.,* 2010).

Laparoscopic Resection of The Liver

Laparoscopic resection was observed first in patients with partial resection of 6 cm segment with focal nodular hyperplasia and wedge resection of 5th segment having colorectal metastases (Gagner *et al.*, 1992). Since then, the number of laparoscopic liver surgery has increased in the last five years. Although there is a doubt about laparoscopic hepatectomy from the oncological perspective, an extended prognosis is necessary to establish the effect of minimally invasive surgery for hepatic malignancies and HCC. It was proposed (Buell *et al.*, 2009) that laparoscopic hepatectomy could be done to those HCC patients with solitary lesions of 5 cm or less in diameter located in the periphery of the segment. Many surgeons opt for minimally invasive liver surgery, especially for HCC patients with cirrhotic liver, as less liver mobilization is required. Less quantity of intravenous fluid is required since, in minimal surgery, the fluid loss is lesser than open liver surgery. As for the outcomes of laparoscopic liver surgery, higher mortality and morbidity have been reported. Although laparoscopic resection should be taken care of depending on the condition and types of tumors, priority should be given to the oncological curative aspect.

Surgical Resection of Re-Occurring HCC

HCC reoccurred in 85 to 90% of patients operated for HCC tumors. Intrahepatic recurrence has been reported to come back in 2 years following primary hepatic resection. In recurrent HCC patients, in the non-appearance of extrahepatic metastases, the best way to treat and increase patients' survival rate is to undergo repeat hepatectomy. Studies show that the repetition of liver resection gives a better prognosis with a 50 to 70% five-year survival rate than patients without surgical intervention. Wu *et al.*, 2000 studied the survival aspect of HCC patients undergoing repeat hepatectomy four times. The results showed that patients undergoing hepatectomy for second and third times, and for the fourth time had shown more remarkable survival than those without recurrent surgery. Repeat hepatectomy is not suitable for patients with impaired liver function with or without multiple intrahepatic tumor recurrence.

Liver Transplantation

For patients with advanced HCC, there are two positive aspects of liver transplantation. In the first case, liver transplantation has shown highly positive results, and the HCC present in the liver could be adequately removed irrespective of liver cirrhosis. For the second case, a continuation of the learning phase should understand how to use and extend the possibilities of liver transplantation in managing advanced HCC.

For patients having HCC, there is a selection criterion which is known as the Milan criteria. It helps in the selection of candidates needing liver transplantation. Patients who fulfilled the Milan criteria showed better survival results than those who did not fulfill the requirements (Kishi *et al.*, 2011). However, Milan criteria are quite restrictive, and liver transplantation is permitted only to a limited number of patients having HCC. Patients with tumors less than 5 cm or more than 3 cm fulfill the Milan criteria and show a reasonable survival rate after liver transplantation.

According to the reports, stage IV HCC patients' liver transplantation showed 20% more of 5-year survival. Presently, there is no scope to identify before undergoing liver transplantation which patient will do well and which patient will not do well upon hepatic transplantation.

Ablation

At the early stage of HCC, local percutaneous ablation is recognized as a potentially curative therapeutic approach. The modalities which are most frequently used are radiofrequency and microwave. Among the two modalities, microwave ablation is preferred over radiofrequency ablation for local ablation therapy. The principal mechanism of ablation is to induce necrosis by transporting heat to the tumor. The reasons behind the superiority of microwave ablation over radiofrequency ablation are as follows: (i) ability of microwave to generate heat through multiple mechanisms that result in superior thermal efficiency of the microwave as compared to radiofrequency, (ii) vulnerability of microwave ablation to “the heat sink effect” (defective thermal ablation near the large blood vessels due to the cooling effect provided by the blood flow) is lesser as compared to radiofrequency counterpart, (iii) high efficacy for giant tumor (3-4cm long), (iv) duration of treatment is shorter for microwave ablation as compared to radiofrequency. A randomized controlled, single-blinded phase II trial with 76 patients was conducted at the four tertiary university centers of Switzerland and France to compare microwave and radiofrequency ablation (Yang *et al.*, 2019). Findings revealed that 6% of 98 lesions in microwave ablation and 12% of 114 lesions in radiofrequency ablation showed tumor progression locally, indicating superior efficacy of the former (Yang *et al.*, 2019; Marrero *et al.*, 2018). Besides microwave and radiofrequency ablation, percutaneous ethanol injection has been utilized in the past, and to date, it has been most frequently used in resource-limited settings. Ethanol injection may be highly preferred for the tumor nodules adjacent to large intrahepatic vessels or bile ducts, thus preventing thermal injury. Cryoablation, which has an efficacy similar to radiofrequency ablation, has also been explored in high-resource settings. Generally, local ablation is ideal for patients ineligible for liver transplantation or hepatic resection due to comorbid conditions or hepatic impairment. Literature has reported the utility of ablation as bridge therapy (Yang *et al.*, 2019), a therapy during waiting time before the transplantation to prevent the tumor's progression.

Palliative Treatment

Various external and internal factors such as tumor size, multiple lesions, metastatic nature, liver function status, organ shortage, and late diagnosis have restricted the curative therapies to a limited group of patients. Further, these limitations lean towards various palliative therapies, which are remarkably more effective for patients under stage B and C of the Barcelona Clinic Liver Cancer (BCLC) class. The objectives of palliative therapies are to escalate survival and improve patients' quality of life (Kumari *et al.*, 2018). Different types of palliative therapies are mentioned below.

Embolizing Therapies for HCC

HCC is vascular, and it shows a strong dependence on the arterial blood supply (75-80%) compared to normal liver. Thus, embolization is the process to obstruct blood flow to cancer cells resulting in the induction of tumor hypoxia, and necrosis. Embolization can be used as the sole therapeutic strategy or combined with chemotherapy/radiotherapy (Kumari *et al.*, 2018).

Transarterial Chemoembolization (TACE)

TACE is recommended for patients at the B/C stage of BCLC and a compensated liver function. This technique is also advised for the patients at the queue of liver transplantation to prevent tumor progression (Otto *et al.*, 2013). TACE is a technique where administration of chemotherapy is done directly to the hepatic artery, and embolization is performed subsequently. The embolizing agents are of two types, such as temporary and permanent embolizing agents. The temporary embolizing agents include gelatin sponge and autologous blood clots, whereas permanent embolizing agents include polyvinyl alcohol, steel coils, and microspheres. Among the various embolizing agents, the gelatin sponge is most extensively used (Wang *et al.*, 2014). The application of TACE without a drug is known as transarterial embolization (TAE), and the purpose of this technique is to embolize arterial supply only. Advancement to the conventional TAE technique gives rise to the birth of drug-eluting bead (DEB)-TACE, which utilizes embolizing particles as a carrier of chemotherapeutic drugs. The most commonly used chemotherapeutics for DEB-TACE are doxorubicin and cisplatin, as reported in the literature (Bruix and Sherman 2011; Luz *et al.,* 2017). This technique performs dual functions such as embolization of the hepatic artery and slow and steady release of chemotherapeutic drugs, increasing tumor cells' length of exposure (Kumari *et al.,* 2018). TACE has been considered as a treatment of choice for patients with multi-focal large lesions without any vascular invasion and extra-hepatic spread. TACE is regarded as a treatment of choice as recommended by the European Association for the Liver (EASL) Study. TACE is well-tolerated since complications related to it are observed in less than 5% of patients, and the complications can be controlled by using analgesics and antiemetics (Clark 2006; Leung *et al.,* 2001).

Radiotherapy

One of the powerful treatment strategies is radiotherapy (also known as radiation therapy), which destroys cancer and shrinks tumors using high doses of radiation. Radiotherapy utilizes high-energy waves or particles, such as x-rays, gamma rays, electron beams, or protons, which result in the destruction or damage of cancer cells. The principal mechanism through which radiotherapy causes cancer cells' death includes the induction of small breaks in DNA within the cells. These DNA splits prevent cancer cells' growth and division and cause them to die. Nearly fifty out of a hundred percent of people have radiotherapy at some point during their cancer treatment. The application of radiotherapy is dependent on factors such as stages and types of cancer, size of the tumor, the position of the tumor within the body, closeness between tumor and normal tissues which are susceptible to radiation, health status, and medical history of the patients, namely, age and whether patients receive other types of cancer treatment at the time of radiotherapy. The external and internal beams are the fundamental modes of radiotherapy.

External Beam Radiotherapy

External beam is the most frequent type of radiation therapy used for cancer treatment. A high-energy beam has been targeted to the tumor from outside the body. The key advantages of these modes are (i) high-energy beam can move around the body without making any contact with the body, (ii) It does not touch the body but can move around the patient, (ii) direct radiation to a specified location of the body from multiple directions (iii) can produce a significantly low impact on normal cells.

Internal Beam Radiotherapy

In Internal beam radiotherapy, the radiation source, either solid or liquid, is located inside the body. Solid source therapy is known as brachytherapy. It directly delivers a high dose of radiation to the tumor and helps nearby spare tissues with seeds, ribbons, or capsules. Brachytherapy is a localized treatment that specifically targets a particular part of the body. Internal radiation therapy comprising of the liquid source is known as systemic therapy. In this type of treatment, treatment travels in the whole body through the blood to precisely identify the cancer cells and finally destroy them.

Radiotherapy Modalities

HCC is one of the leading causes of global mortality. The advancement of technology and improved imaging led to radiotherapy as one of the potent therapeutic modalities in HCC treatment over the last few decades. Radiotherapy can provide better local rates in unresectable HCC, which needs significant vascular involvement and can give a modality to help bridge patients to potential curative transplantation. In metastasis, radiotherapy can possess the potential to provide improved palliation. The applications of the following radioisotopes have been reported for HCC.

(i) Holmium -199 (Ho^{199}), a beta and a minor gamma emitter isotope, has a half-life of 26.8 h. The chitosan complex's potential (Ho^{199}) has been explored either through intratumoral or transarterial approaches. In another phase II study, the authors reported that in the treatment of HCC, transarterial administration of the ^{166}Ho-chitosan complex was highly effective, especially for the patients with 3-5 cm tumors (Sohn *et al.*, 2009). Kim *et al.*, 2006 reported that in a phase IIb clinical trial, 91.7% response rate of percutaneous ^{166}Ho-chitosan injection showed complete tumor necrosis (tumors < 2 cm).

(ii) Iodine -131 (I^{131}), which has a half-life of 8 days, is most prevalently a beta emitter accompanied with a limited potential as a gamma emitter. It has been applied in the form of I^{131}-Lipiodol (Boucher *et al.*, 2007). It was also successfully used for the treatment of non-operable HCC (Lintia-Gaultier *et al.*, 2013). The clinical response was in 17-92% of patients upon intra-arterial administration of ^{131}I-Lipiodol (Lambert *et al.*, 2005).

(iii) The starting information obtained from ^{188}Re and ^{90}Y-labelled conjugates are promising, which make them emerging radiotherapeutic modality

(iv) The therapeutic efficiency of ^{90}Y-labelled microspheres is quite similar compared to that with radiolabelled lipiodol (Lambert *et al.*, 2005).

A growing number of promising findings in the literature have revealed the safety and efficacy of radiotherapy for the treatment of HCC. The radiotherapy approach is viable for tumors of various sizes that are not vulnerable to percutaneous therapy and down-staging tumors before transplantation or surgery.

Three-Dimensional Conformal Radiotherapy (3DCRT)

3DCRT or Three-dimensional conformal radiotherapy is an advanced imaging technique to generate three-dimensional images of tumors and nearby organs and tissues of patients. Radiotherapy reveals significant promise to deliver radical tumor doses to a well-defined liver lesion more effectively and precisely. 3DCRT has been explored as a viable substitute therapy for cirrhotic HCC patients. Conversely, it exhibits limited potential towards different curative approaches such as surgical resection of tumors, liver transplantation, and radiofrequency ablation.

Robertson *et al.* (1997), in an early investigation, reported that combined conformal radiotherapy (RT) and the administration of fluorodeoxyuridine (FdUrd) through hepatic artery resulted in the significant halting of HCC progression that led to elevated survival in patients with unresectable, nondiffuse primary hepatobiliary malignancies (Robertson *et al.*, 1997). Ben-josef *et al.* (2005) reported that high dose focal liver irradiation (60.75 Gy, 1.5-Gy fraction bid) through hepatic artery using floxuridine prolonged the survival of patients with intrahepatic cancers were ineligible for surgical resection. Findings from Mornex *et al.* (2006) confirmed from a phase II study that high dose 3DCRT (66 Gy, 2 Gy/fraction) was highly suitable for the treatment of the cirrhotic patient (small HCC, one nodule < or = 5 cm, or two nodules < or = 3 cm), with promising results. Several positive features such as the global accessibility of three-dimensional conformal radiotherapy, the potential to treat multiple lesions exclusively in a non-invasive manner, and plenty of promising results reported well in the literature (Kouloulias *et al.*, 2013) lends it an attractive therapeutic approach for patients who are ineligible for different curative approaches.

Transarterial Radioembolization (TARE)

TARE is used for the same kind of patients as transarterial chemoembolization (TACE). This technique utilizes intra-arterial delivery of Yttrium (Y90) loaded microsphere or lipiodol labeled with rhenium or iodine (Sacco *et al.*, 2016). Currently, glass-made thermosphere and resin-made SIR (selective internal radiation) spheres are the two fundamental types of microspheres used in TARE.

They have wide variations in embolic powers and activities. TARE is preferred in HCC patients with portal vein thrombosis due to its ability to remove hepatic ischemia upon delivering the local radiation to liver tumors (Cho *et al.,* 2016). Reports in the literature (Cho *et al.,* 2016; Kumari *et al.,* 2018) have mentioned that the utility of microsphere brachytherapy may be explored for the treatment of intermediate and advanced stage HCC where curative treatment has not been recommended. This technique prevents normal hepatic cells' exposure to the toxic effects of radiation by implanting selective radiation sources within the tumor (Kim 2017). Plenty of clinical trials was conducted for the evaluation of this technique. Only a few studies have reported the superiority of radioembolization compared to TACE in terms of a better response and fewer side effects (Ricke *et al.,* 2015; Vilgrain *et al.,* 2014).

Systemic Therapies of HCC

The long latent period associated with HCC results in the initial diagnosis of HCC-patients at the intermediate and advanced stages, thus rendering chemotherapy the only available treatment option. The marginal improvement in survival is observed upon administration of conventional chemotherapeutic agents such as cisplatin, doxorubicin, 5-fluorouracil, and gemcitabine. Further, some randomized trials revealed a mild improvement in response rate upon using the combined chemotherapy. However, there was no change in objective response (Leung *et al.,* 1999; Yeo *et al.,* 2005; Mohamed *et al.,* 2017). Multiple factors are responsible for the poor therapeutic outcome and potentially high side effects of conventional chemotherapeutic agents. Some of the critical elements are multi-drug resistance in HCC tumors, faster clearance rate, low drug concentration in HCC cells (only 5-10% of dose accumulated in normal organs), and non-specific distribution (Zhang *et al.,* 2016; Lo *et al.,* 2008; Han and Park 2008).

The poor therapeutic response associated with traditional chemotherapeutics has set up a platform for exploring multi-kinase inhibitors (MKIs) and immune checkpoint inhibitors as an effective targeted therapy in advanced unresectable HCC. A detailed description of first-line and second-line targeted therapeutics in HCC has been described below

First-line Therapy

Sorafenib

Sorafenib (Nexavar®, Bayer Pharmaceuticals, Berlin, Germany), the first multi-kinase inhibitor, has been approved by the United States Food and Drug Administration (USFDA) as a first-line drug for the treatment of advanced HCC. It prevents the angiogenesis, cellular proliferation, and metastasis upon binding with the various extracellular tyrosine kinases such as vascular endothelial growth factor receptors (VEGFR 2, VEGFR-3, VEGFR1), platelet-derived growth factor receptor β (PDGFR β), and downstream intracellular signaling molecules Raf kinases (B-Raf and C-Raf) and serine/threonine kinases (Al-Rajabi *et al.,* 2015; Fitzmoris *et al.,* 2015). As per the result of Sorafenib Hepatocellular carcinoma Randomized Trial (SHARP) in 2007 and the Asia-Pacific study in 2008, sorafenib showed improvement of median overall survival (OS) of advanced HCC patients (BCLC stage C) by 2.8 months (Keating and Santoro 2009).

The promising results of sorafenib have instigated the researchers to explore several other MKIs. However, in a stretch during 2007-2017, the arena of MKIs witnessed several failed phase III trials such as sunitinib (2015), brivanib (2013), sorafenib plus erlotinib (2015), and linifanib (2015) (Cheng *et al.,* 2013d; Johnson *et al.,* 2013; Zhu *et al.,* 2015). The intensive search of MKIs gave the birth of the two other promising oral MKIs, namely, regorafenib and lenvatinib, which showed promising results in clinical trials in 2017 and 2018, respectively (Kim and Abou-Alfa 2014).

Lenvatinib

The broad-spectrum oral MKI, lenvatinib, has been approved by USFDA as a first-line drug to treat advanced HCC. It targets various tyrosine kinases, namely VEFGR 1-3, fibroblast growth factor 1-4 (FGFR1-4), PDGFR-α, c-Kit, rearranged during transfection (RET) (Kudo *et al.,* 2018). The data of randomized open-label, multinational non-inferiority phase III REFLECT trial (Kudo *et al.,* 2018b) in patients having previously untreated, metastatic or unresectable HCC paved the way for the approval of lenvatinib by USFDA. In a trial on 954 patients randomized 1:1, the patients with body weight≥60 kg received lenvatinib (12 mg/ Kg body weight orally once daily). The patients having bodyweight < 60kg received the drug 8 mg/ Kg body weight daily. Sorafenib (Nexavar®, 400mg orally twice daily) continued until the assessment of the disease progression by radiography or unacceptable toxicity occurred in patients. As per the trial result, lenvatinib was non-inferior but not statistically superior compared to sorafenib in terms of median overall survival (OS). However, it showed significant superiority as compared to sorafenib to improve all secondary endpoints as it resulted in a higher objective response rate (ORR), more prolonged progression-free survival (PFS), and time to progression (TPP) of the disease.

Second-line Therapy

Multi-Target Tyrosine Kinase Inhibitors

Regorafenib

The United States Food and Drug Administration (USFDA) has recommended Regorafenib as a second-line agent for advanced HCC-patients exhibiting tolerance to sorafenib. The fundamental mechanism of the action of regorafenib is to act as inhibitors of multiple targets such as VEGFR1, tyrosine kinase with Ig and epidermal growth factor (EGF) homology domains-2 (TIE-2), PDGFR, fibroblast-derived growth factor receptor (FDGFR), and colony-stimulating factor 1 receptor (CSF1R). It has a similarity in structure and function with sorafenib (Martin *et al.*, 2008). The resource trial data showed that regorafenib resulted in an increase in survival of patients compared to placebo from 7.8 months (in placebo) to 10.6 (after regorafenib treatment). It also caused an increase in progression-free survival from 1.5 months to 3.1 months. Further, patients treated with regorafenib and sorafenib exhibited longer survival (26 months) as compared to the patients who received sorafenib and placebo (19.2 months) (Frennette 2017; Cheng *et al.*, 2017).

Cabozantinib

Cabozantinib, one of the oral multiple tyrosine kinase inhibitors, suppresses angiogenesis, metastasis, and oncogenesis (Yang. *et al.*, 2019; Liu *et al.*, 2019). Cabozantinib's target receptors include VEGFR (1-3), AXL, and c-Met (Huang *et al.*, 2020). The findings of the phase III CELESTIAL trial (Abou-Alfa *et al.*, 2018) revealed that the treatment with cabozantinib resulted in significant improvement in OS as compared to placebo in patients (with advanced HCC) who were undergone treatment with sorafenib previously. The study enrolled 707 patients who were randomly stratified into cabozantinib and placebo groups at a ratio of 2:1. The median OS with cabozantinib and with placebo was found to be 10.2 and 8 months, respectively (hazard ratio (HR)-0.76, confidence interval (CI)-95%, P=0.005). Among the patient, 68% of patients in cabozantinib and 36% in the placebo group reported grade 3 or grade 4 adverse events. Interestingly, the values of hazard ratio of death in HBV-infected HCC patients and HCV-infected HCC patients were found to be 0.69 and 1.11, respectively, indicating better effectivity of cabozantinib second-line drug, especially in HBV-infected HCC patients. However, further studies are required to clarify this correlation aspect.

Ramucirumab

Ramucirumab, a recombinant IgG1 monoclonal antibody, exhibits its potential as an antagonist of VEGFR2. It inhibits VEGF receptor ligands' binding, such as VEGFA, VEGFC, and VEGFD, to the VEGF receptor, thus suppressing its activation. Initially, ramucirumab has been approved for the treatment of gastric cancer (April 21st, 2014), non-small cell lung cancer (December 12th, 2014), and colorectal cancer (29th April 2015) (Yang. *et al.,* 2019; Liu *et al.*, 2019). A multicentre (154 centers from 27 countries) double-blind trial known as the REACH trial, which Andrew X. Zhu led, was conducted to explore the effect of ramucirumab (8mg/kg in every 2 weeks) as a second-line agent *vs.* placebo in 568 patients with advanced progressive HCC and the patients received treatment with sorafenib previously (Yang. *et al.,* 2019; Liu *et al.*, 2019). Findings revealed that OS was superior in the ramucirumab group (9.2 months) than the placebo (7.8 months). Although the difference in OS between ramicirumab and placebo group was not statistically significant, subgroup assessment revealed that OS benefit is significantly better in patients with raised serum AFP concentration 400 ng/ml. Further, REACH-2 study was also conducted based on the previous finding in 292 patients with advanced HCC and serum AFP level $\geq$400 ng/ml enrolled from 92 hospitals, clinics, and medical centers in 20 countries under the leadership of Andrew X. Zhu (Liu *et al.*, 2019; Huang *et al.,* 2020). Among 292 patients, 197 patients were randomly assigned to ramucirumab (8 mg/kg in every two weeks) group and rest (95 patients) belonged to the placebo group revealed that the OS of ramucirumab group was 8.5 months compared to 7.3 months as seen in the placebo group. The performance-free survival (PFS) was significantly superior in the ramucirumab group (2.8 months) in comparison to the placebo group (1.8 months). Interestingly, ramucirumab was well accepted, with a significantly reduced incidence of adverse events and a good safety profile. Based on the agreement of REACH-2 trial with the subgroup analysis REACH trial, which was a pioneer in the arena of phase III trial in biomarker-selected advanced HCC patients, FDA approved ramucirumab as a sole agent in the treatment of HCC patients with serum AFP level $\geq$400 ng/ml and have received prior treatment with sorafenib.

Immune Checkpoint Inhibitor

The advent of MKIs as chemotherapeutics brought a hope that a significant improvement in patients' overall survival with advanced HCC would lead to better therapeutic outcomes. The practical scenario was quite different than expected. There was no substantial improvement in OS and objective response rates (ORR) observed upon administration of MKI alone or in combination. In phase III clinical trials, patients treated with different MKIs exhibited drug-related adverse events (AEs). In 45 to 70% of cases, grade 3 AEs were reported, indicating interruption of therapies or dose reduction. The most common AEs are hand-foot syndrome (HFS), diarrhea, hypertension, fatigue, nausea, vomiting, *etc.* Further, the development of acquired and adaptive resistance against MKIs has also been reported (Zhu *et al.*, 2017; Rotow and Bivana 2017).

The microenvironment of cancer cells allows them to escape from immune surveillance, and multiple mechanisms are involved in immune suppression. The immune checkpoint mechanism and its related molecules are being explored immensely to develop targeted therapy (Keenan *et al.*, 2019; Pardee and Butterfield 2012). Among the battery of molecules involved in the immune checkpoint, programmed death-ligand 1 (PD-L1) (found at the surface of cancer cells and stromal cells), programmed cell death 1 (PD-1), and cytotoxic T lymphocyte-associated protein 4 (CTLA-4) (found on the surface of T cells) play a pivotal role in suppression of T cell activation by cancer cells. Researchers have explored monoclonal antibodies against these ligands. Clinical trials will evaluate their efficacy in various types of malignancies, including HCC (Kudo 2018b; Gong *et al.*, 2018). Considering their potential against HCC, the sincere effort has been taken to develop an antibody against PD-L1 and PD-1, leading to accelerated approval of nivolumab, an anti-PD-1 antibody that showed promising results in phase II clinical trial (Checkmate-040) for the treatment of HCC patients who received sorafenib previously. The administration of sorafenib resulted in a decrease in myeloid-derived suppressor cells (MDSC) and regulatory T-cells (T-reg) levels in spleen, bone marrow, and tumor, leading to an impairment in their function as evidenced in pre-clinical studies in liver cancer models (Kudo 2018b). Further, sorafenib's excessive pruning of tumor vasculature led to aggravating hypoxia in the tumor microenvironment by upregulating the expression of HIF-α, resulting in an increased expression of immune checkpoint molecules such as PD-L1. Thus, the researchers have highlighted the potential of a combination comprising MKIs with immune checkpoint molecules to achieve an improved therapeutic outcome in HCC. Several combinations are on clinical trials (Kudo 2018b; Gong *et al.*, 2018; Wu *et al.*, 2019). Apart from the nivolumab, several other molecules such as tislelizumab, camrelizumab, tremelimumab, durvalumab and their combinations and combinations of immune checkpoints molecules local therapies such as TACE and DEB-TACE are being investigated extensively through clinical trials for the development of powerful therapeutic arsenals against HCC. However, several issues have to be resolved to explore the potential of these immuno-therapeutics in full swing. The key points are immune-related adverse events leading to fatal consequences and variation in responses among the various patients (Kudo 2018b; Gong *et al.*, 2018).

A representation depicting the binding of different FDA-approved targeted therapeutics with their cognate receptors that result in downregulation of oncogenic stimulation is shown in Fig. (**2**).

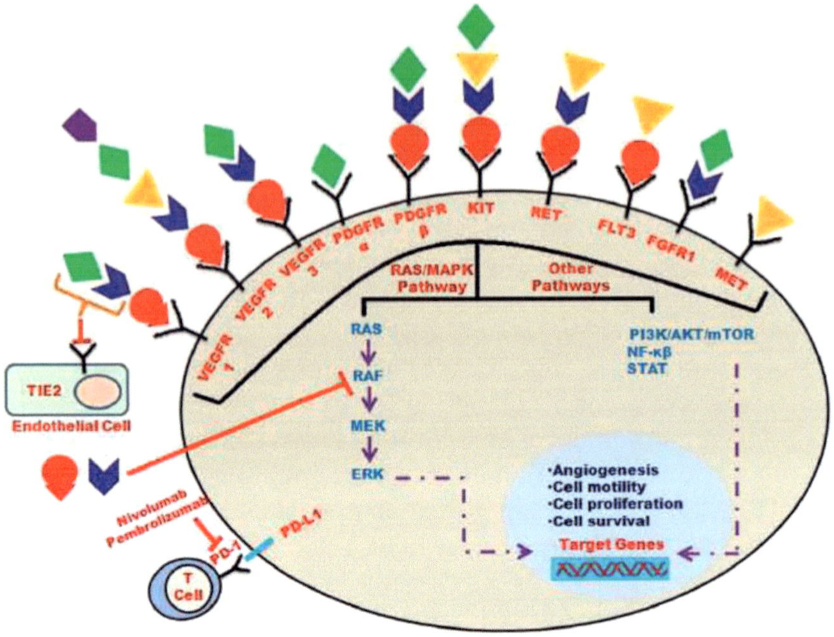

Fig. (2). Schematic representation revealing binding of different multi-kinase inhibitors (MKIs) and immune checkpoint inhibitors with their target receptor resulting in suppression of oncogenic transformation. Red = Sorafenib, blue = Regorafenib, yellow = Cabozantinib, green =Lenvatinib, violet = Ramucirumab.

FUTURE PERSPECTIVES

The past few decades have witnessed some of the most remarkable and significant improvements in the treatment of HCC. Perhaps, ongoing clinical investigations on drugs such as linifanib, vandetanib, oratinib, and dovitinib have prominently potential findings that enable comparatively higher survival rates. Inhibition of immune checkpoints associated with tumor malignancies has raised greater expectations in HCC treatment. Studies have proven that additional support of nutritional supplements and BCAAs provide some control over neoplastic activity in HCC patients. Despite the availability of numerous new drugs currently being tested, only sorafenib has proven to be effective. The research needs to be continued on new medications. Targeted formulations and site-specific nanoformulations with the existing drugs can open up a new avenue in cancer therapy shortly. However, the development in the overall survival of the HCC population significantly depends on the early diagnosis of HCC patients. Additional studies on single/concomitant biomarker(s) are required to provide fast and early detection of HCC to improve survival and tumor regression. Furthermore, reducing drug toxicity and the combination of therapies that affect synergistically will challenge the present way of HCC therapy to the next improved level.

CONCLUSION

The greatest challenge of treating HCC is its late-stage diagnosis, as it often remains asymptomatic at the initial stage. Properly convincing and easily utilizable prognostic and diagnostic markers should be identified for easy diagnosis of HCC at the early stage. Planned regular check-ups of the HCC-prone population's hepatic health with the government or private effort can also help us identify HCC at the early stage. The need for drastic improvisation of medical therapies to treat patients affected by the advanced stages of HCC is extremely important in dealing with this life-threatening neoplasia. The concrete understanding of the effects of drugs and molecular mechanisms for HCC progress can limit the resistance mechanisms of neoplasia against drugs and thus, provide a practical approach to resolve this fatal drug resistance issue. Several modified therapies and immunotherapeutic agents are emerging, and they may potentially substitute sorafenib shortly. Furthermore, the efforts to determine novel therapeutic targets must be continued, along with various combinational therapies, potentially assuring treatment modalities for HCC.

CONSENT FOR PUBLICATION

Not applicable.

CONFLICT OF INTEREST

The authors declare no conflict of interest, financial or otherwise.

ACKNOWLEDGEMENTS

The authors acknowledge the Department of Pharmaceutical Technology, Jadavpur University, Kolkata, India, for providing facilities to write the book chapter.

REFERENCES

Abdel-Aziz, MM, Elshal, MF, Abass, AT, El-Kafrawy, S, Ezzat, S & Abdel-Wahab, M (2016) Comparison of AFP-L3 and p53 antigen concentration with alpha-fetoprotein as serum markers for hepatocellular carcinoma. *Clin Lab,* 62, 1121-9.
[http://dx.doi.org/10.7754/Clin.Lab.2015.151102] [PMID: 27468575]

Abou-Alfa, GK, Meyer, T, Cheng, AL, El-Khoueiry, AB, Rimassa, L, Ryoo, BY, Cicin, I, Merle, P, Chen, Y, Park, JW, Blanc, JF, Bolondi, L, Klümpen, HJ, Chan, SL, Zagonel, V, Pressiani, T, Ryu, MH, Venook, AP, Hessel, C, Borgman-Hagey, AE, Schwab, G & Kelley, RK (2018) Cabozantinib in Patients with Advanced and Progressing Hepatocellular Carcinoma. *N Engl J Med,* 379, 54-63.
[http://dx.doi.org/10.1056/NEJMoa1717002] [PMID: 29972759]

Acharya, SK (2014) Epidemiology of hepatocellular carcinoma in India. *J Clin Exp Hepatol,* 4 (Suppl. 3), S27-33.
[http://dx.doi.org/10.1016/j.jceh.2014.05.013] [PMID: 25755607]

Adhoute, X, Penaranda, G, Bronowicki, JP & Raoul, JL (2015) Usefulness of the HKLC *vs.* the BCLC staging system in a European HCC cohort. *J Hepatol,* 62, 492-3.
[http://dx.doi.org/10.1016/j.jhep.2014.08.035] [PMID: 25194894]

Granito, A, Guidetti, E & Gramantieri, L (2015) c-MET receptor tyrosine kinase as a molecular target in advanced hepatocellular carcinoma. *J Hepatocell Carcinoma,* 2, 29-38.
[PMID: 27508192]

Al-Rajabi, R, Patel, S, Ketchum, NS, Jaime, NA, Lu, TW, Pollock, BH & Mahalingam, D (2015) Comparative dosing and efficacy of sorafenib in hepatocellular cancer patients with varying liver dysfunction. *J Gastrointest Oncol,* 6, 259-67.
[PMID: 26029452]

Ang, CS, Sun, MY, Huitzil-Melendez, DF, Chou, JF, Capanu, M, Jarnagin, W, Fong, Y, Dematteo, RP, D'Angelica, M, Allen, P, Chen, CT, O'Reilly, EM, Weiser, MR & Abou-Alfa, GK (2013) c-MET and HGF mRNA expression in hepatocellular carcinoma: correlation with clinicopathological features and survival. *Anticancer Res,* 33, 3241-5.
[PMID: 23898085]

Antoury, C, Lopez, R, Zein, N, Stoller, JK & Alkhouri, N (2015) Alpha-1 antitrypsin deficiency and the risk of hepatocellular carcinoma in end-stage liver disease. *World J Hepatol,* 7, 1427-32.
[http://dx.doi.org/10.4254/wjh.v7.i10.1427] [PMID: 26052388]

Aravalli, RN, Cressman, ENK & Steer, CJ (2013) Cellular and molecular mechanisms of hepatocellular carcinoma: an update. *Arch Toxicol,* 87, 227-47.
[http://dx.doi.org/10.1007/s00204-012-0931-2] [PMID: 23007558]

Arlt, VM, Stiborova, M & Schmeiser, HH (2002) Aristolochic acid as a probable human cancer hazard in herbal remedies: a review. *Mutagenesis,* 17, 265-77.
[http://dx.doi.org/10.1093/mutage/17.4.265] [PMID: 12110620]

Balkau, B, Kahn, HS, Courbon, D, Eschwège, E & Ducimetière, P (2001) Hyperinsulinemia predicts fatal liver cancer but is inversely associated with fatal cancer at some other sites: the Paris Prospective Study. *Diabetes Care,* 24, 843-9.
[http://dx.doi.org/10.2337/diacare.24.5.843] [PMID: 11347741]

Balogh, J, Victor, D, III, Asham, EH, Burroughs, SG, Boktour, M, Saharia, A, Li, X, Ghobrial, RM & Monsour, HP, Jr (2016) Hepatocellular carcinoma: a review. *J Hepatocell Carcinoma,* 3, 41-53.
[http://dx.doi.org/10.2147/JHC.S61146] [PMID: 27785449]

Baumhoer, D, Tornillo, L, Stadlmann, S, Roncalli, M, Diamantis, EK & Terracciano, LM (2008) Glypican 3 expression in human nonneoplastic, preneoplastic, and neoplastic tissues: a tissue microarray analysis of 4,387 tissue samples. *Am J Clin Pathol,* 129, 899-906.
[http://dx.doi.org/10.1309/HCQWPWD50XHD2DW6] [PMID: 18480006]

Bedossa, P, Peltier, E, Terris, B, Franco, D & Poynard, T (1995) Transforming growth factor-beta 1 (TGF-beta 1) and TGF-beta 1 receptors in normal, cirrhotic, and neoplastic human livers. *Hepatology,* 21, 760-6.
[PMID: 7875675]

Bell, RJA, Rube, HT, Kreig, A, Mancini, A, Fouse, SD, Nagarajan, RP, Choi, S, Hong, C, He, D, Pekmezci, M, Wiencke, JK, Wrensch, MR, Chang, SM, Walsh, KM, Myong, S, Song, JS & Costello, JF (2015) Cancer. The transcription factor GABP selectively binds and activates the mutant TERT promoter in cancer. *Science,* 348, 1036-9.
[http://dx.doi.org/10.1126/science.aab0015] [PMID: 25977370]

Ben-Josef, E, Normolle, D, Ensminger, WD, Walker, S, Tatro, D, Ten Haken, RK, Knol, J, Dawson, LA, Pan, C & Lawrence, TS (2005) Phase II trial of high-dose conformal radiation therapy with concurrent hepatic artery floxuridine for unresectable intrahepatic malignancies. *J Clin Oncol,* 23, 8739-47.
[http://dx.doi.org/10.1200/JCO.2005.01.5354] [PMID: 16314634]

Berasain, C & Avila, MA (2014) The EGFR signalling system in the liver: from hepatoprotection to

hepatocarcinogenesis. *J Gastroenterol,* 49, 9-23.
[http://dx.doi.org/10.1007/s00535-013-0907-x] [PMID: 24318021]

Bergamini, C, Sgarra, C, Trerotoli, P, Lupo, L, Azzariti, A, Antonaci, S & Giannelli, G (2007) Laminin-5 stimulates hepatocellular carcinoma growth through a different function of α6β4 and α3β1 integrins. *Hepatology,* 46, 1801-9.
[http://dx.doi.org/10.1002/hep.21936] [PMID: 17948258]

Bertoli, G, Cava, C & Castiglioni, I (2015) MicroRNAs: new biomarkers for diagnosis, prognosis, therapy prediction and therapeutic tools for breast cancer. *Theranostics,* 5, 1122-43.
[http://dx.doi.org/10.7150/thno.11543] [PMID: 26199650]

Best, J, Bilgi, H, Heider, D, Schotten, C, Manka, P, Bedreli, S, Gorray, M, Ertle, J, van Grunsven, LA & Dechêne, A (2016) The GALAD scoring algorithm based on AFP, AFP-L3, and DCP significantly improves detection of BCLC early stage hepatocellular carcinoma. *Z Gastroenterol,* 54, 1296-305.
[http://dx.doi.org/10.1055/s-0042-119529] [PMID: 27936479]

Biasiolo, A, Trotta, E, Fasolato, S, Ruvoletto, M, Martini, A, Gallotta, A, Fassina, G, Angeli, P, Gatta, A & Pontisso, P (2016) Squamous cell carcinoma antigen-IgM is associated with hepatocellular carcinoma in patients with cirrhosis: A prospective study. *Dig Liver Dis,* 48, 197-202.
[http://dx.doi.org/10.1016/j.dld.2015.10.022] [PMID: 26614642]

Bläker, M, Schmitz, M, Gocht, A, Burghardt, S, Schulz, M, Bröring, DC, Pace, A, Greten, H & De Weerth, A (2004) Differential expression of somatostatin receptor subtypes in hepatocellular carcinomas. *J Hepatol,* 41, 112-8.
[http://dx.doi.org/10.1016/j.jhep.2004.03.018] [PMID: 15246216]

Block, T, Mehta, AS & London, WT (2010) Hepatocellular carcinoma of the liver. *Cancer Biomark,* 9, 375-83.
[http://dx.doi.org/10.3233/CBM-2011-0165] [PMID: 22112485]

Bochud, PY, Bibert, S, Kutalik, Z, Patin, E, Guergnon, J, Nalpas, B, Goossens, N, Kuske, L, Müllhaupt, B, Gerlach, T, Heim, MH, Moradpour, D, Cerny, A, Malinverni, R, Regenass, S, Dollenmaier, G, Hirsch, H, Martinetti, G, Gorgiewski, M, Bourlière, M, Poynard, T, Theodorou, I, Abel, L, Pol, S, Dufour, JF & Negro, F (2012) IL28B alleles associated with poor hepatitis C virus (HCV) clearance protect against inflammation and fibrosis in patients infected with non-1 HCV genotypes. *Hepatology,* 55, 384-94.
[http://dx.doi.org/10.1002/hep.24678] [PMID: 22180014]

Bolt, HM (2005) Vinyl chloride-a classical industrial toxicant of new interest. *Crit Rev Toxicol,* 35, 307-23.
[http://dx.doi.org/10.1080/10408440490915975] [PMID: 15989139]

Boucher, E, Garin, E, Guylligomarc'h, A, Olivié, D, Boudjema, K & Raoul, JL (2007) Intra-arterial injection of iodine-131-labeled lipiodol for treatment of hepatocellular carcinoma. *Radiother Oncol,* 82, 76-82.
[http://dx.doi.org/10.1016/j.radonc.2006.11.001] [PMID: 17141900]

Bowyer, C, Lewis, AL, Lloyd, AW, Phillips, GJ & Macfarlane, WM (2017) Hypoxia as a target for drug combination therapy of liver cancer. *Anticancer Drugs,* 28, 771-80.
[http://dx.doi.org/10.1097/CAD.0000000000000516] [PMID: 28542038]

Breuhahn, K & Schirmacher, P (2008) Reactivation of the insulin-like growth factor-II signaling pathway in human hepatocellular carcinoma. *World J Gastroenterol,* 14, 1690-8.
[http://dx.doi.org/10.3748/wjg.14.1690] [PMID: 18350600]

Bruix, J & Sherman, M (2011) Management of hepatocellular carcinoma: an update. *Hepatology,* 53, 1020-2.
[http://dx.doi.org/10.1002/hep.24199] [PMID: 21374666]

Buckley, AF, Burgart, LJ, Sahai, V & Kakar, S (2008) Epidermal growth factor receptor expression and gene copy number in conventional hepatocellular carcinoma. *Am J Clin Pathol,* 129, 245-51.
[http://dx.doi.org/10.1309/WF10QAAED3PP93BH] [PMID: 18208805]

Budhu, A, Forgues, M, Ye, QH, Jia, HL, He, P, Zanetti, KA, Kammula, US, Chen, Y, Qin, LX, Tang, ZY & Wang, XW (2006) Prediction of venous metastases, recurrence, and prognosis in hepatocellular carcinoma based on a unique immune response signature of the liver microenvironment. *Cancer Cell,* 10, 99-111. [http://dx.doi.org/10.1016/j.ccr.2006.06.016] [PMID: 16904609]

Buell, JF, Cherqui, D, Geller, DA, O'Rourke, N, Iannitti, D, Dagher, I, Koffron, AJ, Thomas, M, Gayet, B, Han, HS, Wakabayashi, G, Belli, G, Kaneko, H, Ker, CG, Scatton, O, Laurent, A, Abdalla, EK, Chaudhury, P, Dutson, E, Gamblin, C, D'Angelica, M, Nagorney, D, Testa, G, Labow, D, Manas, D, Poon, RT, Nelson, H, Martin, R, Clary, B, Pinson, WC, Martinie, J, Vauthey, JN, Goldstein, R, Roayaie, S, Barlet, D, Espat, J, Abecassis, M, Rees, M, Fong, Y, McMasters, KM, Broelsch, C, Busuttil, R, Belghiti, J, Strasberg, S & Chari, RS (2009) The international position on laparoscopic liver surgery: The Louisville Statement, 2008. *Ann Surg,* 250, 825-30.
[http://dx.doi.org/10.1097/SLA.0b013e3181b3b2d8] [PMID: 19916210]

Bunney, TD & Katan, M (2010) Phosphoinositide signalling in cancer: beyond PI3K and PTEN. *Nat Rev Cancer,* 10, 342-52.
[http://dx.doi.org/10.1038/nrc2842] [PMID: 20414202]

Calle, EE, Rodriguez, C, Walker-Thurmond, K & Thun, MJ (2003) Overweight, obesity, and mortality from cancer in a prospectively studied cohort of U.S. adults. *N Engl J Med,* 348, 1625-38.
[http://dx.doi.org/10.1056/NEJMoa021423] [PMID: 12711737]

Cancer council. (2020) Understanding Cancer in the liver A guide for people affected by primary liver cancer or secondary cancer in the liver. https://www.cancervic.org.au/cancer-information/types- of-ancer/liver_cancer/secondary-liver-cancer. Accessed on December 29, 2020.

Cancer incidence in five continents. Available at: http://ci5.iarc. fr/ Accessed on January 11, 2021.

Cancer of the liver italian program (CLIP) investigators (1998) A new prognostic system for hepatocellular carcinoma: a retrospective study of 435 patients: the Cancer of the Liver Italian Program (CLIP) investigators. *Hepatology,* 28, 751-5.
[http://dx.doi.org/10.1002/hep.510280322] [PMID: 9731568]

Capurro, MI, Xiang, YY, Lobe, C & Filmus, J (2005) Glypican-3 promotes the growth of hepatocellular carcinoma by stimulating canonical Wnt signaling. *Cancer Res,* 65, 6245-54.
[http://dx.doi.org/10.1158/0008-5472.CAN-04-4244] [PMID: 16024626]

Cardinale, V, Wang, Y, Carpino, G, Cui, CB, Gatto, M, Rossi, M, Berloco, PB, Cantafora, A, Wauthier, E, Furth, ME, Inverardi, L, Dominguez-Bendala, J, Ricordi, C, Gerber, D, Gaudio, E, Alvaro, D & Reid, L (2011) Multipotent stem/progenitor cells in human biliary tree give rise to hepatocytes, cholangiocytes, and pancreatic islets. *Hepatology,* 54, 2159-72.
[http://dx.doi.org/10.1002/hep.24590] [PMID: 21809358]

Cardinale, V, Wang, Y, Carpino, G, Mendel, G, Alpini, G, Gaudio, E, Reid, LM & Alvaro, D (2012) The biliary tree--a reservoir of multipotent stem cells. *Nat Rev Gastroenterol Hepatol,* 9, 231-40.
[http://dx.doi.org/10.1038/nrgastro.2012.23] [PMID: 22371217]

Casanova-Salas, I, Rubio-Briones, J, Calatrava, A, Mancarella, C, Masiá, E, Casanova, J, Fernández-Serra, A, Rubio, L, Ramírez-Backhaus, M, Armiñán, A, Domínguez-Escrig, J, Martínez, F, García-Casado, Z, Scotlandi, K, Vicent, MJ & López-Guerrero, JA (2014) Identification of miR-187 and miR-182 as biomarkers of early diagnosis and prognosis in patients with prostate cancer treated with radical prostatectomy. *J Urol,* 192, 252-9.
[http://dx.doi.org/10.1016/j.juro.2014.01.107] [PMID: 24518785]

Cha, MY, Kim, CM, Park, YM & Ryu, WS (2004) Hepatitis B virus X protein is essential for the activation of Wnt/beta-catenin signaling in hepatoma cells. *Hepatology,* 39, 1683-93.
[http://dx.doi.org/10.1002/hep.20245] [PMID: 15185310]

Chakraborty, S, Dlie, ZY & Chakraborty, S (2020) Aptamer-functionalized drug nanocarrier improves hepatocellular carcinoma toward normal by targeting neoplastic hepatocytes. *Molecular Therapy Nucleic Acids,* 5, 34-49.

Chan, C, Wang, Y & Chow, PK (2013) Altered binding site selection of p53 transcription cassettes by hepatitis B virus X protein. *Molecular and Cellular Biology,* 485-97.

Chauhan, R & Lahiri, N (2016) Tissue-and serum-associated biomarkers of hepatocellular carcinoma. *Biomark Cancer,* 8 (Suppl. 1), 37-55.
[PMID: 27398029]

Chauhan, SC, Vinayek, N, Maher, DM, Bell, MC, Dunham, KA, Koch, MD, Lio, Y & Jaggi, M (2007) Combined staining of TAG-72, MUC1, and CA125 improves labeling sensitivity in ovarian cancer: antigens for multi-targeted antibody-guided therapy. *J Histochem Cytochem,* 55, 867-75.
[http://dx.doi.org/10.1369/jhc.7A7213.2007] [PMID: 17478446]

Chen, CH, Hu, FC, Huang, GT, Lee, PH, Tsang, YM, Cheng, AL, Chen, DS, Wang, JD & Sheu, JC (2009) Applicability of staging systems for patients with hepatocellular carcinoma is dependent on treatment method--analysis of 2010 Taiwanese patients. *Eur J Cancer,* 45, 1630-9.
[http://dx.doi.org/10.1016/j.ejca.2008.12.025] [PMID: 19157858]

Chen, CJ, Yang, YH, Lin, MH, Lee, CP, Tsan, YT, Lai, MN, Yang, HY, Ho, WC & Chen, PC (2018) Herbal medicine containing aristolochic acid and the risk of hepatocellular carcinoma in patients with hepatitis B virus infection. *Int J Cancer,* 143, 1578-87.
[http://dx.doi.org/10.1002/ijc.31544] [PMID: 29667191]

Chen, JS, Huang, XH, Wang, Q, Huang, JQ, Zhang, LJ, Chen, XL, Lei, J & Cheng, ZX (2013) Sonic hedgehog signaling pathway induces cell migration and invasion through focal adhesion kinase/AKT signaling-mediated activation of matrix metalloproteinase (MMP)-2 and MMP-9 in liver cancer. *Carcinogenesis,* 34, 10-9. a
[http://dx.doi.org/10.1093/carcin/bgs274] [PMID: 22948179]

Chen, K, Huang, YH & Chen, JL (2013) Understanding and targeting cancer stem cells: therapeutic implications and challenges. *Acta Pharmacol Sin,* 34, 732-40. b
[http://dx.doi.org/10.1038/aps.2013.27] [PMID: 23685952]

Chen, KJ, Zhou, L, Xie, HY, Ahmed, TE, Feng, XW & Zheng, SS (2012) Intratumoral regulatory T cells alone or in combination with cytotoxic T cells predict prognosis of hepatocellular carcinoma after resection. *Med Oncol,* 29, 1817-26.
[http://dx.doi.org/10.1007/s12032-011-0006-x] [PMID: 21678026]

Chen, S, Cao, Q, Wen, W & Wang, H (2019) Targeted therapy for hepatocellular carcinoma: Challenges and opportunities. *Cancer Lett,* 460, 1-9.
[http://dx.doi.org/10.1016/j.canlet.2019.114428] [PMID: 31207320]

Chen, W, Dong, J, Haiech, J, Kilhoffer, MC & Zeniou, M (2016) Cancer stem cell quies-cence and plasticity as major challenges in cancer therapy. *Stem Cells Int,* 2016, 1740936.
[http://dx.doi.org/10.1155/2016/1740936] [PMID: 27418931]

Chen, Y, Wong, PP, Sjeklocha, L, Steer, CJ & Sahin, MB (2012) Mature hepatocytes exhibit unexpected plasticity by direct dedifferentiation into liver progenitor cells in culture. *Hepatology,* 55, 563-74.
[http://dx.doi.org/10.1002/hep.24712] [PMID: 21953633]

Chen, YJ, Chien, PH, Chen, WS, Chien, YF, Hsu, YY, Wang, LY, Chen, JY, Lin, CW, Huang, TC, Yu, YL & Huang, WC (2013) Hepatitis B virus-encoded X protein downregulates EGFR expression *via* inducing microRNA-7 in hepatocellular carcinoma cells. *Evid Based Complement Alternat Med,* 2013, 682380. c
[http://dx.doi.org/10.1155/2013/682380] [PMID: 23840262]

Cheng, AL, Kang, YK, Lin, DY, Park, JW, Kudo, M, Qin, S, Chung, HC, Song, X, Xu, J, Poggi, G, Omata, M, Pitman Lowenthal, S, Lanzalone, S, Yang, L, Lechuga, MJ & Raymond, E (2013) Sunitinib *versus* sorafenib in advanced hepatocellular cancer: results of a randomized phase III trial. *J Clin Oncol,* 31, 4067-75. d
[http://dx.doi.org/10.1200/JCO.2012.45.8372] [PMID: 24081937]

Cheng, AL, Finn, RS & Qin, S (2017) Phase III trial of lenvatinib (LEN) *vs* sorafenib (SOR) in first-line treatment of patients (pts) with unresectable hepatocellular carcinoma (uHCC). *J Clin Oncol,* 35, 4001-1.
[http://dx.doi.org/10.1200/JCO.2017.35.15_suppl.4001]

Chevret, S, Trinchet, JC, Mathieu, D, Rached, AA, Beaugrand, M & Chastang, C (1999) A new prognostic classification for predicting survival in patients with hepatocellular carcinoma. Groupe d'Etude et de Traitement du Carcinome Hépatocellulaire. *J Hepatol,* 31, 133-41.
[http://dx.doi.org/10.1016/S0168-8278(99)80173-1] [PMID: 10424293]

Chew, V, Chen, J, Lee, D, Loh, E, Lee, J, Lim, KH, Weber, A, Slankamenac, K, Poon, RT, Yang, H, Ooi, LL, Toh, HC, Heikenwalder, M, Ng, IO, Nardin, A & Abastado, JP (2012) Chemokine-driven lymphocyte infiltration: an early intratumoural event determining long-term survival in resectable hepatocellular carcinoma. *Gut,* 61, 427-38.
[http://dx.doi.org/10.1136/gutjnl-2011-300509] [PMID: 21930732]

Chiba, T, Kita, K, Zheng, YW, Yokosuka, O, Saisho, H, Iwama, A, Nakauchi, H & Taniguchi, H (2006) Side population purified from hepatocellular carcinoma cells harbors cancer stem cell-like properties. *Hepatology,* 44, 240-51.
[http://dx.doi.org/10.1002/hep.21227] [PMID: 16799977]

Cho, YY, Lee, M, Kim, HC, Chung, JW, Kim, YH, Gwak, GY, Bae, SH, Kim, Y, Heo, J & Kim, YJ (2016) Radioembolization is a safe and effective treatment for hepatocellular carcinoma with portal veinthrombosis: a propensity score analysis. *PLoS One,* 11, e0154986.
[http://dx.doi.org/10.1371/journal.pone.0154986] [PMID: 27149067]

Choi, SH & Hwang, SB (2006) Modulation of the transforming growth factor-beta signal transduction pathway by hepatitis C virus nonstructural 5A protein. *J Biol Chem,* 281, 7468-78.
[http://dx.doi.org/10.1074/jbc.M512438200] [PMID: 16407286]

Choo, QL, Richman, KH & Han, JH (1991) Genetic organization and diversity of the hepatitis C virus. *Proceedings of the National Academy of Sciences of the United States of America,* 88, 2451-5.
[http://dx.doi.org/10.1073/pnas.88.6.2451]

Cillo, U, Bassanello, M, Vitale, A, Grigoletto, FA, Burra, P, Fagiuoli, S, D'Amico, F, Ciarleglio, FA, Boccagni, P, Brolese, A, Zanus, G & D'Amico, DF (2004) The critical issue of hepatocellular carcinoma prognostic classification: which is the best tool available? *J Hepatol,* 40, 124-31.
[http://dx.doi.org/10.1016/j.jhep.2003.09.027] [PMID: 14672623]

Cillo, U, Vitale, A, Grigoletto, F, Farinati, F, Brolese, A, Zanus, G, Neri, D, Boccagni, P, Srsen, N, D'Amico, F, Ciarleglio, FA, Bridda, A & D'Amico, DF (2006) Prospective validation of the Barcelona Clinic Liver Cancer staging system. *J Hepatol,* 44, 723-31.
[http://dx.doi.org/10.1016/j.jhep.2005.12.015] [PMID: 16488051]

Clark, TW (2006) Complications of hepatic chemoembolization. *Semin Intervent Radiol,* 23, 119-25.
[http://dx.doi.org/10.1055/s-2006-941442] [PMID: 21326755]

Comunale, MA, Wang, M, Rodemich-Betesh, L, Hafner, J, Lamontagne, A, Klein, A, Marrero, J, Di Bisceglie, AM, Gish, R, Block, T & Mehta, A (2011) Novel changes in glycosylation of serum Apo-J in patients with hepatocellular carcinoma. *Cancer Epidemiol Biomarkers Prev,* 20, 1222-9.
[http://dx.doi.org/10.1158/1055-9965.EPI-10-1047] [PMID: 21467232]

Development of Atlas of cancer in India. Available at: https://www.ncdirindia.org/ncrp/ca/about.aspx Accessed on January 11, 2021.

D'Souza, AA & Devarajan, PV (2015) Asialoglycoprotein receptor mediated hepatocyte targeting - strategies and applications. *J Control Release,* 203, 126-39.
[http://dx.doi.org/10.1016/j.jconrel.2015.02.022] [PMID: 25701309]

Das, T, Patra, F & Mukherjee, B (2010) Effect of antisense oligomer in controlling c-raf.1 overexpression during diethylnitrosamine-induced hepatocarcinogenesis in rat. *Cancer Chemother Pharmacol,* 65, 309-18.
[http://dx.doi.org/10.1007/s00280-009-1035-4] [PMID: 19499222]

De Stefano, F, Chacon, E, Turcios, L, Marti, F & Gedaly, R (2018) Novel biomarkers in hepatocellular carcinoma. *Curr Opin Pharmacol,* 50, 1115-23.
[PMID: 30217732]

Ding, W, You, H, Dang, H, LeBlanc, F, Galicia, V, Lu, SC, Stiles, B & Rountree, CB (2010) Epithelial-t--mesenchymal transition of murine liver tumor cells promotes invasion. *Hepatology,* 52, 945-53. [http://dx.doi.org/10.1002/hep.23748] [PMID: 20564331]

Dolgin, E (2017) The most popular genes in the human genome. *Nature,* 551, 427-31. [http://dx.doi.org/10.1038/d41586-017-07291-9]

Dong, J, Liu, B & Zhu, R (2016) Targeting ROS for cancer therapy. *Chemotherapy: Open Access,* 5, 1-7.

Du, H, Yang, W, Chen, L, Shen, B, Peng, C, Li, H, Ann, DK, Yen, Y & Qiu, W (2012) Emerging role of autophagy during ischemia-hypoxia and reperfusion in hepatocellular carcinoma. *Int J Oncol,* 40, 2049-57. [PMID: 22469951]

Duarte-Salles, T, Misra, S, Stepien, M, Plymoth, A, Muller, D, Overvad, K, Olsen, A, Tjønneland, A, Baglietto, L, Severi, G, Boutron-Ruault, MC, Turzanski-Fortner, R, Kaaks, R, Boeing, H, Aleksandrova, K, Trichopoulou, A, Lagiou, P, Bamia, C, Pala, V, Palli, D, Mattiello, A, Tumino, R, Naccarati, A, Bueno-d--Mesquita, HB, Peeters, PH, Weiderpass, E, Quirós, JR, Agudo, A, Sánchez-Cantalejo, E, Ardanaz, E, Gavrila, D, Dorronsoro, M, Werner, M, Hemmingsson, O, Ohlsson, B, Sjöberg, K, Wareham, NJ, Khaw, KT, Bradbury, KE, Gunter, MJ, Cross, AJ, Riboli, E, Jenab, M, Hainaut, P & Beretta, L (2016) Circulating osteopontin and prediction of hepatocellular carcinoma development in a large European population. *Cancer Prev Res (Phila),* 9, 758-65. [http://dx.doi.org/10.1158/1940-6207.CAPR-15-0434] [PMID: 27339170]

Eguchi, A, Wree, A & Feldstein, AE (2014) Biomarkers of liver cell death. *J Hepatol,* 60, 1063-74. [http://dx.doi.org/10.1016/j.jhep.2013.12.026] [PMID: 24412608]

Eguchi, S, Kanematsu, T, Arii, S, Okazaki, M, Okita, K, Omata, M, Ikai, I, Kudo, M, Kojiro, M, Makuuchi, M, Monden, M, Matsuyama, Y, Nakanuma, Y & Takayasu, K (2008) Comparison of the outcomes between an anatomical subsegmentectomy and a non-anatomical minor hepatectomy for single hepatocellular carcinomas based on a Japanese nationwide survey. *Surgery,* 143, 469-75. [http://dx.doi.org/10.1016/j.surg.2007.12.003] [PMID: 18374043]

Elmberg, M, Hultcrantz, R, Ekbom, A, Brandt, L, Olsson, S, Olsson, R, Lindgren, S, Lööf, L, Stål, P, Wallerstedt, S, Almer, S, Sandberg-Gertzén, H & Askling, J (2003) Cancer risk in patients with hereditary hemochromatosis and in their first-degree relatives. *Gastroenterology,* 125, 1733-41. [http://dx.doi.org/10.1053/j.gastro.2003.09.035] [PMID: 14724826]

Elnaggar, MH, Abushouk, AI, Hassan, AHE, Lamloum, HM, Benmelouka, A, Moatamed, SA, Abd-Elmegeed, H, Attia, S, Samir, A, Amr, N, Johar, D & Zaky, S (2021) Nanomedicine as a putative approach for active targeting of hepatocellular carcinoma. *Semin Cancer Biol,* 69, 91-9. [http://dx.doi.org/10.1016/j.semcancer.2019.08.016] [PMID: 31421265]

Elsamanoudy, AZ, El-Alfy, HA & Neamat-Allah, MA (2016) Dysregulation of signaling pathways plays a role in the development and pathogenesis of hepatocellular carcinoma. *Int J Biochem Res Rev,* 9, 1-24. [http://dx.doi.org/10.9734/IJBCRR/2016/22158]

El-Serag, HB (2012) Epidemiology of viral hepatitis and hepatocellular carcinoma. *Gastroenterology,* 142, 1264-1273.e1. [http://dx.doi.org/10.1053/j.gastro.2011.12.061] [PMID: 22537432]

El-Serag, HB & Rudolph, KL (2007) Hepatocellular carcinoma: epidemiology and molecular carcinogenesis. *Gastroenterology,* 132, 2557-76. [http://dx.doi.org/10.1053/j.gastro.2007.04.061] [PMID: 17570226]

El-Serag, HB, Hampel, H & Javadi, F (2006) The association between diabetes and hepatocellular carcinoma: a systematic review of epidemiologic evidence. *Clin Gastroenterol Hepatol,* 4, 369-80. [http://dx.doi.org/10.1016/j.cgh.2005.12.007] [PMID: 16527702]

Endo, K & Terada, T (2000) Protein expression of CD44 (standard and variant isoforms) in hepatocellular carcinoma: relationships with tumor grade, clinicopathologic parameters, p53 expression, and patient survival. *J Hepatol,* 32, 78-84.

[http://dx.doi.org/10.1016/S0168-8278(00)80192-0] [PMID: 10673070]

Fallot, G, Neuveut, C & Buendia, MA (2012) Diverse roles of hepatitis B virus in liver cancer. *Curr Opin Virol,* 2, 467-73.
[http://dx.doi.org/10.1016/j.coviro.2012.05.008] [PMID: 22722078]

Fang, F, Chang, R & Yang, L (2012) Heat shock factor 1 promotes invasion and metastasis of hepatocellular carcinoma *in vitro* and *in vivo*. *Cancer,* 118, 1782-94.
[http://dx.doi.org/10.1002/cncr.26482] [PMID: 22009757]

Farazi, PA & DePinho, RA (2006) Hepatocellular carcinoma pathogenesis: from genes to environment. *Nat Rev Cancer,* 6, 674-87.
[http://dx.doi.org/10.1038/nrc1934] [PMID: 16929323]

Farinati, F, Rinaldi, M, Gianni, S & Naccarato, R (2000) How should patients with hepatocellular carcinoma be staged? Validation of a new prognostic system. *Cancer,* 89, 2266-73.
[http://dx.doi.org/10.1002/1097-0142(20001201)89:11<2266::AID-CNCR15>3.0.CO;2-0] [PMID: 11147597]

Feng, M, Gao, W, Wang, R, Chen, W, Man, YG, Figg, WD, Wang, XW, Dimitrov, DS & Ho, M (2013) Therapeutically targeting glypican-3 *via* a conformation-specific single-domain antibody in hepatocellular carcinoma. *Proc Natl Acad Sci USA,* 110, E1083-91.
[http://dx.doi.org/10.1073/pnas.1217868110] [PMID: 23471984]

Filmus, J & Selleck, SB (2001) Glypicans: proteoglycans with a surprise. *J Clin Invest,* 108, 497-501.
[http://dx.doi.org/10.1172/JCI200113712] [PMID: 11518720]

Fitzmorris, P, Shoreibah, M, Anand, BS & Singal, AK (2015) Management of hepatocellular carcinoma. *J Cancer Res Clin Oncol,* 141, 861-76.
[http://dx.doi.org/10.1007/s00432-014-1806-0] [PMID: 25158999]

Forner, A, Reig, M & Bruix, J (2018) Hepatocellular carcinoma. *Lancet,* 391, 1301-14.
[http://dx.doi.org/10.1016/S0140-6736(18)30010-2] [PMID: 29307467]

Fouad, SA, Mohamed, NAG, Fawzy, MW & Moustafa, DA (2015) Plasma osteopontin level in chronic liver disease and hepatocellular carcinoma. *Hepat Mon,* 15, e30753.
[http://dx.doi.org/10.5812/hepatmon.30753] [PMID: 26500684]

Fox, SI (2011) *Human physiology* McGraw-Hill, Boston.

Frenette, CT (2017) The role of regorafenib in hepatocellular carcinoma. *Gastroenterol Hepatol (N Y),* 13, 122-4.
[PMID: 28450818]

Friedman, SL (2008) Mechanisms of hepatic fibrogenesis. *Gastroenterology,* 134, 1655-69.
[http://dx.doi.org/10.1053/j.gastro.2008.03.003] [PMID: 18471545]

Gagner, MR & Dubuc, JM (1992) Laparoscopic partial hepatectomy for liver tumor. *Surg Endosc,* 6, 99.

Galun, D, Srdic-Rajic, T, Bogdanovic, A, Loncar, Z & Zuvela, M (2017) Targeted therapy and personalized medicine in hepatocellular carcinoma: drug resistance, mechanisms, and treatment strategies. *J Hepatocell Carcinoma,* 4, 93-103.
[http://dx.doi.org/10.2147/JHC.S106529] [PMID: 28744453]

Gao, P, Li, M, Tian, QB & Liu, DW (2012) Diagnostic performance of des-γ-carboxy prothrombin (DCP) for hepatocellular carcinoma: a bivariate meta-analysis. *Neoplasma,* 59, 150-9.
[http://dx.doi.org/10.4149/neo_2012_020] [PMID: 22248272]

Ghosh, MK, Patra, F, Ghosh, S, Hossain, CM & Mukherjee, B (2014) Antisense oligonucleotides directed against insulin-like growth factor-II messenger ribonucleic acids delay the progress of rat hepatocarcinogenesis. *J Carcinog,* 13, 2.
[PMID: 24737950]

Giannini, E, Risso, D, Botta, F, Romagnoli, P, Malfatti, F, Fumagalli, A, Testa, E, Podestà, E, Chiarbonello,

B, Polegato, S & Testa, R (2004) Prognosis of hepatocellular carcinoma in anti-HCV positive cirrhotic patients: a single-centre comparison amongst four different staging systems. *J Intern Med,* 255, 399-408.
[http://dx.doi.org/10.1046/j.1365-2796.2003.01284.x] [PMID: 14871465]

Giannini, EG, Moscatelli, A, Pellegatta, G, Vitale, A, Farinati, F, Ciccarese, F, Piscaglia, F, Rapaccini, GL, Di Marco, M, Caturelli, E, Zoli, M, Borzio, F, Cabibbo, G, Felder, M, Sacco, R, Morisco, F, Missale, G, Foschi, FG, Gasbarrini, A, Baroni, GS, Virdone, R, Masotto, A & Trevisani, F (2016) Application of the intermediate-stage subclassification to patients with untreated hepatocellular carcinoma. *Am J Gastroenterol,* 111, 70-7.
[http://dx.doi.org/10.1038/ajg.2015.389] [PMID: 26729544]

Giordano, S & Columbano, A (2014) Met as a therapeutic target in HCC: facts and hopes. *J Hepatol,* 60, 442-52.
[http://dx.doi.org/10.1016/j.jhep.2013.09.009] [PMID: 24045150]

Gomaa, AI & Waked, I (2015) Recent advances in multidisciplinary management of hepatocellular carcinoma. *World J Hepatol,* 7, 673-87.
[http://dx.doi.org/10.4254/wjh.v7.i4.673] [PMID: 25866604]

Gong, J, Chehrazi-Raffle, A, Reddi, S & Salgia, R (2018) Development of PD-1 and PD-L1 inhibitors as a form of cancer immunotherapy: a comprehensive review of registration trials and future considerations. *J Immunother Cancer,* 6, 8.
[http://dx.doi.org/10.1186/s40425-018-0316-z] [PMID: 29357948]

Goodison, S, Urquidi, V & Tarin, D (1999) CD44 cell adhesion molecules. *Mol Pathol,* 52, 189-96.
[http://dx.doi.org/10.1136/mp.52.4.189] [PMID: 10694938]

Gouas, D, Shi, H & Hainaut, P (2009) The aflatoxin-induced TP53 mutation at codon 249 (R249S): biomarker of exposure, early detection and target for therapy. *Cancer Lett,* 286, 29-37.
[http://dx.doi.org/10.1016/j.canlet.2009.02.057] [PMID: 19376640]

Gramantieri, L, Giovannini, C, Lanzi, A, Chieco, P, Ravaioli, M, Venturi, A, Grazi, GL & Bolondi, L (2007) Aberrant Notch3 and Notch4 expression in human hepatocellular carcinoma. *Liver Int,* 27, 997-1007.
[http://dx.doi.org/10.1111/j.1478-3231.2007.01544.x] [PMID: 17696940]

Guest, RV, Boulter, L, Kendall, TJ, Minnis-Lyons, SE, Walker, R, Wigmore, SJ, Sansom, OJ & Forbes, SJ (2014) Cell lineage tracing reveals a biliary origin of intrahepatic cholangiocarcinoma. *Cancer Res,* 74, 1005-10.
[http://dx.doi.org/10.1158/0008-5472.CAN-13-1911] [PMID: 24310400]

Gupta, A & Dixon, E (2017) Epidemiology and risk factors: intrahepatic cholangiocarcinoma. *Hepatobiliary Surg Nutr,* 6, 101-4.
[http://dx.doi.org/10.21037/hbsn.2017.01.02] [PMID: 28503557]

Guyton, AC & Hall, JE (2006) *Textbook of Medical Physiology* Elsevier Saunders, Amsterdam.

Hadziyannis, E, Sialevris, K, Georgiou, A & Koskinas, J (2013) Analysis of serum α-fetoprotein-L3% and des-γ carboxyprothrombin markers in cases with misleading hepatocellular carcinoma total α-fetoprotein levels. *Oncol Rep,* 29, 835-9.
[http://dx.doi.org/10.3892/or.2012.2147] [PMID: 23174906]

Han, B, Chao, J & Yao, H (2018) Circular RNA and its mechanisms in disease: From the bench to the clinic. *Pharmacol Ther,* 187, 31-44.
[http://dx.doi.org/10.1016/j.pharmthera.2018.01.010] [PMID: 29406246]

Han, KH & Park, JY (2008) Chemotherapy for advanced hepatocellular carcinoma. *J Gastroenterol Hepatol,* 23, 682-4.
[http://dx.doi.org/10.1111/j.1440-1746.2008.05444.x] [PMID: 18410601]

Han, YN, Xia, SQ, Zhang, YY, Zheng, JH & Li, W (2017) Circular RNAs: A novel type of biomarker and genetic tools in cancer. *Oncotarget,* 8, 64551-63.
[http://dx.doi.org/10.18632/oncotarget.18350] [PMID: 28969093]

Han, YP, Zhou, L, Wang, J, Xiong, S, Garner, WL, French, SW & Tsukamoto, H (2004) Essential role of matrix metalloproteinases in interleukin-1-induced myofibroblastic activation of hepatic stellate cell in collagen. *J Biol Chem,* 279, 4820-8.
[http://dx.doi.org/10.1074/jbc.M310999200] [PMID: 14617627]

Hanaoka, H, Nagaya, T, Sato, K, Nakamura, Y, Watanabe, R, Harada, T, Gao, W, Feng, M, Phung, Y, Kim, I, Paik, CH, Choyke, PL, Ho, M & Kobayashi, H (2015) Glypican-3 targeted human heavy chain antibody as a drug carrier for hepatocellular carcinoma therapy. *Mol Pharm,* 12, 2151-7.
[http://dx.doi.org/10.1021/acs.molpharmaceut.5b00132] [PMID: 25955255]

Hasegawa, K, Kokudo, N, Imamura, H, Matsuyama, Y, Aoki, T, Minagawa, M, Sano, K, Sugawara, Y, Takayama, T & Makuuchi, M (2005) Prognostic impact of anatomic resection for hepatocellular carcinoma. *Ann Surg,* 242, 252-9.
[http://dx.doi.org/10.1097/01.sla.0000171307.37401.db] [PMID: 16041216]

He, G, Dhar, D, Nakagawa, H, Font-Burgada, J, Ogata, H, Jiang, Y, Shalapour, S, Seki, E, Yost, SE, Jepsen, K, Frazer, KA, Harismendy, O, Hatziapostolou, M, Iliopoulos, D, Suetsugu, A, Hoffman, RM, Tateishi, R, Koike, K & Karin, M (2013) Identification of liver cancer progenitors whose malignant progression depends on autocrine IL-6 signaling. *Cell,* 155, 384-96.
[http://dx.doi.org/10.1016/j.cell.2013.09.031] [PMID: 24120137]

He, Q, Cheng, R, Chen, Z, Xiao, X, Xiao, Z, Li, C, Li, B, Zhang, P, Zheng, H & Feng, D (2007) Cell transformation and proteome alteration in QSG7701 cells transfected with hepatitis C virus non-structural protein 3. *Acta Biochim Biophys Sin (Shanghai),* 39, 751-62.
[http://dx.doi.org/10.1111/j.1745-7270.2007.00344.x] [PMID: 17928924]

Henley, SA & Dick, FA (2012) The retinoblastoma family of proteins and their regulatory functions in the mammalian cell division cycle. *Cell Div,* 7, 10.
[http://dx.doi.org/10.1186/1747-1028-7-10] [PMID: 22417103]

Holczbauer, Á, Factor, VM, Andersen, JB, Marquardt, JU, Kleiner, DE, Raggi, C, Kitade, M, Seo, D, Akita, H, Durkin, ME & Thorgeirsson, SS (2013) Modeling pathogenesis of primary liver cancer in lineage-specific mouse cell types. *Gastroenterology,* 145, 221-31.
[http://dx.doi.org/10.1053/j.gastro.2013.03.013] [PMID: 23523670]

Hong, L, Cai, Y, Jiang, M, Zhou, D & Chen, L (2015) The Hippo signaling pathway in liver regeneration and tumorigenesis. *Acta Biochim Biophys Sin (Shanghai),* 47, 46-52.
[http://dx.doi.org/10.1093/abbs/gmu106] [PMID: 25476204]

Hosaka, T, Suzuki, F, Kobayashi, M, Seko, Y, Kawamura, Y, Sezaki, H, Akuta, N, Suzuki, Y, Saitoh, S, Arase, Y, Ikeda, K, Kobayashi, M & Kumada, H (2013) Long-term entecavir treatment reduces hepatocellular carcinoma incidence in patients with hepatitis B virus infection. *Hepatology,* 58, 98-107.
[http://dx.doi.org/10.1002/hep.26180] [PMID: 23213040]

Hoshida, Y, Fuchs, BC & Tanabe, KK (2012) Prevention of hepatocellular carcinoma: potential targets, experimental models, and clinical challenges. *Curr Cancer Drug Targets,* 12, 1129-59.
[PMID: 22873223]

Hsieh, SC, Lin, IH, Tseng, WL, Lee, CH & Wang, JD (2008) Prescription profile of potentially aristolochic acid containing Chinese herbal products: an analysis of National Health Insurance data in Taiwan between 1997 and 2003. *Chin Med,* 3, 13.
[http://dx.doi.org/10.1186/1749-8546-3-13] [PMID: 18945373]

Hsieh, SY, He, JR, Yu, MC, Lee, WC, Chen, TC, Lo, SJ, Bera, R, Sung, CM & Chiu, CT (2011) Secreted ERBB3 isoforms are serum markers for early hepatoma in patients with chronic hepatitis and cirrhosis. *J Proteome Res,* 10, 4715-24.
[http://dx.doi.org/10.1021/pr200519q] [PMID: 21877752]

Hu, H, Gao, L, Wang, C, Li, Y, Ma, H, Chen, L, Qin, J, Liu, B, Liu, Y & Liang, C (2015) Lower serum soluble-EGFR is a potential biomarker for metastasis of HCC demonstrated by N-glycoproteomic analysis. *Discov Med,* 19, 333-41.

[PMID: 26105696]

Huang, A, Yang, XR, Chung, WY, Dennison, AR & Zhou, J (2020) Targeted therapy for hepatocellular carcinoma. *Signal Transduct Target Ther,* 5, 146.
[http://dx.doi.org/10.1038/s41392-020-00264-x] [PMID: 32782275]

Huang, SF, Chang, IC, Hong, CC, Yen, TC, Chen, CL, Wu, CC, Tsai, CC, Ho, MC, Lee, WC, Yu, HC, Shen, YY, Eng, HL, Wang, J, Tseng, HH, Jeng, YM, Yeh, CT, Chen, CL, Chen, PJ & Liaw, YF (2018) Metabolic risk factors are associated with non-hepatitis B non-hepatitis C hepatocellular carcinoma in Taiwan, an endemic area of chronic hepatitis B. *Hepatol Commun,* 2, 747-59.
[http://dx.doi.org/10.1002/hep4.1182] [PMID: 29881825]

Huynh, H, Nguyen, TTT, Chow, KHP, Tan, PH, Soo, KC & Tran, E (2003) Over-expression of the mitogen-activated protein kinase (MAPK) kinase (MEK)-MAPK in hepatocellular carcinoma: its role in tumor progression and apoptosis. *BMC Gastroenterol,* 3, 19.
[http://dx.doi.org/10.1186/1471-230X-3-19] [PMID: 12906713]

Hyodo, I, Mizuno, M, Yamada, G & Tsuji, T (1993) Distribution of asialoglycoprotein receptor in human hepatocellular carcinoma. *Liver,* 13, 80-5.
[http://dx.doi.org/10.1111/j.1600-0676.1993.tb00611.x] [PMID: 8389955]

Ikai, I, Takayasu, K, Omata, M, Okita, K, Nakanuma, Y, Matsuyama, Y, Makuuchi, M, Kojiro, M, Ichida, T, Arii, S & Yamaoka, Y (2006) A modified Japan Integrated Stage score for prognostic assessment in patients with hepatocellular carcinoma. *J Gastroenterol,* 41, 884-92.
[http://dx.doi.org/10.1007/s00535-006-1878-y] [PMID: 17048053]

Ikenoue, T, Terakado, Y, Nakagawa, H, Hikiba, Y, Fujii, T, Matsubara, D, Noguchi, R, Zhu, C, Yamamoto, K, Kudo, Y, Asaoka, Y, Yamaguchi, K, Ijichi, H, Tateishi, K, Fukushima, N, Maeda, S, Koike, K & Furukawa, Y (2017) Corrigendum: A novel mouse model of intrahepatic cholangiocarcinoma induced by liver-specific Kras activation and Pten deletion. *Sci Rep,* 7, 39567.
[http://dx.doi.org/10.1038/srep39567] [PMID: 28045050]

Imamura, H, Matsuyama, Y & Miyagawa, Y (1999) Prognostic significance of anatomical resection and des-γ-carboxy prothrombin in patients with hepatocellular carcinoma. *The British Journal of Surgery,* 86, 1032-8.

Iwatsuki, M, Mimori, K, Yokobori, T, Ishi, H, Beppu, T, Nakamori, S, Baba, H & Mori, M (2010) Epithelial-mesenchymal transition in cancer development and its clinical significance. *Cancer Sci,* 101, 293-9.
[http://dx.doi.org/10.1111/j.1349-7006.2009.01419.x] [PMID: 19961486]

Janssen, HLA, Reesink, HW, Lawitz, EJ, Zeuzem, S, Rodriguez-Torres, M, Patel, K, van der Meer, AJ, Patick, AK, Chen, A, Zhou, Y, Persson, R, King, BD, Kauppinen, S, Levin, AA & Hodges, MR (2013) Treatment of HCV infection by targeting microRNA. *N Engl J Med,* 368, 1685-94.
[http://dx.doi.org/10.1056/NEJMoa1209026] [PMID: 23534542]

Jiang, L, Cheng, Q, Zhang, BH & Zhang, MZ (2015) Circulating microRNAs as biomarkers in hepatocellular carcinoma screening: a validation set from China. *Medicine (Baltimore),* 94, e603.
[http://dx.doi.org/10.1097/MD.0000000000000603] [PMID: 25761179]

Jin, X, Moskophidis, D & Mivechi, NF (2011) Heat shock transcription factor 1 is a key determinant of HCC development by regulating hepatic steatosis and metabolic syndrome. *Cell Metab,* 14, 91-103.
[http://dx.doi.org/10.1016/j.cmet.2011.03.025] [PMID: 21723507]

Jin, Y, Wang, J, Han, J, Luo, D & Sun, Z (2017) MiR-122 inhibits epithelial-mesenchymal transition in hepatocellular carcinoma by targeting Snail1 and Snail2 and suppressing WNT/β-cadherin signaling pathway. *Exp Cell Res,* 360, 210-7.
[http://dx.doi.org/10.1016/j.yexcr.2017.09.010] [PMID: 28890291]

Jin, Y, Wong, YS, Goh, BKP, Chan, CY, Cheow, PC, Chow, PKH, Lim, TKH, Goh, GBB, Krishnamoorthy, TL, Kumar, R, Ng, TP, Chong, SS, Tan, HH, Chung, AYF, Ooi, LLPJ, Chang, JPE, Tan, CK & Lee, CGL (2019) Circulating microRNAs as Potential Diagnostic and Prognostic Biomarkers in Hepatocellular Carcinoma. *Sci Rep,* 9, 10464.

[http://dx.doi.org/10.1038/s41598-019-46872-8] [PMID: 31320713]

Johnson, PJ, Qin, S, Park, JW, Poon, RT, Raoul, JL, Philip, PA, Hsu, CH, Hu, TH, Heo, J, Xu, J, Lu, L, Chao, Y, Boucher, E, Han, KH, Paik, SW, Robles-Aviña, J, Kudo, M, Yan, L, Sobhonslidsuk, A, Komov, D, Decaens, T, Tak, WY, Jeng, LB, Liu, D, Ezzeddine, R, Walters, I & Cheng, AL (2013) Brivanib *versus* sorafenib as first-line therapy in patients with unresectable, advanced hepatocellular carcinoma: results from the randomized phase III BRISK-FL study. *J Clin Oncol,* 31, 3517-24.
[http://dx.doi.org/10.1200/JCO.2012.48.4410] [PMID: 23980084]

Jörs, S, Jeliazkova, P, Ringelhan, M, Thalhammer, J, Dürl, S, Ferrer, J, Sander, M, Heikenwalder, M, Schmid, RM, Siveke, JT & Geisler, F (2015) Lineage fate of ductular reactions in liver injury and carcinogenesis. *J Clin Invest,* 125, 2445-57.
[http://dx.doi.org/10.1172/JCI78585] [PMID: 25915586]

Joshita, S, Umemura, T, Katsuyama, Y, Ichikawa, Y, Kimura, T, Morita, S, Kamijo, A, Komatsu, M, Ichijo, T, Matsumoto, A, Yoshizawa, K, Kamijo, N, Ota, M & Tanaka, E (2012) Association of IL28B gene polymorphism with development of hepatocellular carcinoma in Japanese patients with chronic hepatitis C virus infection. *Hum Immunol,* 73, 298-300.
[http://dx.doi.org/10.1016/j.humimm.2011.12.021] [PMID: 22245236]

Kamiyama, T, Nakanishi, K & Yokoo, H (2010) The impact of anatomical resection for hepatocellular carcinoma that meets the Milan criteria. *The Journal of Surgical Oncology,* 101, 54-60.

Kang, W, Cheng, AS, Yu, J & To, KF (2016) Emerging role of Hippo pathway in gastric and other gastrointestinal cancers. *World J Gastroenterol,* 22, 1279-88.
[http://dx.doi.org/10.3748/wjg.v22.i3.1279] [PMID: 26811664]

Kanwal, R & Gupta, S (2012) Epigenetic modifications in cancer. *Clin Genet,* 81, 303-11.
[http://dx.doi.org/10.1111/j.1399-0004.2011.01809.x] [PMID: 22082348]

Karademir, S (2018) Staging of hepatocellular carcinoma. *Hepatoma Res,* 4, 58.
[http://dx.doi.org/10.20517/2394-5079.2018.40]

Keating, GM & Santoro, A (2009) Sorafenib: a review of its use in advanced hepatocellular carcinoma. *Drugs,* 69, 223-40.
[http://dx.doi.org/10.2165/00003495-200969020-00006] [PMID: 19228077]

Keenan, BP, Fong, L & Kelley, RK (2019) Immunotherapy in hepatocellular carcinoma: the complex interface between inflammation, fibrosis, and the immune response. *J Immunother Cancer,* 7, 267.
[http://dx.doi.org/10.1186/s40425-019-0749-z] [PMID: 31627733]

Kevin, S, Mariappan, B & Selvi, K (2015) Notch signaling in hepatocellular carcinoma: Molecular targeting in an advanced disease. *Hepatoma Res,* 1, 11-8.
[http://dx.doi.org/10.4103/2394-5079.154132]

Kikkawa, Y, Sudo, R, Kon, J, Mizuguchi, T, Nomizu, M, Hirata, K & Mitaka, T (2008) Laminin α 5 mediates ectopic adhesion of hepatocellular carcinoma through integrins and/or Lutheran/basal cell adhesion molecule. *Exp Cell Res,* 314, 2579-90.
[http://dx.doi.org/10.1016/j.yexcr.2008.05.021] [PMID: 18635166]

Kim, HC (2017) Radioembolization for the treatment of hepatocellular carcinoma. *Clin Mol Hepatol,* 23, 109-14.
[http://dx.doi.org/10.3350/cmh.2017.0004] [PMID: 28494530]

Kim, J, Hong, SJ, Park, JY, Park, JH, Yu, YS, Park, SY, Lim, EK, Choi, KY, Lee, EK, Paik, SS, Lee, KG, Wang, HJ, Do, IG, Joh, JW & Kim, DS (2010) Epithelial-mesenchymal transition gene signature to predict clinical outcome of hepatocellular carcinoma. *Cancer Sci,* 101, 1521-8.
[http://dx.doi.org/10.1111/j.1349-7006.2010.01536.x] [PMID: 20331628]

Kim, JK, Han, KH, Lee, JT, Paik, YH, Ahn, SH, Lee, JD, Lee, KS, Chon, CY & Moon, YM (2006) Long-term clinical outcome of phase IIb clinical trial of percutaneous injection with holmium-166/chitosan complex (Milican) for the treatment of small hepatocellular carcinoma. *Clin Cancer Res,* 12, 543-8.

[http://dx.doi.org/10.1158/1078-0432.CCR-05-1730] [PMID: 16428498]

Kim, S & Abou-Alfa, GK (2014) The role of tyrosine kinase inhibitors in hepatocellular carcinoma. *Clin Adv Hematol Oncol,* 12, 36-41.
[PMID: 25000314]

Kishi, Y, Hasegawa, K, Sugawara, Y & Kokudo, N (2011) Hepatocellular carcinoma: current management and future development-improved outcomes with surgical resection. *Int J Hepatol,* 2011, 728103.
[http://dx.doi.org/10.4061/2011/728103] [PMID: 21994868]

Kitai, S, Kudo, M, Minami, Y, Ueshima, K, Chung, H, Hagiwara, S, Inoue, T, Ishikawa, E, Takahashi, S, Asakuma, Y, Haji, S, Osaki, Y, Oka, H, Seki, T, Kasugai, H, Sasaki, Y & Matsunaga, T (2008) A new prognostic staging system for hepatocellular carcinoma: value of the biomarker combined Japan integrated staging score. *Intervirology,* 51 (Suppl. 1), 86-94.
[http://dx.doi.org/10.1159/000122599] [PMID: 18544953]

Kladney, RD, Bulla, GA, Guo, L, Mason, AL, Tollefson, AE, Simon, DJ, Koutoubi, Z & Fimmel, CJ (2000) GP73, a novel Golgi-localized protein upregulated by viral infection. *Gene,* 249, 53-65.
[http://dx.doi.org/10.1016/S0378-1119(00)00136-0] [PMID: 10831838]

Knouse, KA, Wu, J, Whittaker, CA & Amon, A (2014) Single cell sequencing reveals low levels of aneuploidy across mammalian tissues. *Proc Natl Acad Sci USA,* 111, 13409-14.
[http://dx.doi.org/10.1073/pnas.1415287111] [PMID: 25197050]

Koike, Y, Shiratori, Y, Sato, S, Obi, S, Teratani, T, Imamura, M, Yoshida, H, Shiina, S & Omata, M (2001) Des-gamma-carboxy prothrombin as a useful predisposing factor for the development of portal venous invasion in patients with hepatocellular carcinoma: a prospective analysis of 227 patients. *Cancer,* 91, 561-9.
[http://dx.doi.org/10.1002/1097-0142(20010201)91:3<561::AID-CNCR1035>3.0.CO;2-N] [PMID: 11169939]

Kolly, P, Reeves, H, Sangro, B, Knöpfli, M, Candinas, D & Dufour, JF (2016) Assessment of the Hong Kong Liver Cancer Staging System in Europe. *Liver Int,* 36, 911-7.
[http://dx.doi.org/10.1111/liv.13045] [PMID: 26677809]

Komposch, K & Sibilia, M (2015) EGFR Signaling in liver diseases. *Int J Mol Sci,* 17, 30.
[http://dx.doi.org/10.3390/ijms17010030] [PMID: 26729094]

Kong, G, Zhang, J, Zhang, S, Shan, C, Ye, L & Zhang, X (2011) Upregulated microRNA-29a by hepatitis B virus X protein enhances hepatoma cell migration by targeting PTEN in cell culture model. *PLoS One,* 6, e19518.
[http://dx.doi.org/10.1371/journal.pone.0019518] [PMID: 21573166]

Korenaga, M, Wang, T, Li, Y, Showalter, LA, Chan, T, Sun, J & Weinman, SA (2005) Hepatitis C virus core protein inhibits mitochondrial electron transport and increases reactive oxygen species (ROS) production. *J Biol Chem,* 280, 37481-8.
[http://dx.doi.org/10.1074/jbc.M506412200] [PMID: 16150732]

Kouloulias, V, Mosa, E, Georgakopoulos, J, Platoni, K, Brountzos, I, Zygogianni, A, Antypas, C, Kosmidis, P, Mystakidou, K, Tolia, M, Beli, I, Gouliamos, A, Kouvaris, J & Kelekis, N (2013) Three-dimensional conformal radiotherapy for hepatocellular carcinoma in patients unfit for resection, ablation, or chemotherapy: a retrospective study. *ScientificWorldJournal,* 2013, 780141.
[http://dx.doi.org/10.1155/2013/780141] [PMID: 24379750]

Kouroumalis, E, Skordilis, P, Thermos, K, Vasilaki, A, Moschandrea, J & Manousos, ON (1998) Treatment of hepatocellular carcinoma with octreotide: a randomised controlled study. *Gut,* 42, 442-7.
[http://dx.doi.org/10.1136/gut.42.3.442] [PMID: 9577356]

Kudo, M (2018) Management of hepatocellular carcinoma in Japan as a world-leading model. *Liver Cancer,* 7, 134-47.
[http://dx.doi.org/10.1159/000484619] [PMID: 29888204]

Kudo, M, Chung, H & Osaki, Y (2003) Prognostic staging system for hepatocellular carcinoma (CLIP score):

its value and limitations, and a proposal for a new staging system, the Japan Integrated Staging Score (JIS score). *J Gastroenterol,* 38, 207-15.
[http://dx.doi.org/10.1007/s005350300038] [PMID: 12673442]

Kudo, M, Chung, H, Haji, S, Osaki, Y, Oka, H, Seki, T, Kasugai, H, Sasaki, Y & Matsunaga, T (2004) Validation of a new prognostic staging system for hepatocellular carcinoma: the JIS score compared with the CLIP score. *Hepatology,* 40, 1396-405.
[http://dx.doi.org/10.1002/hep.20486] [PMID: 15565571]

Kudo, M, Finn, RS, Qin, S, Han, KH, Ikeda, K, Piscaglia, F, Baron, A, Park, JW, Han, G, Jassem, J, Blanc, JF, Vogel, A, Komov, D, Evans, TRJ, Lopez, C, Dutcus, C, Guo, M, Saito, K, Kraljevic, S, Tamai, T, Ren, M & Cheng, AL (2018) Lenvatinib *versus* sorafenib in first-line treatment of patients with unresectable hepatocellular carcinoma: a randomised phase 3 non-inferiority trial. *Lancet,* 391, 1163-73. b
[http://dx.doi.org/10.1016/S0140-6736(18)30207-1] [PMID: 29433850]

Kumar, A, Acharya, SK, Singh, SP, Saraswat, VA, Arora, A, Duseja, A, Goenka, MK, Jain, D, Kar, P, Kumar, M, Kumaran, V, Mohandas, KM, Panda, D, Paul, SB, Ramachandran, J, Ramesh, H, Rao, PN, Shah, SR, Sharma, H & Thandassery, RB (2014) The Indian National Association for Study of the Liver (INASL) Consensus on Prevention, Diagnosis and Management of Hepatocellular Carcinoma in India: The Puri Recommendations. *J Clin Exp Hepatol,* 4 (Suppl. 3), S3-S26.
[http://dx.doi.org/10.1016/j.jceh.2014.04.003] [PMID: 25755608]

Kumari, R, Sahu, MK, Tripathy, A, Uthansingh, K & Behera, M (2018) Hepatocellular carcinoma treatment: hurdles, advances and prospects. *Hepat Oncol,* 5, HEP08.
[http://dx.doi.org/10.2217/hep-2018-0002] [PMID: 31293776]

Kwun, HJ, Jung, EY, Ahn, JY, Lee, MN & Jang, KL (2001) p53-dependent transcriptional repression of p21(waf1) by hepatitis C virus NS3. *J Gen Virol,* 82, 2235-41.
[http://dx.doi.org/10.1099/0022-1317-82-9-2235] [PMID: 11514734]

Ladju, RB, Pascut, D, Massi, MN, Tiribelli, C & Sukowati, CHC (2017) Aptamer: A potential oligonucleotide nanomedicine in the diagnosis and treatment of hepatocellular carcinoma. *Oncotarget,* 9, 2951-61.
[http://dx.doi.org/10.18632/oncotarget.23359] [PMID: 29416827]

Lai, Q, Iesari, S, Levi Sandri, GB & Lerut, J (2017) Des-gamma-carboxy prothrombin in hepatocellular cancer patients waiting for liver transplant: a systematic review and meta-analysis. *Int J Biol Markers,* 32, e370-4.
[http://dx.doi.org/10.5301/ijbm.5000276] [PMID: 28561879]

Lambert, B & Van de Wiele, C (2005) Treatment of hepatocellular carcinoma by means of radiopharmaceuticals. *Eur J Nucl Med Mol Imaging,* 32, 980-9.
[http://dx.doi.org/10.1007/s00259-005-1859-z] [PMID: 16032439]

Lanaya, H, Natarajan, A & Komposch, K (2014) EGFR has a tumour-promoting role in liver macrophages during hepatocellular carcinoma formation. *Nature Cell Biology,* 16, 971-7.
[http://dx.doi.org/10.1038/ncb3031]

Larsson, SC & Wolk, A (2007) Overweight, obesity and risk of liver cancer: a meta-analysis of cohort studies. *Br J Cancer,* 97, 1005-8.
[http://dx.doi.org/10.1038/sj.bjc.6603932] [PMID: 17700568]

Lee, JS, Heo, J, Libbrecht, L, Chu, IS, Kaposi-Novak, P, Calvisi, DF, Mikaelyan, A, Roberts, LR, Demetris, AJ, Sun, Z, Nevens, F, Roskams, T & Thorgeirsson, SS (2006) A novel prognostic subtype of human hepatocellular carcinoma derived from hepatic progenitor cells. *Nat Med,* 12, 410-6.
[http://dx.doi.org/10.1038/nm1377] [PMID: 16532004]

Lee, KP, Lee, JH & Kim, TS (2010) e Hippo-Salvador pathway restrains hepatic oval cell proliferation, liver size, and liver tumorigenesis. *Proceedings of the National Academy of Sciences U S A,* 8248-53.
[http://dx.doi.org/10.1073/pnas.0912203107]

Lee, RTH, Zhao, Z & Ingham, PW (2016) Hedgehog signalling. *Development,* 143, 367-72.

[http://dx.doi.org/10.1242/dev.120154] [PMID: 26839340]

Lee, WC, Wu, TJ, Chou, HS, Yu, MC, Hsu, PY, Hsu, HY & Wang, CC (2012) The impact of CD4+ CD25+ T cells in the tumor microenvironment of hepatocellular carcinoma. *Surgery,* 151, 213-22. [http://dx.doi.org/10.1016/j.surg.2011.07.029] [PMID: 21975289]

Leonardi, GC, Candido, S, Cervello, M, Nicolosi, D, Raiti, F, Travali, S, Spandidos, DA & Libra, M (2012) The tumor microenvironment in hepatocellular carcinoma (review). *Int J Oncol,* 40, 1733-47. [review]. [PMID: 22447316]

Lerat, H, Higgs, M & Pawlotsky, JM (2011) Animal models in the study of hepatitis C virus-associated liver pathologies. *Expert Rev Gastroenterol Hepatol,* 5, 341-52. [http://dx.doi.org/10.1586/egh.11.14] [PMID: 21651352]

Leung, TW, Tang, AM, Zee, B, Lau, WY, Lai, PB, Leung, KL, Lau, JT, Yu, SC & Johnson, PJ (2002) Construction of the Chinese University Prognostic Index for hepatocellular carcinoma and comparison with the TNM staging system, the Okuda staging system, and the Cancer of the Liver Italian Program staging system: a study based on 926 patients. *Cancer,* 94, 1760-9. [http://dx.doi.org/10.1002/cncr.10384] [PMID: 11920539]

Leung, DA, Goin, JE, Sickles, C, Raskay, BJ & Soulen, MC (2001) Determinants of postembolization syndrome after hepatic chemoembolization. *J Vasc Interv Radiol,* 12, 321-6. [http://dx.doi.org/10.1016/S1051-0443(07)61911-3] [PMID: 11287509]

Leung, TW, Patt, YZ, Lau, WY, Ho, SK, Yu, SC, Chan, AT, Mok, TS, Yeo, W, Liew, CT, Leung, NW, Tang, AM & Johnson, PJ (1999) Complete pathological remission is possible with systemic combination chemotherapy for inoperable hepatocellular carcinoma. *Clin Cancer Res,* 5, 1676-81. [PMID: 10430068]

Levi-Montalcini, R (1987) The nerve growth factor 35 years later. *Science,* 237, 1154-62. [http://dx.doi.org/10.1126/science.3306916] [PMID: 3306916]

Levy, I & Sherman, M (2002) Staging of hepatocellular carcinoma: assessment of the CLIP, Okuda, and Child-Pugh staging systems in a cohort of 257 patients in Toronto. *Gut,* 50, 881-5. [http://dx.doi.org/10.1136/gut.50.6.881] [PMID: 12010894]

Li, H, Wolfe, A, Septer, S, Edwards, G, Zhong, X, Abdulkarim, AB, Ranganathan, S & Apte, U (2012) Deregulation of Hippo kinase signalling in human hepatic malignancies. *Liver Int,* 32, 38-47. a [http://dx.doi.org/10.1111/j.1478-3231.2011.02646.x] [PMID: 22098159]

Li, L, Jin, R, Zhang, X, Lv, F, Liu, L, Liu, D, Liu, K, Li, N & Chen, D (2012) Oncogenic activation of glypican-3 by c-Myc in human hepatocellular carcinoma. *Hepatology,* 56, 1380-90. b [http://dx.doi.org/10.1002/hep.25891] [PMID: 22706665]

Li, M, Zhang, W, Wang, B, Gao, Y, Song, Z & Zheng, QC (2016) Ligand-based targeted therapy: a novel strategy for hepatocellular carcinoma. *Int J Nanomedicine,* 11, 5645-69. [http://dx.doi.org/10.2147/IJN.S115727] [PMID: 27920520]

Li, Q, Liu, G, Shao, D, Wang, J, Yuan, H, Chen, T, Zhai, R, Ni, W & Tai, G (2015) Mucin1 mediates autocrine transforming growth factor beta signaling through activating the c-Jun N-terminal kinase/activator protein 1 pathway in human hepatocellular carcinoma cells. *Int J Biochem Cell Biol,* 59, 116-25. [http://dx.doi.org/10.1016/j.biocel.2014.11.012] [PMID: 25526895]

Li, X, Quon, G, Lipshitz, HD & Morris, Q (2010) Predicting *in vivo* binding sites of RNA-binding proteins using mRNA secondary structure. *RNA,* 16, 1096-107. [http://dx.doi.org/10.1261/rna.2017210] [PMID: 20418358]

Li, YW, Qiu, SJ, Fan, J, Zhou, J, Gao, Q, Xiao, YS & Xu, YF (2011) Intratumoral neutrophils: a poor prognostic factor for hepatocellular carcinoma following resection. *J Hepatol,* 54, 497-505. [http://dx.doi.org/10.1016/j.jhep.2010.07.044] [PMID: 21112656]

Liang, X, Zeng, J, Wang, L, Fang, M, Wang, Q, Zhao, M, Xu, X, Liu, Z, Li, W, Liu, S, Yu, H, Jia, J & Chen, C (2013) Histone demethylase retinoblastoma binding protein 2 is overexpressed in hepatocellular carcinoma

and negatively regulated by hsa-miR-212. *PLoS One,* 8, e69784.
[http://dx.doi.org/10.1371/journal.pone.0069784] [PMID: 23922798]

Lian-Yi, G, Pei, L & Ying, W (2014) Sonic Hedgehog signaling pathway in primary liver cancer cells. *Asian Pac J Trop Med,* 7, 735-8.
[http://dx.doi.org/10.1016/S1995-7645(14)60126-7]

Lin, A, Schildknecht, A, Nguyen, LT & Ohashi, PS (2010) Dendritic cells integrate signals from the tumor microenvironment to modulate immunity and tumor growth. *Immunol Lett,* 127, 77-84.
[http://dx.doi.org/10.1016/j.imlet.2009.09.003] [PMID: 19778555]

Lin, Ci-Ai (2018) Hypoxic microenvironment and hepatocellular carcinoma treatment. *Hepatoma Res,* 4, 1-8.
[http://dx.doi.org/10.20517/2394-5079.2018.27]

Lin, OS, Keeffe, EB, Sanders, GD & Owens, DK (2004) Cost-effectiveness of screening for hepatocellular carcinoma in patients with cirrhosis due to chronic hepatitis C. *Aliment Pharmacol Ther,* 19, 1159-72.
[http://dx.doi.org/10.1111/j.1365-2036.2004.01963.x] [PMID: 15153169]

Lin, XJ, Chong, Y, Guo, ZW, Xie, C, Yang, XJ, Zhang, Q, Li, SP, Xiong, Y, Yuan, Y, Min, J, Jia, WH, Jie, Y, Chen, MS, Chen, MX, Fang, JH, Zeng, C, Zhang, Y, Guo, RP, Wu, Y, Lin, G, Zheng, L & Zhuang, SM (2015) A serum microRNA classifier for early detection of hepatocellular carcinoma: a multicentre, retrospective, longitudinal biomarker identification study with a nested case-control study. *Lancet Oncol,* 16, 804-15.
[http://dx.doi.org/10.1016/S1470-2045(15)00048-0] [PMID: 26088272]

Lindenbach, BD, Evans, MJ, Syder, AJ, Wölk, B, Tellinghuisen, TL, Liu, CC, Maruyama, T, Hynes, RO, Burton, DR, McKeating, JA & Rice, CM (2005) Complete replication of hepatitis C virus in cell culture. *Science,* 309, 623-6.
[http://dx.doi.org/10.1126/science.1114016] [PMID: 15947137]

Lintia-Gaultier, A, Perret, C, Ansquer, C, Eugène, T, Kraeber-Bodéré, F & Frampas, E (2013) Intra-arterial injection of 131I-labeled Lipiodol for advanced hepatocellular carcinoma: a 7 years' experience. *Nucl Med Commun,* 34, 674-81.
[http://dx.doi.org/10.1097/MNM.0b013e32836141a0] [PMID: 23587835]

Liu, CC, Jan, YJ, Ko, BS, Wu, YM, Liang, SM, Chen, SC, Lee, YM, Liu, TA, Chang, TC, Wang, J, Shyue, SK, Sung, LY & Liou, JY (2014) 14-3-3σ induces heat shock protein 70 expression in hepatocellular carcinoma. *BMC Cancer,* 14, 425.
[http://dx.doi.org/10.1186/1471-2407-14-425] [PMID: 24923353]

Liu, PH, Hsu, CY, Hsia, CY, Lee, YH, Su, CW, Huang, YH, Lee, FY, Lin, HC & Huo, TI (2016) Prognosis of hepatocellular carcinoma: Assessment of eleven staging systems. *J Hepatol,* 64, 601-8.
[http://dx.doi.org/10.1016/j.jhep.2015.10.029] [PMID: 26551516]

Liu, S, Ma, L, Huang, W, Shai, Y, Ji, X, Ding, L, Liu, Y, Yu, L & Zhao, S (2006) Decreased expression of the human carbonyl reductase 2 gene HCR2 in hepatocellular carcinoma. *Cell Mol Biol Lett,* 11, 230-41.
[http://dx.doi.org/10.2478/s11658-006-0022-6] [PMID: 16847567]

Liu, Y, Cao, L, Chen, R, Zhou, X, Fan, X, Liang, Y, Jia, R, Wang, H, Liu, G, Guo, Y & Zhao, J (2015) Osteopontin promotes hepatic progenitor cell expansion and tumorigenicity *via* activation of beta-catenin in mice. *Stem Cells,* 33, 3569-80.
[http://dx.doi.org/10.1002/stem.2072] [PMID: 26033745]

Liu, Z, Lin, Y, Zhang, J, Zhang, Y, Li, Y, Liu, Z, Li, Q, Luo, M, Liang, R & Ye, J (2019) Molecular targeted and immune checkpoint therapy for advanced hepatocellular carcinoma. *J Exp Clin Cancer Res,* 38, 447.
[http://dx.doi.org/10.1186/s13046-019-1412-8] [PMID: 31684985]

Liu, ZM, Tseng, HY, Tsai, HW, Su, FC & Huang, HS (2015) Transforming growth factor β-interacting factor-induced malignant progression of hepatocellular carcinoma cells depends on superoxide production from Nox4. *Free Radic Biol Med,* 84, 54-64.
[http://dx.doi.org/10.1016/j.freeradbiomed.2015.03.028] [PMID: 25841779]

Llovet, JM & Bruix, J (2000) Prospective validation of the CLIP score: a new prognostic system for patients with cirrhosis and hepatocellular carcinoma. *Hepatology,* 31, 840-5.
[http://dx.doi.org/10.1053/he.2000.5628] [PMID: 10733537]

Llovet, JM & Bruix, J (2008) Novel advancements in the management of hepatocellular carcinoma in 2008. *J Hepatol,* 48 (Suppl. 1), S20-37.
[http://dx.doi.org/10.1016/j.jhep.2008.01.022] [PMID: 18304676]

Llovet, JM, Brú, C & Bruix, J (1999) Prognosis of hepatocellular carcinoma: the BCLC staging classification. *Semin Liver Dis,* 19, 329-38.
[http://dx.doi.org/10.1055/s-2007-1007122] [PMID: 10518312]

Llovet, JM, Bruix, J, Fuster, J, Castells, A, Garcia-Valdecasas, JC, Grande, L, Franca, A, Brú, C, Navasa, M, Ayuso, MC, Solé, M, Real, MI, Vilana, R, Rimola, A, Visa, J & Rodés, J (1998) Liver transplantation for small hepatocellular carcinoma: the tumor-node-metastasis classification does not have prognostic power. *Hepatology,* 27, 1572-7.
[http://dx.doi.org/10.1002/hep.510270616] [PMID: 9620329]

Llovet, JM, Peña, CEA, Lathia, CD, Shan, M, Meinhardt, G & Bruix, J (2012) Plasma biomarkers as predictors of outcome in patients with advanced hepatocellular carcinoma. *Clin Cancer Res,* 18, 2290-300.
[http://dx.doi.org/10.1158/1078-0432.CCR-11-2175] [PMID: 22374331]

Lo, A, Lin, CT & Wu, HC (2008) Hepatocellular carcinoma cell-specific peptide ligand for targeted drug delivery. *Mol Cancer Ther,* 7, 579-89.
[http://dx.doi.org/10.1158/1535-7163.MCT-07-2359] [PMID: 18347144]

Lokman, NA, Ween, MP, Oehler, MK & Ricciardelli, C (2011) The role of annexin A2 in tumorigenesis and cancer progression. *Cancer Microenviron,* 4, 199-208.
[http://dx.doi.org/10.1007/s12307-011-0064-9] [PMID: 21909879]

Lou, J, Zhang, L, Lv, S, Zhang, C & Jiang, S (2017) Biomarkers for hepatocellular carcinoma. *Biomark Cancer,* 9, 1-9.
[http://dx.doi.org/10.1177/1179299X16684640] [PMID: 28469485]

Luo, D, Wang, Z, Wu, J, Jiang, C & Wu, J (2014) The role of hypoxia inducible factor-1 in hepatocellular carcinoma. *BioMed Res Int,* 2014, 409272.
[http://dx.doi.org/10.1155/2014/409272] [PMID: 25101278]

Luz, JHM, Luz, PM, Martin, HS, Gouveia, HR, Levigard, RB, Nogueira, FD, Rodrigues, BC, de Miranda, TN & Mamede, MH (2017) 'DEB TACE for intermediate and advanced HCC: initial experience in a Brazilian Cancer Center'. *Cancer Imaging,* 17, 5.
[http://dx.doi.org/10.1186/s40644-017-0108-6] [PMID: 28166821]

Ma, S, Chan, KW, Hu, L, Lee, TK, Wo, JY, Ng, IO, Zheng, BJ & Guan, XY (2007) Identification and characterization of tumorigenic liver cancer stem/progenitor cells. *Gastroenterology,* 132, 2542-56.
[http://dx.doi.org/10.1053/j.gastro.2007.04.025] [PMID: 17570225]

Ma, X, Gong, N, Zhong, L, Sun, J & Liang, XJ (2016) Future of nanotherapeutics: Targeting the cellular sub-organelles. *Biomaterials,* 97, 10-21.
[http://dx.doi.org/10.1016/j.biomaterials.2016.04.026] [PMID: 27155363]

Macfarlane, LA & Murphy, PR (2010) MicroRNA: biogenesis, function and role in cancer. *Curr Genomics,* 11, 537-61.
[http://dx.doi.org/10.2174/138920210793175895] [PMID: 21532838]

Maegdefrau, U, Amann, T, Winklmeier, A, Braig, S, Schubert, T, Weiss, TS, Schardt, K, Warnecke, C, Hellerbrand, C & Bosserhoff, AK (2009) Bone morphogenetic protein 4 is induced in hepatocellular carcinoma by hypoxia and promotes tumour progression. *J Pathol,* 218, 520-9.
[http://dx.doi.org/10.1002/path.2563] [PMID: 19431154]

Makuuchi, M, Belghiti, J, Belli, G, Fan, ST, Lau, JW, Ringe, B, Strasberg, SM, Vauthey, JN, Yamaoka, Y & Yamasaki, S (2003) IHPBA concordant classification of primary liver cancer: working group report. *J*

Hepatobiliary Pancreat Surg, 10, 26-30.
[http://dx.doi.org/10.1007/s10534-002-0808-6] [PMID: 12918454]

Makuuchi, M, Kokudo, N, Arii, S, Futagawa, S, Kaneko, S, Kawasaki, S, Matsuyama, Y, Okazaki, M, Okita, K, Omata, M, Saida, Y, Takayama, T & Yamaoka, Y (2008) Development of evidence-based clinical guidelines for the diagnosis and treatment of hepatocellular carcinoma in Japan. *Hepatol Res,* 38, 37-51.
[http://dx.doi.org/10.1111/j.1872-034X.2007.00216.x] [PMID: 18039202]

Makuuchi, M, Thai, BL, Takayasu, K, Takayama, T, Kosuge, T, Gunvén, P, Yamazaki, S, Hasegawa, H & Ozaki, H (1990) Preoperative portal embolization to increase safety of major hepatectomy for hilar bile duct carcinoma: a preliminary report. *Surgery,* 107, 521-7.
[PMID: 2333592]

Mantovani, A, Germano, G, Marchesi, F, Locatelli, M & Biswas, SK (2011) Cancer-promoting tumor-associated macrophages: new vistas and open questions. *Eur J Immunol,* 41, 2522-5.
[http://dx.doi.org/10.1002/eji.201141894] [PMID: 21952810]

Marabita, F, Aghemo, A, De Nicola, S, Rumi, MG, Cheroni, C, Scavelli, R, Crimi, M, Soffredini, R, Abrignani, S, De Francesco, R & Colombo, M (2011) Genetic variation in the interleukin-28B gene is not associated with fibrosis progression in patients with chronic hepatitis C and known date of infection. *Hepatology,* 54, 1127-34.
[http://dx.doi.org/10.1002/hep.24503] [PMID: 21721028]

Marquardt, JU (2016) Deconvolution of the cellular origin in hepatocellular carcinoma: Hepatocytes take the center stage. *Hepatology,* 64, 1020-3.
[http://dx.doi.org/10.1002/hep.28671] [PMID: 27287264]

Marra, M, Sordelli, IM, Lombardi, A, Lamberti, M, Tarantino, L, Giudice, A, Stiuso, P, Abbruzzese, A, Sperlongano, R, Accardo, M, Agresti, M, Caraglia, M & Sperlongano, P (2011) Molecular targets and oxidative stress biomarkers in hepatocellular carcinoma: an overview. *J Transl Med,* 9, 171.
[http://dx.doi.org/10.1186/1479-5876-9-171] [PMID: 21985599]

Marrero, JA, Kudo, M & Bronowicki, JP (2010) The challenge of prognosis and staging for hepatocellular carcinoma. *Oncologist,* 15 (Suppl. 4), 23-33.
[http://dx.doi.org/10.1634/theoncologist.2010-S4-23] [PMID: 21115578]

Marrero, JA, Fontana, RJ, Barrat, A, Askari, F, Conjeevaram, HS, Su, GL & Lok, AS (2005) Prognosis of hepatocellular carcinoma: comparison of 7 staging systems in an American cohort. *Hepatology,* 41, 707-16.
[http://dx.doi.org/10.1002/hep.20636] [PMID: 15795889]

Marrero, JA, Kulik, LM, Sirlin, CB, Zhu, AX, Finn, RS, Abecassis, MM, Roberts, LR & Heimbach, JK (2018) Diagnosis, Staging, and Management of Hepatocellular Carcinoma: 2018 Practice Guidance by the American Association for the Study of Liver Diseases. *Hepatology,* 68, 723-50.
[http://dx.doi.org/10.1002/hep.29913] [PMID: 29624699]

Marsh, JW, Dvorchik, I, Bonham, CA & Iwatsuki, S (2000) Is the pathologic TNM staging system for patients with hepatoma predictive of outcome? *Cancer,* 88, 538-43.
[http://dx.doi.org/10.1002/(SICI)1097-0142(20000201)88:3<538::AID-CNCR7>3.0.CO;2-H] [PMID: 10649244]

Martin, V, Liu, D, Fueyo, J & Gomez-Manzano, C (2008) Tie2: a journey from normal angiogenesis to cancer and beyond. *Histol Histopathol,* 23, 773-80.
[PMID: 18366015]

Massarweh, NN & El-Serag, HB (2017) Epidemiology of hepatocellular carcinoma and intrahepatic cholangiocarcinoma. *Cancer Contr,* 24, 1073274817729245.
[http://dx.doi.org/10.1177/1073274817729245] [PMID: 28975830]

Mathai, AM, Kapadia, MJ, Alexander, J, Kernochan, LE, Swanson, PE & Yeh, MM (2012) Role of Foxp3-positive tumor-infiltrating lymphocytes in the histologic features and clinical outcomes of hepatocellular carcinoma. *Am J Surg Pathol,* 36, 980-6.

[http://dx.doi.org/10.1097/PAS.0b013e31824e9b7c] [PMID: 22446942]

Mathew, J, Hines, JE, Obafunwa, JO, Burr, AW, Toole, K & Burt, AD (1996) CD44 is expressed in hepatocellular carcinomas showing vascular invasion. *J Pathol,* 179, 74-9.
[http://dx.doi.org/10.1002/(SICI)1096-9896(199605)179:1<74::AID-PATH531>3.0.CO;2-E] [PMID: 8691349]

Matsubara, M, Shiraha, H, Kataoka, J, Iwamuro, M, Horiguchi, S, Nishina, S, Takaoka, N, Uemura, M, Takaki, A, Nakamura, S, Kobayashi, Y, Nouso, K & Yamamoto, K (2012) Des-γ-carboxyl prothrombin is associated with tumor angiogenesis in hepatocellular carcinoma. *J Gastroenterol Hepatol,* 27, 1602-8.
[http://dx.doi.org/10.1111/j.1440-1746.2012.07173.x] [PMID: 22554292]

Matsumoto, T, Takai, A, Eso, Y, Kinoshita, K, Manabe, T, Seno, H, Chiba, T & Marusawa, H (2017) 'Proliferating EpCAM-positive ductal cells in the inflamed liver give rise to hepatocellularcarcinoma. *Cancer Res,* 77, 6131-43.
[http://dx.doi.org/10.1158/0008-5472.CAN-17-1800] [PMID: 28951464]

Mazzaferro, V, Regalia, E, Doci, R, Andreola, S, Pulvirenti, A, Bozzetti, F, Montalto, F, Ammatuna, M, Morabito, A & Gennari, L (1996) Liver transplantation for the treatment of small hepatocellular carcinomas in patients with cirrhosis. *N Engl J Med,* 334, 693-9.
[http://dx.doi.org/10.1056/NEJM199603143341104] [PMID: 8594428]

Mekuria, AN & Abdi, AD (2017) Potential molecular targets and drugs for treatment of hepatocellular carcinoma. *J Cancer Sci Ther,* 9, 12.

Mello, SS & Attardi, LD (2018) Deciphering p53 signaling in tumor suppression. *Curr Opin Cell Biol,* 51, 65-72.
[http://dx.doi.org/10.1016/j.ceb.2017.11.005] [PMID: 29195118]

Menon, S, Yecies, JL, Zhang, HH, Howell, JJ, Nicholatos, J, Harputlugil, E, Bronson, RT, Kwiatkowski, DJ & Manning, BD (2012) Chronic activation of mTOR complex 1 is sufficient to cause hepatocellular carcinoma in mice. *Sci Signal,* 5, ra24.
[http://dx.doi.org/10.1126/scisignal.2002739] [PMID: 22457330]

Merlo, LM, Pepper, JW, Reid, BJ & Maley, CC (2006) Cancer as an evolutionary and ecological process. *Nat Rev Cancer,* 6, 924-35.
[http://dx.doi.org/10.1038/nrc2013] [PMID: 17109012]

Meyers, RL, Czauderna, P & Otte, JB (2012) Surgical treatment of hepatoblastoma. *Pediatr Blood Cancer,* 59, 800-8.
[http://dx.doi.org/10.1002/pbc.24220] [PMID: 22887704]

Michalopoulos, GK (2010) Liver regeneration after partial hepatectomy: critical analysis of mechanistic dilemmas. *Am J Pathol,* 176, 2-13.
[http://dx.doi.org/10.2353/ajpath.2010.090675] [PMID: 20019184]

Min, L, He, B & Hui, L (2011) Mitogen-activated protein kinases in hepatocellular carcinoma development. *Semin Cancer Biol,* 21, 10-20.
[http://dx.doi.org/10.1016/j.semcancer.2010.10.011] [PMID: 20969960]

Mittal, S, El-Serag, HB, Sada, YH, Kanwal, F, Duan, Z, Temple, S, May, SB, Kramer, JR, Richardson, PA & Davila, JA (2016) Hepatocellular Carcinoma in the Absence of Cirrhosis in United States Veterans is Associated With Nonalcoholic Fatty Liver Disease. *Clin Gastroenterol Hepatol,* 14, 124-31.e1.
[http://dx.doi.org/10.1016/j.cgh.2015.07.019] [PMID: 26196445]

Mizuguchi, T, Katsuramaki, T, Nobuoka, T, Kawamoto, M, Oshima, H, Kawasaki, H, Kikuchi, H, Shibata, C & Hirata, K (2004) Serum hyaluronate level for predicting subclinical liver dysfunction after hepatectomy. *World J Surg,* 28, 971-6.
[http://dx.doi.org/10.1007/s00268-004-7389-1] [PMID: 15573250]

Mizuno, H, Ogura, M, Saito, Y, Sekine, W, Sano, R, Gotou, T, Oku, T, Itoh, S, Katabami, K & Tsuji, T (2008) Changes in adhesive and migratory characteristics of hepatocellular carcinoma (HCC) cells induced

by expression of α3β1 integrin. *Biochim Biophys Acta,* 1780, 564-70.
[http://dx.doi.org/10.1016/j.bbagen.2007.09.007] [PMID: 17997226]

Mohamed, NK, Hamad, MA, Hafez, MZE, Wooley, KL & Elsabahy, M (2017) Nanomedicine in management of hepatocellular carcinoma: Challenges and opportunities. *Int J Cancer,* 140, 1475-84.
[http://dx.doi.org/10.1002/ijc.30517] [PMID: 27861850]

Mohamed, WS, Omar, MM, Khayri, TM & Fakhr, IM (2008) Assessment of the pro-liferative marker Ki-67 and p53 protein expression in HBV- and HCV-related hepatocellular carcinoma cases in Egypt. *Int J Health Sci (Qassim),* 2, 27-34.
[PMID: 21475468]

Mohammed, MK, Shao, C, Wang, J, Wei, Q, Wang, X, Collier, Z, Tang, S, Liu, H, Zhang, F, Huang, J, Guo, D, Lu, M, Liu, F, Liu, J, Ma, C, Shi, LL, Athiviraham, A, He, TC & Lee, MJ (2016) Wnt/β-catenin signaling plays an ever-expanding role in stem cell self-renewal, tumorigenesis and cancer chemoresistance. *Genes Dis,* 3, 11-40.
[http://dx.doi.org/10.1016/j.gendis.2015.12.004] [PMID: 27077077]

Molina, E & Hernandez, A (2003) Clinical manifestations of primary hepatic angiosarcoma. *Dig Dis Sci,* 48, 677-82.
[http://dx.doi.org/10.1023/A:1022868221670] [PMID: 12741455]

Monsour, HP, Asham, E & McFadden, RS (2013) Hepatocellular carcinoma: the rising tide from east to west a review of epidemiology, screening and tumor markers. *Transl Cancer Res,* 2, 492-506.

Moradpour, D, Compagnon, B, Wilson, BE, Nicolau, C & Wands, JR (1995) Specific targeting of human hepatocellular carcinoma cells by immunoliposomes *in vitro*. *Hepatology,* 22, 1527-37.
[http://dx.doi.org/10.1016/0270-9139(95)90161-2] [PMID: 7590672]

Moreira, AJ, Rodrigues, G, Bona, S, Cerski, CT, Marroni, CA, Mauriz, JL, González-Gallego, J & Marroni, NP (2014) Oxidative stress and cell damage in a model of precancerous lesions and advanced hepatocellular carcinoma in rats. *Toxicol Rep,* 2, 333-40.
[http://dx.doi.org/10.1016/j.toxrep.2014.11.015] [PMID: 28962366]

Mornex, F, Girard, N, Beziat, C, Kubas, A, Khodri, M, Trepo, C & Merle, P (2006) Feasibility and efficacy of high-dose three-dimensional-conformal radiotherapy in cirrhotic patients with small-size hepatocellular carcinoma non-eligible for curative therapies--mature results of the French Phase II RTF-1 trial. *Int J Radiat Oncol Biol Phys,* 66, 1152-8.
[http://dx.doi.org/10.1016/j.ijrobp.2006.06.015] [PMID: 17145534]

Movahedi, K, Laoui, D, Gysemans, C, Baeten, M, Stangé, G, Van den Bossche, J, Mack, M, Pipeleers, D, In't Veld, P, De Baetselier, P & Van Ginderachter, JA (2010) Different tumor microenvironments contain functionally distinct subsets of macrophages derived from Ly6C(high) monocytes. *Cancer Res,* 70, 5728-39.
[http://dx.doi.org/10.1158/0008-5472.CAN-09-4672] [PMID: 20570887]

Mu, H, Lin, KX, Zhao, H, Xing, S, Li, C, Liu, F, Lu, HZ, Zhang, Z, Sun, YL, Yan, XY, Cai, JQ & Zhao, XH (2014) Identification of biomarkers for hepatocellular carcinoma by semiquantitative immunocytochemistry. *World J Gastroenterol,* 20, 5826-38.
[http://dx.doi.org/10.3748/wjg.v20.i19.5826] [PMID: 24914343]

Mu, X, Español-Suñer, R, Mederacke, I, Affò, S, Manco, R, Sempoux, C, Lemaigre, FP, Adili, A, Yuan, D, Weber, A, Unger, K, Heikenwälder, M, Leclercq, IA & Schwabe, RF (2015) Hepatocellular carcinoma originates from hepatocytes and not from the progenitor/biliary compartment. *J Clin Invest,* 125, 3891-903.
[http://dx.doi.org/10.1172/JCI77995] [PMID: 26348897]

Mueller, L, Goumas, FA, Affeldt, M, Sandtner, S, Gehling, UM, Brilloff, S, Walter, J, Karnatz, N, Lamszus, K, Rogiers, X & Broering, DC (2007) Stromal fibroblasts in colorectal liver metastases originate from resident fibroblasts and generate an inflammatory microenvironment. *Am J Pathol,* 171, 1608-18.
[http://dx.doi.org/10.2353/ajpath.2007.060661] [PMID: 17916596]

Munakata, T, Nakamura, M, Liang, Y, Li, K & Lemon, SM (2005) Down-regulation of the retinoblastoma tumor suppressor by the hepatitis C virus NS5B RNA-dependent RNA polymerase. *Proc Natl Acad Sci USA,*

102, 18159-64.
[http://dx.doi.org/10.1073/pnas.0505605102] [PMID: 16332962]

Nafee, AM & Pasha, HF (2012) Clinical significance of serum clusterin as a biomarker for evaluating diagnosis and metastasis potential of viral-related hepatocellular carcinoma. *Clinical Biochemistry,* 45, 1070-4.

Nakamura, S, Muro, H, Suzuki, S, Sakaguchi, T, Konno, H, Baba, S & Syed, AS (1997) Immunohistochemical studies on endothelial cell phenotype in hepatocellular carcinoma. *Hepatology,* 26, 407-15.
[http://dx.doi.org/10.1002/hep.510260222] [PMID: 9252152]

Nam, HJ & van Deursen, JM (2014) Cyclin B2 and p53 control proper timing of centrosome separation. *Nat Cell Biol,* 16, 538-49.
[http://dx.doi.org/10.1038/ncb2952] [PMID: 24776885]

Zheng, N, Wei, W & Wang, Z (2016) Emerging roles of FGF signaling in hepatocellular carcinoma. *Transl Cancer Res,* 5, 1-6.
[PMID: 27226954]

Naugler, WE & Karin, M (2008) The wolf in sheep's clothing: the role of interleukin-6 in immunity, inflammation and cancer. *Trends Mol Med,* 14, 109-19. b
[http://dx.doi.org/10.1016/j.molmed.2007.12.007] [PMID: 18261959]

Naugler, WE & Karin, M (2008) NF-kappaB and cancer-identifying targets and mechanisms. *Curr Opin Genet Dev,* 18, 19-26. a
[http://dx.doi.org/10.1016/j.gde.2008.01.020] [PMID: 18440219]

Nault, JC (2014) Molecular determinants of prognosis in hepatocellular carcinoma. *J Clin Transl Hepatol,* 2, 31-6.
[PMID: 26357615]

Nault, JC, Mallet, M, Pilati, C, Calderaro, J, Bioulac-Sage, P, Laurent, C, Laurent, A, Cherqui, D, Balabaud, C & Zucman-Rossi, J (2013) High frequency of telomerase reverse-transcriptase promoter somatic mutations in hepatocellular carcinoma and preneoplastic lesions. *Nat Commun,* 4, 2218.
[http://dx.doi.org/10.1038/ncomms3218] [PMID: 23887712]

Neuman, MG, Malnick, S, Maor, Y, Nanau, RM, Melzer, E, Ferenci, P, Seitz, HK, Mueller, S, Mell, H, Samuel, D, Cohen, LB, Kharbanda, KK, Osna, NA, Ganesan, M, Thompson, KJ, McKillop, IH, Bautista, A, Bataller, R & French, SW (2015) Alcoholic liver disease: Clinical and translational research. *Exp Mol Pathol,* 99, 596-610.
[http://dx.doi.org/10.1016/j.yexmp.2015.09.001] [PMID: 26342547]

Ng, AW, Poon, SL & Huang, MN (2017) Aristolochic acids and their derivatives are widely implicated in liver cancers in Taiwan and throughout Asia. *Science translational medicine,* 9, 6446.

Norton, PA, Comunale, MA, Krakover, J, Rodemich, L, Pirog, N, D'Amelio, A, Philip, R, Mehta, AS & Block, TM (2008) N-linked glycosylation of the liver cancer biomarker GP73. *J Cell Biochem,* 104, 136-49.
[http://dx.doi.org/10.1002/jcb.21610] [PMID: 18004786]

Notas, G, Kolios, G, Mastrodimou, N, Kampa, M, Vasilaki, A, Xidakis, C, Castanas, E, Thermos, K & Kouroumalis, E (2004) Cortistatin production by HepG2 human hepatocellular carcinoma cell line and distribution of somatostatin receptors. *J Hepatol,* 40, 792-8.
[http://dx.doi.org/10.1016/j.jhep.2004.01.016] [PMID: 15094227]

O'Beirne, J, Farzaneh, F & Harrison, PM (2010) Generation of functional CD8+ T cells by human dendritic cells expressing glypican-3 epitopes. *J Exp Clin Cancer Res,* 29, 48.
[http://dx.doi.org/10.1186/1756-9966-29-48] [PMID: 20465843]

Okamura, N, Yoshida, M, Shibuya, A, Sugiura, H, Okayasu, I & Ohbu, M (2005) Cellular and stromal characteristics in the scirrhous hepatocellular carcinoma: comparison with hepatocellular carcinomas and intrahepatic cholangiocarcinomas. *Pathol Int,* 55, 724-31.

[http://dx.doi.org/10.1111/j.1440-1827.2005.01891.x] [PMID: 16271085]

Okuda, K, Ohtsuki, T, Obata, H, Tomimatsu, M, Okazaki, N, Hasegawa, H, Nakajima, Y & Ohnishi, K (1985) Natural history of hepatocellular carcinoma and prognosis in relation to treatment. Study of 850 patients. *Cancer,* 56, 918-28.
[http://dx.doi.org/10.1002/1097-0142(19850815)56:4<918::AID-CNCR2820560437>3.0.CO;2-E] [PMID: 2990661]

Otto, G, Schuchmann, M, Hoppe-Lotichius, M, Heise, M, Weinmann, A, Hansen, T & Pitton, MP (2013) How to decide about liver transplantation in patients with hepatocellular carcinoma: size and number of lesions or response to TACE? *J Hepatol,* 59, 279-84.
[http://dx.doi.org/10.1016/j.jhep.2013.04.006] [PMID: 23587474]

Pardee, AD & Butterfield, LH (2012) Immunotherapy of hepatocellular carcinoma: Unique challenges and clinical opportunities. *OncoImmunology,* 1, 48-55.
[http://dx.doi.org/10.4161/onci.1.1.18344] [PMID: 22720211]

Park, EJ, Lee, JH, Yu, GY, He, G, Ali, SR, Holzer, RG, Osterreicher, CH, Takahashi, H & Karin, M (2010) Dietary and genetic obesity promote liver inflammation and tumorigenesis by enhancing IL-6 and TNF expression. *Cell,* 140, 197-208.
[http://dx.doi.org/10.1016/j.cell.2009.12.052] [PMID: 20141834]

Park, JW, Chen, M, Colombo, M, Roberts, LR, Schwartz, M, Chen, PJ, Kudo, M, Johnson, P, Wagner, S, Orsini, LS & Sherman, M (2015) Global patterns of hepatocellular carcinoma management from diagnosis to death: the BRIDGE Study. *Liver Int,* 35, 2155-66.
[http://dx.doi.org/10.1111/liv.12818] [PMID: 25752327]

Patel, YC (1999) Somatostatin and its receptor family. *Front Neuroendocrinol,* 20, 157-98.
[http://dx.doi.org/10.1006/frne.1999.0183] [PMID: 10433861]

Reports, PBCR http://www.ncrpindia. org/Reports/PBCR_2006_2008.aspx

P, Polakis (2012) Wnt signaling in cancer. *Cold Spring Harbor perspectives in biology,* 4, a008052.

Pollak, M (2012) The insulin and insulin-like growth factor receptor family in neoplasia: an update. *Nat Rev Cancer,* 12, 159-69.
[http://dx.doi.org/10.1038/nrc3215] [PMID: 22337149]

Pons, F, Varela, M & Llovet, JM (2005) Staging systems in hepatocellular carcinoma. *HPB (Oxford),* 7, 35-41.
[http://dx.doi.org/10.1080/13651820410024058] [PMID: 18333159]

Poon, RTP, Ho, JWY, Tong, CSW, Lau, C, Ng, IO & Fan, ST (2004) Prognostic significance of serum vascular endothelial growth factor and endostatin in patients with hepatocellular carcinoma. *Br J Surg,* 91, 1354-60.
[http://dx.doi.org/10.1002/bjs.4594] [PMID: 15376182]

Pozzan, C, Cardin, R, Piciocchi, M, Cazzagon, N, Maddalo, G, Vanin, V, Giacomin, A, Pontisso, P, Cillo, U & Farinati, F (2014) Diagnostic and prognostic role of SCCA-IgM serum levels in hepatocellular carcinoma (HCC). *J Gastroenterol Hepatol,* 29, 1637-44.
[http://dx.doi.org/10.1111/jgh.12576] [PMID: 24635038]

Qin, L (2014) Osteopontin is a promoter for hepatocellular carcinoma metastasis: a summary of 10 years of studies. *Front Med,* 8, 24-32.
[http://dx.doi.org/10.1007/s11684-014-0312-8] [PMID: 24464486]

Qin, W, Cao, ZY & Liu, SY (2020) Recent advances regarding tumor microenvironment and immunotherapy in hepatocellular carcinoma. *Hepatoma Res,* 6, 24.
[http://dx.doi.org/10.20517/2394-5079.2020.04]

Quaglia, A (2018) Hepatocellular carcinoma: a review of diagnostic challenges for the pathologist. *J Hepatocell Carcinoma,* 5, 99-108.

[http://dx.doi.org/10.2147/JHC.S159808] [PMID: 30519546]

Quan, S, Wang, Y, Zhou, A, Kumar, P & Narain, R (2015) Galactose-based thermosensitive nanogels for targeted drug delivery of iodoazomycin arabinofuranoside (IAZA) for theranostic management of hypoxic hepa¬tocellular carcinoma. *Biomacromolecules,* 16, 1978-86.
[http://dx.doi.org/10.1021/acs.biomac.5b00576] [PMID: 25996799]

Rabe, C, Lenz, M, Schmitz, V, Pilz, T, Fimmers, R, Sauerbruch, T & Caselmann, WH (2003) An independent evaluation of modern prognostic scores in a central European cohort of 120 patients with hepatocellular carcinoma. *Eur J Gastroenterol Hepatol,* 15, 1305-15.
[http://dx.doi.org/10.1097/00042737-200312000-00009] [PMID: 14624154]

Ramaiah, SK & Rittling, S (2008) Pathophysiological role of osteopontin in hepatic inflammation, toxicity, and cancer. *Toxicol Sci,* 103, 4-13.
[http://dx.doi.org/10.1093/toxsci/kfm246] [PMID: 17890765]

Ranjan, K & Pathak, C (2016) FADD regulates NF-κB activation and promotes ubiquitination of cFLIPL to induce apoptosis. *Sci Rep,* 6, 22787.
[http://dx.doi.org/10.1038/srep22787] [PMID: 26972597]

Rasi, G, Serafino, A, Bellis, L, Lonardo, MT, Andreola, F, Zonfrillo, M, Vennarecci, G, Pierimarchi, P, Sinibaldi Vallebona, P, Ettorre, GM, Santoro, E & Puoti, C (2007) Nerve growth factor involvement in liver cirrhosis and hepatocellular carcinoma. *World J Gastroenterol,* 13, 4986-95.
[http://dx.doi.org/10.3748/wjg.v13.i37.4986] [PMID: 17854142]

Reddy, JK & Rao, MS (2006) Lipid metabolism and liver inflammation. II. Fatty liver disease and fatty acid oxidation. *Am J Physiol Gastrointest Liver Physiol,* 290, G852-8.
[http://dx.doi.org/10.1152/ajpgi.00521.2005] [PMID: 16603729]

Reya, T, Morrison, SJ, Clarke, MF & Weissman, IL (2001) Stem cells, cancer, and cancer stem cells. *Nature,* 414, 105-11.
[http://dx.doi.org/10.1038/35102167] [PMID: 11689955]

Reynaert, H, Rombouts, K, Vandermonde, A, Urbain, D, Kumar, U, Bioulac-Sage, P, Pinzani, M, Rosenbaum, J & Geerts, A (2004) Expression of somatostatin receptors in normal and cirrhotic human liver and in hepatocellular carcinoma. *Gut,* 53, 1180-9.
[http://dx.doi.org/10.1136/gut.2003.036053] [PMID: 15247189]

Ricke, J, Bulla, K, Kolligs, F, Peck-Radosavljevic, M, Reimer, P, Sangro, B, Schott, E, Schütte, K, Verslype, C, Walecki, J & Malfertheiner, P (2015) Safety and toxicity of radioembolization plus Sorafenib in advanced hepatocellular carcinoma: analysis of the European multicentre trial SORAMIC. *Liver Int,* 35, 620-6.
[http://dx.doi.org/10.1111/liv.12622] [PMID: 24930619]

Ricke, J, Bulla, K, Kolligs, F, Peck-Radosavljevic, M, Reimer, P, Sangro, B, Schott, E, Schütte, K, Verslype, C, Walecki, J & Malfertheiner, P (2015) Safety and toxicity of radioembolization plus Sorafenib in advanced hepatocellular carcinoma: analysis of the European multicentre trial SORAMIC. *Liver Int,* 35, 620-6.
[http://dx.doi.org/10.1111/liv.12622] [PMID: 24930619]

Robertson, JM, Lawrence, TS, Andrews, JC, Walker, S, Kessler, ML & Ensminger, WD (1997) Long-term results of hepatic artery fluorodeoxyuridine and conformal radiation therapy for primary hepatobiliary cancers. *Int J Radiat Oncol Biol Phys,* 37, 325-30.
[http://dx.doi.org/10.1016/S0360-3016(96)00528-7] [PMID: 9069303]

Rosenquist, TA & Grollman, AP (2016) Mutational signature of aristolochic acid: Clue to the recognition of a global disease. *DNA Repair (Amst),* 44, 205-11.
[http://dx.doi.org/10.1016/j.dnarep.2016.05.027] [PMID: 27237586]

Roskams, T & Kojiro, M (2010) Pathology of early hepatocellular carcinoma: conventional and molecular diagnosis. *Semin Liver Dis,* 30, 17-25.
[http://dx.doi.org/10.1055/s-0030-1247129] [PMID: 20175030]

Roskams, TA, Libbrecht, L & Desmet, VJ (2003) Progenitor cells in diseased human liver. *Semin Liver Dis,*

23, 385-96.
[http://dx.doi.org/10.1055/s-2004-815564] [PMID: 14722815]

Roskoski, R, Jr (2010) RAF protein-serine/threonine kinases: structure and regulation. *Biochem Biophys Res Commun,* 399, 313-7.
[http://dx.doi.org/10.1016/j.bbrc.2010.07.092] [PMID: 20674547]

Rotow, J & Bivona, TG (2017) Understanding and targeting resistance mechanisms in NSCLC. *Nat Rev Cancer,* 17, 637-58.
[http://dx.doi.org/10.1038/nrc.2017.84] [PMID: 29068003]

Rusyn, I & Lemon, SM (2014) Mechanisms of HCV-induced liver cancer: what did we learn from in vitro and animal studies? *Cancer Lett,* 345, 210-5.
[http://dx.doi.org/10.1016/j.canlet.2013.06.028] [PMID: 23871966]

Sabatini, DM (2006) mTOR and cancer: insights into a complex relationship. *Nat Rev Cancer,* 6, 729-34.
[http://dx.doi.org/10.1038/nrc1974] [PMID: 16915295]

Sacco, R, Conte, C, Tumino, E, Parisi, G, Marceglia, S, Metrangolo, S, Eggenhoffner, R, Bresci, G, Cabibbo, G & Giacomelli, L (2016) Transarterial radioembolization for hepatocellular carcinoma: a review. *J Hepatocell Carcinoma,* 3, 25-9.
[http://dx.doi.org/10.2147/JHC.S50359] [PMID: 27574589]

Saha, SK, Parachoniak, CA, Ghanta, KS, Fitamant, J, Ross, KN, Najem, MS, Gurumurthy, S, Akbay, EA, Sia, D, Cornella, H, Miltiadous, O, Walesky, C, Deshpande, V, Zhu, AX, Hezel, AF, Yen, KE, Straley, KS, Travins, J, Popovici-Muller, J, Gliser, C, Ferrone, CR, Apte, U, Llovet, JM, Wong, KK, Ramaswamy, S & Bardeesy, N (2014) Mutant IDH inhibits HNF-4α to block hepatocyte differentiation and promote biliary cancer. *Nature,* 513, 110-4.
[http://dx.doi.org/10.1038/nature13441] [PMID: 25043045]

Saito-Diaz, K, Chen, TW, Wang, X, Thorne, CA, Wallace, HA, Page-McCaw, A & Lee, E (2013) The way Wnt works: components and mechanism. *Growth Factors,* 31, 1-31.
[http://dx.doi.org/10.3109/08977194.2012.752737] [PMID: 23256519]

Salomao, M, Yu, WM, Brown, RS, Jr, Emond, JC & Lefkowitch, JH (2010) Steatohepatitic hepatocellular carcinoma (SH-HCC): a distinctive histological variant of HCC in hepatitis C virus-related cirrhosis with associated NAFLD/NASH. *Am J Surg Pathol,* 34, 1630-6.
[http://dx.doi.org/10.1097/PAS.0b013e3181f31caa] [PMID: 20975341]

Sanker, J, Selvakumar, G & Suguna, L (2019) Epithelial and Mesenchymal Transition Pathway (EMT) and Hepatocellular Carcinoma: A Mini Review. *Clin Oncol,* 4, 1617.

Sano, K, Takayama, T, Murakami, K, Saiki, I & Makuuchi, M (2003) Overexpression of retinoic acid receptor alpha in hepatocellular carcinoma. *Clin Cancer Res,* 9, 3679-83.
[PMID: 14506158]

Sarasin, FP, Giostra, E & Hadengue, A (1996) Cost-effectiveness of screening for detection of small hepatocellular carcinoma in western patients with Child-Pugh class A cirrhosis. *Am J Med,* 101, 422-34.
[http://dx.doi.org/10.1016/S0002-9343(96)00197-0] [PMID: 8873514]

Scaggiante, B, Farra, R & Dapas, B (2016) Aptamer targeting of the elongation factor 1A impairs hepatocarcinoma cells viability and potentiates bortezomib and idarubicin effects. *International Journal of Pharmaceutics,* 506, 268-79.

Schmitz, KJ, Wohlschlaeger, J, Lang, H, Sotiropoulos, GC, Malago, M, Steveling, K, Reis, H, Cicinnati, VR, Schmid, KW & Baba, HA (2008) Activation of the ERK and AKT signalling pathway predicts poor prognosis in hepatocellular carcinoma and ERK activation in cancer tissue is associated with hepatitis C virus infection. *J Hepatol,* 48, 83-90.
[http://dx.doi.org/10.1016/j.jhep.2007.08.018] [PMID: 17998146]

Scholzen, T & Gerdes, J (2000) The Ki-67 protein: from the known and the unknown. *J Cell Physiol,* 182, 311-22.

[http://dx.doi.org/10.1002/(SICI)1097-4652(200003)182:3<311::AID-JCP1>3.0.CO;2-9] [PMID: 10653597]

Schrader, J & Iredale, JP (2011) The inflammatory microenvironment of HCC - the plot becomes complex. *J Hepatol,* 54, 853-5.
[http://dx.doi.org/10.1016/j.jhep.2010.12.014] [PMID: 21185341]

Schwartz, JM & Reinus, JF (2012) Prevalence and natural history of alcoholic liver disease. *Clin Liver Dis,* 16, 659-66.
[http://dx.doi.org/10.1016/j.cld.2012.08.001] [PMID: 23101975]

Severi, T, van Malenstein, H, Verslype, C & van Pelt, JF (2010) Tumor initiation and progression in hepatocellular carcinoma: risk factors, classification, and therapeutic targets. *Acta Pharmacol Sin,* 31, 1409-20.
[http://dx.doi.org/10.1038/aps.2010.142] [PMID: 20953207]

Shang, S, Plymoth, A, Ge, S, Feng, Z, Rosen, HR, Sangrajrang, S, Hainaut, P, Marrero, JA & Beretta, L (2012) Identification of osteopontin as a novel marker for early hepatocellular carcinoma. *Hepatology,* 55, 483-90.
[http://dx.doi.org/10.1002/hep.24703] [PMID: 21953299]

Sharma, AK, Kumar, S, Chashoo, G, Saxena, AK & Pandey, AK (2014) Cell cycle inhibitory activity of Piper longum against A549 cell line and its protective effect against metal-induced toxicity in rats. *Indian J Biochem Biophys,* 51, 358-64.
[PMID: 25630105]

Shen, Q, Fan, J, Yang, XR, Tan, Y, Zhao, W, Xu, Y, Wang, N, Niu, Y, Wu, Z, Zhou, J, Qiu, SJ, Shi, YH, Yu, B, Tang, N, Chu, W, Wang, M, Wu, J, Zhang, Z, Yang, S, Gu, J, Wang, H & Qin, W (2012) Serum DKK1 as a protein biomarker for the diagnosis of hepatocellular carcinoma: a large-scale, multicentre study. *Lancet Oncol,* 13, 817-26.
[http://dx.doi.org/10.1016/S1470-2045(12)70233-4] [PMID: 22738799]

Shen, S, Lin, Y, Yuan, X, Shen, L, Chen, J, Chen, L, Qin, L & Shen, B (2016) Biomarker MicroRNAs for diagnosis, prognosis and treatment of hepatocellular carcinoma: a functional survey and comparison. *Sci Rep,* 6, 38311.
[http://dx.doi.org/10.1038/srep38311] [PMID: 27917899]

Shin, S, Wangensteen, KJ, Teta-Bissett, M, Wang, YJ, Mosleh-Shirazi, E, Buza, EL, Greenbaum, LE & Kaestner, KH (2016) Genetic lineage tracing analysis of the cell of origin of hepatotoxin-induced liver tumors in mice. *Hepatology,* 64, 1163-77.
[http://dx.doi.org/10.1002/hep.28602] [PMID: 27099001]

Shouval, D (2002) HCC: what's the score. *Gut,* 50, 749-50.
[http://dx.doi.org/10.1136/gut.50.6.749] [PMID: 12010872]

Si, MW, Thorson, JA, Lauwers, GY, DalCin, P & Furman, J (2004) Hepatocellular lymphoepithelioma-like carcinoma associated with epstein barr virus: a hitherto unrecognized entity. *Diagn Mol Pathol,* 13, 183-9.
[http://dx.doi.org/10.1097/01.pas.0000124336.90615.8d] [PMID: 15322431]

Sia, D, Villanueva, A, Friedman, SL & Llovet, JM (2017) Liver cancer cell of origin, molecular class, and effects on patient prognosis. *Gastroenterology,* 152, 745-61.
[http://dx.doi.org/10.1053/j.gastro.2016.11.048] [PMID: 28043904]

Singh, AK, Kumar, R & Pandey, AK (2018) Hepatocellular Carcinoma: Causes, Mechanism of Progression and Biomarkers. *Curr Chem Genomics Transl Med,* 12, 9-26.
[http://dx.doi.org/10.2174/2213988501812010009] [PMID: 30069430]

Singh, S, Chakraborty, S, Bonthu, N, Radio, S, Hussain, SM & Sasson, A (2013) Combined hepatocellular cholangiocarcinoma: a case report and review of literature. *Dig Dis Sci,* 58, 2114-23.
[http://dx.doi.org/10.1007/s10620-013-2585-1] [PMID: 23397471]

Sohn, JH, Choi, HJ, Lee, JT, Lee, JD, Kim, JH, Moon, YM, Park, K, Park, KB, Kim, E & Yoo, NC (2009) Phase II study of transarterial holmium-166-chitosan complex treatment in patients with a single, large

hepatocellular carcinoma. *Oncology,* 76, 1-9.
[http://dx.doi.org/10.1159/000173735] [PMID: 19018149]

Sohn, JH, Duran, R, Zhao, Y, Fleckenstein, F, Chapiro, J, Sahu, S, Schernthaner, RE, Qian, T, Lee, H, Zhao, L, Hamilton, J, Frangakis, C, Lin, M, Salem, R & Geschwind, JF (2017) Validation of the Hong Kong Liver Cancer Staging System in determining prognosis of the North American patients following intra-arterial therapy. *Clin Gastroenterol Hepatol,* 15, 746-755.e4.
[http://dx.doi.org/10.1016/j.cgh.2016.10.036] [PMID: 27847278]

Song, J, Qu, Z, Guo, X, Zhao, Q, Zhao, X, Gao, L, Sun, K, Shen, F, Wu, M & Wei, L (2009) Hypoxia-induced autophagy contributes to the chemoresistance of hepatocellular carcinoma cells. *Autophagy,* 5, 1131-44.
[http://dx.doi.org/10.4161/auto.5.8.9996] [PMID: 19786832]

Stanger, BZ (2015) Cellular homeostasis and repair in the mammalian liver. *Annu Rev Physiol,* 77, 179-200.
[http://dx.doi.org/10.1146/annurev-physiol-021113-170255] [PMID: 25668020]

Sterling, RK, Jeffers, L, Gordon, F, Venook, AP, Reddy, KR, Satomura, S, Kanke, F, Schwartz, ME & Sherman, M (2009) Utility of Lens culinaris agglutinin-reactive fraction of alpha-fetoprotein and des-gamm--carboxy prothrombin, alone or in combination, as biomarkers for hepatocellular carcinoma. *Clin Gastroenterol Hepatol,* 7, 104-13.
[http://dx.doi.org/10.1016/j.cgh.2008.08.041] [PMID: 18849011]

Su, ZX, Zhao, J, Rong, ZH, Geng, WM, Wu, YG & Qin, CK (2014) Upregulation of microRNA-25 associates with prognosis in hepatocellular carcinoma. *Diagn Pathol,* 9, 47.
[http://dx.doi.org/10.1186/1746-1596-9-47] [PMID: 24593846]

Subramaniam, S, Kelley, RK & Venook, Ap (2013) A review of hepatocellular carcinoma (HCC) staging systems. *Chinese Clinical Oncology,* 2, 33-1-12.

Sukowati, CH, Anfuso, B, Torre, G, Francalanci, P, Crocè, LS & Tiribelli, C (2013) The expression of CD90/Thy-1 in hepatocellular carcinoma: an *in vivo* and *in vitro* study. *PLoS One,* 8, e76830.
[http://dx.doi.org/10.1371/journal.pone.0076830] [PMID: 24116172]

Sun, Y, Gao, G, Cai, J, Wang, Y, Qu, X, He, L, Liu, F, Zhang, Y, Lin, K, Ma, S, Yang, X, Qian, X & Zhao, X (2013) Annexin A2 is a discriminative serological candidate in early hepatocellular carcinoma. *Carcinogenesis,* 34, 595-604.
[http://dx.doi.org/10.1093/carcin/bgs372] [PMID: 23188673]

Sung, WK, Zheng, H, Li, S, Chen, R, Liu, X, Li, Y, Lee, NP, Lee, WH, Ariyaratne, PN, Tennakoon, C, Mulawadi, FH, Wong, KF, Liu, AM, Poon, RT, Fan, ST, Chan, KL, Gong, Z, Hu, Y, Lin, Z, Wang, G, Zhang, Q, Barber, TD, Chou, WC, Aggarwal, A, Hao, K, Zhou, W, Zhang, C, Hardwick, J, Buser, C, Xu, J, Kan, Z, Dai, H, Mao, M, Reinhard, C, Wang, J & Luk, JM (2012) Genome-wide survey of recurrent HBV integration in hepatocellular carcinoma. *Nat Genet,* 44, 765-9.
[http://dx.doi.org/10.1038/ng.2295] [PMID: 22634754]

Han, SX, Bai, E, Jin, GH, He, CC, Guo, XJ, Wang, LJ, Li, M, Ying, X & Zhu, Q (2014) Expression and clinical significance of YAP, TAZ, and AREG in hepatocellular carcinoma. *J Immunol Res,* 2014, 261365.
[http://dx.doi.org/10.1155/2014/261365] [PMID: 24860833]

Szklaruk, J, Silverman, PM & Charnsangavej, C (2003) Imaging in the diagnosis, staging, treatment, and surveillance of hepatocellular carcinoma. *AJR Am J Roentgenol,* 180, 441-54.
[http://dx.doi.org/10.2214/ajr.180.2.1800441] [PMID: 12540450]

Tacke, RS, Tosello-Trampont, A & Nguyen, V (2011) Extracellular hepatitis C virus core protein activates STAT3 in human monocytes/macrophages/dendritic cells via an IL-6 autocrine pathway. *Journal of Biological Chemistry,* 286, 10847-55.

Tangkijvanich, P, Tosukhowong, P, Bunyongyod, P, Lertmaharit, S, Hanvivatvong, O, Kullavanijaya, P & Poovorawan, Y (1999) Alpha-L-fucosidase as a serum marker of hepatocellular carcinoma in Thailand. *Southeast Asian J Trop Med Public Health,* 30, 110-4.

[PMID: 10695798]

Tanimizu, N, Nakamura, Y, Ichinohe, N, Mizuguchi, T, Hirata, K & Mitaka, T (2013) Hepatic biliary epithelial cells acquire epithelial integrity but lose plasticity to differentiate into hepatocytes in vitro during development. *J Cell Sci,* 126, 5239-46.
[PMID: 24046446]

Tansel, A, Katz, LH, El-Serag, HB, Thrift, AP, Parepally, M, Shakhatreh, MH & Kanwal, F (2017) Incidence and determinants of hepatocellular carcinoma in autoimmunehepatitis: a systematic review and meta-analysis. *Clin Gastroenterol Hepatol,* 15, 1207-1217.e4.
[http://dx.doi.org/10.1016/j.cgh.2017.02.006] [PMID: 28215616]

Tarlow, BD, Pelz, C, Naugler, WE, Wakefield, L, Wilson, EM, Finegold, MJ & Grompe, M (2014) Bipotential adult liver progenitors are derived from chronically injured mature hepatocytes. *Cell Stem Cell,* 15, 605-18.
[http://dx.doi.org/10.1016/j.stem.2014.09.008] [PMID: 25312494]

Terris, B, Cavard, C & Perret, C (2010) EpCAM, a new marker for cancer stem cells in hepatocellular carcinoma. *J Hepatol,* 52, 280-1.
[http://dx.doi.org/10.1016/j.jhep.2009.10.026] [PMID: 20006402]

Thambi, T, Deepagan, VG, Yoon, HY, Han, HS, Kim, SH, Son, S, Jo, DG, Ahn, CH, Suh, YD, Kim, K, Kwon, IC, Lee, DS & Park, JH (2014) Hypoxia-responsive polymeric nanoparticles for tumor-targeted drug delivery. *Biomaterials,* 35, 1735-43.
[http://dx.doi.org/10.1016/j.biomaterials.2013.11.022] [PMID: 24290696]

Thapa, B, Kumar, P, Zeng, H & Narain, R (2015) Asialoglycoprotein receptor-mediated gene delivery to hepatocytes using galactosylated polymers. *Biomacromolecules,* 16, 3008-20.
[http://dx.doi.org/10.1021/acs.biomac.5b00906] [PMID: 26258607]

Thiery, JP, Acloque, H, Huang, RY & Nieto, MA (2009) Epithelial-mesenchymal transitions in development and disease. *Cell,* 139, 871-90.
[http://dx.doi.org/10.1016/j.cell.2009.11.007] [PMID: 19945376]

Tian, Y, Yang, W, Song, J, Wu, Y & Ni, B (2013) Hepatitis B virus X protein-induced aberrant epigenetic modifications contributing to human hepatocellular carcinoma pathogenesis. *Mol Cell Biol,* 33, 2810-6.
[http://dx.doi.org/10.1128/MCB.00205-13] [PMID: 23716588]

Tokushige, K, Hashimoto, E, Yatsuji, S, Tobari, M, Taniai, M, Torii, N & Shiratori, K (2010) Prospective study of hepatocellular carcinoma in nonalcoholic steatohepatitis in comparison with hepatocellular carcinoma caused by chronic hepatitis C. *J Gastroenterol,* 45, 960-7.
[http://dx.doi.org/10.1007/s00535-010-0237-1] [PMID: 20376504]

Torbenson, M (2012) Fibrolamellar carcinoma: 2012 update. *Scientifica (Cairo),* 2012, 743790.
[http://dx.doi.org/10.6064/2012/743790] [PMID: 24278737]

Tortorella, S & Karagiannis, TC (2014) Transferrin receptor-mediated endocytosis: a useful target for cancer therapy. *J Membr Biol,* 247, 291-307.
[http://dx.doi.org/10.1007/s00232-014-9637-0] [PMID: 24573305]

Toyoda, H, Kumada, T, Kiriyama, S, Sone, Y, Tanikawa, M, Hisanaga, Y, Yamaguchi, A, Isogai, M, Kaneoka, Y & Washizu, J (2005) Comparison of the usefulness of three staging systems for hepatocellular carcinoma (CLIP, BCLC, and JIS) in Japan. *Am J Gastroenterol,* 100, 1764-71.
[http://dx.doi.org/10.1111/j.1572-0241.2005.41943.x] [PMID: 16086713]

Trachootham, D, Alexandre, J & Huang, P (2009) Targeting cancer cells by ROS-mediated mechanisms: a radical therapeutic approach? *Nat Rev Drug Discov,* 8, 579-91.
[http://dx.doi.org/10.1038/nrd2803] [PMID: 19478820]

Treiber, G, Wex, T, Röcken, C, Fostitsch, P & Malfertheiner, P (2006) Impact of biomarkers on disease survival and progression in patients treated with octreotide for advanced hepatocellular carcinoma. *J Cancer Res Clin Oncol,* 132, 699-708.

[http://dx.doi.org/10.1007/s00432-006-0118-4] [PMID: 16835748]

Trerè, D, Fiume, L, De Giorgi, LB, Di Stefano, G, Migaldi, M & Derenzini, M (1999) The asialoglycoprotein receptor in human hepatocellular carcinomas: its expression on proliferating cells. *Br J Cancer,* 81, 404-8. [http://dx.doi.org/10.1038/sj.bjc.6690708] [PMID: 10507763]

Tros de Ilarduya, C & Düzgüneş, N (2013) Delivery of therapeutic nucleic acids *via* transferrin and transferrin receptors: lipoplexes and other carriers. *Expert Opin Drug Deliv,* 10, 1583-91. [http://dx.doi.org/10.1517/17425247.2013.837447] [PMID: 24050263]

Tsai, JF, Jeng, JE & Chuang, WL (2012) Dickkopf-1 and hepatocellular carcinoma. *Lancet Oncol,* 13, e410. [http://dx.doi.org/10.1016/S1470-2045(12)70416-3] [PMID: 23026825]

Tsai, WC, Hsu, SD, Hsu, CS, Lai, TC, Chen, SJ, Shen, R, Huang, Y, Chen, HC, Lee, CH, Tsai, TF, Hsu, MT, Wu, JC, Huang, HD, Shiao, MS, Hsiao, M & Tsou, AP (2012) MicroRNA-122 plays a critical role in liver homeostasis and hepatocarcinogenesis. *J Clin Invest,* 122, 2884-97. [http://dx.doi.org/10.1172/JCI63455] [PMID: 22820290]

Tumanova, U & Shchegolev, A (2015) Angiogenesis in hepatocellular carcinoma. *Biol Bull Rev,* 5, 568-78. [http://dx.doi.org/10.1134/S2079086415060080]

Turati, F, Galeone, C, Rota, M, Pelucchi, C, Negri, E, Bagnardi, V, Corrao, G, Boffetta, P & La Vecchia, C (2014) Alcohol and liver cancer: a systematic review and meta-analysis of prospective studies. *Ann Oncol,* 25, 1526-35. [http://dx.doi.org/10.1093/annonc/mdu020] [PMID: 24631946]

Ueno, S, Tanabe, G, Sako, K, Hiwaki, T, Hokotate, H, Fukukura, Y, Baba, Y, Imamura, Y & Aikou, T (2001) Discrimination value of the new western prognostic system (CLIP score) for hepatocellular carcinoma in 662 Japanese patients. Cancer of the Liver Italian Program. *Hepatology,* 34, 529-34. [http://dx.doi.org/10.1053/jhep.2001.27219] [PMID: 11526539]

Umemura, A, He, F, Taniguchi, K, Nakagawa, H, Yamachika, S, Font-Burgada, J, Zhong, Z, Subramaniam, S, Raghunandan, S, Duran, A, Linares, JF, Reina-Campos, M, Umemura, S, Valasek, MA, Seki, E, Yamaguchi, K, Koike, K, Itoh, Y, Diaz-Meco, MT, Moscat, J & Karin, M (2016) p62, Upregulated during Preneoplasia, Induces Hepatocellular Carcinogenesis by Maintaining Survival of Stressed HCC-Initiating Cells. *Cancer Cell,* 29, 935-48. [http://dx.doi.org/10.1016/j.ccell.2016.04.006] [PMID: 27211490]

van Malenstein, H, Gevaert, O, Libbrecht, L, Daemen, A, Allemeersch, J, Nevens, F, Van Cutsem, E, Cassiman, D, De Moor, B, Verslype, C & van Pelt, J (2010) A seven-gene set associated with chronic hypoxia of prognostic importance in hepatocellular carcinoma. *Clin Cancer Res,* 16, 4278-88. [http://dx.doi.org/10.1158/1078-0432.CCR-09-3274] [PMID: 20592013]

Vauthey, JN, Lauwers, GY, Esnaola, NF, Do, KA, Belghiti, J, Mirza, N, Curley, SA, Ellis, LM, Regimbeau, JM, Rashid, A, Cleary, KR & Nagorney, DM (2002) Simplified staging for hepatocellular carcinoma. *J Clin Oncol,* 20, 1527-36. [http://dx.doi.org/10.1200/JCO.2002.20.6.1527] [PMID: 11896101]

Valero, V, III, Pawlik, TM & Anders, RA (2015) Emerging role of Hpo signaling and YAP in hepatocellular carcinoma. *J Hepatocell Carcinoma,* 2, 69-78. [PMID: 27508196]

Vilgrain, V, Abdel-Rehim, M, Sibert, A, Ronot, M, Lebtahi, R, Castéra, L & Chatellier, G (2014) Radioembolisation with yttrium 90 microspheres *versus* sorafenib for treatment of advanced hepatocellular carcinoma (SARAH): study protocol for a randomised controlled trial. *Trials,* 15, 474. [http://dx.doi.org/10.1186/1745-6215-15-474] [PMID: 25472660]

Villanueva, A, Alsinet, C, Yanger, K, Hoshida, Y, Zong, Y, Toffanin, S, Rodriguez-Carunchio, L, Solé, M, Thung, S, Stanger, BZ & Llovet, JM (2012) Notch signaling is activated in human hepatocellular carcinoma and induces tumor formation in mice. *Gastroenterology,* 143, 1660-1669.e7. [http://dx.doi.org/10.1053/j.gastro.2012.09.002] [PMID: 22974708]

Villanueva, A, Chiang, DY, Newell, P, Peix, J, Thung, S, Alsinet, C, Tovar, V, Roayaie, S, Minguez, B, Sole, M, Battiston, C, Van Laarhoven, S, Fiel, MI, Di Feo, A, Hoshida, Y, Yea, S, Toffanin, S, Ramos, A, Martignetti, JA, Mazzaferro, V, Bruix, J, Waxman, S, Schwartz, M, Meyerson, M, Friedman, SL & Llovet, JM (2008) Pivotal role of mTOR signaling in hepatocellular carcinoma. *Gastroenterology,* 135, 1972-1983, 1983.e1-1983.e11.
[http://dx.doi.org/10.1053/j.gastro.2008.08.008] [PMID: 18929564]

Villari, D, Caruso, R, Grosso, M, Vitarelli, E, Righi, M & Barresi, G (2002) Hep Par 1 in gastric and bowel carcinomas: an immunohistochemical study. *Pathology,* 34, 423-6.
[http://dx.doi.org/10.1080/003130202100009333] [PMID: 12408340]

Visvader, JE & Lindeman, GJ (2008) Cancer stem cells in solid tumours: accumulating evidence and unresolved questions. *Nat Rev Cancer,* 8, 755-68.
[http://dx.doi.org/10.1038/nrc2499] [PMID: 18784658]

Waisberg, J & Saba, GT (2015) Wnt-/-β-catenin pathway signaling in human hepatocellular carcinoma. *World J Hepatol,* 7, 2631-5.
[http://dx.doi.org/10.4254/wjh.v7.i26.2631] [PMID: 26609340]

Wakai, T, Shirai, Y, Sakata, J, Korita, PV, Ajioka, Y & Hatakeyama, K (2011) Surgical outcomes for hepatocellular carcinoma in nonalcoholic fatty liver disease. *J Gastrointest Surg,* 15, 1450-8.
[http://dx.doi.org/10.1007/s11605-011-1540-8] [PMID: 21512848]

Wang, F, Jing, X, Li, G, Wang, T, Yang, B, Zhu, Z, Gao, Y, Zhang, Q, Yang, Y, Wang, Y, Wang, P & Du, Z (2012) Foxp3+ regulatory T cells are associated with the natural history of chronic hepatitis B and poor prognosis of hepatocellular carcinoma. *Liver Int,* 32, 644-55.
[http://dx.doi.org/10.1111/j.1478-3231.2011.02675.x] [PMID: 22118340]

Wang, H, Gao, Z, Liu, X, Agarwal, P, Zhao, S, Conroy, DW, Ji, G, Yu, J, Jaroniec, CP, Liu, Z, Lu, X, Li, X & He, X (2018) Targeted production of reactive oxygen species in mitochondria to overcome cancer drug resistance. *Nat Commun,* 9, 562.
[http://dx.doi.org/10.1038/s41467-018-02915-8] [PMID: 29422620]

Wang, K, Guo, W, Li, N, Shi, J, Zhang, C, Lau, WY, Wu, M & Cheng, S (2014) Alpha-1-fucosidase as a prognostic indicator for hepatocellular carcinoma following hepatectomy: a large-scale, long-term study. *Br J Cancer,* 110, 1811-9.
[http://dx.doi.org/10.1038/bjc.2014.102] [PMID: 24569461]

Wang, M, Xiao, J, Jiang, J & Qin, R (2011) CD133 and ALDH may be the molecular markers of cholangiocarcinoma stem cells. *Int J Cancer,* 128, 1996-7.
[http://dx.doi.org/10.1002/ijc.25519] [PMID: 20568110]

Wang, S, Zhang, C, Wang, G, Cheng, B, Wang, Y, Chen, F, Chen, Y, Feng, M & Xiong, B (2016) 'Aptamer-mediated transparent biocompatible nanostructured surfaces for hepotocellular circulating tumor cells enrichment. *Theranostics,* 6, 1877-86.
[http://dx.doi.org/10.7150/thno.15284] [PMID: 27570557]

Wang, SB, Cheng, YN, Cui, SX, Zhong, JL, Ward, SG, Sun, LR, Chen, MH, Kokudo, N, Tang, W & Qu, XJ (2009) Des-gamma-carboxy prothrombin stimulates human vascular endothelial cell growth and migration. *Clin Exp Metastasis,* 26, 469-77.
[http://dx.doi.org/10.1007/s10585-009-9246-y] [PMID: 19263229]

Wang, Z, Zhang, G, Wu, J & Jia, M (2013) Adjuvant therapy for hepatocellular carcinoma: current situation and prospect. *Drug Discov Ther,* 7, 137-43.
[http://dx.doi.org/10.5582/ddt.2013.v7.4.137] [PMID: 24071575]

Weber, GF (2011) The cancer biomarker osteopontin: combination with other markers. *Cancer Genomics Proteomics,* 8, 263-88.
[PMID: 22086896]

Weigel, PH (1981) Evidence that the hepatic asialoglycoprotein receptor is internalized during endocytosis

and that receptor recycling can be uncoupled from endocytosis at low temperature. *Biochem Biophys Res Commun,* 101, 1419-25.
[http://dx.doi.org/10.1016/0006-291X(81)91605-3] [PMID: 6272785]

Weigel, PH & Oka, JA (1982) Endocytosis and degradation mediated by the asialoglycoprotein receptor in isolated rat hepatocytes. *J Biol Chem,* 257, 1201-7.
[http://dx.doi.org/10.1016/S0021-9258(19)68175-5] [PMID: 6276377]

Welzel, TM, Graubard, BI, Quraishi, S, Zeuzem, S, Davila, JA, El-Serag, HB & McGlynn, KA (2013) Population-attributable fractions of risk factors for hepatocellular carcinoma in the United States. *Am J Gastroenterol,* 108, 1314-21.
[http://dx.doi.org/10.1038/ajg.2013.160] [PMID: 23752878]

Weng, MW, Lee, HW, Choi, B, Wang, HT, Hu, Y, Mehta, M, Desai, D, Amin, S, Zheng, Y & Tang, MS (2017) AFB1 hepatocarcinogenesis is *via* lipid peroxidation that inhibits DNA repair, sensitizes mutation susceptibility and induces aldehyde-DNA adducts at p53 mutational hotspot codon 249. *Oncotarget,* 8, 18213-26.
[http://dx.doi.org/10.18632/oncotarget.15313] [PMID: 28212554]

West, J, Card, TR, Aithal, GP & Fleming, KM (2017) Risk of hepatocellular carcinoma among individuals with different aetiologies of cirrhosis: a population-based cohort study. *Aliment Pharmacol Ther,* 45, 983-90.
[http://dx.doi.org/10.1111/apt.13961] [PMID: 28144999]

White, DL, Kanwal, F & El-Serag, HB (2012) Association between nonalcoholic fatty liver disease and risk for hepatocellular cancer, based on systematic review. *Clin Gastroenterol Hepatol,* 10, 1342-1359.e2.
[http://dx.doi.org/10.1016/j.cgh.2012.10.001] [PMID: 23041539]

Wilson, B, Ozturk, M, Takahashi, H, Motté, P, Kew, M, Isselbacher, KJ & Wands, JR (1988) Cell-surface changes associated with transformation of human hepatocytes to the malignant phenotype. *Proc Natl Acad Sci USA,* 85, 3140-4.
[http://dx.doi.org/10.1073/pnas.85.9.3140] [PMID: 2834734]

Wilson, GK, Tennant, DA & McKeating, JA (2014) Hypoxia inducible factors in liver disease and hepatocellular carcinoma: current understanding and future directions. *J Hepatol,* 61, 1397-406.
[http://dx.doi.org/10.1016/j.jhep.2014.08.025] [PMID: 25157983]

Wong, VW, Yu, J, Cheng, AS, Wong, GL, Chan, HY, Chu, ES, Ng, EK, Chan, FK, Sung, JJ & Chan, HL (2009) High serum interleukin-6 level predicts future hepatocellular carcinoma development in patients with chronic hepatitis B. *Int J Cancer,* 124, 2766-70.
[http://dx.doi.org/10.1002/ijc.24281] [PMID: 19267406]

Wu, CC, Hsieh, SR, Chen, JT, Ho, WL, Lin, MC, Yeh, DC, Liu, TJ & P'eng, FK (2000) An appraisal of liver and portal vein resection for hepatocellular carcinoma with tumor thrombi extending to portal bifurcation. *Arch Surg,* 135, 1273-9.
[http://dx.doi.org/10.1001/archsurg.135.11.1273] [PMID: 11074879]

Wu, SD, Ma, YS, Fang, Y, Liu, LL, Fu, D & Shen, XZ (2012) Role of the microenvironment in hepatocellular carcinoma development and progression. *Cancer Treat Rev,* 38, 218-25.
[http://dx.doi.org/10.1016/j.ctrv.2011.06.010] [PMID: 21763074]

Wu, X, Gu, Z, Chen, Y, Chen, B, Chen, W, Weng, L & Liu, X (2019) Application of PD-1 blockade in cancer Immunotherapy. *Comput Struct Biotechnol J,* 17, 661-74.
[http://dx.doi.org/10.1016/j.csbj.2019.03.006] [PMID: 31205619]

Xie, Z, Choong, PF, Poon, LF, Zhou, J, Khng, J, Jasinghe, VJ, Palaniyandi, S & Chen, CS (2008) Inhibition of CD44 expression in hepatocellular carcinoma cells enhances apoptosis, chemosensitivity, and reduces tumorigenesis and invasion. *Cancer Chemother Pharmacol,* 62, 949-57.
[http://dx.doi.org/10.1007/s00280-008-0684-z] [PMID: 18259754]

Xiong, Q, Lee, GY, Ding, J, Li, W & Shi, J (2018) Biomedical applications of mRNA nanomedicine. *Nano Res,* 11, 5281-309.

[http://dx.doi.org/10.1007/s12274-018-2146-1] [PMID: 31007865]

Xue, F, Higgs, BW, Huang, J, Morehouse, C, Zhu, W, Yao, X, Brohawn, P, Xiao, Z, Sebastian, Y, Liu, Z, Xia, Y, Shen, D, Kuziora, M, Dong, Z, Han, H, Gu, Y, Gu, J, Xia, Q & Yao, Y (2015) HERC5 is a prognostic biomarker for post-liver transplant recurrent human hepatocellular carcinoma. *J Transl Med,* 13, 379. [http://dx.doi.org/10.1186/s12967-015-0743-2] [PMID: 26653219]

Yamagamim, H, Moriyama, M, Matsumura, H, Aoki, H, Shimizu, T, Saito, T, Kaneko, M, Shioda, A, Tanaka, N & Arakawa, Y (2002) Serum concentrations of human hepatocyte growth factor is a useful indicator for predicting the occurrence of hepatocellular carcinomas in C-viral chronic liver diseases. *Cancer,* 95, 824-34. [http://dx.doi.org/10.1002/cncr.10732] [PMID: 12209727]

Yamamoto, M, Takasaki, K, Ohtsubo, T, Katsuragawa, H, Fukuda, C & Katagiri, S (2001) Effectiveness of systematized hepatectomy with Glisson's pedicle transection at the hepatic hilus for small nodular hepatocellular carcinoma: retrospective analysis. *Surgery,* 130, 443-8. [http://dx.doi.org/10.1067/msy.2001.116406] [PMID: 11562668]

Yamamoto, S, Schulze, KL & Bellen, HJ (2014) Introduction to Notch signaling. *Mol Biol,* 1187, 1-14. [http://dx.doi.org/10.1007/978-1-4939-1139-4_1] [PMID: 25053477]

Yamashita, T, Honda, M, Nakamoto, Y, Baba, M, Nio, K, Hara, Y, Zeng, SS, Hayashi, T, Kondo, M, Takatori, H, Yamashita, T, Mizukoshi, E, Ikeda, H, Zen, Y, Takamura, H, Wang, XW & Kaneko, S (2013) Discrete nature of EpCAM+ and CD90+ cancer stem cells in human hepatocellular carcinoma. *Hepatology,* 57, 1484-97. [http://dx.doi.org/10.1002/hep.26168] [PMID: 23174907]

Yan, W, Chang, Y, Liang, X, Cardinal, JS, Huang, H, Thorne, SH, Monga, SP, Geller, DA, Lotze, MT & Tsung, A (2012) High-mobility group box 1 activates caspase-1 and promotes hepatocellular carcinoma invasiveness and metastases. *Hepatology,* 55, 1863-75. [http://dx.doi.org/10.1002/hep.25572] [PMID: 22234969]

Yan, Y, Zuo, X & Wei, D (2015) 'Concise review: emerging role of CD44 in cancer stem cells: a promising biomarker and therapeutic target. *Stem Cells Transl Med,* 4, 1033-43. [http://dx.doi.org/10.5966/sctm.2015-0048] [PMID: 26136504]

Yang, JD, Hainaut, P, Gores, GJ, Amadou, A, Plymoth, A & Roberts, LR (2019) A global view of hepatocellular carcinoma: trends, risk, prevention and management. *Nat Rev Gastroenterol Hepatol,* 16, 589-604. [http://dx.doi.org/10.1038/s41575-019-0186-y] [PMID: 31439937]

Yang, F, Yin, Y, Wang, F, Wang, Y, Zhang, L, Tang, Y & Sun, S (2010) miR-17-5p Promotes migration of human hepatocellular carcinoma cells through the p38 mitogen-activated protein kinase-heat shock protein 27 pathway. *Hepatology,* 51, 1614-23. [http://dx.doi.org/10.1002/hep.23566] [PMID: 20209605]

Yang, JD & Roberts, LR (2010) Hepatocellular carcinoma: A global view. *Nat Rev Gastroenterol Hepatol,* 7, 448-58. [http://dx.doi.org/10.1038/nrgastro.2010.100] [PMID: 20628345]

Yang, JD, Ahmed Mohammed, H, Harmsen, WS, Enders, F, Gores, GJ & Roberts, LR (2017) Recent Trends in the Epidemiology of Hepatocellular Carcinoma in Olmsted County, Minnesota: A US Population-based Study. *J Clin Gastroenterol,* 51, 742-8. [http://dx.doi.org/10.1097/MCG.0000000000000810] [PMID: 28445235]

Yang, JD, Gyedu, A, Afihene, MY, Duduyemi, BM, Micah, E, Kingham, TP, Nyirenda, M, Nkansah, AA, Bandoh, S, Duguru, MJ, Okeke, EN, Kouakou-Lohoues, MJ, Abdo, A, Awuku, YA, Ajayi, AO, Omonisi, AE, Ocama, P, Malu, AO, Mustapha, S, Okonkwo, U, Kooffreh-Ada, M, Debes, JD, Onyekwere, C, Ekere, F, Rufina, I & Roberts, LR (2015) Hepatocellular carcinoma occurs at an earlier age in Africans, particularly in Association With Chronic Hepatitis B. *Am J Gastroenterol,* 110, 1629-31. [http://dx.doi.org/10.1038/ajg.2015.289] [PMID: 26618430]

Yang, JD, Mohamed, EA, Aziz, AO, Shousha, HI, Hashem, MB, Nabeel, MM, Abdelmaksoud, AH, Elbaz, TM, Afihene, MY, Duduyemi, BM, Ayawin, JP, Gyedu, A, Lohouès-Kouacou, MJ, Ndam, AW, Moustafa, EF, Hassany, SM, Moussa, AM, Ugiagbe, RA, Omuemu, CE, Anthony, R, Palmer, D, Nyanga, AF, Malu, AO, Obekpa, S, Abdo, AE, Siddig, AI, Mudawi, HM, Okonkwo, U, Kooffreh-Ada, M, Awuku, YA, Nartey, YA, Abbew, ET, Awuku, NA, Otegbayo, JA, Akande, KO, Desalegn, HM, Omonisi, AE, Ajayi, AO, Okeke, EN, Duguru, MJ, Davwar, PM, Okorie, MC, Mustapha, S, Debes, JD, Ocama, P, Lesi, OA, Odeghe, E, Bello, R, Onyekwere, C, Ekere, F, Igetei, R, Mah'moud, MA, Addissie, B, Ali, HM, Gores, GJ, Topazian, MD & Roberts, LR (2017) Characteristics, management, and outcomes of patients with hepatocellular carcinoma in Africa: a multicountry observational study from the Africa Liver Cancer Consortium. *Lancet Gastroenterol Hepatol,* 2, 103-11. a
[http://dx.doi.org/10.1016/S2468-1253(16)30161-3] [PMID: 28403980]

Yang, JD, Nakamura, I & Roberts, LR (2011) The tumor microenvironment in hepatocellular carcinoma: current status and therapeutic targets. *Semin Cancer Biol,* 21, 35-43.
[http://dx.doi.org/10.1016/j.semcancer.2010.10.007] [PMID: 20946957]

Yang, T, Lin, C, Zhai, J, Shi, S, Zhu, M, Zhu, N, Lu, JH, Yang, GS & Wu, MC (2012) Surgical resection for advanced hepatocellular carcinoma according to Barcelona Clinic Liver Cancer (BCLC) staging. *J Cancer Res Clin Oncol,* 138, 1121-9.
[http://dx.doi.org/10.1007/s00432-012-1188-0] [PMID: 22402598]

Yang, Y, Nagano, H, Ota, H, Morimoto, O, Nakamura, M, Wada, H, Noda, T, Damdinsuren, B, Marubashi, S, Miyamoto, A, Takeda, Y, Dono, K, Umeshita, K, Nakamori, S, Wakasa, K, Sakon, M & Monden, M (2007) Patterns and clinicopathologic features of extrahepatic recurrence of hepatocellular carcinoma after curative resection. *Surgery,* 141, 196-202.
[http://dx.doi.org/10.1016/j.surg.2006.06.033] [PMID: 17263976]

Yang, ZF, Ho, DW, Ng, MN, Lau, CK, Yu, WC, Ngai, P, Chu, PW, Lam, CT, Poon, RT & Fan, ST (2008) Significance of CD90+ cancer stem cells in human liver cancer. *Cancer Cell,* 13, 153-66.
[http://dx.doi.org/10.1016/j.ccr.2008.01.013] [PMID: 18242515]

Yao, Z, Luo, J, Hu, K, Lin, J, Huang, H, Wang, Q, Zhang, P, Xiong, Z, He, C, Huang, Z, Liu, B & Yang, Y (2017) ZKSCAN1 gene and its related circular RNA (circZKSCAN1) both inhibit hepatocellular carcinoma cell growth, migration, and invasion but through different signaling pathways. *Mol Oncol,* 11, 422-37.
[http://dx.doi.org/10.1002/1878-0261.12045] [PMID: 28211215]

Yapali, S & Tozun, N (2018) Epidemiology and viral risk factors for hepatocellular carcinoma in the Eastern Mediterranean countries. *Hepatoma Res,* 4, 24.
[http://dx.doi.org/10.20517/2394-5079.2018.57]

Yau, T, Tang, VY, Yao, TJ, Fan, ST, Lo, CM & Poon, RT (2014) Development of Hong Kong Liver Cancer staging system with treatment stratification for patients with hepatocellular carcinoma. *Gastroenterology,* 146, 1691-700.e3.
[http://dx.doi.org/10.1053/j.gastro.2014.02.032] [PMID: 24583061]

Yeo, W, Mok, TS, Zee, B, Leung, TW, Lai, PB, Lau, WY, Koh, J, Mo, FK, Yu, SC, Chan, AT, Hui, P, Ma, B, Lam, KC, Ho, WM, Wong, HT, Tang, A & Johnson, PJ (2005) A randomized phase III study of doxorubicin *versus* cisplatin/interferon alpha-2b/doxorubicin/fluorouracil (PIAF) combination chemotherapy for unresectable hepatocellular carcinoma. *J Natl Cancer Inst,* 97, 1532-8.
[http://dx.doi.org/10.1093/jnci/dji315] [PMID: 16234567]

Yin, S, Li, J, Hu, C, Chen, X, Yao, M, Yan, M, Jiang, G, Ge, C, Xie, H, Wan, D, Yang, S, Zheng, S & Gu, J (2007) CD133 positive hepatocellular carcinoma cells possess high capacity for tumorigenicity. *Int J Cancer,* 120, 1444-50.
[http://dx.doi.org/10.1002/ijc.22476] [PMID: 17205516]

Yoon, SK (2018) Molecular mechanism of hepatocellular carcinoma. *Hepatoma Res,* 4, 42.
[http://dx.doi.org/10.20517/2394-5079.2018.23]

Yoshimoto, S, Loo, TM, Atarashi, K, Kanda, H, Sato, S, Oyadomari, S, Iwakura, Y, Oshima, K, Morita, H,

Hattori, M, Honda, K, Ishikawa, Y, Hara, E & Ohtani, N (2013) Obesity-induced gut microbial metabolite promotes liver cancer through senescence secretome. *Nature,* 499, 97-101.
[http://dx.doi.org/10.1038/nature12347] [PMID: 23803760]

Younossi, ZM, Blissett, D, Blissett, R, Henry, L, Stepanova, M, Younossi, Y, Racila, A, Hunt, S & Beckerman, R (2016) The economic and clinical burden of nonalcoholic fatty liver disease in the United States and Europe. *Hepatology,* 64, 1577-86.
[http://dx.doi.org/10.1002/hep.28785] [PMID: 27543837]

Younossi, ZM, Koenig, AB, Abdelatif, D, Fazel, Y, Henry, L & Wymer, M (2016) Global epidemiology of nonalcoholic fatty liver disease-Meta-analytic assessment of prevalence, incidence, and outcomes. *Hepatology,* 64, 73-84.
[http://dx.doi.org/10.1002/hep.28431] [PMID: 26707365]

Yu, GY, He, G, Li, CY, Tang, M, Grivennikov, S, Tsai, WT, Wu, MS, Hsu, CW, Tsai, Y, Wang, LH & Karin, M (2012) Hepatic expression of HCV RNA-dependent RNA polymerase triggers innate immune signaling and cytokine production. *Mol Cell,* 48, 313-21.
[http://dx.doi.org/10.1016/j.molcel.2012.07.032] [PMID: 22959272]

Yu, H, Pardoll, D & Jove, R (2009) STATs in cancer inflammation and immunity: a leading role for STAT3. *Nat Rev Cancer,* 9, 798-809.
[http://dx.doi.org/10.1038/nrc2734] [PMID: 19851315]

Yu, R, Xiang, X, Tan, Z, Zhou, Y, Wang, H & Deng, G (2016) Efficacy of PIVKA-II in prediction and early detection of hepatocellular carcinoma: a nested case-control study in Chinese patients. *Sci Rep,* 6, 35050.
[http://dx.doi.org/10.1038/srep35050] [PMID: 27731353]

Yu, T, Tang, B & Sun, X (2017) Development of Inhibitors Targeting Hypoxia-Inducible Factor 1 and 2 for Cancer Therapy. *Yonsei Med J,* 58, 489-96.
[http://dx.doi.org/10.3349/ymj.2017.58.3.489] [PMID: 28332352]

Yu, Z, Ye, S, Hu, G, Lv, M, Tu, Z, Zhou, K & Li, Q (2015) The RAF-MEK-ERK pathway: targeting ERK to overcome obstacles to effective cancer therapy. *Future Med Chem,* 7, 269-89.
[http://dx.doi.org/10.4155/fmc.14.143] [PMID: 25826360]

Zender, S, Nickeleit, I, Wuestefeld, T, Sörensen, I, Dauch, D, Bozko, P, El-Khatib, M, Geffers, R, Bektas, H, Manns, MP, Gossler, A, Wilkens, L, Plentz, R, Zender, L & Malek, NP (2013) A critical role for notch signaling in the formation of cholangiocellular carcinomas. *Cancer Cell,* 23, 784-95.
[http://dx.doi.org/10.1016/j.ccr.2013.04.019] [PMID: 23727022]

Zhang, H, Yao, M & Wu, W (2015) 'Up-regulation of annexin A2 expression predicates advanced clinicopathological features and poor prognosis in hepatocellular carcinoma. *Tumour Biol,* 37, 211-6.
[http://dx.doi.org/10.1007/s13277-015-3678-6] [PMID: 26189841]

Zhang, L, Yang, L, Liu, X, Chen, W, Chang, L, Chen, L, Loera, S, Chu, P, Huang, WC, Liu, YR & Yen, Y (2013) MicroRNA-657 promotes tumorigenesis in hepatocellular carcinoma by targeting transducin-like enhancer protein 1 through nuclear factor kappa B pathways. *Hepatology,* 57, 1919-30.
[http://dx.doi.org/10.1002/hep.26162] [PMID: 23175432]

Zhang, T, Zhang, J, You, X, Liu, Q, Du, Y, Gao, Y, Shan, C, Kong, G, Wang, Y, Yang, X, Ye, L & Zhang, X (2012) Hepatitis B virus X protein modulates oncogene Yes-associated protein by CREB to promote growth of hepatoma cells. *Hepatology,* 56, 2051-9.
[http://dx.doi.org/10.1002/hep.25899] [PMID: 22707013]

Zhang, X, Ng, HLH, Lu, A, Lin, C, Zhou, L, Lin, G, Zhang, Y, Yang, Z & Zhang, H (2016) Drug delivery system targeting advanced hepatocellular carcinoma: Current and future. *Nanomedicine,* 12, 853-69.
[http://dx.doi.org/10.1016/j.nano.2015.12.381] [PMID: 26772424]

Zhang, Y, Deng, ZS, Liao, MM, Wang, N, Zhang, XQ, Yu, HY & Zhang, YD (2012) Tumor associated glycoprotein-72 is a novel marker for poor survival in hepatocellular carcinoma. *Pathol Oncol Res,* 18, 911-6.
[http://dx.doi.org/10.1007/s12253-012-9521-0] [PMID: 22434316]

Zhang, Y, Yang, B, Du, Z, Bai, T, Gao, YT, Wang, YJ, Lou, C, Wang, FM & Bai, Y (2012) Aberrant methylation of SPARC in human hepatocellular carcinoma and its clinical implication. *World J Gastroenterol,* 18, 2043-52.
[http://dx.doi.org/10.3748/wjg.v18.i17.2043] [PMID: 22563191]

Zheng, W, Yao, M & Sai, W (2015) Diagnostic and prognostic significance of secre¬tory clusterin expression in patients with hepatocellular carcinoma. *Tumour Biol,* 37, 1-12.
[PMID: 26432328]

Zhu, AX, Rosmorduc, O, Evans, TR, Ross, PJ, Santoro, A, Carrilho, FJ, Bruix, J, Qin, S, Thuluvath, PJ, Llovet, JM, Leberre, MA, Jensen, M, Meinhardt, G & Kang, YK (2015) SEARCH: a phase III, randomized, double-blind, placebo-controlled trial of sorafenib plus erlotinib in patients with advanced hepatocellular carcinoma. *J Clin Oncol,* 33, 559-66.
[http://dx.doi.org/10.1200/JCO.2013.53.7746] [PMID: 25547503]

Zhu, J, Liu, S, Ye, F, Shen, Y, Tie, Y, Zhu, J, Jin, Y, Zheng, X, Wu, Y & Fu, H (2014) The long noncoding RNA expression profile of hepatocellular carcinoma identified by microarray analysis. *PLoS One,* 9, e101707.
[http://dx.doi.org/10.1371/journal.pone.0101707] [PMID: 25025236]

Zhu, K, Dai, Z & Zhou, J (2013) Biomarkers for hepatocellular carcinoma: progression in early diagnosis, prognosis, and personalized therapy. *Biomark Res,* 1, 10.
[http://dx.doi.org/10.1186/2050-7771-1-10] [PMID: 24252133]

Zhu, R, Yang, J, Xu, L, Dai, W, Wang, F, Shen, M, Zhang, Y, Zhang, H, Chen, K, Cheng, P, Wang, C, Zheng, Y, Li, J, Lu, J, Zhou, Y, Wu, D & Guo, C (2014) Diagnostic performance of des-gamma-carboxy prothrombin for hepatocellular carcinoma: a metaanalysis. *Gastroenterol Res Pract,* 2014, 529314.
[http://dx.doi.org/10.1155/2014/529314] [PMID: 25165471]

Zhu, WW, Guo, JJ, Guo, L, Jia, HL, Zhu, M, Zhang, JB, Loffredo, CA, Forgues, M, Huang, H, Xing, XJ, Ren, N, Dong, QZ, Zhou, HJ, Ren, ZG, Zhao, NQ, Wang, XW, Tang, ZY, Qin, LX & Ye, QH (2013) Evaluation of midkine as a diagnostic serum biomarker in hepatocellular carcinoma. *Clin Cancer Res,* 19, 3944-54.
[http://dx.doi.org/10.1158/1078-0432.CCR-12-3363] [PMID: 23719264]

Zhu, YZ, Zhu, R, Fan, J, Pan, Q, Li, H, Chen, Q & Zhu, HG (2010) Hepatitis B virus X protein induces hypermethylation of p16(INK4A) promoter *via* DNA methyltransferases in the early stage of HBV-associated hepatocarcinogenesis. *J Viral Hepat,* 17, 98-107.
[http://dx.doi.org/10.1111/j.1365-2893.2009.01156.x] [PMID: 19732323]

Zhu, Z, Wilson, AT, Gopalakrishna, K, Brown, KE, Luxon, BA & Schmidt, WN (2010) Hepatitis C virus core protein enhances Telomerase activity in Huh7 cells. *J Med Virol,* 82, 239-48.
[http://dx.doi.org/10.1002/jmv.21644] [PMID: 20029802]

Zimmerman, RL, Burke, MA, Young, NA, Solomides, CC & Bibbo, M (2001) Diagnostic value of hepatocyte paraffin 1 antibody to discriminate hepatocellular carcinoma from metastatic carcinoma in fine-needle aspiration biopsies of the liver. *Cancer,* 93, 288-91.
[http://dx.doi.org/10.1002/cncr.9043] [PMID: 11507703]

Ziol, M, Poté, N, Amaddeo, G, Laurent, A, Nault, JC, Oberti, F, Costentin, C, Michalak, S, Bouattour, M, Francoz, C, Pageaux, GP, Ramos, J, Decaens, T, Luciani, A, Guiu, B, Vilgrain, V, Aubé, C, Derman, J, Charpy, C, Zucman-Rossi, J, Barget, N, Seror, O, Ganne-Carrié, N, Paradis, V & Calderaro, J (2018) Macrotrabecular-massive hepatocellular carcinoma: A distinctive histological subtype with clinical relevance. *Hepatology,* 68, 103-12.
[http://dx.doi.org/10.1002/hep.29762] [PMID: 29281854]

CHAPTER 2

Hepatocellular Carcinoma and Therapeutic Challenges

Somenath Datta[1,*]

[1] *Duke Molecular Physiology Institute (DMPI), Duke University School of Medicine, Durham, North Carolina, USA*

Abstract: Hepatocellular carcinoma (HCC) is the most common primary hepatic malignancy and accounts for more than 90% of liver cancers. Despite HBV vaccination programs and targeted therapies, the global burden of HCC is still increasing. Early diagnosis of HCC has been crucial for selecting the best curative treatment options and improving overall patient survival. Despite several advancements in surveillance programs and diagnostic strategies, most HCC cases are still diagnosed at the late stages when most of the current therapeutics become ineffective, making HCC one of the main reasons for cancer-related deaths. Enormous heterogeneity in HCC poses the most prominent challenges for scientists and physicians in designing perfect staging systems and therapeutic selection for HCC patients. Although several HCC therapeutic advancements have come up in the past decade, the current status is far from satisfactory. At present, HCC therapeutics are struggling with several challenges: a shortage of human donors for transplantation, drug resistance, lack of standard operating protocol for immunotherapy, *etc.* Some clinical trials using single or combination therapies are currently underway, hoping to overcome some of these challenges. Constant improvement in HCC therapeutic strategies and prevention measures provides optimism for further advancement in the coming future.

Keywords: Cirrhosis, Early diagnosis, Hepatocellular carcinoma (HCC), Immuno checkpoints, Immunotherapy, Multi-kinase inhibitors (MKIs), Nanoparticle, Prognostic assessments, Systemic therapy, Transplantation.

INTRODUCTION

Hepatocellular carcinoma (HCC) is a significant public health concern and is the most predominant primary liver cancer. Globally, HCC is the 5th most common neoplasm and 3rd leading cause of cancer-related mortality (Wang and Wang, 2019). Worldwide, the numbers of new HCC cases are continuously increasing annually (3-9%) (Velazquez *et al.*, 2003). In 2000, the global estimated number of

* **Corresponding author Somenath Datta:** Duke Molecular Physiology Institute (DMPI), Duke University School of Medicine, Duke University, North Carolina, USA; E-mail: somenath.datta@duke.edu

HCC cases was 625,000, and due to the high mortality rate of this cancer, the occurrence rate was almost equal to the mortality rate. According to World Health Organization, there will be more than one million liver cancer-related deaths in 2030 (https://www.who.int/healthinfo/global_burden_disease/projections/en/). More than 80% of these HCC cases belong to developing countries, and the male to female ratio is 2.4 to 1 (Parkin, 2001). In 2008, the American Cancer Society estimated 18,000 deaths in HCC in the United States and showed a strong male preponderance (Jemal *et al.*, 2007, Siegel *et al.*, 2013). HCC patients without any underlying liver disease are sporadic. The major risk factor for the development of HCC is liver cirrhosis, which commonly occurs due to chronic infection with hepatitis B virus (HBV) and hepatitis C virus (HCV), excessive consumption of alcohol, presence of non-alcoholic fatty liver disease (NAFLD), *etc.* (Tinkle and Haas-Kogan, 2012) (Fig. **1**). Studies from different parts of the world have shown that around 75%-80% of HCC cases are due to chronic viral infection (HBV: 50%-55% and HCV: 25%-30%) (Lu *et al.*, 2006a, Lu *et al.*, 2006b). Due to its higher prevalence rate, HBV outweighs HCV as the most critical risk factor for the development of HCC. A report suggested that the proportion of HCC cases attributable to HBV infection was 16% in the USA, 18% in Western Europe, 51% in Eastern Europe, and 65% in China and the Far East regions (Bharadwaj *et al.*, 2013). Other factors associated with HCC development are presence of liver fibrosis, higher viral load, viral genotype (HBV/C; HBV/D1), diabetes, male sex, older-age, exposure to aflatoxins, and a family history of HCC (Datta *et al.*, 2018, Datta *et al.*, 2014, Yang *et al.*, 2011) (Fig. **1**).

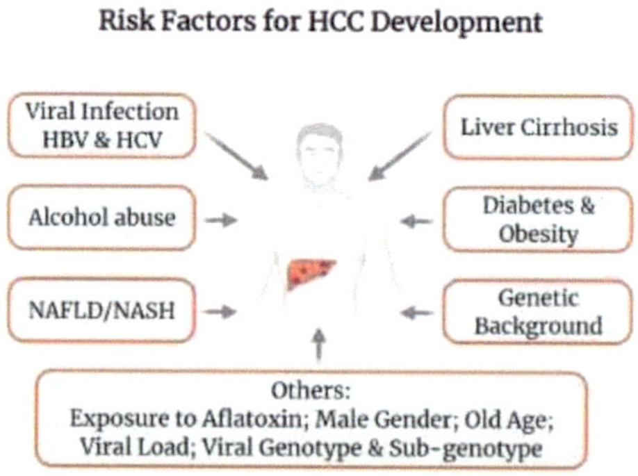

Fig. (1). Schematic diagram showing risk factors for the development of HCC.

The simplest way to prevent HCC-related death is to avoid its risk factors. Nationwide vaccination programs against HBV and broad uses of direct-acting anti-HCV agents are more likely changing the etiologic landscape of HCC (Villanueva, 2019, Forner *et al.*, 2018). However, the increasing rate of NAFLD and excessive obesity and metabolic disorders enhance HCC development risk, imposing a possible future burden of liver cancer in Western countries (Younossi *et al.*, 2019). Although the recent CONCORD-3 data published in Lancet showed an increase in survival trends for most cancers because of early diagnosis and treatment, minimal changes were observed in liver cancer survival during a period of 20 years, from 1995 to 2014 (Allemani *et al.*, 2018, Anwanwan *et al.*, 2020). The present chapter highlights the therapeutic challenges of HCC from diagnosis to therapy precisely.

HCC SURVEILLANCE AND DIAGNOSIS

The development of HCC is a multistep-complex process involving an underlying repetitive cycle of chronic hepatic damage followed by regeneration and repair. Cumulative accumulation of different somatic mutations and epigenetic, transcriptomic, and metabolic alterations make a unique molecular fingerprint for each HCC, explaining enormous clinical and molecular heterogeneity among HCC cases (Marquardt *et al.*, 2015, Zucman-Rossi *et al.*, 2015). Early-stage diagnosis of HCC is crucial for the selection of proper curative treatments and improved patient survival. Despite several advanced surveillance programs globally, the detection efficiency of early-stage HCC is very low and challenging, mainly because most of the early stages are asymptomatic. Current surveillance imaging techniques are often unaffordable to most patients. Early-stage diagnosis of HCC results in a good prognosis with 5-year survival for more than 70% of patients. In contrast, late-stage diagnosis, which generally happens in most cases, results in less than 16% overall 5-year survival rate (Jemal *et al.*, 2007, Siegel *et al.*, 2013). In more than 15% of HCC cases, the extrahepatic metastatic spread has been in lungs, lymph nodes, bones, adrenals, and brain at the time of diagnosis, indicating the urgent need to diagnose HCC in the beginning stages (Uka *et al.*, 2007, Katyal *et al.*, 2000, Choi *et al.*, 2009, Yoon *et al.*, 2007). According to the American Association for the Study of the Liver Disease (AASLD) guideline, every cirrhotic and high-risk chronic HBV patient should undertake screening with liver ultrasound imaging every six months. Diagnosis of HCC using multi-phase computed tomography (CT) and dynamic magnetic resonance imaging (MRI) is currently going on based on AASLD and the European Association for the Study of the Liver (EASL) guideline. For the detection of HCC, these techniques focused on arterial phase enhancement or vascular shift during malignant transformation of hepatocytes (Bruix *et al.*, 2011, European Association for the Study of the Liver 2012, Barr and Hussain, 2014, Willatt *et al.*, 2008). This pattern of imaging characteristics has 66-82% sensitivity and more than 90% specificity for the diagnosis of HCC in patients with cirrhotic liver and larger nodule size (>1cm in diameter) (Roberts *et al.*, 2018). For patients without cirrhosis and those with no conclusive imaging patterns observed in liver nodules, the diagnosis mainly depends on histologic analysis of liver biopsies.

The utilization of immunological markers such as HSP70, glypican 3, and glutamine synthetase increases the diagnosis accuracy of HCC, especially for patients with small nodule sizes (Tremosini *et al*., 2012). Besides the imaging techniques, elevated serum alpha-fetoprotein (AFP) level (>500mcg/L) has been routinely used as a biomarker for HCC, despite its lower sensitivity and specificity (Farinati *et al*., 2006, Tangkijvanich *et al*., 2000, Wu, 1990). Since only a small population of early-stage HCC shows elevated AFP levels, this marker becomes more valuable as a prognostic factor after HCC surgery (Charriere *et al*., 2016). Besides, des-gamma-carboxy-prothrombin (DCP) is also commonly used as a potential biomarker for HCC in Asian countries (Lok *et al*., 2010). Unfortunately, there are no robust and readily available surveillance programs or diagnosis techniques to detect HCC in its early stages.

CURRENT HCC THERAPEUTICS AND THEIR CHALLENGES

Importance of Staging Systems and Their Challenges in Prognostic Assessments

Management of HCC is a complex process and involves multidisciplinary strategies where patient management is performed by hepatologists, hepatobiliary surgeons, oncologists, pathologists, interventional radiologists, and nursing specialists. Because most HCC patients have underlying liver diseases, the actual benefits of HCC treatment should be balanced between the possible harm from the therapeutic interventions and prognostic evaluation of a patient, including the tumor burden and the degree of liver dysfunction. Staging systems are commonly used for the predictive assessment of HCC patients and are very important for determining therapy. Because of its unique characteristics and enormous heterogeneity, it is very challenging to use the standard cancer staging strategies for HCC. Although several scoring or staging systems have been proposed from different parts of the world, the most relevant systems are the Barcelona Clinic Liver Cancer (BCLC) system, Tumour, Node, Metastasis (TNM) staging, Cancer of the Liver Italian Program, Japanese Integrated Staging, Taipei Integrated Scoring System, and Hong Kong Liver Cancer Staging System (Forner *et al*., 2014a, Yau *et al*., 2014). Among them, the BCLC method has been extensively validated, modified with updated evidence, and most widely applied since its introduction in 1999 (Llovet *et al*., 1999, Villanueva, 2019, Forner *et al*., 2018). The main advantage of this BCLC system is its unique way of providing staging-based therapeutics guidelines (Marrero *et al*., 2010) (Fig. **2**). According to the most recently updated version of the BCLC system, patients with very early and early stages, BCLC O/BCLC A (HCC with a single or up to 3 nodules, ≤3 cm diameter, and preserved liver function) could be candidates for hepatic resection, transplantation, or ablation. Patients with intermediate-stage BCLC B (multinodular HCC with preserved liver function) can benefit from transarterial chemoembolization (TACE) (Fig. **2**). For advanced-stage BCLC C (HCC with portal invasion, extrahepatic spread and preserved liver function) HCC patients, systemic treatments, *i.e.*, tyrosine kinase inhibitors sorafenib and regorafenib, are recommended for prolonging survival. End-stage BCLC D patients (HCC with poor liver function and cancer-related symptoms) require supportive care and are not recommended for liver transplantation because of poor prognosis (Fig. **2**). Although the BCLC system is most popular and widely accepted as one of the best HCC staging systems, it also has some limitations. As discussed above, in this staging system, TACE treatment is only recommended for patients with the intermediate stage (BCLC B).

In contrast, surgical resections and systemic treatments are only recommended for early stages (BCLC O/BCLC A) and advanced stages (BCLC C), respectively. These guidelines are not followed in many cases because of tremendous heterogeneity among HCC patients, mainly in the intermediate stage B (BCLC B). Studies have shown that in many HCC cases of the BCLC B stage, the prognosis and suitability of TACE treatment vary (Barman *et al.*, 2014, Hsu *et al.*, 2013). Emerging evidence also shows that surgical intervention, which is only recommended for early-stage disease, may have better long-term outcomes for intermediate-stage HCC patients than TACE treatment (Zhong *et al.*, 2013). These limitations of the BCLC staging system need to be corrected or modified, making it more flexible for treating heterogeneous HCC populations. Multiple groups are currently working on subclassification of BCLC staging and scoring systems to improve patient selection and survival and overall HCC management (Sieghart *et al.*, 2015, Forner *et al.*, 2014, Bolondi *et al.*, 2012, Barman and Su, 2016).

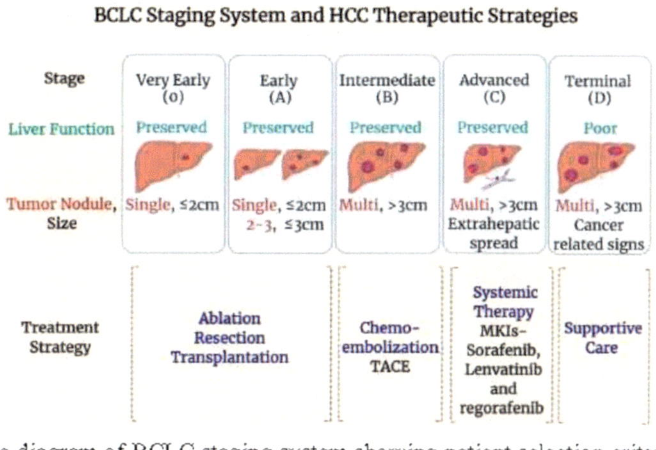

Fig. (2). Schematic diagram of BCLC staging system showing patient selection criteria and recommended treatment options.

Surgical Resection and Liver Transplantation: Challenges in HCC Therapeutics

At present, hepatic resection and liver transplantation are the two therapeutic options that provide the only fortuitous for long-term cure of HCC patients. Surgical resection is generally recommended for non-cirrhotic HCC patients and, in some cases, for cirrhotic early-stage HCC patients with minimal to well-compensated hepatic function. A surgical resection is an option for less than 18% of HCC patients, as 85%-90% of HCC patients have underlying chronic liver disease or cirrhotic liver (Hung, 2005). For HCC patients with decompensated cirrhotic liver, surgical resection is not a good choice because of the increased risk of postoperative liver failure and death (Hung, 2005, Duffy *et al*., 2007). In those cases, liver transplantation is considered a better treatment option. Careful evaluation of compensated cirrhotic-HCC patients is crucial to avoid any treatment-related hurdles and accomplish long-term patient survival. In Asian countries such as Japan, indocyanine green retention rate is generally used for the selection of appropriate candidates (Kokudo *et al*., 2015), whereas in Europe and the USA, clinically significant portal hypertension (CSPH; hepatic vein pressure gradient > 10 mm Hg) and bilirubin content are the variables (European Association for the Study of the Liver, 2012, Boleslawski *et al*., 2012, Roayaie *et al*., 2015). There was a 5-year postoperative survival rate of 70% among patients with normal bilirubin and without CSPH, whereas survival was reduced to 50% or less when patients had both adverse variables (Ishizawa *et al*., 2008). Increasing tumor size and vascular invasion are also risk predictors for poor prognosis (European Association for the Study of the Liver, 2012, Bruix *et al*., 2005, Pawlik *et al*., 2005). Besides these factors, patients with multinodular HCC commonly experienced poor outcomes with less than 29.9% postoperative survival at 5-year, compared to patients with solitary HCC, where the 5-year postoperative survival rate is 58.4% (Pawlik *et al*., 2005, Wang *et al*., 2008). Although 5-year postoperative survival rate can reach up to 70%, surgical resection was limited by early recurrences. Studies have found about 50-60% recurrence rate after 5-years of surgery even in very early HCC patients with no microvascular invasion, and in the majority of the cases (~80%), the recurrences were intrahepatic with lesser chances for repeat resection (Poon *et al*., 2007, Llovet and Bruix, 2003, Imamura *et al*., 2003, Roayaie *et al*., 2011). Although the use of vitamin K2, retinoids, transarterial ^{131}I-lipiodol, and interferon has shown some promising results, there is no efficacy in chemoembolization and systemic use therapy to improve the postoperative recurrence rate (Lu *et al*., 2014). Despite these limitations, surgical resection still remains a strongly recommended therapeutic option, especially for non-cirrhotic HCC patients.

Liver transplantation is the best option for HCC patients with underlying chronic liver disease or cirrhosis as it tackles both problems. The Milan criteria have been the most popularly used benchmark for HCC patient selection, offering the best post-transplantation survival rate. Greater than 70% 5-year post-transplantation survival with less than 10-15% recurrence rate can be achieved following the Milan criteria, *i.e.*, solitary tumor ≤5 cm in size or up to 3 nodules with ≤3 cm in size, without vascular invasion or extrahepatic spread (Mazzaferro *et al.*, 1996). Modification of the Milan criteria using AFP level and tumor volume rather than tumor size and the number has been found with improved predictive value for liver transplantation (Duvoux *et al.*, 2012, Toso *et al.*, 2015). The main limitation of liver transplantation is the shortage of human donors. During the waiting period that arises due to donor shortage, some tumors might progress beyond the patient selection criteria for transplantation, impairing the therapy effectiveness. However, the proposal of living donor liver transplantation (LDLT) may increase the liver donor (European Association for the Study of the Liver, 2012, Bruix *et al.*, 2005). In cases where the waiting time exceeds six months, locoregional therapies are optional in slowing down the tumor progression during waiting for a donor (Sapisochin and Bruix, 2017). Furthermore, continuous reevaluation of patient selection criteria is essential for prioritizing the sickest patients on the waiting list.

Non-surgical Therapies: Locoregional Therapies and Their Challenges

Percutaneous Ablation

Locoregional therapies like percutaneous ablation (PA) are most valuable when surgical resection or liver transplantation is impossible for early-stage HCC patients (BCLC O/BCLC A stage patients). Patients waiting for a donor's liver for more than 6 months are also suggested for locoregional therapies to delay the tumor progression. Two types of percutaneous ablations, thermal and chemical, are more commonly used. In thermal ablation, cancer cells are destroyed by temperature modifications through ultrasound, microwaves, or radiofrequency treatment. In contrast, chemical ablation destroys cancer cells by injecting chemicals (*e.g.*, ethanol/acetic acid) directly into the tumor. Better disease control and patient outcomes have been reported in radiofrequency ablation than chemical ablation by percutaneous ethanol injection (Breen and Lencioni, 2015, Germani *et al.*, 2010). The main limitation of percutaneous ablation is increased local recurrence rate (33%-43%) at 3-years after treatment (Lencioni *et al.*, 2004).

Trans-Arterial Therapies

According to the BCLC staging system, patients with the intermediate stage (BCLC/B) are generally considered for trans-arterial therapies such as transarterial chemoembolization (TACE). In the TACE process, the hepatic artery which supplies blood to the tumor is blocked and delivered with chemotherapeutic agents such as doxorubicin and cisplatin. Obstruction of hepatic artery-induced tumor necrosis due to ischemia and the chemotherapeutic agents enhanced the antitumor activity. Although TACE is widely used for the treatment of intermediate stages HCC, some randomized controlled trials have reported unsatisfactory benefits in patient survival by using chemotherapeutic agents compared to untreated patients (Bruix *et al.*, 1998, Pelletier *et al.*, 1990). Furthermore, several studies have demonstrated enhanced intrahepatic and extrahepatic metastases and reduced patient survival after TACE therapy (Lencioni, 2012, Jiang *et al.*, 2007). Although TACE therapy did not harm the adjacent non-tumor tissues because their blood supply is through the portal vein, severe side effects and cytotoxicity due to arterial blockage and effects of antitumor drugs have been reported. Moreover, TACE therapy also resulted in multidrug resistance (MDR) due to increased expression of ABC transporter proteins of efflux pumps and abnormal p53 functions that lead to drug-resistant tumor cells (Arancia *et al.*, 2001, Dart *et al.*, 2004, Gimenez-Bonafe *et al.*, 2009).

Systemic Therapies and Their Challenges

As most HCC cases are diagnosed in the advanced stages, hepatic resection or transplantation and locoregional TACE treatment have been found ineffective in overall patient survival (Forner *et al.*, 2018). The traditional chemotherapeutics such as treatment with 5-FU, cisplatin, and doxorubicin have not been offering any promising success for treating advanced stages of HCC. In 2007, FDA approved sorafenib, a multikinase inhibitor (MKIs), as the first systemic drug for the treatment of advanced-stage HCC. A survival benefit of about three months was reported by Sorafenib HCC Assessment Randomized Protocol (SHARP) trial (Llovet *et al.*, 2008). Since then, several clinical trials have been conducted on different targeted drugs. The FDA has approved three MKIs, sorafenib, regorafenib, and lenvatinib, as the first or second therapy line for patients with advanced-stage HCC (Dhanasekaran *et al.*, 2019). Besides MKIs, several clinical trials on immunotherapy have been conducted or are still going on (Zheng *et al.*, 2013, Gao *et al.*, 2014).

Multi-kinase Inhibitors (MKIs) and Challenges with Drug Resistance

Sorafenib inhibits cancer cell proliferation by blocking kinases involved in the Ras/Raf/MEK/ERK signaling pathway. Sorafenib also blocks tumor angiogenesis by targeting VEGFR-2/3, PDGFRβ, c-Kit, FLT-3 and other tyrosine kinases (Chen *et al.*, 2015, Thabut *et al.*, 2011, Kohga *et al.*, 2010, Wilhelm *et al.*, 2004, Wilhelm *et al.*, 2006, Tanaka and Arii, 2012). The SHARP trial showed a 3-

month prolonged survival of HCC patients using sorafenib and has opened a promising window for the treatment of advanced HCC patients (Llovet *et al.*, 2008, Cheng *et al.*, 2019). After several failed trials between the year 2008 to 2017 (Cheng *et al.*, 2013, Johnson *et al.*, 2013, Zhu *et al.*, 2017, Cainap *et al.*, 2015), another two-promising oral MKIs, regorafenib, and lenvatinib have been discovered (Andre *et al.*, 2013, Pavlakis *et al.*, 2016). Although sorafenib, regorafenib, and lenvatinib have shown promising results in various advanced HCC treatment trials, the overall outcomes are not satisfactory. A large number of patients' pool has been shown unresponsive to sorafenib treatment, but with severe side effects (diarrhea, weight loss, hypertension, abdominal pain, *etc.*) and drug resistance (Wilhelm *et al.*, 2006). Both innate and acquired drug resistance are associated with sorafenib resistance (Zhu *et al.*, 2017, Rotow and Bivona, 2017). At present, the main challenge is to develop new therapeutic strategies to overcome the drug-resistance events. The key to winning this challenge is to uncover the mechanism of sorafenib resistance.

Current Challenges with Drug-resistance

Gene mutations and dysregulation of gene expression significantly contribute to tumor progression. Epidermal growth factor receptor (EGFR) is a member of the receptor tyrosine kinase family and is frequently observed at a higher level in HCC (Ito *et al.*, 2001), suggesting its possible contribution to HCC development or progression and therapy. Activation of the EGFR pathway in HCC cells is also a proven determinant of sorafenib resistance (Ezzoukhry *et al.*, 2012, Blivet-Van Eggelpoel *et al.*, 2012). Interestingly, some EGFR mutations have been identified within more than half of HCC cases and play an important role in constitutive activation of multiple downstream oncogenic signaling pathways such as MAPK, PI3K-AKT, and JAK signaling, which ultimately influence cancer cells to resist MKIs (Ito *et al.*, 2001, Buckley *et al.*, 2008, Yarden and Sliwkowski, 2001). Studies have shown that EGFR- and mTOR-mediated downstream activation of PI3K/Akt/mTOR cascade can promote HCC metastasis and drug resistance (Ling *et al.*, 2017). Furthermore, inhibition of these downstream pathways enhances sorafenib sensitivity to HCC cells (Han *et al.*, 2015).

Cancer stem cells (CSCs) are a small population of highly malignant cells within solid tumors. Growing evidence proved the significant contribution of CSCs in cancer cell chemoresistance (Zhao *et al.*, 2014). Nanog is a biomarker of CSCs in HCC and is involved in the self-renewal process of CSCs. HCC with Nanog-positive CSCs has lower sensitivity to sorafenib (Shan *et al.*, 2012). These findings indicate the importance of CSC markers detection during the evaluation of sorafenib response in HCC patients. Wnt-β-catenin signaling pathway plays an important role in the induction of the self-renewal process of hepatic CSCs.

Dysregulation of this signaling pathway has been reported to promote drug resistance during chemotherapy and altered β-catenin gene (*CTNNB1*) expression has been reported in about 23-36% of HCC cases (Lachenmayer *et al.*, 2012, Harding and Abou-Alfa, 2014), suggesting the possible mechanism of sorafenib-resistance in these subtypes of HCC patients. Shp2 and a novel long-noncoding RNA (lncRNA), THOR, have been recently reported as an activator of the Wnt---catenin signaling pathway (Xiang *et al.*, 2017, Cheng *et al.*, 2019). These studies indicate that HCC patients with low expression of those genes might get benefit from sorafenib treatment.

In a subset of HCC patients, KRAS mutations have been identified. KRAS is an isoform of the RAS protein family, which are the common upstream mediators of sorafenib targeted signaling pathways such as PI3K/Akt/mTOR cascade (Wilhelm *et al.*, 2004, Calvisi *et al.*, 2006, Delire and Starkel, 2015, Gao *et al.*, 2015a). Interestingly, combination therapy using sorafenib and KRAS inhibitors has shown improved sorafenib sensitivity and overall antitumor effects in HCC, indicating another potential therapeutic strategy to deal with drug-resistance HCC (Dietrich *et al.*, 2018). Combination therapy with sorafenib and other drugs, like rapamycin or aspirin, could also potentiate sorafenib sensitivity to HCC cells by disrupting the mTOR pathway (Sun *et al.*). Identifying biomarkers is very important for selecting patients who might be more sensitive and benefit from systematic therapy. Moreover, choosing combination therapy with downstream signaling inhibitors and MKIs is also a potential option for systematic treatment for advanced-stage HCC.

In summary, to overcome MKIs resistance:

a) The tumor heterogeneity between individual patients and intra-tumor heterogeneity should be considered during drug selection for advanced HCC patients.

b) High-throughput genomics and proteomics analysis should be used to screen the genetic background and phenotype of HCC patients. It will guide the selection of combination therapy and avoid drug resistance.

c) Finally, patient-derived models like liver cancer-derived organoids (Broutier *et al.*, 2017) could monitor drug sensitivity and possible drug resistance during MKIs therapy. It will guide in designing the sequential therapy to avoid drug resistance in HCC patients.

Current Immunotherapies and Their Challenges

Irrespective of etiology, about 90% of HCC develops under the background of chronic liver disease, caused by a repetitive cycle of chronic inflammation and hepatic damage following hepatic regeneration and repair through induction of hepatic fibrogenesis. Hepatic fibrogenesis, subsequently through multiple stages of liver fibrosis, leads to liver cirrhosis, which often ends up in HCC. The liver is a central immunomodulator that tightly maintains immunotolerance within the human body. Dysfunction of the liver-controlled immunological network is the main underlying event of chronic liver disease and hepatocarcinogenesis (Ringelhan *et al.*, 2018). Thus, immunotherapies emerge as a potential strategy to modulate or activate the immunological network against cancer cells in HCC patients. In 2013, cancer immunotherapy had been designated as 'the breakthrough of the year' by Science because of the exceptional progress in the field of chimeric antigen receptor (CAR)-modified T (CAR-T) cells and immune checkpoint inhibitors (Couzin-Frankel, 2013). CAR-T cells are genetically engineered T-cells carrying chimeric antigen receptor that provides the T-cells a new ability to target a specific tumor-associated antigen. Glypican-3 (GPC3) has been detected in 72% of HCC cases. In contrast, this antigen is undetectable in normal and cirrhotic liver cells (Capurro *et al.*, 2003), making it a potential target antigen for CAR-T cells. Although antibody-based therapy against GPC3 in HCC did not show promising data (Abou-Alfa *et al.*, 2016, Gao *et al.*, 2015b, Feng *et al.*, 2013, Sawada *et al.*, 2012), the use of CAR-T cells targeting GPC3 has shown prolonged survival of HCC-xenograft mice *in* vivo (Gao *et al.*, 2014). Furthermore, the development of CAR-T cells targeting GPC3 and ASGR1, a liver tissue-specific protein, resulted in higher antitumor action and overall survival by increasing the on-target specificity of CAR-T cells (Chen *et al.*, 2017). Increased antitumor activity has been observed by dual-targeted CAR-T cells, co-expressing GPC3 and PD1-CH3 fusion protein (Pan *et al.*, 2018). A recent study using CAR-T cells targeting CD133, a surface marker of cancer stem cells (CSCs) including HCC, has shown effective therapeutic potential in CD133-positive and advanced-stage HCC patients (Wang *et al.*, 2018). Although GPC3 specific CAR-T cells showed promising results in various studies, further studies and validations in clinical trials are needed to finally approve GPC3 specific CAR-T cells as a novel immunotherapy for HCC patients. Several other CAR-T cell-based therapies against HCC are currently under investigation (Chen *et al.*, 2018) to discover the most effective targets or combination of targets for CAR-T cell-mediated targeted treatment for advanced-stage HCC patients.

Cancer cells can be recognized and destroyed by modulating the activity of the immune system. Immune checkpoints responsible for immunosuppression during tumor progression have been used as a target to enhance the immune system against cancer cells. Programmed cell death protein 1 (PD-1) is a cell surface protein expressed on several immune cells like active CD8+ and CD4+ T-cells, B-cells, Treg cells, NK cells, *etc.* (Greten and Sangro, 2017, Gao *et al.*, 2009).

The binding of PD-1 with its ligand PD-L1 leads to an inhibition of T-cell activity and suppresses the antitumor activity of immune cells (Greten and Sangro, 2017, Gao *et al.*, 2009). Based on promising data from a phase-II trial, FDA recently approved Nivolumab, an anti-PD1 monoclonal antibody, as the second line of agent for the treatment of advanced-HCC (El-Khoueiry *et al.*, 2017). Combination therapy of Nivolumab with Y-90 radioembolization showed an increasing antitumor effect (Wehrenberg-Klee *et al.*, 2018). In a case study, pembrolizumab, a PD-1 inhibitor treatment, showed a positive outcome in metastatic HCC cases that were irresponsive to sorafenib treatment (Truong *et al.*, 2016). Tumor progression and recurrence are directly associated with the expression level of PD-L1. HCC patients with higher PD-L1 levels have a poor prognosis than patients with low levels of PD-L1 (Greten and Sangro, 2017, Gao *et al.*, 2009). The FDA has approved Anti-PD-L1 antibodies such as Atezolizumab, Avelumab, and Durvalumab to treat much cancer, excluding HCC (Ribas and Wolchok, 2018). Several other PD-1 and PD-L1 inhibitors, including Atezolizumab, Avelumab, and Durvalumab, are currently on clinical trials for HCC therapy (www.clinicaltrials.gov). Inhibitors to other checkpoint proteins such as CTLA-4 (Tremelimumab and Ipilimumab) (Sangro *et al.*, 2013, Duffy *et al.*, 2017), TIM3 (anti-TIM3 antibody TSR-022), LAG-3, GITR, *etc.* have also been found to be associated with HCC progression (Xu *et al.*, 2018). Many clinical trials for HCC therapy have been registered using combination therapy using PD-1/PD-L1 inhibitors along with the inhibitors of other proteins such as Tremelimumab (NCT03298451), Ipilimumab (NCT01658878)), TSR-022 (NCT03680508), *etc.*

At present most of the novel immune therapeutic approaches are on clinical trials to treat HCC patients. Like MKIs, currently, immune therapeutics are also facing several challenges during the treatment of heterogeneous HCC patient populations. Because of several various cell-based immunotherapies, there is a need for a standard operating protocol to prepare immune agents such as the source of immune cells, culture methods, dose optimization, delivery route, *etc.* For other issues, optimizing clinical immunotherapeutic protocols such as length of treatment and optimal patient selection to get the best benefits from therapy without any major side effects like autoimmunity are also required.

Nanotechnology-Based HCC Therapeutics: Current Opportunities and Challenges

Nanotechnology has provided scientists with a tool to improve and enhance the effectiveness of anti-cancer therapeutics. The use of several nano carrier-based drug delivery systems allows an appropriate amount of drug delivery for the best antitumor effect, lowers the chances of toxicity due to drug overdose, extends release-time of drugs, thereby allowing longer availability of the medication after a single dose, and increases the specificity of the drug targeting HCC cells. Selective delivery of chemotherapeutic drugs using fluorescent silica nanoparticles has confirmed their improved outcome during HCC therapy (Ballout *et al.*, 2018, Xia *et al.*, 2017). As discussed in the systemic therapy section, one of the significant challenges in systemic therapy is drug resistance development due to efflux pumps. These issues have been challenged using lipid nanoparticles that allow sustained release of drugs such as doxorubicin and enhanced sensitivity and cytotoxicity (Zhao *et al.*, 2015). Currently, combination therapies have been identified as more effective for HCC treatment. Thus, the codelivery of multiple drugs using nanoparticles like mesoporous silica nanoparticles (MSNs) can be tremendously useful, getting significant antitumor activity, as demonstrated by Zhao *et al.*, 2017 (Zhao *et al.*, 2017). Recently, a clinical trial for HCC therapy has been started using NBTXR3 (a nanoparticle formulation of hafnium oxide crystals, activated by SBRT). The patients within the trial are experiencing positive outcomes without any drug-related toxicity (NCT02721056). Nanoparticles are also a promising tool for cancer diagnoses, such as in detecting cancer-associated biomarkers like AFP in the case of HCC, circulating tumor cells, and DNA (Jia *et al.*, 2017, Zhang *et al.*, 2019). Several promising nanotechnology-based cancer diagnostic approaches have been developed, but only a few of those proceeded to clinical trials (Muthu and Feng, 2013).

There are several challenges that need to be addressed for the progression of nanotechnology from bench to bedside for cancer patients. The first challenge is to obtain reliable and quantitively detectable data. The nanoparticle-based detection system can be affected by several factors such as non-specific binding, the formation of aggregates, and unfavorable detection conditions (Lin *et al.*, 2011). Extensive validation of the nanoparticle-based assays' reliability and reproducibility needs to be done in a large pool of clinical samples for progression into clinical applications. Secondly, because nanoparticles are produced in multiple batches, massive data changes have been detected by comparing batch-to-batch variations. Another challenge is to develop nanoparticle-based devices that will be highly sensitive, user-friendly, and cost-efficient. Designing novel nanoparticles for *in vivo* imaging without any possible toxicity is another major challenge. Several factors, like nanoparticles shape, size, surface chemistry, biodistribution, biodegradability, and pharmacokinetics, should be considered in designing nanoparticles with or without a reduced level of toxicity.

HCC THERAPEUTICS: FUTURE PERSPECTIVES AND CONCLUSION

In the past ten years, considerable development has been achieved for HCC therapeutics. At present, HCC patients can benefit from updated therapeutic approaches that improve patient overall survival and outcomes irrespective of disease stages at the time of diagnosis. Constant improvement in the field of HCC therapy provides optimism for further advancement in therapeutic approaches. However, several areas in HCC therapeutics are still under development for better therapeutic outcomes. In the coming future, there will be several new options of combination therapies for HCC treatment, which are currently under investigation or in clinical trials. A finding of much-improved treatment combination for individual patients from heterogeneous HCC populations will be one of the significant challenges for scientists and physicians. However, the empowerment of precision medicine can be achieved by detailed molecular profiling of novel therapeutic drugs and prognosis predictors. "Prevention is Better than Cure" is also applicable for HCC management. HBV and HCV infection prevention through HBV vaccination and direct-acting antiviral treatment for HCV are the best strategies to decrease HCC related mortality rates. The establishment of healthy lifestyles such as regular exercise, healthy food consumption, and reducing alcohol abuse also significantly lower HCC incidence.

CONSENT FOR PUBLICATION

Not applicable.

CONFLICT OF INTEREST

The author declares no conflict of interest, financial or otherwise.

ACKNOWLEDGEMENT

Declared none.

REFERENCES

Abou-Alfa, GK, Puig, O, Daniele, B, Kudo, M, Merle, P, Park, JW, Ross, P, Peron, JM, Ebert, O, Chan, S, Poon, TP, Colombo, M, Okusaka, T, Ryoo, BY, Minguez, B, Tanaka, T, Ohtomo, T, Ukrainskyj, S, Boisserie, F, Rutman, O, Chen, YC, Xu, C, Shochat, E, Jukofsky, L, Reis, B, Chen, G, Di Laurenzio, L, Lee, R & Yen, CJ (2016) Randomized phase II placebo controlled study of codrituzumab in previously treated patients with advanced hepatocellular carcinoma. *J Hepatol,* 65, 289-95.
[http://dx.doi.org/10.1016/j.jhep.2016.04.004] [PMID: 27085251]

Allemani, C, Matsuda, T, Di Carlo, V, Harewood, R, Matz, M, Nikšić, M, Bonaventure, A, Valkov, M, Johnson, CJ, Estève, J, Ogunbiyi, OJ, Azevedo E Silva, G, Chen, WQ, Eser, S, Engholm, G, Stiller, CA, Monnereau, A, Woods, RR, Visser, O, Lim, GH, Aitken, J, Weir, HK, Coleman, MP & Group, CW (2018) Global surveillance of trends in cancer survival 2000-14 (CONCORD-3): analysis of individual records for 37 513 025 patients diagnosed with one of 18 cancers from 322 population-based registries in 71 countries. *Lancet,* 391, 1023-75.
[http://dx.doi.org/10.1016/S0140-6736(17)33326-3] [PMID: 29395269]

André, T, Raymond, E & de Gramont, A (2013) Regorafenib for metastatic colorectal cancer. *Lancet,* 381, 1536-7.
[http://dx.doi.org/10.1016/S0140-6736(13)60975-7] [PMID: 23642693]

Anwanwan, D, Singh, SK, Singh, S, Saikam, V & Singh, R (2020) Challenges in liver cancer and possible treatment approaches. *Biochim Biophys Acta Rev Cancer,* 1873, 188314.
[http://dx.doi.org/10.1016/j.bbcan.2019.188314] [PMID: 31682895]

Arancia, G, Molinari, A, Calcabrini, A, Meschini, S & Cianfriglia, M (2001) Intracellular P-glycoprotein in multidrug resistant tumor cells. *Ital J Anat Embryol,* 106 (Suppl. 1), 59-68.
[PMID: 11729998]

Ballout, F, Habli, Z, Rahal, ON, Fatfat, M & Gali-Muhtasib, H (2018) Thymoquinone-based nanotechnology for cancer therapy: promises and challenges. *Drug Discov Today,* 23, 1089-98.
[http://dx.doi.org/10.1016/j.drudis.2018.01.043] [PMID: 29374534]

Barman, PM, Sharma, P, Krishnamurthy, V, Willatt, J, McCurdy, H, Moseley, RH & Su, GL (2014) Predictors of mortality in patients with hepatocellular carcinoma undergoing transarterial chemoembolization. *Dig Dis Sci,* 59, 2821-5.
[http://dx.doi.org/10.1007/s10620-014-3247-7] [PMID: 24973040]

Barman, PM & Su, GL (2016) Limitations of the barcelona clinic liver cancer staging system with a focus on transarterial chemoembolization as a key modality for treatment of hepatocellular carcinoma. *Clin Liver Dis (Hoboken),* 7, 32-5.
[http://dx.doi.org/10.1002/cld.530] [PMID: 31041024]

Barr, DC & Hussain, HK (2014) MR imaging in cirrhosis and hepatocellular carcinoma. *Magn Reson Imaging Clin N Am,* 22, 315-35.
[http://dx.doi.org/10.1016/j.mric.2014.04.006] [PMID: 25086932]

Bharadwaj, M, Roy, G, Dutta, K, Misbah, M, Husain, M & Hussain, S (2013) Tackling hepatitis B virus-associated hepatocellular carcinoma--the future is now. *Cancer Metastasis Rev,* 32, 229-68.
[http://dx.doi.org/10.1007/s10555-012-9412-6] [PMID: 23114844]

Blivet-Van Eggelpoël, MJ, Chettouh, H, Fartoux, L, Aoudjehane, L, Barbu, V, Rey, C, Priam, S, Housset, C, Rosmorduc, O & Desbois-Mouthon, C (2012) Epidermal growth factor receptor and HER-3 restrict cell response to sorafenib in hepatocellular carcinoma cells. *J Hepatol,* 57, 108-15.
[http://dx.doi.org/10.1016/j.jhep.2012.02.019] [PMID: 22414764]

Boleslawski, E, Petrovai, G, Truant, S, Dharancy, S, Duhamel, A, Salleron, J, Deltenre, P, Lebuffe, G, Mathurin, P & Pruvot, FR (2012) Hepatic venous pressure gradient in the assessment of portal hypertension before liver resection in patients with cirrhosis. *Br J Surg,* 99, 855-63.
[http://dx.doi.org/10.1002/bjs.8753] [PMID: 22508371]

Bolondi, L, Burroughs, A, Dufour, JF, Galle, PR, Mazzaferro, V, Piscaglia, F, Raoul, JL & Sangro, B (2012) Heterogeneity of patients with intermediate (BCLC B) Hepatocellular Carcinoma: proposal for a subclassification to facilitate treatment decisions. *Semin Liver Dis,* 32, 348-59.
[PMID: 23397536]

Breen, DJ & Lencioni, R (2015) Image-guided ablation of primary liver and renal tumours. *Nat Rev Clin Oncol,* 12, 175-86.
[http://dx.doi.org/10.1038/nrclinonc.2014.237] [PMID: 25601446]

Broutier, L, Mastrogiovanni, G, Verstegen, MM, Francies, HE, Gavarró, LM, Bradshaw, CR, Allen, GE, Arnes-Benito, R, Sidorova, O, Gaspersz, MP, Georgakopoulos, N, Koo, BK, Dietmann, S, Davies, SE, Praseedom, RK, Lieshout, R, IJzermans, JNM, Wigmore, SJ, Saeb-Parsy, K, Garnett, MJ, van der Laan, LJ & Huch, M (2017) Human primary liver cancer-derived organoid cultures for disease modeling and drug screening. *Nat Med,* 23, 1424-35.
[http://dx.doi.org/10.1038/nm.4438] [PMID: 29131160]

Bruix, J, Llovet, JM, Castells, A, Montañá, X, Brú, C, Ayuso, MC, Vilana, R & Rodés, J (1998) Transarterial embolization *versus* symptomatic treatment in patients with advanced hepatocellular carcinoma: results of a randomized, controlled trial in a single institution. *Hepatology,* 27, 1578-83.
[http://dx.doi.org/10.1002/hep.510270617] [PMID: 9620330]

Bruix, J & Sherman, M (2011) Management of hepatocellular carcinoma: an update. *Hepatology,* 53, 1020-2. [http://dx.doi.org/10.1002/hep.24199] [PMID: 21374666]

Bruix, J & Sherman, M (2005) Management of hepatocellular carcinoma. *Hepatology,* 42, 1208-36. [http://dx.doi.org/10.1002/hep.20933] [PMID: 16250051]

Buckley, AF, Burgart, LJ, Sahai, V & Kakar, S (2008) Epidermal growth factor receptor expression and gene copy number in conventional hepatocellular carcinoma. *Am J Clin Pathol,* 129, 245-51. [http://dx.doi.org/10.1309/WF10QAAED3PP93BH] [PMID: 18208805]

Cainap, C, Qin, S, Huang, WT, Chung, IJ, Pan, H, Cheng, Y, Kudo, M, Kang, YK, Chen, PJ, Toh, HC, Gorbunova, V, Eskens, FA, Qian, J, McKee, MD, Ricker, JL, Carlson, DM & El-Nowiem, S (2015) Linifanib *versus* Sorafenib in patients with advanced hepatocellular carcinoma: results of a randomized phase III trial. *J Clin Oncol,* 33, 172-9.
[http://dx.doi.org/10.1200/JCO.2013.54.3298] [PMID: 25488963]

Calvisi, DF, Ladu, S, Gorden, A, Farina, M, Conner, EA, Lee, JS, Factor, VM & Thorgeirsson, SS (2006) Ubiquitous activation of Ras and Jak/Stat pathways in human HCC. *Gastroenterology,* 130, 1117-28. [http://dx.doi.org/10.1053/j.gastro.2006.01.006] [PMID: 16618406]

Capurro, M, Wanless, IR, Sherman, M, Deboer, G, Shi, W, Miyoshi, E & Filmus, J (2003) Glypican-3: a novel serum and histochemical marker for hepatocellular carcinoma. *Gastroenterology,* 125, 89-97. [http://dx.doi.org/10.1016/S0016-5085(03)00689-9] [PMID: 12851874]

Charrière, B, Maulat, C, Suc, B & Muscari, F (2016) Contribution of alpha-fetoprotein in liver transplantation for hepatocellular carcinoma. *World J Hepatol,* 8, 881-90.
[http://dx.doi.org/10.4254/wjh.v8.i21.881] [PMID: 27478538]

Chen, C, Li, K, Jiang, H, Song, F, Gao, H, Pan, X, Shi, B, Bi, Y, Wang, H, Wang, H & Li, Z (2017) Development of T cells carrying two complementary chimeric antigen receptors against glypican-3 and asialoglycoprotein receptor 1 for the treatment of hepatocellular carcinoma. *Cancer Immunol Immunother,* 66, 475-89.
[http://dx.doi.org/10.1007/s00262-016-1949-8] [PMID: 28035433]

Chen, J, Jin, R, Zhao, J, Liu, J, Ying, H, Yan, H, Zhou, S, Liang, Y, Huang, D, Liang, X, Yu, H, Lin, H & Cai, X (2015) Potential molecular, cellular and microenvironmental mechanism of sorafenib resistance in hepatocellular carcinoma. *Cancer Lett,* 367, 1-11.
[http://dx.doi.org/10.1016/j.canlet.2015.06.019] [PMID: 26170167]

Chen, Y, e, CY, Gong, ZW, Liu, S, Wang, ZX, Yang, YS & Zhang, XW (2018) Chimeric antigen receptor-engineered T-cell therapy for liver cancer. *Hepatobiliary Pancreat Dis Int,* 17, 301-9.
[http://dx.doi.org/10.1016/j.hbpd.2018.05.005] [PMID: 29861325]

Cheng, AL, Kang, YK, Lin, DY, Park, JW, Kudo, M, Qin, S, Chung, HC, Song, X, Xu, J, Poggi, G, Omata, M, Pitman Lowenthal, S, Lanzalone, S, Yang, L, Lechuga, MJ & Raymond, E (2013) Sunitinib *versus* sorafenib in advanced hepatocellular cancer: results of a randomized phase III trial. *J Clin Oncol,* 31, 4067-75.
[http://dx.doi.org/10.1200/JCO.2012.45.8372] [PMID: 24081937]

Cheng, Z, Lei, Z, Yang, P, Si, A, Xiang, D, Zhou, J & Hüser, N (2019) Long non-coding RNA THOR promotes liver cancer stem cells expansion *via* β-catenin pathway. *Gene,* 684, 95-103.
[http://dx.doi.org/10.1016/j.gene.2018.10.051] [PMID: 30359743]

Choi, HJ, Cho, BC, Sohn, JH, Shin, SJ, Kim, SH, Kim, JH & Yoo, NC (2009) Brain metastases from hepatocellular carcinoma: prognostic factors and outcome: brain metastasis from HCC. *J Neurooncol,* 91, 307-13.
[http://dx.doi.org/10.1007/s11060-008-9713-3] [PMID: 18949445]

Couzin-Frankel, J (2013) Breakthrough of the year 2013. Cancer immunotherapy. *Science,* 342, 1432-3. [http://dx.doi.org/10.1126/science.342.6165.1432] [PMID: 24357284]

Dart, DA, Picksley, SM, Cooper, PA, Double, JA & Bibby, MC (2004) The role of p53 in the chemotherapeutic responses to cisplatin, doxorubicin and 5-fluorouracil treatment. *Int J Oncol,* 24, 115-25. [http://dx.doi.org/10.3892/ijo.24.1.115] [PMID: 14654948]

Datta, S, Dasgupta, D, Ghosh, A, Ghosh, S, Manna, A, Datta, S, Chatterjee, M, Chowdhury, A & Banerjee, S (2018) Oncogenic potential of hepatitis B virus subgenotype D1 surpasses D3: significance in the development of hepatocellular carcinoma. *Carcinogenesis,* 39, 283-92. [http://dx.doi.org/10.1093/carcin/bgx145] [PMID: 29228221]

Datta, S, Roychoudhury, S, Ghosh, A, Dasgupta, D, Ghosh, A, Chakraborty, BC, Ray, S, Gupta, S, Santra, AK, Datta, S, Das, K, Dhali, GK, Chowdhury, A & Banerjee, S (2014) Distinct distribution pattern of hepatitis B virus genotype C and D in liver tissue and serum of dual genotype infected liver cirrhosis and hepatocellular carcinoma patients. *PLoS One,* 9, e102573. [http://dx.doi.org/10.1371/journal.pone.0102573] [PMID: 25032957]

Delire, B & Stärkel, P (2015) The Ras/MAPK pathway and hepatocarcinoma: pathogenesis and therapeutic implications. *Eur J Clin Invest,* 45, 609-23. [http://dx.doi.org/10.1111/eci.12441] [PMID: 25832714]

Dhanasekaran, R, Nault, JC, Roberts, LR & Zucman-Rossi, J (2019) Genomic Medicine and Implications for Hepatocellular Carcinoma Prevention and Therapy. *Gastroenterology,* 156, 492-509. [http://dx.doi.org/10.1053/j.gastro.2018.11.001] [PMID: 30404026]

Dietrich, P, Koch, A, Fritz, V, Hartmann, A, Bosserhoff, AK & Hellerbrand, C (2018) Wild type Kirsten rat sarcoma is a novel microRNA-622-regulated therapeutic target for hepatocellular carcinoma and contributes to sorafenib resistance. *Gut,* 67, 1328-41. [http://dx.doi.org/10.1136/gutjnl-2017-315402] [PMID: 29275358]

Duffy, AG, Ulahannan, SV, Makorova-Rusher, O, Rahma, O, Wedemeyer, H, Pratt, D, Davis, JL, Hughes, MS, Heller, T, ElGindi, M, Uppala, A, Korangy, F, Kleiner, DE, Figg, WD, Venzon, D, Steinberg, SM, Venkatesan, AM, Krishnasamy, V, Abi-Jaoudeh, N, Levy, E, Wood, BJ & Greten, TF (2017) Tremelimumab in combination with ablation in patients with advanced hepatocellular carcinoma. *J Hepatol,* 66, 545-51. [http://dx.doi.org/10.1016/j.jhep.2016.10.029] [PMID: 27816492]

Duffy, JP, Vardanian, A, Benjamin, E, Watson, M, Farmer, DG, Ghobrial, RM, Lipshutz, G, Yersiz, H, Lu, DS, Lassman, C, Tong, MJ, Hiatt, JR & Busuttil, RW (2007) Liver transplantation criteria for hepatocellular carcinoma should be expanded: a 22-year experience with 467 patients at UCLA. *Ann Surg,* 246, 502-9. [http://dx.doi.org/10.1097/SLA.0b013e318148c704] [PMID: 17717454]

Duvoux, C, Roudot-Thoraval, F, Decaens, T, Pessione, F, Badran, H, Piardi, T, Francoz, C, Compagnon, P, Vanlemmens, C, Dumortier, J, Dharancy, S, Gugenheim, J, Bernard, PH, Adam, R, Radenne, S, Muscari, F, Conti, F, Hardwigsen, J, Pageaux, GP, Chazouillères, O, Salame, E, Hilleret, MN, Lebray, P, Abergel, A, Debette-Gratien, M, Kluger, MD, Mallat, A, Azoulay, D & Cherqui, D (2012) Liver transplantation for hepatocellular carcinoma: a model including α-fetoprotein improves the performance of Milan criteria. *Gastroenterology,* 143, 986-94.e3. [http://dx.doi.org/10.1053/j.gastro.2012.05.052] [PMID: 22750200]

El-Khoueiry, AB, Sangro, B, Yau, T, Crocenzi, TS, Kudo, M, Hsu, C, Kim, TY, Choo, SP, Trojan, J, Welling, THR, Meyer, T, Kang, YK, Yeo, W, Chopra, A, Anderson, J, Dela Cruz, C, Lang, L, Neely, J, Tang, H, Dastani, HB & Melero, I (2017) Nivolumab in patients with advanced hepatocellular carcinoma (CheckMate 040): an open-label, non-comparative, phase 1/2 dose escalation and expansion trial. *Lancet,* 389, 2492-502. [http://dx.doi.org/10.1016/S0140-6736(17)31046-2] [PMID: 28434648]

European Association For The Study Of The Liver; (2012) European Organisation For Research And Treatment Of Cancer (2012) EASL-EORTC clinical practice guidelines: management of hepatocellular carcinoma. *J Hepatol,* 56, 908-43. [http://dx.doi.org/10.1016/j.jhep.2011.12.001] [PMID: 22424438]

Ezzoukhry, Z, Louandre, C, Trécherel, E, Godin, C, Chauffert, B, Dupont, S, Diouf, M, Barbare, JC, Mazière, JC & Galmiche, A (2012) EGFR activation is a potential determinant of primary resistance of hepatocellular carcinoma cells to sorafenib. *Int J Cancer,* 131, 2961-9.

[http://dx.doi.org/10.1002/ijc.27604] [PMID: 22514082]

Farinati, F, Marino, D, De Giorgio, M, Baldan, A, Cantarini, M, Cursaro, C, Rapaccini, G, Del Poggio, P, Di Nolfo, MA, Benvegnù, L, Zoli, M, Borzio, F, Bernardi, M & Trevisani, F (2006) Diagnostic and prognostic role of alpha-fetoprotein in hepatocellular carcinoma: both or neither? *Am J Gastroenterol,* 101, 524-32.
[http://dx.doi.org/10.1111/j.1572-0241.2006.00443.x] [PMID: 16542289]

Feng, M, Gao, W, Wang, R, Chen, W, Man, YG, Figg, WD, Wang, XW, Dimitrov, DS & Ho, M (2013) Therapeutically targeting glypican-3 *via* a conformation-specific single-domain antibody in hepatocellular carcinoma. *Proc Natl Acad Sci USA,* 110, E1083-91.
[http://dx.doi.org/10.1073/pnas.1217868110] [PMID: 23471984]

Forner, A, Díaz-González, A, Liccioni, A & Vilana, R (2014) Prognosis prediction and staging. *Best Pract Res Clin Gastroenterol,* 28, 855-65. a
[http://dx.doi.org/10.1016/j.bpg.2014.08.002] [PMID: 25260313]

Forner, A, Gilabert, M, Bruix, J & Raoul, JL (2014) Treatment of intermediate-stage hepatocellular carcinoma. *Nat Rev Clin Oncol,* 11, 525-35. b
[http://dx.doi.org/10.1038/nrclinonc.2014.122] [PMID: 25091611]

Forner, A, Reig, M & Bruix, J (2018) Hepatocellular carcinoma. *Lancet,* 391, 1301-14.
[http://dx.doi.org/10.1016/S0140-6736(18)30010-2] [PMID: 29307467]

Gao, H, Li, K, Tu, H, Pan, X, Jiang, H, Shi, B, Kong, J, Wang, H, Yang, S, Gu, J & Li, Z (2014) Development of T cells redirected to glypican-3 for the treatment of hepatocellular carcinoma. *Clin Cancer Res,* 20, 6418-28.
[http://dx.doi.org/10.1158/1078-0432.CCR-14-1170] [PMID: 25320357]

Gao, JJ, Shi, ZY, Xia, JF, Inagaki, Y & Tang, W (2015) Sorafenib-based combined molecule targeting in treatment of hepatocellular carcinoma. *World J Gastroenterol,* 21, 12059-70. a
[http://dx.doi.org/10.3748/wjg.v21.i42.12059] [PMID: 26576091]

Gao, Q, Wang, XY, Qiu, SJ, Yamato, I, Sho, M, Nakajima, Y, Zhou, J, Li, BZ, Shi, YH, Xiao, YS, Xu, Y & Fan, J (2009) Overexpression of PD-L1 significantly associates with tumor aggressiveness and postoperative recurrence in human hepatocellular carcinoma. *Clin Cancer Res,* 15, 971-9.
[http://dx.doi.org/10.1158/1078-0432.CCR-08-1608] [PMID: 19188168]

Gao, W, Tang, Z, Zhang, YF, Feng, M, Qian, M, Dimitrov, DS & Ho, M (2015) Immunotoxin targeting glypican-3 regresses liver cancer *via* dual inhibition of Wnt signalling and protein synthesis. *Nat Commun,* 6, 6536. b
[http://dx.doi.org/10.1038/ncomms7536] [PMID: 25758784]

Germani, G, Pleguezuelo, M, Gurusamy, K, Meyer, T, Isgrò, G & Burroughs, AK (2010) Clinical outcomes of radiofrequency ablation, percutaneous alcohol and acetic acid injection for hepatocelullar carcinoma: a meta-analysis. *J Hepatol,* 52, 380-8.
[http://dx.doi.org/10.1016/j.jhep.2009.12.004] [PMID: 20149473]

Giménez-Bonafé, P, Tortosa, A & Pérez-Tomás, R (2009) Overcoming drug resistance by enhancing apoptosis of tumor cells. *Curr Cancer Drug Targets,* 9, 320-40.
[http://dx.doi.org/10.2174/156800909788166600] [PMID: 19442052]

Greten, TF & Sangro, B (2017) Targets for immunotherapy of liver cancer. *J Hepatol,* S0168-8278(17)32287-0.
[PMID: 28923358]

Han, T, Xiang, DM, Sun, W, Liu, N, Sun, HL, Wen, W, Shen, WF, Wang, RY, Chen, C, Wang, X, Cheng, Z, Li, HY, Wu, MC, Cong, WM, Feng, GS, Ding, J & Wang, HY (2015) PTPN11/Shp2 overexpression enhances liver cancer progression and predicts poor prognosis of patients. *J Hepatol,* 63, 651-60.
[http://dx.doi.org/10.1016/j.jhep.2015.03.036] [PMID: 25865556]

Harding, JJ & Abou-Alfa, GK (2014) Treating advanced hepatocellular carcinoma: How to get out of first gear. *Cancer,* 120, 3122-30.

[http://dx.doi.org/10.1002/cncr.28850] [PMID: 24898783]

Hsu, CY, Lee, YH, Hsia, CY, Huang, YH, Su, CW, Lin, HC, Lee, RC, Chiou, YY, Lee, FY & Huo, TI (2013) Performance status in patients with hepatocellular carcinoma: determinants, prognostic impact, and ability to improve the Barcelona Clinic Liver Cancer system. *Hepatology,* 57, 112-9.
[http://dx.doi.org/10.1002/hep.25950] [PMID: 22806819]

Hung, H (2005) Treatment modalities for hepatocellular carcinoma. *Curr Cancer Drug Targets,* 5, 131-8.
[http://dx.doi.org/10.2174/1568009053202063] [PMID: 15810877]

Imamura, H, Matsuyama, Y, Tanaka, E, Ohkubo, T, Hasegawa, K, Miyagawa, S, Sugawara, Y, Minagawa, M, Takayama, T, Kawasaki, S & Makuuchi, M (2003) Risk factors contributing to early and late phase intrahepatic recurrence of hepatocellular carcinoma after hepatectomy. *J Hepatol,* 38, 200-7.
[http://dx.doi.org/10.1016/S0168-8278(02)00360-4] [PMID: 12547409]

Ishizawa, T, Hasegawa, K, Aoki, T, Takahashi, M, Inoue, Y, Sano, K, Imamura, H, Sugawara, Y, Kokudo, N & Makuuchi, M (2008) Neither multiple tumors nor portal hypertension are surgical contraindications for hepatocellular carcinoma. *Gastroenterology,* 134, 1908-16.
[http://dx.doi.org/10.1053/j.gastro.2008.02.091] [PMID: 18549877]

Ito, Y, Takeda, T, Sakon, M, Tsujimoto, M, Higashiyama, S, Noda, K, Miyoshi, E, Monden, M & Matsuura, N (2001) Expression and clinical significance of erb-B receptor family in hepatocellular carcinoma. *Br J Cancer,* 84, 1377-83.
[http://dx.doi.org/10.1054/bjoc.2000.1580] [PMID: 11355950]

Jemal, A, Siegel, R, Ward, E, Murray, T, Xu, J & Thun, MJ (2007) Cancer statistics, 2007. *CA Cancer J Clin,* 57, 43-66.
[http://dx.doi.org/10.3322/canjclin.57.1.43] [PMID: 17237035]

Jia, S, Zhang, R, Li, Z & Li, J (2017) Clinical and biological significance of circulating tumor cells, circulating tumor DNA, and exosomes as biomarkers in colorectal cancer. *Oncotarget,* 8, 55632-45.
[http://dx.doi.org/10.18632/oncotarget.17184] [PMID: 28903450]

Jiang, H, Meng, Q, Tan, H, Pan, S, Sun, B, Xu, R & Sun, X (2007) Antiangiogenic therapy enhances the efficacy of transcatheter arterial embolization for hepatocellular carcinomas. *Int J Cancer,* 121, 416-24.
[http://dx.doi.org/10.1002/ijc.22655] [PMID: 17330237]

Johnson, PJ, Qin, S, Park, JW, Poon, RT, Raoul, JL, Philip, PA, Hsu, CH, Hu, TH, Heo, J, Xu, J, Lu, L, Chao, Y, Boucher, E, Han, KH, Paik, SW, Robles-Aviña, J, Kudo, M, Yan, L, Sobhonslidsuk, A, Komov, D, Decaens, T, Tak, WY, Jeng, LB, Liu, D, Ezzeddine, R, Walters, I & Cheng, AL (2013) Brivanib *versus* sorafenib as first-line therapy in patients with unresectable, advanced hepatocellular carcinoma: results from the randomized phase III BRISK-FL study. *J Clin Oncol,* 31, 3517-24.
[http://dx.doi.org/10.1200/JCO.2012.48.4410] [PMID: 23980084]

Katyal, S, Oliver, JH, III, Peterson, MS, Ferris, JV, Carr, BS & Baron, RL (2000) Extrahepatic metastases of hepatocellular carcinoma. *Radiology,* 216, 698-703.
[http://dx.doi.org/10.1148/radiology.216.3.r00se24698] [PMID: 10966697]

Kohga, K, Takehara, T, Tatsumi, T, Ishida, H, Miyagi, T, Hosui, A & Hayashi, N (2010) Sorafenib inhibits the shedding of major histocompatibility complex class I-related chain A on hepatocellular carcinoma cells by down-regulating a disintegrin and metalloproteinase 9. *Hepatology,* 51, 1264-73.
[http://dx.doi.org/10.1002/hep.23456] [PMID: 20099300]

Kokudo, N, Hasegawa, K, Akahane, M, Igaki, H, Izumi, N, Ichida, T, Uemoto, S, Kaneko, S, Kawasaki, S, Ku, Y, Kudo, M, Kubo, S, Takayama, T, Tateishi, R, Fukuda, T, Matsui, O, Matsuyama, Y, Murakami, T, Arii, S, Okazaki, M & Makuuchi, M (2015) Evidence-based Clinical Practice Guidelines for Hepatocellular Carcinoma: The Japan Society of Hepatology 2013 update (3rd JSH-HCC Guidelines). *Hepatol Res,* 45, 45.
[http://dx.doi.org/10.1111/hepr.12464] [PMID: 25625806]

Lachenmayer, A, Alsinet, C, Savic, R, Cabellos, L, Toffanin, S, Hoshida, Y, Villanueva, A, Minguez, B, Newell, P, Tsai, HW, Barretina, J, Thung, S, Ward, SC, Bruix, J, Mazzaferro, V, Schwartz, M, Friedman, SL & Llovet, JM (2012) Wnt-pathway activation in two molecular classes of hepatocellular carcinoma and

experimental modulation by sorafenib. *Clin Cancer Res,* 18, 4997-5007.
[http://dx.doi.org/10.1158/1078-0432.CCR-11-2322] [PMID: 22811581]

Lencioni, R (2012) Management of hepatocellular carcinoma with transarterial chemoembolization in the era of systemic targeted therapy. *Crit Rev Oncol Hematol,* 83, 216-24.
[http://dx.doi.org/10.1016/j.critrevonc.2011.10.008] [PMID: 22142656]

Lencioni, R, Cioni, D, Crocetti, L & Bartolozzi, C (2004) Percutaneous ablation of hepatocellular carcinoma: state-of-the-art. *Liver Transpl,* 10 (Suppl. 1), S91-7.
[http://dx.doi.org/10.1002/lt.20043] [PMID: 14762847]

Lin, YW, Huang, CC & Chang, HT (2011) Gold nanoparticle probes for the detection of mercury, lead and copper ions. *Analyst (Lond),* 136, 863-71.
[http://dx.doi.org/10.1039/C0AN00652A] [PMID: 21157604]

Ling, S, Song, L, Fan, N, Feng, T, Liu, L, Yang, X, Wang, M, Li, Y, Tian, Y, Zhao, F, Liu, Y, Huang, Q, Hou, Z, Xu, F, Shi, L & Li, Y (2017) Combination of metformin and sorafenib suppresses proliferation and induces autophagy of hepatocellular carcinoma *via* targeting the mTOR pathway. *Int J Oncol,* 50, 297-309.
[http://dx.doi.org/10.3892/ijo.2016.3799] [PMID: 27959383]

Llovet, JM, Brú, C & Bruix, J (1999) Prognosis of hepatocellular carcinoma: the BCLC staging classification. *Semin Liver Dis,* 19, 329-38.
[http://dx.doi.org/10.1055/s-2007-1007122] [PMID: 10518312]

Llovet, JM & Bruix, J (2003) Systematic review of randomized trials for unresectable hepatocellular carcinoma: Chemoembolization improves survival. *Hepatology,* 37, 429-42.
[http://dx.doi.org/10.1053/jhep.2003.50047] [PMID: 12540794]

Llovet, JM, Ricci, S, Mazzaferro, V, Hilgard, P, Gane, E, Blanc, JF, de Oliveira, AC, Santoro, A, Raoul, JL, Forner, A, Schwartz, M, Porta, C, Zeuzem, S, Bolondi, L, Greten, TF, Galle, PR, Seitz, JF, Borbath, I, Häussinger, D, Giannaris, T, Shan, M, Moscovici, M, Voliotis, D, Bruix, J & Group, SIS (2008) Sorafenib in advanced hepatocellular carcinoma. *N Engl J Med,* 359, 378-90.
[http://dx.doi.org/10.1056/NEJMoa0708857] [PMID: 18650514]

Lok, AS, Sterling, RK, Everhart, JE, Wright, EC, Hoefs, JC, Di Bisceglie, AM, Morgan, TR, Kim, HY, Lee, WM, Bonkovsky, HL & Dienstag, JL (2010) Des-gamma-carboxy prothrombin and alpha-fetoprotein as biomarkers for the early detection of hepatocellular carcinoma. *Gastroenterology,* 138, 493-502.
[http://dx.doi.org/10.1053/j.gastro.2009.10.031] [PMID: 19852963]

Lu, LC, Cheng, AL & Poon, RT (2014) Recent advances in the prevention of hepatocellular carcinoma recurrence. *Semin Liver Dis,* 34, 427-34.
[http://dx.doi.org/10.1055/s-0034-1394141] [PMID: 25369304]

Lu, SN, Su, WW, Yang, SS, Chang, TT, Cheng, KS, Wu, JC, Lin, HH, Wu, SS, Lee, CM, Changchien, CS, Chen, CJ, Sheu, JC, Chen, DS & Chen, CH (2006) Secular trends and geographic variations of hepatitis B virus and hepatitis C virus-associated hepatocellular carcinoma in Taiwan. *Int J Cancer,* 119, 1946-52. a
[http://dx.doi.org/10.1002/ijc.22045] [PMID: 16708389]

Lu, SN, Wang, JH, Liu, SL, Hung, CH, Chen, CH, Tung, HD, Chen, TM, Huang, WS, Lee, CM, Chen, CC & Changchien, CS (2006) Thrombocytopenia as a surrogate for cirrhosis and a marker for the identification of patients at high-risk for hepatocellular carcinoma. *Cancer,* 107, 2212-22. b
[http://dx.doi.org/10.1002/cncr.22242] [PMID: 17019738]

Marquardt, JU, Andersen, JB & Thorgeirsson, SS (2015) Functional and genetic deconstruction of the cellular origin in liver cancer. *Nat Rev Cancer,* 15, 653-67.
[http://dx.doi.org/10.1038/nrc4017] [PMID: 26493646]

Marrero, JA, Kudo, M & Bronowicki, JP (2010) The challenge of prognosis and staging for hepatocellular carcinoma. *Oncologist,* 15 (Suppl. 4), 23-33.
[http://dx.doi.org/10.1634/theoncologist.2010-S4-23] [PMID: 21115578]

Mazzaferro, V, Regalia, E, Doci, R, Andreola, S, Pulvirenti, A, Bozzetti, F, Montalto, F, Ammatuna, M,

Morabito, A & Gennari, L (1996) Liver transplantation for the treatment of small hepatocellular carcinomas in patients with cirrhosis. *N Engl J Med,* 334, 693-9.
[http://dx.doi.org/10.1056/NEJM199603143341104] [PMID: 8594428]

Muthu, MS & Feng, SS (2013) Theranostic liposomes for cancer diagnosis and treatment: current development and pre-clinical success. *Expert Opin Drug Deliv,* 10, 151-5.
[http://dx.doi.org/10.1517/17425247.2013.729576] [PMID: 23061654]

Pan, Z, Di, S, Shi, B, Jiang, H, Shi, Z, Liu, Y, Wang, Y, Luo, H, Yu, M, Wu, X & Li, Z (2018) Increased antitumor activities of glypican-3-specific chimeric antigen receptor-modified T cells by coexpression of a soluble PD1-CH3 fusion protein. *Cancer Immunol Immunother,* 67, 1621-34.
[http://dx.doi.org/10.1007/s00262-018-2221-1] [PMID: 30078052]

Parkin, DM (2001) Global cancer statistics in the year 2000. *Lancet Oncol,* 2, 533-43.
[http://dx.doi.org/10.1016/S1470-2045(01)00486-7] [PMID: 11905707]

Pavlakis, N, Sjoquist, KM, Martin, AJ, Tsobanis, E, Yip, S, Kang, YK, Bang, YJ, Alcindor, T, O'Callaghan, CJ, Burnell, MJ, Tebbutt, NC, Rha, SY, Lee, J, Cho, JY, Lipton, LR, Wong, M, Strickland, A, Kim, JW, Zalcberg, JR, Simes, J & Goldstein, D (2016) Regorafenib for the Treatment of Advanced Gastric Cancer (INTEGRATE): A Multinational Placebo-Controlled Phase II Trial. *J Clin Oncol,* 34, 2728-35.
[http://dx.doi.org/10.1200/JCO.2015.65.1901] [PMID: 27325864]

Pawlik, TM, Delman, KA, Vauthey, JN, Nagorney, DM, Ng, IO, Ikai, I, Yamaoka, Y, Belghiti, J, Lauwers, GY, Poon, RT & Abdalla, EK (2005) Tumor size predicts vascular invasion and histologic grade: Implications for selection of surgical treatment for hepatocellular carcinoma. *Liver Transpl,* 11, 1086-92.
[http://dx.doi.org/10.1002/lt.20472] [PMID: 16123959]

Pelletier, G, Roche, A, Ink, O, Anciaux, ML, Derhy, S, Rougier, P, Lenoir, C, Attali, P & Etienne, JP (1990) A randomized trial of hepatic arterial chemoembolization in patients with unresectable hepatocellular carcinoma. *J Hepatol,* 11, 181-4.
[http://dx.doi.org/10.1016/0168-8278(90)90110-D] [PMID: 2174933]

Poon, RT, Lau, C, Pang, R, Ng, KK, Yuen, J & Fan, ST (2007) High serum vascular endothelial growth factor levels predict poor prognosis after radiofrequency ablation of hepatocellular carcinoma: importance of tumor biomarker in ablative therapies. *Ann Surg Oncol,* 14, 1835-45.
[http://dx.doi.org/10.1245/s10434-007-9366-z] [PMID: 17406950]

Ribas, A & Wolchok, JD (2018) Cancer immunotherapy using checkpoint blockade. *Science,* 359, 1350-5.
[http://dx.doi.org/10.1126/science.aar4060] [PMID: 29567705]

Ringelhan, M, Pfister, D, O'Connor, T, Pikarsky, E & Heikenwalder, M (2018) The immunology of hepatocellular carcinoma. *Nat Immunol,* 19, 222-32.
[http://dx.doi.org/10.1038/s41590-018-0044-z] [PMID: 29379119]

Roayaie, S, Bassi, D, Tarchi, P, Labow, D & Schwartz, M (2011) Second hepatic resection for recurrent hepatocellular cancer: a Western experience. *J Hepatol,* 55, 346-50.
[http://dx.doi.org/10.1016/j.jhep.2010.11.026] [PMID: 21147184]

Roayaie, S, Jibara, G, Tabrizian, P, Park, JW, Yang, J, Yan, L, Schwartz, M, Han, G, Izzo, F, Chen, M, Blanc, JF, Johnson, P, Kudo, M, Roberts, LR & Sherman, M (2015) The role of hepatic resection in the treatment of hepatocellular cancer. *Hepatology,* 62, 440-51.
[http://dx.doi.org/10.1002/hep.27745] [PMID: 25678263]

Roberts, LR, Sirlin, CB, Zaiem, F, Almasri, J, Prokop, LJ, Heimbach, JK, Murad, MH & Mohammed, K (2018) Imaging for the diagnosis of hepatocellular carcinoma: A systematic review and meta-analysis. *Hepatology,* 67, 401-21.
[http://dx.doi.org/10.1002/hep.29487] [PMID: 28859233]

Rotow, J & Bivona, TG (2017) Understanding and targeting resistance mechanisms in NSCLC. *Nat Rev Cancer,* 17, 637-58.
[http://dx.doi.org/10.1038/nrc.2017.84] [PMID: 29068003]

Sangro, B, Gomez-Martin, C, de la Mata, M, Iñarrairaegui, M, Garralda, E, Barrera, P, Riezu-Boj, JI, Larrea, E, Alfaro, C, Sarobe, P, Lasarte, JJ, Pérez-Gracia, JL, Melero, I & Prieto, J (2013) A clinical trial of CTLA-4 blockade with tremelimumab in patients with hepatocellular carcinoma and chronic hepatitis C. *J Hepatol,* 59, 81-8.
[http://dx.doi.org/10.1016/j.jhep.2013.02.022] [PMID: 23466307]

Sapisochin, G & Bruix, J (2017) Liver transplantation for hepatocellular carcinoma: outcomes and novel surgical approaches. *Nat Rev Gastroenterol Hepatol,* 14, 203-17.
[http://dx.doi.org/10.1038/nrgastro.2016.193] [PMID: 28053342]

Sawada, Y, Yoshikawa, T, Nobuoka, D, Shirakawa, H, Kuronuma, T, Motomura, Y, Mizuno, S, Ishii, H, Nakachi, K, Konishi, M, Nakagohri, T, Takahashi, S, Gotohda, N, Takayama, T, Yamao, K, Uesaka, K, Furuse, J, Kinoshita, T & Nakatsura, T (2012) Phase I trial of a glypican-3-derived peptide vaccine for advanced hepatocellular carcinoma: immunologic evidence and potential for improving overall survival. *Clin Cancer Res,* 18, 3686-96.
[http://dx.doi.org/10.1158/1078-0432.CCR-11-3044] [PMID: 22577059]

Shan, J, Shen, J, Liu, L, Xia, F, Xu, C, Duan, G, Xu, Y, Ma, Q, Yang, Z, Zhang, Q, Ma, L, Liu, J, Xu, S, Yan, X, Bie, P, Cui, Y, Bian, XW & Qian, C (2012) Nanog regulates self-renewal of cancer stem cells through the insulin-like growth factor pathway in human hepatocellular carcinoma. *Hepatology,* 56, 1004-14.
[http://dx.doi.org/10.1002/hep.25745] [PMID: 22473773]

Siegel, R, Naishadham, D & Jemal, A (2013) Cancer statistics, 2013. *CA Cancer J Clin,* 63, 11-30.
[http://dx.doi.org/10.3322/caac.21166] [PMID: 23335087]

Sieghart, W, Hucke, F & Peck-Radosavljevic, M (2015) Transarterial chemoembolization: modalities, indication, and patient selection. *J Hepatol,* 62, 1187-95.
[http://dx.doi.org/10.1016/j.jhep.2015.02.010] [PMID: 25681552]

Sun, D, Liu, H, Dai, X, Zheng, X, Yan, J, Wei, R, Fu, X, Huang, M, Shen, A, Huang, X, Ding, J & Geng, M (2017) Aspirin disrupts the mTOR-Raptor complex and potentiates the anti-cancer activities of sorafenib *via* mTORC1 inhibition. *Cancer Lett,* 406, 105-15.
[http://dx.doi.org/10.1016/j.canlet.2017.06.029] [PMID: 28687354]

Tanaka, S & Arii, S (2012) Molecular targeted therapies in hepatocellular carcinoma. *Semin Oncol,* 39, 486-92.
[http://dx.doi.org/10.1053/j.seminoncol.2012.05.005] [PMID: 22846865]

Tangkijvanich, P, Anukulkarnkusol, N, Suwangool, P, Lertmaharit, S, Hanvivatvong, O, Kullavanijaya, P & Poovorawan, Y (2000) Clinical characteristics and prognosis of hepatocellular carcinoma: analysis based on serum alpha-fetoprotein levels. *J Clin Gastroenterol,* 31, 302-8.
[http://dx.doi.org/10.1097/00004836-200012000-00007] [PMID: 11129271]

Thabut, D, Routray, C, Lomberk, G, Shergill, U, Glaser, K, Huebert, R, Patel, L, Masyuk, T, Blechacz, B, Vercnocke, A, Ritman, E, Ehman, R, Urrutia, R & Shah, V (2011) Complementary vascular and matrix regulatory pathways underlie the beneficial mechanism of action of sorafenib in liver fibrosis. *Hepatology,* 54, 573-85.
[http://dx.doi.org/10.1002/hep.24427] [PMID: 21567441]

Tinkle, CL & Haas-Kogan, D (2012) Hepatocellular carcinoma: natural history, current management, and emerging tools. *Biologics,* 6, 207-19.
[PMID: 22904613]

Toso, C, Meeberg, G, Hernandez-Alejandro, R, Dufour, JF, Marotta, P, Majno, P & Kneteman, NM (2015) Total tumor volume and alpha-fetoprotein for selection of transplant candidates with hepatocellular carcinoma: A prospective validation. *Hepatology,* 62, 158-65.
[http://dx.doi.org/10.1002/hep.27787] [PMID: 25777590]

Tremosini, S, Forner, A, Boix, L, Vilana, R, Bianchi, L, Reig, M, Rimola, J, Rodríguez-Lope, C, Ayuso, C, Solé, M & Bruix, J (2012) Prospective validation of an immunohistochemical panel (glypican 3, heat shock protein 70 and glutamine synthetase) in liver biopsies for diagnosis of very early hepatocellular carcinoma.

Gut, 61, 1481-7.
[http://dx.doi.org/10.1136/gutjnl-2011-301862] [PMID: 22287594]

Truong, P, Rahal, A & Kallail, KJ (2016) Metastatic Hepatocellular Carcinoma Responsive to Pembrolizumab. *Cureus,* 8, e631.
[PMID: 27433410]

Uka, K, Aikata, H, Takaki, S, Shirakawa, H, Jeong, SC, Yamashina, K, Hiramatsu, A, Kodama, H, Takahashi, S & Chayama, K (2007) Clinical features and prognosis of patients with extrahepatic metastases from hepatocellular carcinoma. *World J Gastroenterol,* 13, 414-20.
[http://dx.doi.org/10.3748/wjg.v13.i3.414] [PMID: 17230611]

Velázquez, RF, Rodríguez, M, Navascués, CA, Linares, A, Pérez, R, Sotorríos, NG, Martínez, I & Rodrigo, L (2003) Prospective analysis of risk factors for hepatocellular carcinoma in patients with liver cirrhosis. *Hepatology,* 37, 520-7.
[http://dx.doi.org/10.1053/jhep.2003.50093] [PMID: 12601348]

Villanueva, A (2019) Hepatocellular Carcinoma. Reply. *N Engl J Med,* 381, e2. [Reply].
[http://dx.doi.org/10.1056/NEJMc1906565] [PMID: 31269387]

Wang, BW, Mok, KT, Liu, SI, Chou, NH, Tsai, CC, Chen, IS, Yeh, MH & Chen, YC (2008) Is hepatectomy beneficial in the treatment of multinodular hepatocellular carcinoma? *J Formos Med Assoc,* 107, 616-26.
[http://dx.doi.org/10.1016/S0929-6646(08)60179-5] [PMID: 18678545]

Wang, L & Wang, FS (2019) Clinical immunology and immunotherapy for hepatocellular carcinoma: current progress and challenges. *Hepatol Int,* 13, 521-33.
[http://dx.doi.org/10.1007/s12072-019-09967-y] [PMID: 31352593]

Wang, Y, Chen, M, Wu, Z, Tong, C, Dai, H, Guo, Y, Liu, Y, Huang, J, Lv, H, Luo, C, Feng, KC, Yang, QM, Li, XL & Han, W (2018) CD133-directed CAR T cells for advanced metastasis malignancies: A phase I trial. *OncoImmunology,* 7, e1440169.
[http://dx.doi.org/10.1080/2162402X.2018.1440169] [PMID: 29900044]

Wehrenberg-Klee, E, Goyal, L, Dugan, M, Zhu, AX & Ganguli, S (2018) Y-90 Radioembolization Combined with a PD-1 Inhibitor for Advanced Hepatocellular Carcinoma. *Cardiovasc Intervent Radiol,* 41, 1799-802.
[http://dx.doi.org/10.1007/s00270-018-1993-1] [PMID: 29845347]

Wilhelm, S, Carter, C, Lynch, M, Lowinger, T, Dumas, J, Smith, RA, Schwartz, B, Simantov, R & Kelley, S (2006) Discovery and development of sorafenib: a multikinase inhibitor for treating cancer. *Nat Rev Drug Discov,* 5, 835-44.
[http://dx.doi.org/10.1038/nrd2130] [PMID: 17016424]

Wilhelm, SM, Carter, C, Tang, L, Wilkie, D, McNabola, A, Rong, H, Chen, C, Zhang, X, Vincent, P, McHugh, M, Cao, Y, Shujath, J, Gawlak, S, Eveleigh, D, Rowley, B, Liu, L, Adnane, L, Lynch, M, Auclair, D, Taylor, I, Gedrich, R, Voznesensky, A, Riedl, B, Post, LE, Bollag, G & Trail, PA (2004) BAY 43-9006 exhibits broad spectrum oral antitumor activity and targets the RAF/MEK/ERK pathway and receptor tyrosine kinases involved in tumor progression and angiogenesis. *Cancer Res,* 64, 7099-109.
[http://dx.doi.org/10.1158/0008-5472.CAN-04-1443] [PMID: 15466206]

Willatt, JM, Hussain, HK, Adusumilli, S & Marrero, JA (2008) MR Imaging of hepatocellular carcinoma in the cirrhotic liver: challenges and controversies. *Radiology,* 247, 311-30.
[http://dx.doi.org/10.1148/radiol.2472061331] [PMID: 18430871]

Wu, JT (1990) Serum alpha-fetoprotein and its lectin reactivity in liver diseases: a review. *Ann Clin Lab Sci,* 20, 98-105.
[PMID: 1691611]

Xia, Q, Li, L & Zhao, L (2017) Silica nanoparticle-based dual-responsive nanoprodrug system for liver cancer therapy. *Exp Ther Med,* 14, 2071-7.
[http://dx.doi.org/10.3892/etm.2017.4768] [PMID: 28962126]

Xiang, D, Cheng, Z, Liu, H, Wang, X, Han, T, Sun, W, Li, X, Yang, W, Chen, C, Xia, M, Liu, N, Yin, S, Jin,

G, Lee, T, Dong, L, Hu, H, Wang, H & Ding, J (2017) Shp2 promotes liver cancer stem cell expansion by augmenting β-catenin signaling and predicts chemotherapeutic response of patients. *Hepatology,* 65, 1566-80. [http://dx.doi.org/10.1002/hep.28919] [PMID: 28059452]

Xu, F, Jin, T, Zhu, Y & Dai, C (2018) Immune checkpoint therapy in liver cancer. *J Exp Clin Cancer Res,* 37, 110.
[http://dx.doi.org/10.1186/s13046-018-0777-4] [PMID: 29843754]

Yang, HI, Yuen, MF, Chan, HL, Han, KH, Chen, PJ, Kim, DY, Ahn, SH, Chen, CJ, Wong, VW & Seto, WK (2011) Risk estimation for hepatocellular carcinoma in chronic hepatitis B (REACH-B): development and validation of a predictive score. *Lancet Oncol,* 12, 568-74.
[http://dx.doi.org/10.1016/S1470-2045(11)70077-8] [PMID: 21497551]

Yarden, Y & Sliwkowski, MX (2001) Untangling the ErbB signalling network. *Nat Rev Mol Cell Biol,* 2, 127-37.
[http://dx.doi.org/10.1038/35052073] [PMID: 11252954]

Yau, T, Tang, VY, Yao, TJ, Fan, ST, Lo, CM & Poon, RT (2014) Development of Hong Kong Liver Cancer staging system with treatment stratification for patients with hepatocellular carcinoma. *Gastroenterology,* 146, 1691-700.e3.
[http://dx.doi.org/10.1053/j.gastro.2014.02.032] [PMID: 24583061]

Yoon, KT, Kim, JK, Kim, DY, Ahn, SH, Lee, JD, Yun, M, Rha, SY, Chon, CY & Han, KH (2007) Role of 18F-fluorodeoxyglucose positron emission tomography in detecting extrahepatic metastasis in pretreatment staging of hepatocellular carcinoma. *Oncology,* 72 (Suppl. 1), 104-10.
[http://dx.doi.org/10.1159/000111715] [PMID: 18087190]

Younossi, Z, Stepanova, M, Ong, JP, Jacobson, IM, Bugianesi, E, Duseja, A, Eguchi, Y, Wong, VW, Negro, F, Yilmaz, Y, Romero-Gomez, M, George, J, Ahmed, A, Wong, R, Younossi, I, Ziayee, M & Afendy, A (2019) Nonalcoholic Steatohepatitis Is the Fastest Growing Cause of Hepatocellular Carcinoma in Liver Transplant Candidates. *Clin Gastroenterol Hepatol,* 17, 748-755.e3.
[http://dx.doi.org/10.1016/j.cgh.2018.05.057] [PMID: 29908364]

Zhang, Y, Li, M, Gao, X, Chen, Y & Liu, T (2019) Nanotechnology in cancer diagnosis: progress, challenges and opportunities. *J Hematol Oncol,* 12, 137.
[http://dx.doi.org/10.1186/s13045-019-0833-3] [PMID: 31847897]

Zhao, D, Zhai, B, He, C, Tan, G, Jiang, X, Pan, S, Dong, X, Wei, Z, Ma, L, Qiao, H, Jiang, H & Sun, X (2014) Upregulation of HIF-2α induced by sorafenib contributes to the resistance by activating the TGF-α/EGFR pathway in hepatocellular carcinoma cells. *Cell Signal,* 26, 1030-9.
[http://dx.doi.org/10.1016/j.cellsig.2014.01.026] [PMID: 24486412]

Zhao, R, Li, T, Zheng, G, Jiang, K, Fan, L & Shao, J (2017) Simultaneous inhibition of growth and metastasis of hepatocellular carcinoma by co-delivery of ursolic acid and sorafenib using lactobionic acid modified and pH-sensitive chitosan-conjugated mesoporous silica nanocomplex. *Biomaterials,* 143, 1-16.
[http://dx.doi.org/10.1016/j.biomaterials.2017.07.030] [PMID: 28755539]

Zhao, X, Chen, Q, Liu, W, Li, Y, Tang, H, Liu, X & Yang, X (2014) Codelivery of doxorubicin and curcumin with lipid nanoparticles results in improved efficacy of chemotherapy in liver cancer. *Int J Nanomedicine,* 10, 257-70.
[PMID: 25565818]

Zheng, L, Yang, W, Wu, F, Wang, C, Yu, L, Tang, L, Qiu, B, Li, Y, Guo, L, Wu, M, Feng, G, Zou, D & Wang, H (2013) Prognostic significance of AMPK activation and therapeutic effects of metformin in hepatocellular carcinoma. *Clin Cancer Res,* 19, 5372-80.
[http://dx.doi.org/10.1158/1078-0432.CCR-13-0203] [PMID: 23942093]

Zhong, JH, Xiang, BD, Gong, WF, Ke, Y, Mo, QG, Ma, L, Liu, X & Li, LQ (2013) Comparison of long-term survival of patients with BCLC stage B hepatocellular carcinoma after liver resection or transarterial chemoembolization. *PLoS One,* 8, e68193.
[http://dx.doi.org/10.1371/journal.pone.0068193] [PMID: 23874536]

Zhu, YJ, Zheng, B, Wang, HY & Chen, L (2017) New knowledge of the mechanisms of sorafenib resistance in liver cancer. *Acta Pharmacol Sin,* 38, 614-22.
[http://dx.doi.org/10.1038/aps.2017.5] [PMID: 28344323]

Zucman-Rossi, J, Villanueva, A, Nault, JC & Llovet, JM (2015) Genetic Landscape and Biomarkers of Hepatocellular Carcinoma. *Gastroenterology,* 149, 1226-1239.e4.
[http://dx.doi.org/10.1053/j.gastro.2015.05.061] [PMID: 26099527]

CHAPTER 3

Nanoformulations and Their Therapeutic Advantages

D. Nedra Karunaratne[1,*], **Thusini D. Wijerathne**[1], **Nuwanthi P. Katuwavila**[2] and **Geethi K. Pamunuwa**[3]

[1] *Department of Chemistry, University of Peradeniya, Peradeniya, Sri Lanka*

[2] *Faculty of Engineering and Science, National School of Business Management, Mahenwatte, Pitipana, Homagama, Sri Lanka*

[3] *Department of Horticulture and Landscape Gardening, Faculty of Agriculture and Plantation Management, Wayamba University of Sri Lanka, Makandura, Gonawila, Sri Lanka*

Abstract: Cancer therapy involves nanomedicine, which can provide a plethora of advantages unattainable *via* conventional medicine as the materials of nano-level exhibit unique physicochemical and biological properties. Both cancer therapy and cancer therapy research utilize nanoformulations based on liposomes, polymeric nanoparticles, solid lipid nanoparticles, metal nanoparticles, dendrimers, and nanoemulsions for facilitating high specificity negating off-target toxicity, prolonged-release maintaining drug concentration and reducing dosing frequency, increased solubilization and absorption, and penetration of impermeable barriers. The entrée to this chapter is thus made with a brief description of nanomedicine, which is followed by a description of the designing of nanoformulations for therapeutics. Explanations on the types and advantages of nanoformulations are also given. The second section of the chapter describes nanoformulations as therapeutics for cancer, explaining the different targeting strategies and novel approaches involving nanoparticles. Like numerous other cancers, nanoformulations are researched extensively in therapy for hepatocellular carcinoma, the second leading cause of cancer-related deaths. The final section of the chapter deals with the therapeutic advantages of nanoformulations in hepatocellular carcinoma. The prominent nanomaterials investigated in hepatocellular carcinoma therapy include nanoparticles of biopolymers, nanoparticles of artificial biodegradable polymers, metallic nanoparticles, carbon nanotubes, and mesoporous nanoparticles. Targeting of drug-loaded nanoparticles is achieved in therapy for hepatocellular carcinoma *via* passive targeting and/or active targeting. A key milestone in hepatocellular carcinoma therapy is the approval of the drug Zinostatin stimalamer, an emulsion-based formulation, by the Japanese Ministry of Labour, Health, and Welfare.

* **Corresponding author Nedra Karunaratne:** Department of Chemistry, University of Peradeniya, Peradeniya, Sri Lanka; E-mail: nedrak@pdn.ac.ik

Biswajit Mukherjee (Ed.)

Keywords: Active targeting, Bioavailability, Biodegradable, Cancer, Chemotherapy, Controlled release, Dendrimers, Emulsions, Hepatocellular carcinoma, Immunoliposomes, Liposomes, Metal nanoparticles nanoformulations, Nano-medicine, Nanoparticles, Passive targeting, Polymeric nanoparticles, Solid lipid nanoparticles, Therapeutics, Targeted delivery.

INTRODUCTION

Brief Introduction to Nanomedicine

Healthcare and the application of medical practice date back to ancient times and early civilizations. Medicine involves the prevention of illness, restoration of health, and diagnosis and treatment of ailments. When nanotechnology applications are used for diagnosis (nanobiosensors), drug delivery (nanoparticles and nanomaterials), and treatment based on nanodevices, imaging techniques, *etc.* (Zhou *et al.*, 2019), that branch of medical applications is called nanomedicine (Karunaratne, 2007). The positive side of nanomedicine deals with the premise that nano-based applications provide a service above the standard conventional methods of medicine. The unique properties, both physicochemical and biological at the nanolevel, have proved nanomedicine to afford conventionally unknown benefits. Thus, many reports based on the nano-level advantages have been documented (Yetisgin *et al.*, 2020).

Many of the reported research on nanomedicine are concerned with drug delivery. Therapeutic advantages of nanoformulations are observed when drugs are delivered to the disease site by targeting or improving the bioavailability of the drug to make it more effective. The importance of formulating drugs at the nano level is discussed in the following sections.

Designing Nanoformulations for Therapeutics

In the past decade, nanoformulations of various drugs took center stage with claims for improved delivery and efficacy due to properties at the nano level. Some of the salient features are the ability to target specific tissues (Jafari *et al.*, 2012), impart biodegradability, increase bioavailability (Yallapu *et al.*, 2015), protect the drug in harsh environments, particularly in the gastrointestinal tract (GIT), and overcome biological barriers (Khan *et al.*, 2018).

The design of nanoformulations must consider the mode of delivery, type of drug, and the carrier to be utilized. Oral administration is a widespread and sought-after drug administration route since it is convenient, non-invasive, economical, and independent of specific medical requirements (Khosa *et al.*, 2018; Kermanizadeh *et al.*, 2018). Oral delivery requires nanoformulation to resist the gastric environment and safely deliver the drug cargo to the intended delivery site. Therefore, the formulation must be resilient to the pH changes and the enzymes encountered throughout the GIT. Nanocarriers facilitate the delivery of drug molecules to target sites in the gastrointestinal tract despite the harsh environment (Plapied *et al.*, 2011). Encapsulation of drug molecules in nanocarriers protects them from enzymatic and chemical degradation in the GIT, enhances the absorption in the intestine to reach the bloodstream, facilitates targeted delivery, and also controls the release of drug molecules (Reinholz *et al.*, 2018). Once the drug-loaded nanocarrier is in the intestine, it either releases drug molecules for intestinal absorption, or the entire particle has to pass several cell barriers to reach the bloodstream and then the targeted cells (Reinholz *et al.*, 2018). Crossing intestinal epithelial cells to reach lamina propia and the endothelial cell layer of blood vessels to reach blood vessel lumen are some challenges for nanocarriers to overcome (Reinholz *et al.*, 2018). Therefore, the successful delivery of orally administered therapeutic nanocarriers to targeted cells may be affected by the type, size, composition, and surface modifications of the nanoparticle. For instance, the degradation of liposomes in the gastrointestinal tract is facilitated by the presence of bile salts (Rhee and Mansour, 2011). Modifying the liposome surface with polyethylene glycol (PEG) has imparted some resistance to degradation (Rhee and Mansour, 2011). Regarding orally administered polymeric nanoparticles, chitosan has gained popularity as a natural polymeric material that possesses the ability to increase permeability in the intestine by opening tight junctions (Plapied *et al.*, 2011). Likewise, drug formulations intended for colon cancer need to avoid the harsh conditions of the stomach and upper intestine by avoiding degradation and absorption until they reach the colon (Banerjee *et al.*, 2017).

On the other hand, the efficacy of topical delivery formulations depends on the penetrability of the dermal barrier. *The stratum corneum* of the epidermis is an obstacle for skin administration of drugs since it limits drug permeation (Zhang *et al.*, 2013). The nature of the dermal cells and the epidermal cell composition requires special consideration and the polarity of the drug being delivered when selecting the suitable carrier. For optimum drug encapsulation, combined with its full release, both carrier, and drug compatibilities should be considered. In skin cancers and other skin-related diseases, dermal administration of drugs holds higher efficacy than oral and parenteral delivery (Sala *et al.*, 2018). Transdermal drug delivery attracts more interest since those drug particles are not subjected to "first-pass" metabolism and can be achieved with less toxic side effects (Sala *et al.*, 2018). Designing suitable nanocarriers enhance the permeation of drugs through the intact skin.

The ability of nanoformulations to increase the bioavailability of poorly water-soluble drugs is of particular interest (Karunaratne *et al.*, 2017). Several carriers have enabled improved absorption of less soluble drugs through encapsulation in delivery vehicles. Polymer-based delivery vehicles may be polysaccharides, proteins, or synthetic biodegradable polymers. Similarly, lipid carriers have also shown improved drug performance as liposomal or solid lipid nanoparticle vehicles (Wang *et al.*, 2018). Other types of carriers based on metal nanoparticles (Hu *et al.*, 2018), dendrimers (Yousef *et al.*, 2018), and peptides (Karunaratne *et al.*, 2015) are also documented.

The importance of designing nanoformulations is elaborated by Ling *et al.* (2014) in their formulation of a pH-sensitive nano-formulated triptolide targeted toward hepatocellular carcinoma. Here they have labeled the polymer vehicle with a tumor-targeting ligand and formulated a pH-sensitive release of the drug from the carrier. The fact that targeting the drug to a specific site reduces the load of drug required and avoids absorption or degradation at other locations before reaching its target is elaborated by Banerjee *et al.* (2017). More examples of drug targeting in hepatocellular carcinoma are discussed in the section 'Mechanism of action of nanoformulations in hepatocellular carcinoma.'

Finally, for maximum results from the designed nanoformulation, the therapeutic advantage should be based on the disease being treated. When delivering drugs to the brain, the nanoformulation must be designed to permeate through the blood-brain barrier (BBB) and deliver the drug in the optimum concentration. The lipidic nature of the BBB favors nonpolar carrier materials, and many of these drugs are formulated in lipid carriers (liposomes, micelles) or polymer nanoparticles (Khan *et al.*, 2018). Saha *et al.* (2020) prepared liposomes that could entrap both siRNA and paclitaxel to transport these drugs across the BBB. The use of amphetamine as the targeting ligand was exploited by conjugating it to the lipids to enable the liposomes to target brain tumors (Saha *et al.*, 2020).

Therefore, the success of therapeutic nanoformulation depends on careful design strategies to ensure safe passage to the intended target tissues.

Types of Therapeutic Nanoformulations

Nanoformulations are available in various forms. Polymer nanoformulations, metal nanoformulations, solid lipid nanoformulations, and microemulsions are a few of them. A comprehensive account of various types of nanoformulations such as peptide carriers, lipid carriers, immunoliposomes, mixed systems like ferri-liposomes, dendrimers, and polymer-carriers is explicitly explained by Jafari *et al.* (2012). Delivery systems based on lipids, including pH-sensitive and targeting liposomes, nanostructured lipid carriers, solid lipid nanoparticles, and lipid-polymer hybrid nanoparticles, are described by Yingchoncharoen *et al.* (2016). A list of different types of nanoformulations is depicted in Table **1**.

Table 1. Applications and composition of different types of nanoformulations.

Type of Nanoformulation	Application	Carrier	References
Lipid- liposome	Delivery of doxorubicin (Doxil, Myocet), daunorubicin (DaunoXome), Marqibo and DepoCyt	Phospholipids/ sphingolipids	Yingchoncharoen *et al.*, (2016)
Lipid emulsions	Drug delivery through microemulsions and SMEDDS	Lipid	Yan *et al.* (2019a)
Lipid- immunoliposomes	Targeting with antibody linked liposomes	Lipid conjugated with antibodies	Wang *et al.*, (2018); Alavizadeh *et al.*, (2016)
Polymer	Nanoformulations based on natural or synthetic polymer materials for improved delivery	Galactosylated polypeptide (PGLG-b-PLGA) nanoplatforms, dextran-dox nanoparticles, chitosan, PLGL, PEG-PLA	Wang *et al.*, (2019); Devulapally *et al.*, (2016).
Metal nanoparticles	Metal nanoparticle - chemotherapy drug conjugates	Gold nanoparticles, silver nanoparticles	Paino *et al.*, (2012); Zhu *et al.*, (2016).
Mesoporous silica nanoparticles	Drug delivery to tumors	Silica nanoparticles decorated with folic acid	Lu *et al.* (2012)
Nanogels	Drug loaded nanogel for drug delivery	Chitosan nanogels for colorectal drug delivery. Alginate coated chitosan nanogel	Feng *et al.* (2015), El-Feky *et al.*, (2017).
Dendrimers	Targeted dendrimers, Drug conjugated dendrimers	Asialoglycoprotein receptor-targeted PAMAM, PAMAM with conjugated drug	Yousef *et al.*, (2018); Kuruvilla *et al.*, (2017)

PAMAM = Poly(amidoamine), SMEDDS = self-microemulsifying drug delivery system, PGLG-b-PLGA = galactosylated polypeptide, PLGL = poly(lactic-co-glycolide), PEG-PLA polyethylene glycol-polylactide.

Targeted Delivery Applications

Nanoparticle drug delivery systems, as opposed to conventional dosing, possess several advantages. One of the many positive advantages is targeted delivery to specific tissues. It is a technique where the nanoformulation is designed to carry the drug to its target site. The benefits are the precise delivery of the drug at the disease center resulting in the lower dose required to avoid side effects and provide a constant dosage at the targeted site. The carrier is modified such that receptors recognize it at the target site. It enables the drug-carrying nanoparticle to be taken up only by the cells having the specific receptor. This type of delivery is termed active delivery as opposed to passive targeting, in which the nanoparticles without a targeting ligand accumulate at the tumor site due to leaky vasculature at the site and enhanced permeability and retention (EPR effect) (Yetisgin *et al.*, 2020), or due to coating the nanoparticle to increase its circulation time. Active targeting requires modification of the nanoparticle carrier by conjugating the targeting ligand to the matrix (Fig. **1**). For example, immunoliposomes are prepared by conjugating antibodies to the liposomes in order to selectively target cells presenting the antigen (Wang *et al.*, 2018). The work of Yousef *et al.* (2018) describes the linking of the targeting ligand galactosamine to polyamidoamine (PAMAM) dendrimers to target an anticancer curcumin derivative (CDF) to hepatocellular carcinoma (HCC). The HCC cells overexpress asialoglycoprotein receptors having a high binding affinity to galactosamine (Yousef *et al.*, 2018). Mesoporous silica nanoparticles (MSN) can release drug molecules at target sites when modified such that drug release is triggered by a stimulus (Wang *et al.*, 2015). Here, the release of the drug is sensitive to the factors such as external pH, temperature, redox potential, and enzymes. They used macrocyclic β-cyclodextrin (β-CD) to act as a capping agent on previously attached stalks on modified MSN where acidic medium caused a weakening of the interactions between β-CD and stalk to release the drug molecules (Wang *et al.*, 2015). Further, surface modification with hyaluronic acid facilitates both targeting and controlled release of drugs since hyaluronic acid binds to CD-44 receptors on cancer cells and enzymatic degradation with hyaluronidase-1, drug release takes place (Wang *et al.*, 2015).

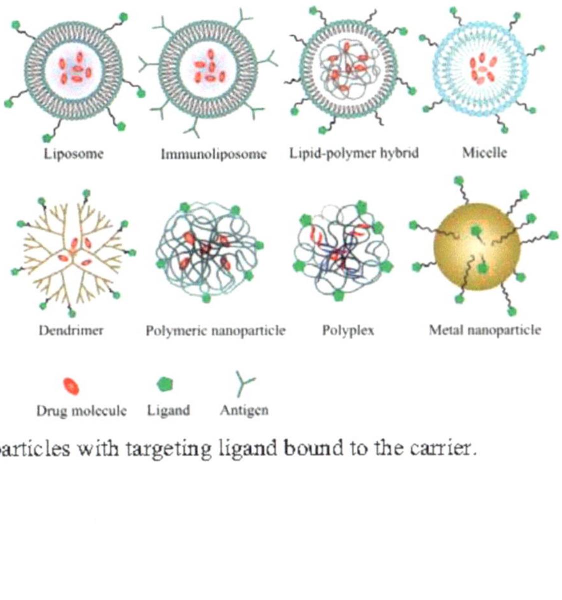

Fig. (1). Types of nanoparticles with targeting ligand bound to the carrier.

Advantages of Nanoformulations

The many pluses of nanoformulations are described by Xu *et al.* (2015). The most important characteristics of any formulation are the benefit afforded to the patient in terms of alleviating the disease symptoms and the ease of administration of the dose. With that in mind, the following advantages of nanoformulations over conventional drugs are addressed below.

A Methods of administration

B Increased solubility and absorption

C Delivery to target tissues

D Maintaining a steady drug concentration in the system

E Penetration of impermeable barriers

Methods of Administration

Commonly used methods of administration such as oral, parental, and ocular routes have issues related to poor solubility of drugs resulting in unfavorable pharmacokinetics, which render them less efficacious. However, nanoformulations, with their small size in the nano- or submicron-range, ability to improve the solubility of drugs through encapsulation, and ease of administration through many of the conventional routes have given new life to some less effective conventional methods for delivery of therapeutic formulations. By changing the delivery matrix (carriers), many of the obstacles faced in delivery through conventional routes have been overcome. Though high in therapeutic potential in many diseases, curcumin is hampered in oral delivery due to its low solubility, physicochemical instability, poor bioavailability, rapid metabolism, and poor pharmacokinetics. Thus, the advantages of curcumin nanoformulations are reviewed extensively by Yallapu *et al.* (2015), where successful delivery through various nanoformulations is elaborated.

In the area of lung diseases, challenges arise due to drugs administered by oral and parenteral delivery routes undergoing first-pass chemical modification in the liver, poor biodistribution, limitations of absorption in the GIT, among other barriers reducing drug delivery at the destination site. The nanoformulations compatible with inhalation as the delivery route are suggested by Lim *et al.* (2016). The polymeric nanoparticles displayed improved pharmacokinetics and better aqueous solubility and properties related to protection from endogenous factors (hydrolytic and enzymatic degradation) and increased bioavailability. However, the authors expressed concern regarding the uptake of the nanoparticles by alveolar macrophages and the presence of sputum, increasing the internalization of particles into epithelial cells (Lim *et al.*, 2016).

Another challenge in the effective delivery of drugs, overcoming the harsh conditions of the upper GI tract, is in colon delivery (Banerjee *et al.*, 2017). Colon cancer is treated by chemotherapy resulting in unfavorable effects of drug toxicity, poor absorption, and degradation of the drug in the transition through the GI tract. To enable the drug to reach the colon safely, nanoformulations with targeting ability resulting in site-specific delivery have been formulated (Banerjee *et al.*, 2017).

In the case of hepatic delivery, drugs used for the treatment of HCC must overcome the first-pass metabolism. As such, targeted delivery to the cancerous cells has been designed. Nanoformulations may be delivered to tumor cells overexpressing cell surface receptors by active targeting or passive targeting *via* the enhanced permeation and retention (EPR) effect (Varshosaz and Farzan, 2015). It is reported that nanoparticle-based drug delivery systems can raise the efficacy of therapeutic drugs in HCC treatment in terms of targeted delivery, enhanced circulation time, increased bioavailability, and reduced toxicity (Devulapally *et al.*, 2016; Ling *et al.*, 2014)

Increased Solubility and Absorption

One of the greatest advantages of a successful drug candidate is its solubility. The low solubility of drug molecules exerts various drawbacks regarding the efficacy of therapeutic treatments, such as limiting the absorption of orally administered hydrophobic drugs in the GIT. Encapsulation of less soluble drugs, especially hydrophobic drugs, in nanoparticles, can increase drug solubility and bioavailability (Wais *et al.*, 2016). Nanocarriers, for instance, liposomes, can accommodate both hydrophilic and hydrophobic drug particles. Increased solubility enhances drug absorption, bioavailability, and tissue accessibility. Several nanotechnological strategies to improve solubility are reviewed by Karunaratne *et al.* (2017). Other than nanosizing the drug, this review elaborates on solubilization techniques, including nanocrystal colloidal delivery systems, self-emulsifying drugs, micelles, liposomes, emulsions, solid lipid nanoparticles, and drug complexes with carriers such as cyclodextrins, calixarenes, and dendrimers (Karunaratne *et al.*, 2017).

Delivery to Target Tissues

A significant advantage in optimizing drug efficacy is in targeting the site of action. Targeting reduces the loss of drug/drug activity during the transport from the absorption site to the target site and lowers the dose of administration of the drug. Nanocarrier systems used to target delivery of therapeutic agents reduce side effects and the frequency of dosing while improving efficiency. Recently, several accounts of nanoformulations designed for targeted drug delivery of various anticancer drugs have emerged. The section on 'targeted delivery applications' has already touched this area briefly. Further, accounts of the advantages of targeted delivery systems will be covered under 'Nanoformulation targeting strategies.'

Maintaining a Steady Drug Concentration in the System

Nanoformulations that have been engineered for controlled or sustained release of drugs can deliver a steady drug concentration over time. In conventional drugs, the drug enters the systemic circulation and usually remains for a short period after dosage. In a sustained and controlled release, the drug is released in small amounts over a prolonged period (Fig. **2**).

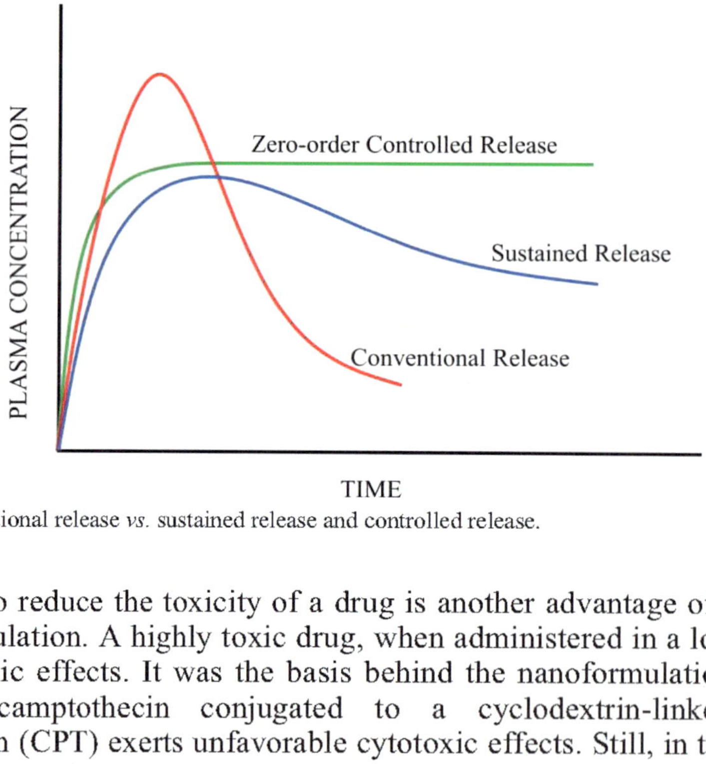

Fig. (2). Conventional release *vs.* sustained release and controlled release.

The ability to reduce the toxicity of a drug is another advantage of a controlled release formulation. A highly toxic drug, when administered in a low dose, may not exert toxic effects. It was the basis behind the nanoformulation CRLX101 containing camptothecin conjugated to a cyclodextrin-linked polymer. Camptothecin (CPT) exerts unfavorable cytotoxic effects. Still, in the CRLX101 nanoformulation, the controlled release of CPT inside the cells lowers its toxicity to the cells and renders it safe for use (Kuruvilla *et al.*, 2017).

Once the drug-loaded nanoparticle enters the bloodstream, there is a possibility for phagocytosis and filtration. The binding of proteins to the surface and aggregation influences the recognition of the nanocarrier by the immune system.

The introduction of protective barriers on nanoparticles can extend the circulation time, thus increasing the therapeutic efficiency. Surface modifications to generate surface hindrance, altering the hydrodynamic volume effects, and introducing charge repulsions can prevent nanoparticles from aggregating and rapid clearance (Rhee and Mansour, 2011). Nanocarriers with polyethylene glycol (PEG) modified surfaces have shown a considerable increase in blood circulation time due to the reduced aggregation as well as reduced interactions between the nanoparticle and the opsonizing proteins. The use of liposomes for therapeutic applications has shown successful results due to their high biocompatibility and biodegradability. However, liposomes are subjected to rapid clearance from the blood. Surface coating of the liposome with hydrophilic polymer or glycolipid introduces a spatial barrier towards other nearby molecules (Immordino *et al.*, 2006).

Penetrating Impermeable Barriers

One of the most significant challenges in delivering drugs to the brain is the blood-brain barrier (BBB), impermeable to most polar drugs. However, nanoformulations have shown impressive advantages in delivering drugs to the brain over conventional drug formulations. In addition to penetrating the lipidic membrane of the BBB, the drugs need to evade the efflux pumps to exert their full therapeutic effect on brain tissues and brain tumors. Thus, polymeric nanoparticles and lipidic nanocarriers such as liposomes, solid lipid nanoparticles (SLNs) and micelles, have been investigated for their ability to penetrate and deliver drugs to the brain (Jain, 2012). The mechanisms of transport of drugs to the brain and the progress made in drug delivery *via* polymeric nanoparticles and lipid-based nanocarriers and dendrimers, carbon nanotubes, nanogels, and other nanoformulations are elegantly discussed by Khan *et al.* (2018).

The dermal barrier can be a challenge to the delivery of active agents in skin formulations. The *stratum corneum* is the outermost epidermal layer, consisting of a lipid bilayer consisting of sphingolipids and free sterols (Leite-Silva *et al.*, 2012). Passive diffusion of the active substance (drug) takes place *via* the transcellular, intercellular, and appendageal routes (Sala *et al.*, 2018). Thus, small molecules and lipophilic drugs can permeate this barrier, while most other polar drugs cannot be used in transdermal delivery. Permeation enhancers have been used to increase the solubility to allow penetration across the *stratum corneum*. In recent years, nano-delivery systems based on liposomes and lipid carriers have shown potential to penetrate the *stratum corneum* by interacting with the targeted cells of the skin, leading to a prolonged release of drugs (Rhee and Mansour, 2011). Transfersomes, which have surfactants in addition to phospholipids, possess more penetration ability than conventional liposomes, mainly consisting of phospholipids and steroids, due to their increased deformability of the structure (Chenthamara *et al.*, 2019). Ethosomes, which consist of phospholipids, surfactants, water, and ethanol, have a high capability for penetration since ethanol permeates the *stratum corneum* (Chenthamara *et al.*, 2019). The permeation of α-tocopherol through pig ear skin was shown to increase by 4.3 fold when encapsulated in liposomes and incorporated in an emulsion (average permeation 5.26%) over the incorporation of free α-tocopherol in the emulsion (average permeation 1.21%), demonstrating the enhanced permeability of liposomes over free drug (Karunaratne *et al.*, 2014).

APPLICATIONS OF NANOFORMULATIONS IN CANCER THERAPY

Nanoformulations as Therapeutics in Cancer Treatment

Cancer, being a malignant non-communicable disease of which survivors are scarce, has become a prime focus in the health sector worldwide. Sadly, cancer patients and cancer survivors suffer from numerous harmful side effects due to the administration of therapies – chemotherapy and radiotherapy – as part of currently available cancer treatment. Thus, a quest to find novel, more advanced, and reliable therapies posing no or less harmful side effects for cancer patients has recently been intensified globally. Nanoformulations have become the desired therapeutic agents among the numerous therapeutics available for cancer treatment, as they stand out in many aspects.

The utilization of nanoformulations in cancer treatment is indeed advantageous due to numerous factors, as described previously. The nanoformulations currently utilized or under investigation for cancer treatment today include liposomes, polymeric nanoparticles, metal nanoparticles, dendrimers, and emulsions. The applications of those nanoformulations in cancer therapy are described in the following subsections.

Liposomes

Liposomes are spheres made up of one or more lipid bilayers entrapping an aqueous component in the interior hence able to deliver both water-soluble species entrapped in the aqueous interior (Pamunuwa *et al.*, 2015) and lipid-soluble species embedded in the lipid bilayer (Nwokwu *et al.*, 2017). Strikingly, it is the principal drug delivery vehicle used in cancer therapy that is explored not only for delivering drugs but also for delivering genes and immunotherapy (Kiaie *et al.*, 2020). Numerous modifications to conventional liposomes have been investigated, and, interestingly, multiple improvements have sometimes shown ameliorated properties.

Conventional Liposomes

Conventional liposomes made primarily of phospholipids and cholesterol have been explored. They have shown encouraging results as delivery vehicles of numerous anticancer/antitumor agents according to both *in vitro* and *in vivo* investigations. For example, nanoliposomal gedunin induced apoptosis in human non-small-cell lung cancer (NCI-H292) cells (Nwokwu *et al.*, 2017). Conventional liposomes carrying curcumin have shown promising results, including anticancer effects against lung cancer, according to an *in vivo* study conducted utilizing rat models (Zhang *et al.*, 2018). Besides, numerous other liposomal anticancer agents such as resveratrol (Summerlin *et al.*, 2015), lycopene (Mirahmadi *et al.*, 2020), and betulinic acid (Mullauer *et al.*, 2011) have shown increased anticancer properties compared to their free counterparts. Interestingly, certain anticancer drug formulations currently being used in therapy are also conventional liposomes.

Stealth Liposomes

Stealth liposomes show increased circulation time in the blood because those vesicles are capable of decreasing their uptake by the mononuclear phagocyte system. The surface of those vesicles is usually modified with molecules such as poly(ethylene glycol) (PEG). Numerous studies are being carried out to further explore their capacity as drug delivery vehicles, and some are already approved as drugs while others are in clinical trials. Doxil and Caelyx, of which the active agent is doxorubicin, are approved medications used to treat Kaposi's sarcoma. The lipid composition of these stealth liposomes comprises hydrogenated soy phosphatidylcholine, cholesterol, and poly(ethylene glycol) harbored on 1,2-distearoyl-sn-glycero-3-phosphoethanolamine. SPI-077 is another formulation with the same lipid composition as Doxil. Its active agent is cisplatin, and it is used in clinical trials treating head and neck cancer and lung cancer. Apart from the PEGylated formulations, formulations such as LipoplatinTM of which the active agent is cisplatin, and S-CKD602 of which the active agent is a camptothecin analog intended to treat several cancers, with no PEGylation have shown to function as stealth liposomes (Immordino *et al.*, 2006; Daraee *et al.*, 2016).

Immunoliposomes

Immunoliposomes comprise antibodies attached to their surface for specific targeting applications. In addition to the surface of liposomes, attachment of antibodies is carried out to the ends of PEG molecules of stealth liposomes (Golkar *et al.*, 2016). Immunoliposomes have shown efficient delivery of numerous drugs used in cancer therapy. An *in vitro* study carried out using nanoliposomal docetaxel, which is used to treat prostate cancer, has shown increased uptake by EGFR (epidermal growth factor receptor)-expressing cancer cells due to the presence of surface anti EGFR antibodies of the liposomes (Eloy *et al.*, 2020). Also, ovarian cancer cells overexpressing CD44 were targeted successfully with glycosylated paclitaxel encapsulated immunoliposomes (Khayrani *et al.*, 2019). Likewise, numerous other cancer cells, including breast cancer cells and lung cancer cells, have been successfully targeted with immunoliposomes (Khan *et al.*, 2020; Lu *et al.*, 2019).

Thermosensitive Liposomes

Thermosensitive liposome, whose structure is sensitive to mild hyperthermia, is extensively researched in cancer therapy. Interestingly, mild hyperthermia is coupled with chemotherapy in cancer treatment regardless of any involvement of thermosensitive liposomes because the EPR effect is facilitated due to thermal treatment. The three types of thermosensitive liposomes: traditional thermosensitive liposomes of which the lipids undergo phase transition upon a favorable hyperthermal treatment, lysolipid-containing thermosensitive liposomes of which lysolipids render the liposomes more easily destabilized, and polymer-modified thermosensitive liposomes of which the incorporated polymers undergo structural changes in response to thermal treatment, have been investigated in cancer therapy (Bi *et al.*, 2019). Dai and coworkers showed that PEGylated targeted thermosensitive liposomes comprising a novel phase-changing material which is a combination of fatty acids, *i.e.*, lauric acid and stearic acid, can be used to deliver doxorubicin to HeLa tumor of a mouse model and that the tumor can be suppressed effectively using mild hyperthermal treatment with thermosensitive liposomes (Dai *et al.*, 2019). Mo and coauthors also reported that a burst release of cargo, *i.e.*, doxorubicin, is achievable at 42 °C using polymer-based thermosensitive liposomes showing stability at normal physiological temperature 37 °C (Mo *et al.*, 2019).

pH-Sensitive Liposomes

pH-sensitive liposomes become destabilized in acidic media, releasing their drug cargo while being stable in the physiological pH of 7.4. Anticancer drugs can be selectively delivered to the tumor/ cancer tissues of low pH, exploiting this property of pH sensitivity of liposomes (Fan *et al.*, 2017). For instance, estrone-anchored pH-sensitive liposomes showed higher cytotoxicity against ER-positive MCF-7 breast carcinoma cells than liposomes exhibiting no pH sensitivity. Further, pH-sensitive liposomes exhibited a more remarkable ability to suppress breast tumor growth in mice relative to liposomes showing no pH sensitivity and free drug doxorubicin (Paliwal *et al.*, 2012). The anticancer drugs used in the formulation of pH-sensitive liposomes for intended cancer therapeutic applications are many and include methotrexate, cytosine-β-D-arabinofuranoside, and doxorubicin (Karanth and Murthy, 2007).

Photosensitive Liposomes

Photosensitive liposomes that release the encapsulated drugs resulting from photo-induced reactions of lipids have also been explored for cancer therapy (Chen *et al.*, 2020). While photosensitive liposomes are a promising drug delivery vehicle for superficial skin cancers, these vesicles have been investigated for a few other cancers, including gastric cancer. For instance, Namiki and co-authors reported that photosensitive stealth liposomes showed much lower LC80 than their non-photosensitive counterparts against gastric cancer cell lines and destroyed tumor tissue in murine models, with much less recurrent rates (Namiki *et al.*, 2004).

Cationic Liposomes

Cationic liposomes have been evaluated mainly for the delivery of nucleic acids for cancer therapy. They have shown selectivity towards tumor vascular endothelial cells showing promise towards antivascular and antiangiogenic therapies of the lungs and liver following intravenous administration (Dass and Choong, 2006). Usually, nucleic acid delivery *via* cationic liposomes is integrated with dual delivery or combination therapy in cancer therapy research (Jose *et al.*, 2018; Lin *et al.*, 2016).

Commercial Liposomal Anticancer Products

The commercial liposomal anticancer products include Doxil, which is used to treat Kaposi's sarcoma, recurrent ovarian cancer, and breast cancer; Depocyt, a formulation used to treat neoplastic and lymphomatous meningitis; DaunoXome which is used to treat Kaposi's sarcoma; Myocet which is used to treat breast cancer; Impact for the treatment of osteosarcoma; Marqibo which is used to treat metastatic malignant uveal melanoma, and OnivydeTM which is used to treat metastatic adenocarcinoma of the pancreas (Kiaie *et al.*, 2020). The principles used in developing commercial liposomal anticancer drugs are worth highlighting as most cases involve multiple principles for enhanced effectiveness. Doxil is a PEGylated liposome formulation made of phospholipids of high melting temperatures (Tm). The liposomes are long circulating in the intact form in the human plasma after intravenous administration. Doxorubicin, the active agent of Doxil, is loaded into the preformed liposomes *via* active loading utilizing a transmembrane ammonium ion gradient where the ammonium ion concentration inside the liposomes is much higher than that in the medium outside to yield a high ratio of drug to lipid, which leads to an increased drug concentration at the target site achieving high therapeutic efficacy.

Further, the liposomes are made small enough to be approximately 100 nm in diameter; therefore, extravasation through leaky vasculature of tumor issues (EPR effect) enables passive targeting of the nanoliposomes after intravenous administration (Barenholz, 2012). DaunoXome, of which the active substance is daunorubicin, is a nanoliposomal formulation made of lipids of transition temperatures higher than the physiological temperatures to remain intact in the body. A decrease in the lipid membrane permeability is achieved through introducing cholesterol in the membrane. Also, amassing of nanoliposomes in the tumors due to the EPR effect is improved by fabricating nanoliposomes of diameters less than 100 nm (Forssen, 1997). DepoCyt, of which the active substance is cytarabine, is not a nanoformulation but a micro liposomal formulation consisting of multivesicular liposomes. Interestingly, sustained-release properties of these liposomes improve the therapeutic efficacy of the active substance in patients with neoplastic meningitis (Murry and Blaney, 2000). Myocet, of which the active substance is doxorubicin, is formulated as non-PEGylated nanoliposomes of diameter 190 nm, thus exhibiting a much longer circulating half-life than free drug in the plasma. The liposome is made of phosphatidylcholine and cholesterol for reducing the drug leakage from the liposome. The liposomes accumulate in the targeted site minimizing cardiac toxicity due to the small size (Leonard *et al.*, 2009). Mepact, of which the active substance is mifamurtide, is formulated as multilamellar vesicles with diameters less than 100 nm. Functioning as an immunostimulant, it targets macrophages of the reticuloendothelial system. Marqibo, of which the active substance is vincristine, is prepared as nanoliposomes of diameter 100 nm capable of passively targeting the site of action *via* EPR (Alphandéry *et al.*, 2015). OnivydeTM, a nanoliposomal formulation containing the anticancer drug irinotecan, is prepared through active loading of its drug cargo using sucrose octasulfate, enabling very high encapsulation efficiency and stability. The circulatory time and efficacy of nanoliposomal irinotecan have been shown to be much higher than those of free irinotecan (Zhang, 2016a).

Apart from the liposomal anticancer drug delivery systems already in the market, numerous potential liposomal anticancer drugs are in clinical trials. Some of those formulations include LEP-ETU, of which the drug is paclitaxel for breast, ovarian, and lung cancers; EndoTAG-1, of which the drug is paclitaxel for breast and pancreatic cancers; SPI-077, of which the drug is cis-platin and its analogs for lung, head, and neck cancers; and LEM-ETU, a mitoxantrone formulation targeted for numerous cancers, including ovarian and breast cancers (Fan and Zhang, 2013).

Polymeric Nanoparticles

Nanoparticles of size 10-1000 nm fabricated using natural or artificial polymers either by encapsulating the active agents in the particles or by conjugating the active agents on the surface constitute polymeric nanoparticles in this context (El-Say and El-Sawy, 2017). The nanoparticles must be fabricated utilizing biocompatible polymers. Also, they need to be biodegradable, forming simple harmless molecules that can be excreted from the body quickly without posing toxicity issues to the patient (Torchilin, 2005). Like with most anticancer drug delivery vehicles, polymeric nanoparticles facilitate increased dissolution and bioavailability, increased *in vivo* circulation, and increased stability of the drugs. The mechanisms through which drug release takes place from polymeric nanoparticles are swelling, diffusion, degradation, and erosion, and the release mechanisms are often matrix dependent (Pamunuwa *et al.*, 2020; Parveen and Sahoo, 2008). Most frequently researched polymers utilized for the fabrication of polymeric nanoparticles encapsulated with anticancer agents include poly lactic-co-glycolic acid (PLGA), polylactic acid (PLA), poly ε-caprolactone (PCL), chitosan and human serum albumin (HSA) (El-Say and El-Sawy, 2017). Cancer therapeutic applications of some of those polymers are briefly discussed below.

PLGA, a synthetic biodegradable polymer, is used in the nanoencapsulation of diverse anticancer agents such as doxorubicin, curcumin, 5-fluorouracil, vincristine sulfate, and cisplatin, and nano-delivery of those anticancer agents to many cancer cell lines or tumors have shown positive results (Cao *et al.*, 2019; Aki *et al.*, 2016; El-Hammadi *et al.*, 2017; Zhang *et al.*, 2016b; Domínguez-Ríos *et al.*, 2019). For instance, PLGA nanoparticles have shown sustained release of encapsulated 5-fluorouracil, which exhibited higher toxicity than free drug against breast cancer cells (MCF -7) and colon cancer cells (HT-29) (El-Hammadi *et al.*, 2017). In addition to drugs, nucleic acids such as siRNAs have been delivered to several cancer cells, including prostate and lung, *via* PLGA particles (Hasan *et al.*, 2012; Zhang *et al.*, 2016c). Interestingly, PLGA nanoparticles have shown promise in targeted delivery utilizing both the EPR effect and ligand-receptor binding that will be discussed in the following sections.

Chitosan, a natural carbohydrate-based biodegradable polymer, has been investigated for therapy for numerous cancers, including pancreatic, liver, colorectal, lung, and breast. Anticancer agents encapsulated in chitosan nanoparticles are many and include paclitaxel, gemcitabine, tamoxifen, and protoporphyrin IX (Babu *et al.*, 2017; Parsian *et al.*, 2016; Guan *et al.*, 2012; Chanphai *et al.*, 2019; Fu *et al.*, 2016). Chitosan nanoparticles have shown many attributes desirable in cancer therapy. For instance, chitosan nanoparticles encapsulated with tamoxifen exhibited pH-dependent controlled release and improved cytotoxicity against MCF-7 human breast cancer cells (Vivek *et al.*, 2013). As with numerous other polymeric nanoparticles, chitosan nanoparticles can be utilized in targeted delivery, reducing off-target damages (Yadav *et al.*, 2020).

Human serum albumin, a plasma protein known for favorable drug-binding properties, has been explored for therapy against numerous cancers, including colon, prostate, and breast (Qu *et al.*, 2016; Saleh *et al.*, 2019; Sharma *et al.*, 2017). Among the many anticancer agents deliverable *via* human serum albumin nanoparticles are doxorubicin, noscapine, cabazitaxel, paclitaxel, and siRNA (Anhorn *et al.*, 2008; Sebak *et al.*, 2010; Sun *et al.*, 2019; Lomis *et al.*, 2016; Abbasi *et al.*, 2011). Like with many other protein nanoparticles, human serum albumin nanoparticles upon surface modification have exhibited targeted delivery of their drug cargo (Saleh *et al.*, 2019).

Solid Lipid Nanoparticles

Solid lipid nanoparticles, nanospheres of lipids encapsulating bioactive agents, have shown numerous favorable properties as anticancer drug delivery vehicles against malignancies, including colorectal, lung, cervical, and breast cancers (Smith *et al.*, 2020; Soni *et al.*, 2016; Wang *et al.*, 2017; Liu *et al.*, 2017). The anticancer agents loaded in solid lipid nanoparticles are many and include camptothecin, cholesteryl butyrate, doxorubicin, paclitaxel, and retinoic acid. The anticancer agent encapsulated solid lipid nanoparticles have exhibited increased stability, favorable drug biodistribution, and enhanced pharmacokinetics. Other important applications of solid lipid nanoparticles explored by numerous researchers include gene delivery, targeted drug delivery to tumor tissues, and combinational therapy (Wong *et al.*, 2007).

Metal Nanoparticles

Metal nanoparticles are explored not only as therapeutic agents but also as diagnostic tools. Metal nanoparticles such as iron nanoparticles, gold nanoparticles, titanium dioxide nanoparticles, zinc oxide nanoparticles, cesium oxide nanoparticles, silver nanoparticles, silicone nanoparticles, and copper nanoparticles are used in cancer therapy. Iron nanoparticles generate cytotoxicity in the presence of oscillating magnetic fields or near-infrared radiation through reactive oxygen species. Posing minimal effect on normal cells, iron nanoparticles exhibit therapeutic effects against a number of cancers and tumors, including brain, prostate, and lung tumors/cancers. When combined with ionizing radiation, gold nanoparticles have shown toxicity against breast cancer and adenocarcinoma. Likewise, other metal nanoparticles have exhibited efficacy against separate cancers/cancer cell lines. In addition to delivering anticancer drugs, metal nanoparticles may be utilized in the delivery of nucleic acids. Also, they can be used in hyperthermia and radiotherapy (Sharma *et al.*, 2018). Notably, metal nanoparticles may be used in the site-specific delivery of anticancer agents to cancer cells (Sadhukhan *et al.*, 2019).

Dendrimers

Dendrimers are macromolecular spheres with multiple branches. Active substances can be attached to the surface or loaded in the interior of the dendrimers that are explored extensively for both cancer therapy and diagnosis (Chauhan, 2018). Many dendrimers with encapsulated anticancer drugs have exhibited positive results against numerous cancers. For example, polyamidoamine based dendrimers carrying doxorubicin have shown efficacy against lung metastasis. Further, those vehicles carrying paclitaxel or docetaxel have shown positive results against breast cancer. Numerous nucleic acids loaded in dendrimers also have been investigated for cancer therapy. For instance, polyamidoamine based dendrimers carrying siBCL-2 have been explored for ovarian cancer therapy, while those carrying IFN-β have been investigated against malignant glioma. Likewise, dendrimers based on other polymers, including poly-L-lysine and poly(propylene imine), have shown promising results as nucleic acid carriers for cancer therapy (Mendes *et al.*, 2017). To further increase the therapeutic efficacy of the loaded drugs, the surface of the dendrimers can be easily functionalized to facilitate site-specific delivery of the cargo (Chauhan, 2018).

Emulsions

Nanoemulsions, emulsions with the droplet size in the nanometer range, are mainly explored in cancer therapy due to their characteristic features being beneficial for this purpose. For example, they show a large surface area, charged surface, and relatively high half-life of circulation. They can be used in both active targetings using ligands and passive targeting, using the EPR effect due to the small size of droplets. Further, enhancement of solubility and stability of poorly water-soluble bioactive agents/drugs is achieved utilizing oil-in-water emulsions. Nanoemulsions are investigated for cancer therapy of various cancers. Nanoemulsions with encapsulated active agents such as lycopene, myrisplatin, didodecyl methotrexate, paclitaxel, and curcumin have shown positive results against colon cancer, ovarian cancer, leukemia, lung cancer, and prostate cancer, respectively. Clinical trials are also being carried out using nanoemulsions with encapsulated 5-aminolevulinic acid or curcumin (Sánchez-López *et al.*, 2019). In addition, nanoemulsions have shown promise in combating multi-drug resistance in cancer. For instance, vitamin E-based nanoemulsions carrying paclitaxel have shown success in reversing multi-drug resistance shown by ovarian carcinoma cells (Zheng *et al*., 2016). In addition to nanoemulsions, microemulsions whose diameters are also in the nanometer range (Karunaratne *et al*., 2017) have also been evaluated for the delivery of anticancer agents. For example, celecoxib and tamoxifen citrate are two drugs delivered to breast cancer cells using microemulsions (Dehghani *et al*., 2017; Mojeiko *et al*., 2019).

Nanoformulation Targeting Strategies

Passive Targeting

Targeting of anticancer drugs is achievable utilizing enhanced permeation and retention (EPR) effect where the drug carriers of sufficiently small size accumulate passively at tumor tissues consisting of leaky vasculature. The diameter of the drug delivery vehicles needs to be in the range of 100 – 200 nm, and the delivery vehicles should exhibit a prolonged circulatory half-life in the blood following intravenous administration. As lymphatic drainage lacks the tumor tissues, the accumulated delivery vehicles reside in the tumor interstitium for a comparatively extended period, allowing the drug concentration to increase to effective levels. Strategies for enhancing the EPR effects have also been explored by numerous researchers (Park *et al*., 2019). Liposomes and polymeric nanoparticles are prominent drug delivery vehicles that have shown passive drug targeting based on the EPR effect (Kalyane *et al*., 2019).

The conventional liposomes are taken up rapidly by the reticuloendothelial system following systemic administration, which constitutes a significant downside shown by those vesicles. A successful strategy to overcome this issue is to utilize stealth liposomes either of small size and/or with poly-(ethylene glycol) chains on their surface (Nosova *et al*., 2019). Interestingly, PEGylated liposomes show a half-life greater than 40 h, enabling the drug carriers to accumulate in the tumor tissues showing much lower off-target accumulation (Maruyama, 2011). Data enabling comparison of therapeutic indices of two commercially available therapeutic formulations and free drug, doxorubicin, were reported by Huwyler and coauthors (Huwyler, 2008). The formulations were PEGylated liposomes with encapsulated doxorubicin (Doxil/Caelyx) and conventional liposomes with encapsulated doxorubicin (Myocet). Doxil/Caelyx exhibiting long circulatory and EPR effects has shown minimal off-target interactions and site avoidance imposing minimum cardiotoxicity. In brief, improved efficacy and diminished toxicity have contributed to the increased therapeutic index of Doxil/Caelyx (Maruyama, 2011). Although passive targeting and active targeting are discussed under different sections in this book chapter, it must be emphasized that most anticancer agent delivery vehicles amalgamate both of those targeting strategies for altered biodistribution and enhanced pharmacokinetics.

Like liposomes, polymeric nanoparticles have been used in passive tumor targeting based on the EPR effect facilitated by the small size and long circulation half-life. For instance, paclitaxel attached to albumin nanoparticles has shown an enhanced anticancer effect in murine models (Kinoshita *et al.*, 2017). Also, poly lactic-co-glycolic acid (PLGA) nanoparticles, which are the center of focus for anticancer drug delivery vehicle development, have displayed passive targeting of numerous bioactive agents showing anticancer activity nucleic acids. The anticancer agents encapsulated in PLGA nanoparticles include dexamethasone, paclitaxel, vincristine sulfate, camptothecin, doxorubicin, cisplatin, and curcumin, and their efficacy has been investigated against many cancers such as breast, ovarian, lung, and head and neck (Acharya and Sahoo, 2011). Interestingly, PEGylation of PLGA nanoparticles has shown increased circulation half-life (Acharya and Sahoo, 2011). PEGylated nanoparticles of diameters in the range of 10 – 40 nm are considered ideal for efficient passive targeting *via* the EPR effect, avoiding renal clearance (Stylianopoulos, 2013). Many polymeric nanoparticles bearing anticancer drugs show combined passive and active targeting facilitating more favorable biodistribution and improved pharmacokinetics (Masood, 2016).

Active Targeting

Active targeting in cancer therapy is based mainly on the premise that functionalizing the drug carrier surface with ligands will enable site-specific delivery of the agents possessing anticancer activities to the malignant tissues. Examples of ligands used in targeted delivery are monoclonal antibodies, antibody fragments, peptides, aptamers, and small molecules. The key advantages of active targeting *via* nanoparticles in cancer therapy include: greater amassing of the nanoparticles in the target tissue, increased cellular uptake of the nanoparticles, augmented therapeutic efficacy of the bioactive agents, and reduced toxicity. Interestingly, both active targeting and passive targeting are used in cancer therapy (Kue *et al.*, 2016; Wakaskar, 2017). Applications of various ligands in active targeting in experimental cancer therapy are briefly discussed below.

Antibodies and Antibody Fragments

Although antibodies were attached to non-PEGylated liposomes in the early days, PEGylated liposomes with encapsulated anticancer agents are utilized in the preparation of sterically stabilized immunoliposomes today to combine the advantages of increased circulation time with targeted delivery. In fact, PEGylated liposomes are usually attached with antibodies at the end of PEG molecules, thereby facilitating ligand binding with minimal steric hindrance from the PEG chains (Golkar *et al.*, 2016). Interestingly, numerous reports highlight that the therapeutic efficacy of sterically stabilized immunoliposomes may be higher than sterically stabilized liposomes despite the fact that their accumulation in the tumor tissues is comparable. This increased efficacy of sterically stabilized immunoliposomes is ascribed to their enhanced cellular uptake in the tumor tissues. However, there are instances that the therapeutic efficacy of immunoliposomes is independent of cellular intake but dependent on drug release (Torchilin, 2008). Examples of antibody modified immunoliposomes investigated to target tumor tissues include the antibody OC-125 attached liposomes loaded with methotrexate-ϒ-aspartate or 5-fluoroorotate for targeting human ovarian cancer cells (Straubinger *et al.* 1998) and the monoclonal nucleosome specific 2C5 antibody (mAb 2C5) attached long-circulating liposomes loaded with doxorubicin for targeting numerous tumor cells (Lukyanov *et al.*, 2004). Some other antibodies used for targeting cancer/tumor cells include an anti-HER2 antibody, anti-CD19 antibody, anti-CD20 antibody, and anti-MT1-MMP antibody. Fab fragments of antibodies are in certain instances used to avoid the cytotoxicity triggered by whole antibodies and to achieve more prolonged circulation. Examples of antibody fragments used include fab′ fragments of anti-GD2 antibodies and fab′ fragments of the monoclonal antibody C225 to target the epidermal growth factor receptor and a variant of it (Torchilin, 2008). The surfaces of polymeric nanoparticles, like liposomes, can be modified with antibodies or antibody fragments for active targeting of anticancer drugs to cancer/tumor cells to yield higher efficacy. For instance, cetuximab-conjugated PLGA nanoparticles loaded with paclitaxel palmitate have shown increased anticancer efficacy against lung cancer cells (Shargh *et al.*, 2016).

Other Ligands

Nanoparticles can be attached to numerous ligands apart from antibody fragments and antibodies to facilitate site-specific delivery of anticancer agents in cancer therapy. The tumor/ cancer cells overexpress specific receptors on their surfaces, and the ligands showing high affinity to those receptors are used for modifying the surfaces of nanoparticles. The ligands include proteins, small molecules, and aptamers, among others. For instance, liposomes to which transferrin protein-ligand is attached are used to deliver siRNA to tumors and to deliver oxaliplatin in the case of gastroesophageal adenocarcinoma. The target in this instance is the transferrin receptor, which is overexpressed on cancer cells, facilitating receptor-mediated internalization of nanoparticles, including nanoliposomes. Also, nanoparticles have been attached to protein kinase N3 to target siRNA to solid tumors (Xu *et al.*, 2015). In addition to proteins, small molecules such as folate have been used in targeted cancer therapy. For instance, folate receptors overexpressed in cancer cells have been targeted by formulating a PLGA-PE--folate conjugate to deliver disulfiram (Fasehee *et al.*, 2016). Examples of aptamer functionalized nanoparticles investigated to deliver anticancer agents include PLGA-PEG nanoparticles to deliver cis-platin to prostate cancer cells (Dhar *et al.*, 2008) and human serum albumin nanoparticles of curcumin to breast cancer cells (Saleh *et al.*, 2019). Notably, numerous therapeutic agents in clinical trials target anticancer agents to tumor/cancer cells *via* ligand-receptor interactions (Xu *et al.*, 2015).

Other Nanoparticle-Based Strategies for Cancer Therapy

Dual Delivery

Cancer therapy utilizes dual delivery to yield synergistic effects of anticancer agents or to overcome drug resistance. Interestingly, several examples show that nanoparticle-mediated dual delivery has demonstrated positive outcomes in cancer therapy. For example, a pluronic P85–polyethylenimine/D-α-tocopheryl polyethylene glycol micellar system has been used for dual delivery of small hairpin RNA and sorafenib to drug-resistant hepatocellular carcinoma cells, which then exhibited inhibition of both tumor growth and angiogenesis (Shen *et al.*, 2014). Also, the resensitizing effect on ovarian cancer cells has been achieved by dual delivery of paclitaxel and a permeability glycoprotein inhibitor (Zhang *et al.*, 2016d). Further, dual delivery of doxorubicin and Bcl-2-regulating siRNA to prostate cancer cells where the drug and siRNA exhibited synergy has been achieved *via* a polyplex conjugated with an aptamer (Kim *et al.*, 2010). An example of dual delivery of cytokines with drugs includes the dual delivery of tumor necrosis factor-related apoptosis-inducing ligand (TRAIL) and paclitaxel *via* cationic micelles to breast cancer cells, which showed increased cytotoxicity (Lee *et al.*, 2011). Cancer therapy utilizes nucleic acids and cytokines, and antibodies in dual delivery, which facilitates mainly targeted delivery followed by increased internalization, improving the pharmacokinetics of the drugs. This phenomenon was explained under active targeting (Jang *et al.*, 2016).

Triggered Cancer Therapy

An innovative approach for anticancer agent delivery is triggered cancer therapy utilizing stimuli such as light, magnetic field, and ultrasound. For instance, photo-inducible nanoparticles attached to the anticancer agent camptothecin have been incorporated in hydrogels, which, upon illumination, released the drug into the malignant cells (Shah *et al.*, 2014). Further, doxorubicin and paclitaxel are among the drugs deliverable using magnetic field responsive nanoparticles, while doxorubicin and mitoxantrone are among the drugs deliverable using ultrasound responsive nanoparticles (Jang *et al.*, 2016). Recently, targeted delivery *via* P-selectin coupled with microwave triggered drug release of doxorubicin for hepatocellular carcinoma was reported (Xu *et al*., 2019). In general, the triggered release has a high potential of increasing the therapeutic efficacy of chemotherapy.

THERAPEUTIC ADVANTAGES OF NANOFORMULATIONS IN HEPATOCELLULAR CARCINOMA

Nanoformulations for Hepatocellular Carcinoma

Hepatocellular carcinoma, a common form of liver cancer, has gained the second place as the cause of death of cancer patients (Torre *et al*., 2015). HCC mutually relates to some health issues such as alcoholic cirrhosis, non-alcoholic fatty liver disease, or hepatitis C virus (HCV) infection and has a tendency of presenting in persons with past records of these diseases (Tsuchiya *et al*., 2015). Most patients are diagnosed after the metastasis phase is reached since it does not show specific symptoms in many of the patients (Balogh *et al*., 2016). The lack of efficient tools for diagnosis and the scarcity of available appropriate treatments are combining factors for increasing the mortality rate of HCC (Baig *et al*., 2019). The patient's condition and profile determine the type of treatment among the various types of available treatments, namely, surgical resection, ablation, liver transplantation, transarterial chemoembolization (TACE), radiotherapy, chemotherapy, and combination therapy (Dimitroulis *et al*., 2017). Various limitations accompany the traditional therapies. Several examples that hamper the existing conventional treatment of HCC are, increasing resistance regarding chemotherapy, radiotherapy with side effects, facilitating cancer metastasis mistakenly by surgery, and immunosuppressive therapy due to transplantation (Baig *et al*., 2019). Scientific research in the domain of HCC has exponentially increased recently through exploring various innovative approaches. Nanotechnology is a promising technology that recently gained more attention in cancer diagnosis and treatment, especially with nanotechnological ongoing advances. A wide range of nanoformulations has been adapted to achieve desired therapeutic efficacy of HCC (Baig *et al*., 2019).

Types of Nanoformulations

As previously described elsewhere, the structures of nanoformulations researched in the field of HCC can be categorized as polymers, lipids, inorganics such as metal nanoparticles, ceramic nanoparticles, and biomacromolecules. Moreover, the combination of different materials to develop more efficient and specific delivery systems has also been investigated. One notable property of albumin is its natural drug binding ability and ubiquitous presence in various tissues. This feature makes albumin an efficient drug carrier (Hoogenboezem & Duvall, 2018).

Zhou *et al*. observed a distinct synergic effect on the destruction of HCC cells in the combined treatment of paclitaxel complexed to albumin compared to taxane drugs alone. It was evident from the results gained from the study performed with a xenograft model of HCC in which superior inhibition and lower cytotoxicity values were observed (Zhou *et al*., 2011). In a study reported by Li *et al*., it was shown that bovine serum albumin nanoparticles could improve drug dispersal of sodium ferrulate into the liver. In contrast, sustained release from the nanoparticles occurred due to covalent crosslinking by glutaraldehyde (Li *et al*., 2008). Liposomes consisting of vesicles made-up of nontoxic, amphiphilic phospholipids and cholesterol are safe, highly biocompatible, and have an exceptional ability in cellular internalization (Bozzuto & Molinari, 2015). These liposomes have been extensively researched as carriers of chemotherapeutics for various malignancies, including HCC (Yingchoncharoen *et al*., 2016). The synergic clinical effectiveness of gemcitabine and pegylated liposomal doxorubicin has been proven by Lombardi *et al*. (Lombardi *et al*., 2011). Poon and Borys documented the potential usage of Lyso-thermosensitive liposomal doxorubicin, the first heat-activated liposomal formulation, as an effective therapeutic for HCC patients when used with radiofrequency ablation (Poon and Borys, 2009).

Many natural origin polymers possess excellent properties required of drug carriers, namely, multifunctionality, biocompatibility, and specially biodegradability. They may be structurally developed for loading various drugs, making them into versatile carriers. According to a study reported by Qi *et al*., chitosan nanoparticles of size around 40 nm and high surface charge demonstrated *in vitro* antitumor activity, which was both dose and time-dependent on an HCC cell line. They resulted in improved *in vivo* tumor inhibitory effects (Qi *et al*., 2007). The high viscosity and low solubility of high molecular weight chitosan at physiological pH may be overcome by low molecular weight chitosan (LMWC). Galactosylation of LMWC afforded increased doxorubicin entrapment, resulting in excellent *in vitro* antitumor activity on HCC (Jain and Jain, 2010). Dextran is another natural water-soluble branched homopolysaccharide approved by the United States Food and Drug administration (Anirudhan and Binusreejayan, 2016). Curcumin, which is considered a suitable candidate for treating liver diseases, was encapsulated into glycyrrhetinic acid, a liver targeting ligand, incorporated onto dextran to make a safer, efficient liver targeting therapy with increased cytotoxicity over pure curcumin (Anirudhan and Binusreejayan, 2016). Another study reports the usage of magnetic nanoparticles coated with dextran for early diagnosis and effective treatment. In this study, crocin-coated magnetic nanoparticles modified with dextran showed an enhanced *in vitro* and *in vivo* cytotoxicity against HepG2 cells (El-Kharrag *et al*., 2017).

Apart from naturally occurring polysaccharides, the usage of synthetic biodegradable polymers such as PLGA, PCL, and polyhydroxy butyrate (PHB), and their copolymers have been documented as drug delivery systems. Promising anticancer properties of curcumin entrapped PLGA nanocarriers against HCC have been reported by Ghosh *et al.* (2012), considering their apoptotic effect on cancerous cells. Polyethyleneimine-coated PLGA nanoparticles are commonly used for their positive charge to entrap negatively charged moieties such as miRNA. This enhanced gene therapy method was adopted by Liang et al., to induce apoptosis in HepG2 cells (Liang *et al.*, 2011).

Metallic nanoparticles, especially gold and silver, have been explored in a wide array of biomedical applications due to their characteristic physical and chemical properties in their nanoscale and their biocompatibility (Yaqoob *et al.*, 2020). Apart from the known antibacterial activity of silver nanoparticles, it also exhibits an anticancer activity (Buttacavoli *et al.*, 2018). According to Ahmadian *et al.*, silver nanoparticles could be an effective chemotherapeutic agent to treat HCC since it induces the formation of reactive oxygen species in liver hepatocellular adenocarcinoma cell lines and also induces cell apoptosis (Ahmadian *et al.*, 2018). Gold nanoparticles which are 20 nm in diameter, show inherent antiangiogenesis properties by binding to heparin-binding pro-angiogenic growth factors such as VEGF165 and bFGF, thereby inhibiting their activity (Saeed *et al.*, 2019). Conjugating the drugs such as cisplatin, doxorubicin, capecitabine, ribavirin to gold nanoparticles demonstrated increased exposure of drugs to cancer cells and reduced chemoresistance of the cells (Tomuleasa *et al.*, 2012).

Carbon nanotubes (CNTs) are hollow fibrous carbon molecules that have been extensively researched for various applications. They are now being applied to the biomedicine field, particularly as nanocarriers to deliver drugs because of their high aspect ratio, large surface area, ability to chemically functionalize, and size stability at the nano-scale (Hwang *et al.*, 2017). Regardless of the contradictory results in terms of possible cytotoxicity of carbon nanotubes, the use of CNTs as drug carriers is slowly advancing (Yan *et al.*, 2019b). Single-walled carbon nanotubes modified with chitosan and folic acid, a targeting ligand, were loaded with doxorubicin and studied for cytotoxicity against HCC SMMC-7721 cell lines. The results indicated excellent stability of the drug-loaded system in physiological conditions and effective cytotoxicity against the cell lines (Ji *et al.*, 2012).

Mesoporous silica nanoparticles are another type of nanocarrier gaining more attention from researchers in drug delivery applications. The unique properties of these nanoparticles, such as the ability of surface modification, good bio-compatibility, easy macroscale synthesis, cost-effective nanoparticle production, definite and controlled size, porosity, morphological features, and stability, have made them more supportive in drug delivery applications (Mehmood *et al.*, 2017). Ashley and coworkers have developed peptide-targeted mesoporous silica nanoparticles decorated lipid bilayers capable of targeting peptides to deliver small interfering RNA which can bind to HCC to cause apoptosis in tumor cells (Ashley *et al.*, 2012).

Mechanism of Action of Nanoformulations in Hepatocellular Carcinoma

All nanoformulations, as mentioned above, have different mechanisms to serve as efficient drug delivery vehicles. By controlling the chemistries of building materials, the therapeutic efficacy can be intensified. By optimizing the properties, the permeability through barriers (Blanco *et al.*, 2015), increased drug loading, protection of the drug from degradation, enhanced cellular uptake (Salatin *et al.*, 2017), targeted delivery, and reduced damage to healthy cells can be achieved (Mohamed *et al.*, 2017). The loading of drugs in nanoparticles, the distribution of the chemotherapeutic at the cancer site, and the mechanism of action to fight against the barriers of efficient therapeutic approaches in HCC have been documented after several preclinical studies (Mohamed *et al.*, 2017).

Accumulation of drugs at the specific cancerous site is achieved by the targeting, which can be either passive or active. Passive targeting occurs *via* the EPR (enhanced permeability and retention) effect, while active targeting is achieved by surface modification of the nanomaterial. The receptor-mediated endocytosis (Li *et al.*, 2016) is the best approach of active targeting for HCC due to the overexpression of some proteins and molecules on the hepatocellular carcinoma cells over normal cells (Li *et al.*, 2016). The asialoglycoprotein receptor (ASGPR), being the highest expressed compared to extrahepatic cells, has gained the attention of many researchers (Li *et al.*, 2016). In particular, modifying the nanoparticle surface with galactose (Gal) residues imparts a high binding affinity to ASGPR (Ma *et al.*, 2015). Frisch *et al.* have developed a lipoplex decorated by triantennary galactosyl ligand to carry the gene and obtained efficiently targeted gene transfection in HCC (Li *et al.*, 2016). Apart from the Gal moiety-based active targeting, the following groups of molecules are also being utilized (Li *et al.*, 2016).

Vitamin Based Active Targeting

Vitamins are one of the main requirements for the survival of living cells. However, due to their rapid proliferation, tumor cells require specific vitamins such as folate, retinoic acid, and biotin (Li *et al.*, 2016) in excess compared to the normal cells. Specific receptors overexpress to increase vitamin uptake, and these receptors can be used for active targeting. The folate receptor is an overexpressed glycosylphosphatidylinositol glycoprotein present on most cancerous cell membranes having a high selective affinity for folic acid (Liu *et al.*, 2016). Therefore, the natural ligand of folate receptor, folic acid, has been widely researched as a targeting moiety for receptor-mediated endocytosis. A study done by Liu and coworkers has proven the enhanced targeting effect and antitumor potency with diacid metabolite of norcantharidin-loaded folic acid-modified polyethylene-glycolated liposome system (Liu *et al.*, 2016).

Antibody-Based Active Targeting

Antibodies are a group of glycoproteins that act as the most critical defense mechanism in vertebral animals. A nanoparticle conjugated with an antibody that combines the antibody's specific and selective recognition ability with an antigen on the tumor surface is an enhanced targeting delivery strategy for HCC (Goodall *et al.*, 2015). As a new and effective therapy for HCC, Jin *et al.* researched doxorubicin-loaded poly(D, L-lactic-co-glycolic acid)-poly(ethylene glycol) micelles conjugated to the bivalent HAb18 F(ab′)2 antibody fragment. Specific molecular targeting and higher uptake by HCC were observed by these coworkers (Jin *et al.*, 2010).

Peptide-Based Active Targeting

Targeting tumor cells by peptides is one of the best strategies for targeted drug delivery to cancer sites. The tripeptide Arg-Gly-Asp (RGD) is an effective targeting motif to several tumor cells *via* the RGD peptide's ability to recognize integrin $\alpha v\beta 3$ (Nieberler *et al.*, 2017). Paclitaxel-loaded RGD modified liposomes developed by Chen *et al.* showed improved targeting and therapeutic efficacy in HepG2 cells compared with paclitaxel-loaded liposomes without RGD modification (Chen *et al.*, 2015).

Aptamer Mediated Active Targeting

Aptamers having similar functionality to protein antibodies are composed of either single-stranded DNA or short RNA, which are able to fold into the 3D conformation and bind to the targets (Sun and Zu, 2015). Pilapong developed a magnetic nanoparticle-aptamer theranostic probe for both treatment and imaging purposes. His coworkers utilized doxorubicin-loaded carboxymethyl cellulose decorated magnetic nanoparticles conjugated with the targeting moiety DNA-based EpCAM aptamer. The *in vitro* studies proved that this smart theranostic probe had efficient MR imaging with better selectivity and higher intracellular uptake over free doxorubicin (Pilapong *et al.*, 2014).

Stimuli-responsive nanocarriers can remotely control the navigation, distribution, and releasing of the entrapped drug from the carriers at the specific site. Stimuli can be either internal (pH, tumor microenvironment) or external (magnetic field, ultrasound, radiofrequency ablation, microwaves). The slightly acidic nature of the tumor microenvironment has been utilized by Wang *et al.* to enhance the antitumor and antiangiogenic effect against HCC using methotrexate and combretastatin A4 entrapped pH-sensitive pullulan nanoparticles (Wang *et al.*, 2013). Several thermosensitive liposomal formulations have been utilized to treat HCC and were more effective than conventional liposomal formulations (Bi *et al.*, 2019).

Key Milestones

At present, a considerable number of nanoformulations for cancer therapy are either approved or in the clinical trial process by the US FDA (Bobo *et al.*, 2016). An approved nanoformulation for HCC is yet to emerge. However, The Japanese Ministry of Labour, Health and Welfare approved a nano-drug for HCC treatment in 1994 after phase 1 and 2 trials (Ishii *et al.*, 2003). This drug, Zinostatin stimalamer, which is a lipidol emulsion, is synthesized by a copolymer of styrene-maleic acid entrapped with the protein neocarzinostatin having an anti-tumor activity (Ishii *et al.*, 2003).

Limitations

The toxicity reduction of the entrapped drug has been the focus of nanoformulations used in drug delivery. However, the possible toxicity of the carrier has not been evaluated in most of the documented findings. Nanoparticles are not flawless. There are drawbacks, primarily due to no common feature other than nano size. Hence, individual particles have to be monitored for their possible toxicity. This toxicity can arise due to various factors, mainly the surface structure, particle size, chemical composition, surrounding environment, *etc.* (Sharifi *et al.*, 2016). Shape and size changes may cause adverse interactions either chemically or physically (Sukhanova *et al.*, 2018). Further, due to the chemical reactivity, nanoparticles could stimulate oxidative stress and inflammation, causing damages to DNA, protein, and membranes leading to toxicity (Khanna *et al.*, 2015; Yu *et al.*, 2020). Once these nanoparticles enter the body, they have the possibility of gaining access to cell organelles, blood-brain barrier, capillary tubes, and cell membrane crossing (Behzadi *et al.*, 2017).

Further, nanoparticles can cause adverse effects to the blood and cardiovascular system depending on their charge. Cationic nanoparticles can initiate blood clotting and hemolysis, while anionic nanoparticles are relatively non-toxic (Harpe *et al.*, 2019). Thus the employment of nanoparticles in cancer therapy requires extensive study and clinical trials to ensure the safety of the nanoformulations.

CONCLUSION

Nanoformulations have been tried out in various forms and sizes and with a variety of carriers to harness the advantages of the nano platform in affording better delivery to the target sites. Several types of cancers have been treated in many ways by applying nanoformulations to overcome each of the difficulties in the delivery regimen. Nanoformulations have an added advantage in the fact that they could penetrate barriers that may be impervious to some drugs. The unique advantages of nanoformulations are the ability to reduce toxicity, increase bioavailability and solubility, increase circulation time, and provide steady drug concentrations through controlled or sustained-release formulations. Besides, the ability to home in on the intended delivery site by passive or active targeting enables nanoformulations to be superior to conventional therapeutics. Nanoformulations that have been designed for the treatment of HCC, keeping the above beneficial factors in mind, overcome the first-pass metabolism and deliver the drugs to the hepatocytes. Increased expression of specific receptors on cancerous hepatocytes has enabled the precision delivery of targeted nanoformulations to the disease site.

CONSENT FOR PUBLICATION

Not applicable.

CONFLICT OF INTEREST

The authors declare no conflict of interest, financial or otherwise.

ACKNOWLEDGEMENT

Declared none.

REFERENCES

Abbasi, S, Paul, A & Prakash, S (2011) Investigation of siRNA-loaded polyethylenimine-coated human serum albumin nanoparticle complexes for the treatment of breast cancer. *Cell Biochem Biophys,* 61, 277-87. [http://dx.doi.org/10.1007/s12013-011-9201-9] [PMID: 21556941]

Acharya, S & Sahoo, SK (2011) PLGA nanoparticles containing various anticancer agents and tumour delivery by EPR effect. *Adv Drug Deliv Rev,* 63, 170-83. [http://dx.doi.org/10.1016/j.addr.2010.10.008] [PMID: 20965219]

Ahmadian, E, Dizaj, S M, Rahimpour, E, Hasanzadeh, A & Eftekhari, A (2018) Effect of silver nanoparticles in the induction of apoptosis on human hepatocellular carcinoma (HepG2) cell line *Materials Science and Engineering C* Elsevier 465-71.

Aki, MA, Kartal-Hodzic, A, Oksanen, T, Ismael, HR, Afouna, MM, Yliperttula, M, Samy, AM & Viitala, T

(2016) 'Factorial design formulation optimization and *in vitro* characterization of curcumin-loaded PLGA nanoparticles for colon delivery'. *J Drug Deliv Sci Technol,* 32, 10-20.
[http://dx.doi.org/10.1016/j.jddst.2016.01.007]

Alavizadeh, SH, Soltani, F & Ramezani, M (2016) 'Recent advances in Immunoliposome-based Cancer therapy'. *Curr Pharmacol Rep,* 2, 129-41.
[http://dx.doi.org/10.1007/s40495-016-0056-z]

Alphandéry, E, Grand-Dewyse, P, Lefèvre, R, Mandawala, C & Durand-Dubief, M (2015) Cancer therapy using nanoformulated substances: scientific, regulatory and financial aspects. *Expert Rev Anticancer Ther,* 15, 1233-55.
[http://dx.doi.org/10.1586/14737140.2015.1086647] [PMID: 26402250]

Anhorn, MG, Wagner, S, Kreuter, J, Langer, K & von Briesen, H (2008) Specific targeting of HER2 overexpressing breast cancer cells with doxorubicin-loaded trastuzumab-modified human serum albumin nanoparticles. *Bioconjug Chem,* 19, 2321-31.
[http://dx.doi.org/10.1021/bc8002452] [PMID: 18937508]

Anirudhan, TS & Binusreejayan, (2016) Dextran based nanosized carrier for the controlled and targeted delivery of curcumin to liver cancer cells. *Elsevier B,* 88, 222-35.
[http://dx.doi.org/10.1016/j.ijbiomac.2016.03.040] [PMID: 27012895]

Arya, G, Vandana, M, Acharya, S & Sahoo, SK (2011) Enhanced antiproliferative activity of Herceptin (HER2)-conjugated gemcitabine-loaded chitosan nanoparticle in pancreatic cancer therapy. *Nanomedicine,* 7, 859-70.
[http://dx.doi.org/10.1016/j.nano.2011.03.009] [PMID: 21550422]

Ashley, CE, Carnes, EC, Epler, KE, Padilla, DP, Phillips, GK, Castillo, RE, Wilkinson, DC, Wilkinson, BS, Burgard, CA, Kalinich, RM, Townson, JL, Chackerian, B, Willman, CL, Peabody, DS, Wharton, W & Brinker, CJ (2012) Delivery of small interfering RNA by peptide-targeted mesoporous silica nanoparticle-supported lipid bilayers. *ACS Nano,* 6, 2174-88.
[http://dx.doi.org/10.1021/nn204102q] [PMID: 22309035]

Babu, A, Amreddy, N, Muralidharan, R, Pathuri, G, Gali, H, Chen, A, Zhao, YD, Munshi, A & Ramesh, R (2017) 'Chemodrug delivery using integrin-targeted PLGA-Chitosan nanoparticle for lung cancer therapy'. *Sci Rep,* 7, 1-17.
[http://dx.doi.org/10.1038/s41598-017-15012-5] [PMID: 28127051]

Baig, B, Halim, SA, Farrukh, A, Greish, Y & Amin, A (2019) Current status of nanomaterial-based treatment for hepatocellular carcinoma. *Biomedicine and Pharmacotherapy Elsevier,* 116, 108852.
[http://dx.doi.org/10.1016/j.biopha.2019.108852] [PMID: 30999152]

Balogh, J, Iii, DV, Gordon, S, Li, X, Ghobrial, RM & Monsour, JrHP (2016) Hepatocellular carcinoma: a review. *J Hepatocell Carcinoma,* 3, 41-53.
[http://dx.doi.org/10.2147/JHC.S61146] [PMID: 27785449]

Banerjee, A, Pathak, S, Subramanium, VD, G, D, Murugesan, R & Verma, RS (2017) Strategies for targeted drug delivery in treatment of colon cancer: current trends and future perspectives. *Drug Discov Today,* 22, 1224-32.
[http://dx.doi.org/10.1016/j.drudis.2017.05.006] [PMID: 28545838]

Barenholz, Y (2012) Doxil®--the first FDA-approved nano-drug: lessons learned. *J Control Release,* 160, 117-34.
[http://dx.doi.org/10.1016/j.jconrel.2012.03.020] [PMID: 22484195]

Behzadi, S, Serpooshan, V, Tao, W, Hamaly, MA, Alkawareek, MY, Dreaden, EC, Brown, D, Alkilany, AM, Farokhzad, OC & Mahmoudi, M (2017) Cellular uptake of nanoparticles: journey inside the cell. *Royal Society of Chemistry,* 46, 4218-44.
[http://dx.doi.org/10.1039/C6CS00636A] [PMID: 28585944]

Bi, H, Xue, J, Jiang, H, Gao, S, Yang, D, Fang, Y & Shi, K (2019) Current developments in drug delivery with thermosensitive liposomes *Asian journal of pharmaceutical sciences,* 14, 365-79.

[http://dx.doi.org/10.1016/j.ajps.2018.07.006]

Blanco, E, Shen, H & Ferrari, M (2015) *'Principles of nanoparticle design for overcoming biological barriers to drug delivery', Nature Biotechnology* Nature Publishing Group 941-51.

Bobo, D, Robinson, KJ, Islam, J, Thurecht, KJ & Corrie, SR (2016) Nanoparticle-Based Medicines: A Review of FDA-Approved Materials and Clinical Trials to Date. *Pharm Res,* 33, 2373-87. [http://dx.doi.org/10.1007/s11095-016-1958-5] [PMID: 27299311]

Bozzuto, G & Molinari, A (2015) Liposomes as nanomedical devices. *Int J Nanomedicine,* 10, 975-99. [http://dx.doi.org/10.2147/IJN.S68861] [PMID: 25678787]

Buttacavoli, M, Albanese, NN, Di Cara, G, Alduina, R, Faleri, C, Gallo, M, Pizzolanti, G, Gallo, G, Feo, S, Baldi, F & Cancemi, P (2017) Anticancer activity of biogenerated silver nanoparticles: an integrated proteomic investigation. *Oncotarget,* 9, 9685-705. [http://dx.doi.org/10.18632/oncotarget.23859] [PMID: 29515763]

Cao, D, Zhang, X, Akabar, MD, Luo, Y, Wu, H, Ke, X & Ci, T (2019) Liposomal doxorubicin loaded PLGA-PEG-PLGA based thermogel for sustained local drug delivery for the treatment of breast cancer. *Artif Cells Nanomed Biotechnol,* 47, 181-91. [http://dx.doi.org/10.1080/21691401.2018.1548470] [PMID: 30686051]

Chanphai, P, Thomas, TJ & Tajmir-Riahi, HA (2019) Design of functionalized folic acid-chitosan nanoparticles for delivery of tetracycline, doxorubicin, and tamoxifen. *J Biomol Struct Dyn,* 37, 1000-6. [http://dx.doi.org/10.1080/07391102.2018.1445559] [PMID: 29478377]

Chauhan, AS (2018) 'Dendrimers for drug delivery'. *Molecules,* 23, 938. [http://dx.doi.org/10.3390/molecules23040938] [PMID: 29670005]

Chen, L, Liu, Y, Wang, W & Liu, K (2015) Effect of integrin receptor-targeted liposomal paclitaxel for hepatocellular carcinoma targeting and therapy. *Oncol Lett,* 10, 77-84. [http://dx.doi.org/10.3892/ol.2015.3242] [PMID: 26170980]

Chen, W, Goldys, EM & Deng, W (2020) Light-induced liposomes for cancer therapeutics. *Prog Lipid Res,* 79, 101052. [http://dx.doi.org/10.1016/j.plipres.2020.101052] [PMID: 32679153]

Chenthamara, D, Subramaniam, S, Ramakrishnan, SG, Krishnaswamy, S, Essa, MM, Lin, FH & Qoronfleh, MW (2019) Therapeutic efficacy of nanoparticles and routes of administration. *Biomater Res,* 23, 20. [http://dx.doi.org/10.1186/s40824-019-0166-x] [PMID: 31832232]

Dai, Y, Su, J, Wu, K, Ma, W, Wang, B, Li, M, Sun, P, Shen, Q, Wang, Q & Fan, Q (2019) 'Multifunctional thermosensitive liposomes based on natural phase-change material: near-infrared light-triggered drug release and multimodal imaging-guided cancer combination therapy'. *ACS Appl Mater Interfaces,* 11, 10540-53. [http://dx.doi.org/10.1021/acsami.8b22748] [PMID: 30807086]

Dass, CR & Choong, PF (2006) Selective gene delivery for cancer therapy using cationic liposomes: *in vivo* proof of applicability. *J Control Release,* 113, 155-63. [http://dx.doi.org/10.1016/j.jconrel.2006.04.009] [PMID: 16764960]

Dehghani, F, Farhadian, N, Golmohammadzadeh, S, Biriaee, A, Ebrahimi, M & Karimi, M (2017) Preparation, characterization and in-vivo evaluation of microemulsions containing tamoxifen citrate anti-cancer drug. *Eur J Pharm Sci,* 96, 479-89. [http://dx.doi.org/10.1016/j.ejps.2016.09.033] [PMID: 27693298]

Daraee, H, Etemadi, A, Kouhi, M, Alimirzalu, S & Akbarzadeh, A (2016) Application of liposomes in medicine and drug delivery. *Artif Cells Nanomed Biotechnol,* 44, 381-91. [http://dx.doi.org/10.3109/21691401.2014.953633] [PMID: 25222036]

Devulapally, R, Foygel, K, Sekar, TV, Willmann, JK & Paulmurugan, R (2016) 'Gemcitabine and antisense-microRNA co-encapsulated PLGA PEG polymer nanoparticles for hepatocellular carcinoma therapy'. *ACS Appl Mater Interfaces,* 8, 33412-22.

[http://dx.doi.org/10.1021/acsami.6b08153] [PMID: 27960411]

Dhar, S, Gu, FX, Langer, R, Farokhzad, OC & Lippard, SJ (2008) Targeted delivery of cisplatin to prostate cancer cells by aptamer functionalized Pt(IV) prodrug-PLGA-PEG nanoparticles. *Proc Natl Acad Sci USA,* 105, 17356-61.
[http://dx.doi.org/10.1073/pnas.0809154105] [PMID: 18978032]

Dimitroulis, D, Damaskos, C, Valsami, S, Davakis, S, Garmpis, N, Spartalis, E, Athanasiou, A, Moris, D, Sakellariou, S, Kykalos, S, Tsourouflis, G, Garmpi, A, Delladetsima, I, Kontzoglou, K & Kouraklis, G (2017) From diagnosis to treatment of hepatocellular carcinoma: An epidemic problem for both developed and developing world. *World J Gastroenterol,* 23, 5282-94.
[http://dx.doi.org/10.3748/wjg.v23.i29.5282] [PMID: 28839428]

Domínguez-Ríos, R, Sánchez-Ramírez, DR, Ruiz-Saray, K, Oceguera-Basurto, PE, Almada, M, Juárez, J, Zepeda-Moreno, A, Del Toro-Arreola, A, Topete, A & Daneri-Navarro, A (2019) Cisplatin-loaded PLGA nanoparticles for HER2 targeted ovarian cancer therapy. *Colloids Surf B Biointerfaces,* 178, 199-207.
[http://dx.doi.org/10.1016/j.colsurfb.2019.03.011] [PMID: 30856589]

El-Feky, GS, El-Banna, ST, El-Bahy, GS, Abdelrazek, EM & Kamal, M (2017) Alginate coated chitosan nanogel for the controlled topical delivery of Silver sulfadiazine. *Carbohydr Polym,* 177, 194-202.
[http://dx.doi.org/10.1016/j.carbpol.2017.08.104] [PMID: 28962758]

El-Hammadi, MM, Delgado, ÁV, Melguizo, C, Prados, JC & Arias, JL (2017) Folic acid-decorated and PEGylated PLGA nanoparticles for improving the antitumour activity of 5-fluorouracil. *Int J Pharm,* 516, 61-70.
[http://dx.doi.org/10.1016/j.ijpharm.2016.11.012] [PMID: 27825867]

El-Kharrag, R, Amin, A, Hisaindee, S, Greish, Y & Karam, SM (2017) Development of a therapeutic model of precancerous liver using crocin-coated magnetite nanoparticles. *Int J Oncol,* 50, 212-22.
[http://dx.doi.org/10.3892/ijo.2016.3769] [PMID: 27878253]

Eloy, JO, Ruiz, A, de Lima, FT, Petrilli, R, Raspantini, G, Nogueira, KAB, Santos, E, de Oliveira, CS, Borges, JC, Marchetti, JM, Al-Jamal, WT & Chorilli, M (2020) EGFR-targeted immunoliposomes efficiently deliver docetaxel to prostate cancer cells. *Colloids Surf B Biointerfaces,* 194, 111185.
[http://dx.doi.org/10.1016/j.colsurfb.2020.111185] [PMID: 32574928]

El-Say, KM & El-Sawy, HS (2017) Polymeric nanoparticles: Promising platform for drug delivery. *Int J Pharm,* 528, 675-91.
[http://dx.doi.org/10.1016/j.ijpharm.2017.06.052] [PMID: 28629982]

Fan, Y & Zhang, Q (2013) 'Development of liposomal formulations: From concept to clinical investigations'. *Asian Journal of Pharmaceutical Sciences,* 8, 81-7.
[http://dx.doi.org/10.1016/j.ajps.2013.07.010]

Fan, Y, Chen, C, Huang, Y, Zhang, F & Lin, G (2017) Study of the pH-sensitive mechanism of tumor-targeting liposomes. *Colloids Surf B Biointerfaces,* 151, 19-25.
[http://dx.doi.org/10.1016/j.colsurfb.2016.11.042] [PMID: 27940165]

Fasehee, H, Dinarvand, R, Ghavamzadeh, A, Esfandyari-Manesh, M, Moradian, H, Faghihi, S & Ghaffari, SH (2016) Delivery of disulfiram into breast cancer cells using folate-receptor-targeted PLGA-PEG nanoparticles: *in vitro* and *in vivo* investigations. *J Nanobiotechnology,* 14, 32.
[http://dx.doi.org/10.1186/s12951-016-0183-z] [PMID: 27102110]

Feng, C, Li, J, Kong, M, Liu, Y, Cheng, XJ, Li, Y, Park, HJ & Chen, XG (2015) Surface charge effect on mucoadhesion of chitosan based nanogels for local anti-colorectal cancer drug delivery. *Colloids Surf B Biointerfaces,* 128, 439-47.
[http://dx.doi.org/10.1016/j.colsurfb.2015.02.042] [PMID: 25769283]

Forssen, EA (1997) 'The design and development of DaunoXome® for solid tumor targeting *in vivo*'. *Adv Drug Deliv Rev,* 24, 133-50.
[http://dx.doi.org/10.1016/S0169-409X(96)00453-X]

Fu, S, Xia, J & Wu, J (2016) 'Functional chitosan nanoparticles in cancer treatment'. *J Biomed Nanotechnol,* 12, 1585-603.
[http://dx.doi.org/10.1166/jbn.2016.2228] [PMID: 29341581]

Ghosh, D, Choudhury, ST, Ghosh, S, Mandal, AK, Sarkar, S, Ghosh, A, Saha, KD & Das, N (2012) Nanocapsulated curcumin: oral chemopreventive formulation against diethylnitrosamine induced hepatocellular carcinoma in rat. *Elsevier Ireland Ltd,* 195, 206-14.
[http://dx.doi.org/10.1016/j.cbi.2011.12.004] [PMID: 22197969]

Golkar, N, Tamaddon, AM & Samani, SM (2016) Effect of lipid composition on incorporation of trastuzumab-PEG-lipid into nanoliposomes by post-insertion method: physicochemical and cellular characterization. *J Liposome Res,* 26, 113-25.
[PMID: 26023889]

Goodall, S, Jones, ML & Mahler, S (2015) Monoclonal antibody-targeted polymeric nanoparticles for cancer therapy - future prospects. *J Chem Technol Biotechnol,* 90, 1169-76.
[http://dx.doi.org/10.1002/jctb.4555]

Guan, M, Zhou, Y, Zhu, QL, Liu, Y, Bei, YY, Zhang, XN & Zhang, Q (2012) N-trimethyl chitosan nanoparticle-encapsulated lactosyl-norcantharidin for liver cancer therapy with high targeting efficacy. *Nanomedicine,* 8, 1172-81.
[http://dx.doi.org/10.1016/j.nano.2012.01.009] [PMID: 22321383]

Hasan, W, Chu, K, Gullapalli, A, Dunn, SS, Enlow, EM, Luft, JC, Tian, S, Napier, ME, Pohlhaus, PD, Rolland, JP & DeSimone, JM (2012) Delivery of multiple siRNAs using lipid-coated PLGA nanoparticles for treatment of prostate cancer. *Nano Lett,* 12, 287-92.
[http://dx.doi.org/10.1021/nl2035354] [PMID: 22165988]

de la Harpe, KM, Kondiah, PPD, Choonara, YE, Marimuthu, T, du Toit, LC & Pillay, V (2019) The Hemocompatibility of Nanoparticles: A Review of Cell-Nanoparticle Interactions and Hemostasis. *Cells,* 8, 1-25.
[http://dx.doi.org/10.3390/cells8101209] [PMID: 31591302]

Hoogenboezem, EN & Duvall, CL (2018) Harnessing albumin as a carrier for cancer therapies. *Adv Drug Deliv Rev,* 130, 73-89.
[http://dx.doi.org/10.1016/j.addr.2018.07.011] [PMID: 30012492]

Hu, M, Ai, X, Wang, Z, Zhang, Z, Cheong, H, Zhang, W, Lin, J, Li, J, Yang, H & Xing, B (2018) 'Nanoformulation of metal complexes: Intelligent stimuli-responsive platforms for precision therapeutics'. *Nano Res,* 11, 5474-98.
[http://dx.doi.org/10.1007/s12274-018-2138-1]

Huwyler, J, Drewe, J & Krähenbuhl, S (2008) Tumor targeting using liposomal antineoplastic drugs. *Int J Nanomedicine,* 3, 21-9.
[http://dx.doi.org/10.2147/IJN.S1253] [PMID: 18488413]

Hwang, Y, Park, SH & Lee, JW (2017) Applications of functionalized carbon nanotubes for the therapy and diagnosis of cancer. *Polymers (Basel),* 9, 1-26.
[http://dx.doi.org/10.3390/polym9010013] [PMID: 30970690]

Immordino, ML, Dosio, F & Cattel, L (2006) Stealth liposomes: review of the basic science, rationale, and clinical applications, existing and potential. *Int J Nanomedicine,* 1, 297-315.
[PMID: 17717971]

Ishii, H, Furuse, J, Nagase, M, Maru, Y, Yoshino, M & Hayashi, T (2003) A phase I study of hepatic arterial infusion chemotherapy with zinostatin stimalamer alone for hepatocellular carcinoma. *Jpn J Clin Oncol,* 33, 570-3.
[http://dx.doi.org/10.1093/jjco/hyg106] [PMID: 14711981]

Jafari, M, Zargar, B, Soltani, M, Karunaratne, DN, Ingalls, B & Chen, P (2012) Intelligent drug delivery systems for cancer therapy. in Biomedical Materials and Diagnostic Devices In: Ashutosh, Tiwari, Murugan,

Ramalingam, Hisatoshi, Kobayashi, Anthony, P.F. Turner, (Eds.), Wiley-Scrivener Publishing LLC.

Jain, KK (2012) Nanobiotechnology-based strategies for crossing the blood-brain barrier. *Nanomedicine (Lond),* 7, 1225-33.
[http://dx.doi.org/10.2217/nnm.12.86] [PMID: 22931448]

Jain, NK & Jain, SK (2010) Development and *in vitro* characterization of galactosylated low molecular weight chitosan nanoparticles bearing doxorubicin. *AAPS PharmSciTech,* 11, 686-97.
[http://dx.doi.org/10.1208/s12249-010-9422-z] [PMID: 20414758]

Jang, B, Kwon, H, Katila, P, Lee, SJ & Lee, H (2016) Dual delivery of biological therapeutics for multimodal and synergistic cancer therapies. *Adv Drug Deliv Rev,* 98, 113-33.
[http://dx.doi.org/10.1016/j.addr.2015.10.023] [PMID: 26654747]

Ji, Z, Lin, G, Lu, Q, Meng, L, Shen, X, Dong, L, Fu, C & Zhang, X (2012) Targeted therapy of SMMC-7721 liver cancer *in vitro* and *in vivo* with carbon nanotubes based drug delivery system. *J Colloid Interface Sci,* 365, 143-9.
[http://dx.doi.org/10.1016/j.jcis.2011.09.013] [PMID: 21974923]

Jin, C, Qian, N, Zhao, W, Yang, W, Bai, L, Wu, H, Wang, M, Song, W & Dou, K (2010) Improved therapeutic effect of DOX-PLGA-PEG micelles decorated with bivalent fragment HAb18 F(ab')(2) for hepatocellular carcinoma. *Biomacromolecules,* 11, 2422-31.
[http://dx.doi.org/10.1021/bm1005992] [PMID: 20831277]

Jose, A, Labala, S, Ninave, KM, Gade, SK & Venuganti, VVK (2018) 'Effective skin cancer treatment by topical co-delivery of curcumin and STAT3 siRNA using cationic liposomes'. *AAPS PharmSciTech,* 19, 166-75.
[http://dx.doi.org/10.1208/s12249-017-0833-y] [PMID: 28639178]

Kalyane, D, Raval, N, Maheshwari, R, Tambe, V, Kalia, K & Tekade, RK (2019) Employment of enhanced permeability and retention effect (EPR): Nanoparticle-based precision tools for targeting of therapeutic and diagnostic agent in cancer. *Mater Sci Eng C,* 98, 1252-76.
[http://dx.doi.org/10.1016/j.msec.2019.01.066] [PMID: 30813007]

Karanth, H & Murthy, RSR (2007) pH-sensitive liposomes--principle and application in cancer therapy. *J Pharm Pharmacol,* 59, 469-83.
[http://dx.doi.org/10.1211/jpp.59.4.0001] [PMID: 17430630]

Karunaratne, DN (2007) 'Nanotechnology in medicine'. *J Natl Sci Found Sri Lanka,* 35, 149-52.
[http://dx.doi.org/10.4038/jnsfsr.v35i3.2012]

Karunaratne, DN, Ariyarathna, IR, Welideniya, D, Siriwardhana, A, Gunasekera, D & Karunaratne, V (2017) 'Nanotechnological strategies to improve water solubility of commercially available drugs'. *Curr Nanomed,* 7, 84-110.
[http://dx.doi.org/10.2174/2468187307666161227171349]

Karunaratne, DN, Dassanayake, AC, Pamunuwa, KMGK & Karunaratne, V (2014) 'Improved skin permeability of dl□α□tocopherol in topical macroemulsions'. *Int J Pharm Pharm Sci,* 6, 53-7.

Karunaratne, DN, Jafari, M, Ranatunge, RJKU & Siriwardene, A (2015) 'Natural carriers for siRNA delivery'. *Curr Pharm Des,* 21, 4527-8.
[http://dx.doi.org/10.2174/138161282131151013185528] [PMID: 26362643]

Karunaratne, DN, Pamunuwa, G & Ranatunga, U (2017) *Properties and uses of microemulsions* IntechOpen, Croatia 3-14.
[http://dx.doi.org/10.5772/63187]

Kermanizadeh, A, Powell, LG, Stone, V & Møller, P (2018) Nanodelivery systems and stabilized solid-drug nanoparticles for orally administered medicine: current landscape. *Int J Nanomedicine,* 13, 7575-605.
[http://dx.doi.org/10.2147/IJN.S177418] [PMID: 30510419]

Khan, A, Aljarbou, AN, Aldebasi, YH, Allemailem, KS, Alsahli, MA, Khan, S, Alruwetei, AM & Khan, MA (2020) Fatty Acid Synthase (FASN) siRNA-Encapsulated-Her-2 Targeted Fab'-Immunoliposomes for Gene

Silencing in Breast Cancer Cells. *Int J Nanomedicine,* 15, 5575-89.
[http://dx.doi.org/10.2147/IJN.S256022] [PMID: 32801705]

Khan, AR, Yang, X, Fu, M & Zhai, G (2018) Recent progress of drug nanoformulations targeting to brain. *J Control Release,* 291, 37-64.
[http://dx.doi.org/10.1016/j.jconrel.2018.10.004] [PMID: 30308256]

Khanna, P, Ong, C, Bay, BH & Baeg, GH (2015) Nanotoxicity: An interplay of oxidative stress, inflammation and cell death. *Nanomaterials (Basel),* 5, 1163-80.
[http://dx.doi.org/10.3390/nano5031163] [PMID: 28347058]

Khayrani, AC, Mahmud, H, Oo, AKK, Zahra, MH, Oze, M, Du, J, Alam, MJ, Afify, SM, Quora, HAA, Shigehiro, T, Calle, AS, Okada, N, Seno, A, Fujita, K, Hamada, H, Seno, Y, Mandai, T & Seno, M (2019) Targeting Ovarian Cancer Cells Overexpressing CD44 with Immunoliposomes Encapsulating Glycosylated Paclitaxel. *Int J Mol Sci,* 20, 1042.
[http://dx.doi.org/10.3390/ijms20051042] [PMID: 30818864]

Khosa, A, Reddi, S & Saha, RN (2018) Nanostructured lipid carriers for site-specific drug delivery. *Biomed Pharmacother,* 103, 598-613.
[http://dx.doi.org/10.1016/j.biopha.2018.04.055] [PMID: 29677547]

Kiaie, SH, Mojarad-Jabali, S, Khaleseh, F, Allahyari, S, Taheri, E, Zakeri-Milani, P & Valizadeh, H (2020) Axial pharmaceutical properties of liposome in cancer therapy: Recent advances and perspectives. *Int J Pharm,* 581, 119269.
[http://dx.doi.org/10.1016/j.ijpharm.2020.119269] [PMID: 32234427]

Kim, E, Jung, Y, Choi, H, Yang, J, Suh, JS, Huh, YM, Kim, K & Haam, S (2010) Prostate cancer cell death produced by the co-delivery of Bcl-xL shRNA and doxorubicin using an aptamer-conjugated polyplex. *Biomaterials,* 31, 4592-9.
[http://dx.doi.org/10.1016/j.biomaterials.2010.02.030] [PMID: 20206379]

Kinoshita, R, Ishima, Y, Chuang, VTG, Nakamura, H, Fang, J, Watanabe, H, Shimizu, T, Okuhira, K, Ishida, T, Maeda, H, Otagiri, M & Maruyama, T (2017) Improved anticancer effects of albumin-bound paclitaxel nanoparticle *via* augmentation of EPR effect and albumin-protein interactions using S-nitrosated human serum albumin dimer. *Biomaterials,* 140, 162-9.
[http://dx.doi.org/10.1016/j.biomaterials.2017.06.021] [PMID: 28651144]

Kue, CS, Kamkaew, A, Burgess, K, Kiew, LV, Chung, LY & Lee, HB (2016) 'Small molecules for active targeting in cancer'. *Med Res Rev,* 36, 494-575.
[http://dx.doi.org/10.1002/med.21387] [PMID: 26992114]

Kuruvilla, SP, Tiruchinapally, G, Crouch, AC, ElSayed, MEH & Greve, JM (2017) Dendrimer-doxorubicin conjugates exhibit improved anticancer activity and reduce doxorubicin-induced cardiotoxicity in a murine hepatocellular carcinoma model. *PLoS One,* 12, e0181944.
[http://dx.doi.org/10.1371/journal.pone.0181944] [PMID: 28829785]

Lee, AL, Wang, Y, Pervaiz, S, Fan, W & Yang, YY (2011) Synergistic anticancer effects achieved by co-delivery of TRAIL and paclitaxel using cationic polymeric micelles. *Macromol Biosci,* 11, 296-307.
[http://dx.doi.org/10.1002/mabi.201000332] [PMID: 21154473]

Leite-Silva, VR, De Almeida, MM, Fradin, A, Grice, JE & Roberts, MS (2012) 'Delivery of drugs applied topically to the skin'. *Expert Rev Dermatol,* 7, 383-97.
[http://dx.doi.org/10.1586/edm.12.32]

Leonard, RCF, Williams, S, Tulpule, A, Levine, AM & Oliveros, S (2009) Improving the therapeutic index of anthracycline chemotherapy: focus on liposomal doxorubicin (Myocet). *Breast,* 18, 218-24.
[http://dx.doi.org/10.1016/j.breast.2009.05.004] [PMID: 19656681]

Li, FQ, Su, H, Wang, J, Liu, JY, Zhu, QG, Fei, YB, Pan, YH & Hu, JH (2008) Preparation and characterization of sodium ferulate entrapped bovine serum albumin nanoparticles for liver targeting. *Int J Pharm,* 349, 274-82.

[http://dx.doi.org/10.1016/j.ijpharm.2007.08.001] [PMID: 17870261]

Li, M, Zhang, W, Wang, B, Gao, Y, Song, Z & Zheng, QC (2016) Ligand-based targeted therapy: a novel strategy for hepatocellular carcinoma. *Int J Nanomedicine,* 11, 5645-69.
[http://dx.doi.org/10.2147/IJN.S115727] [PMID: 27920520]

Liang, GF, Zhu, YL, Sun, B, Hu, FH, Tian, T, Li, SC & Xiao, ZD (2011) 'PLGA-based gene delivering nanoparticle enhance suppression effect of miRNA in HePG2 cells', *Nanoscale Research Letters. Springer Open Ltd,* 6, 1-9.

Lim, YH, Tiemann, KM, Hunstad, DA, Elsabahy, M & Wooley, KL (2016) Polymeric nanoparticles in development for treatment of pulmonary infectious diseases. *Wiley Interdiscip Rev Nanomed Nanobiotechnol,* 8, 842-71.
[http://dx.doi.org/10.1002/wnan.1401] [PMID: 27016134]

Lin, Q, Mao, KL, Tian, FR, Yang, JJ, Chen, PP, Xu, J, Fan, ZL, Zhao, YP, Li, WF, Zheng, L, Zhao, YZ & Lu, CT (2016) Brain tumor-targeted delivery and therapy by focused ultrasound introduced doxorubicin-loaded cationic liposomes. *Cancer Chemother Pharmacol,* 77, 269-80.
[http://dx.doi.org/10.1007/s00280-015-2926-1] [PMID: 26666650]

Ling, D, Xia, H, Park, W, Hackett, MJ, Song, C, Na, K, Hui, KM & Hyeon, T (2014) pH-sensitive nanoformulated triptolide as a targeted therapeutic strategy for hepatocellular carcinoma. *ACS Nano,* 8, 8027-39.
[http://dx.doi.org/10.1021/nn502074x] [PMID: 25093274]

Liu, B, Han, L, Liu, J, Han, S, Chen, Z & Jiang, L (2017) Co-delivery of paclitaxel and TOS-cisplatin *via* TAT-targeted solid lipid nanoparticles with synergistic antitumor activity against cervical cancer. *Int J Nanomedicine,* 12, 955-68.
[http://dx.doi.org/10.2147/IJN.S115136] [PMID: 28203075]

Liu, MC, Liu, L, Wang, XR, Shuai, WP, Hu, Y, Han, M & Gao, JQ (2016) Folate receptor-targeted liposomes loaded with a diacid metabolite of norcantharidin enhance antitumor potency for H22 hepatocellular carcinoma both *in vitro* and *in vivo*. *Int J Nanomedicine,* 11, 1395-412.
[http://dx.doi.org/10.2147/IJN.S96862] [PMID: 27110110]

Lombardi, G, Zustovich, F, Farinati, F, Cillo, U, Vitale, A, Zanus, G, Donach, M, Farina, M, Zovato, S & Pastorelli, D (2011) Pegylated liposomal doxorubicin and gemcitabine in patients with advanced hepatocellular carcinoma: results of a phase 2 study. *Cancer,* 117, 125-33.
[http://dx.doi.org/10.1002/cncr.25578] [PMID: 21058409]

Lomis, N, Westfall, S, Farahdel, L, Malhotra, M, Shum-Tim, D & Prakash, S (2016) 'Human serum albumin nanoparticles for use in cancer drug delivery: process optimization and *in vitro* characterization'. *Nanomaterials (Basel),* 6, 116.
[http://dx.doi.org/10.3390/nano6060116] [PMID: 28335244]

Lu, J, Li, Z, Zink, JI & Tamanoi, F (2012) *In vivo* tumor suppression efficacy of mesoporous silica nanoparticles-based drug-delivery system: enhanced efficacy by folate modification. *Nanomedicine,* 8, 212-20.
[http://dx.doi.org/10.1016/j.nano.2011.06.002] [PMID: 21703996]

Lu, X, Liu, S, Han, M, Yang, X, Sun, K, Wang, H, Mu, H, Du, Y, Wang, A, Ni, L & Zhang, C (2019) Afatinib-loaded immunoliposomes functionalized with cetuximab: A novel strategy targeting the epidermal growth factor receptor for treatment of non-small-cell lung cancer. *Int J Pharm,* 560, 126-35.
[http://dx.doi.org/10.1016/j.ijpharm.2019.02.001] [PMID: 30742982]

Lukyanov, AN, Elbayoumi, TA, Chakilam, AR & Torchilin, VP (2004) Tumor-targeted liposomes: doxorubicin-loaded long-circulating liposomes modified with anti-cancer antibody. *J Control Release,* 100, 135-44.
[http://dx.doi.org/10.1016/j.jconrel.2004.08.007] [PMID: 15491817]

Ma, Y, Chen, H, Su, S, Wang, T, Zhang, C, Fida, G, Cui, S, Zhao, J & Gu, Y (2015) Galactose as broad ligand for multiple tumor imaging and therapy. *J Cancer,* 6, 658-70.

[http://dx.doi.org/10.7150/jca.11647] [PMID: 26078797]

Masood, F (2016) Polymeric nanoparticles for targeted drug delivery system for cancer therapy. *Mater Sci Eng C,* 60, 569-78.
[http://dx.doi.org/10.1016/j.msec.2015.11.067] [PMID: 26706565]

Maeda, H (1992) 'The tumor blood vessel as an ideal target for macromolecular anticancer agents'. *J Control Release,* 19, 315-24.
[http://dx.doi.org/10.1016/0168-3659(92)90086-7]

Maruyama, K (2011) Intracellular targeting delivery of liposomal drugs to solid tumors based on EPR effects. *Adv Drug Deliv Rev,* 63, 161-9.
[http://dx.doi.org/10.1016/j.addr.2010.09.003] [PMID: 20869415]

Mehmood, A, Ghafar, H, Yaqoob, S, Gohar, UF & Ahmad, B (2017) Mesoporous Silica Nanoparticles: A Review. *J Dev Drugs,* 06, 174.
[http://dx.doi.org/10.4172/2329-6631.1000174]

Mendes, LP, Pan, J & Torchilin, VP (2017) 'Dendrimers as nanocarriers for nucleic acid and drug delivery in cancer therapy'. *Molecules,* 22, 1401.
[http://dx.doi.org/10.3390/molecules22091401]

Mirahmadi, M, Azimi-Hashemi, S, Saburi, E, Kamali, H, Pishbin, M & Hadizadeh, F (2020) Potential inhibitory effect of lycopene on prostate cancer. *Biomed Pharmacother,* 129, 110459.
[http://dx.doi.org/10.1016/j.biopha.2020.110459] [PMID: 32768949]

Mo, Y, Du, H, Chen, B, Liu, D, Yin, Q, Yan, Y, Wang, Z, Wan, F, Qi, T, Wang, Y, Zhang, Q & Wang, Y (2019) Quick-Responsive Polymer-Based Thermosensitive Liposomes for Controlled Doxorubicin Release and Chemotherapy. *ACS Biomater Sci Eng,* 5, 2316-29.
[http://dx.doi.org/10.1021/acsbiomaterials.9b00343] [PMID: 33405782]

Mohamed, NK, Hamad, MA, Hafez, MZE, Wooley, KL & Elsabahy, M (2017) Nanomedicine in management of hepatocellular carcinoma: Challenges and opportunities. *Int J Cancer,* 140, 1475-84.
[http://dx.doi.org/10.1002/ijc.30517] [PMID: 27861850]

Mojeiko, G, de Brito, M, Salata, GC & Lopes, LB (2019) Combination of microneedles and microemulsions to increase celecoxib topical delivery for potential application in chemoprevention of breast cancer. *Int J Pharm,* 560, 365-76.
[http://dx.doi.org/10.1016/j.ijpharm.2019.02.011] [PMID: 30772460]

Mullauer, FB, van Bloois, L, Daalhuisen, JB, Ten Brink, MS, Storm, G, Medema, JP, Schiffelers, RM & Kessler, JH (2011) Betulinic acid delivered in liposomes reduces growth of human lung and colon cancers in mice without causing systemic toxicity. *Anticancer Drugs,* 22, 223-33.
[http://dx.doi.org/10.1097/CAD.0b013e3283421035] [PMID: 21263311]

Murry, DJ & Blaney, SM (2000) Clinical pharmacology of encapsulated sustained-release cytarabine. *Ann Pharmacother,* 34, 1173-8.
[http://dx.doi.org/10.1345/aph.19347] [PMID: 11054987]

Namiki, Y, Namiki, T, Date, M, Yanagihara, K, Yashiro, M & Takahashi, H (2004) Enhanced photodynamic antitumor effect on gastric cancer by a novel photosensitive stealth liposome. *Pharmacol Res,* 50, 65-76.
[http://dx.doi.org/10.1016/j.phrs.2003.12.015] [PMID: 15082031]

Nieberler, M, Reuning, U, Reichart, F, Notni, J, Wester, HJ, Schwaiger, M, Weinmüller, M, Räder, A, Steiger, K & Kessler, H (2017) Exploring the role of RGD-recognizing integrins in cancer. *Cancers (Basel),* 9, 1-33.
[http://dx.doi.org/10.3390/cancers9090116] [PMID: 28869579]

Nosova, AS, Koloskova, OO, Nikonova, AA, Simonova, VA, Smirnov, VV, Kudlay, D & Khaitov, MR (2019) Diversity of PEGylation methods of liposomes and their influence on RNA delivery. *MedChemComm,* 10, 369-77.
[http://dx.doi.org/10.1039/C8MD00515J] [PMID: 31015904]

Nwokwu, CDU, Samarakoon, SR, Karunaratne, DN, Katuvawila, NP, Pamunuwa, GK, Ediriweera, MK & Tennekoon, KH (2017) 'Induction of apoptosis in response to improved gedunin by liposomal nano-encapsulation in human non-small-cell lung cancer (NCI-H292) cell line'. *Trop J Pharm Res,* 16, 2079-87. [http://dx.doi.org/10.4314/tjpr.v16i9.6]

Paino, IMM, Marangoni, VS, de Oliveira, RdeC, Antunes, LMG & Zucolotto, V (2012) Cyto and genotoxicity of gold nanoparticles in human hepatocellular carcinoma and peripheral blood mononuclear cells. *Toxicol Lett,* 215, 119-25. [http://dx.doi.org/10.1016/j.toxlet.2012.09.025] [PMID: 23046612]

Paliwal, SR, Paliwal, R, Pal, HC, Saxena, AK, Sharma, PR, Gupta, PN, Agrawal, GP & Vyas, SP (2012) Estrogen-anchored pH-sensitive liposomes as nanomodule designed for site-specific delivery of doxorubicin in breast cancer therapy. *Mol Pharm,* 9, 176-86. [http://dx.doi.org/10.1021/mp200439z] [PMID: 22091702]

Pamunuwa, G, Anjalee, N, Kukulewa, D, Edirisinghe, C, Shakoor, F & Karunaratne, DN (2020) *Tailoring of release properties of folic acid encapsulated nanoparticles via changing alginate and pectin composition in the matrix* Carbohydrate Polymer Technologies and Applications 100008.

Pamunuwa, KMGK, Bandara, CJ, Karunaratne, V & Karunaratne, DN (2015) 'Optimization of a liposomal delivery system for the highly antioxidant methanol extract of stem-bark of Schumacheria castaneifolia Vahl'. *J Chem Pharm Res,* 7, 1236-45.

Park, J, Choi, Y, Chang, H, Um, W, Ryu, JH & Kwon, IC (2019) 'Alliance with EPR effect: Combined strategies to improve the EPR effect in the tumor microenvironment'. *Theranostics,* 9, 8073-90. [http://dx.doi.org/10.7150/thno.37198] [PMID: 31754382]

Parsian, M, Unsoy, G, Mutlu, P, Yalcin, S, Tezcaner, A & Gunduz, U (2016) Loading of Gemcitabine on chitosan magnetic nanoparticles increases the anti-cancer efficacy of the drug. *Eur J Pharmacol,* 784, 121-8. [http://dx.doi.org/10.1016/j.ejphar.2016.05.016] [PMID: 27181067]

Parveen, S & Sahoo, SK (2008) Polymeric nanoparticles for cancer therapy. *J Drug Target,* 16, 108-23. [http://dx.doi.org/10.1080/10611860701794353] [PMID: 18274932]

Pilapong, C, Sitthichai, S, Thongtem, S & Thongtem, T (2014) Smart magnetic nanoparticle-aptamer probe for targeted imaging and treatment of hepatocellular carcinoma. *Elsevier B,* 473, 469-74. [http://dx.doi.org/10.1016/j.ijpharm.2014.07.036] [PMID: 25089503]

Plapied, L, Duhem, N, des Rieux, A & Préat, V (2011) 'Fate of polymeric nanocarriers for oral drug delivery'. *Curr Opin Colloid Interface Sci,* 16, 228-37. [http://dx.doi.org/10.1016/j.cocis.2010.12.005]

Poon, RTP & Borys, N (2009) Lyso-thermosensitive liposomal doxorubicin: a novel approach to enhance efficacy of thermal ablation of liver cancer. *Expert Opin Pharmacother,* 10, 333-43. [http://dx.doi.org/10.1517/14656560802677874] [PMID: 19236203]

Qi, L, Xu, Z & Chen, M (2007) *In vitro* and *in vivo* suppression of hepatocellular carcinoma growth by chitosan nanoparticles. *Eur J Cancer,* 43, 184-93. [http://dx.doi.org/10.1016/j.ejca.2006.08.029] [PMID: 17049839]

Qu, N, Lee, RJ, Sun, Y, Cai, G, Wang, J, Wang, M, Lu, J, Meng, Q, Teng, L, Wang, D & Teng, L (2016) Cabazitaxel-loaded human serum albumin nanoparticles as a therapeutic agent against prostate cancer. *Int J Nanomedicine,* 11, 3451-9. [http://dx.doi.org/10.2147/IJN.S105420] [PMID: 27555767]

Reinholz, J, Landfester, K & Mailänder, V (2018) The challenges of oral drug delivery *via* nanocarriers. *Drug Deliv,* 25, 1694-705. [http://dx.doi.org/10.1080/10717544.2018.1501119] [PMID: 30394120]

Rhee, YS & Mansour, HM (2011) 'Nanopharmaceuticals I: nanocarrier systems in drug delivery'. *Int J Nanotechnol,* 8, 84-114.

[http://dx.doi.org/10.1504/IJNT.2011.037172]

Saeed, B A, Lim, V, Yusof, N A, Khor, K Z, Rahman, H S & Samad, N A (2019) Antiangiogenic properties of nanoparticles: A systematic review *International Journal of Nanomedicine*Dove Medical Press Ltd. 5135-5146 10.2147/IJN.S199974

Sadhukhan, P, Kundu, M, Chatterjee, S, Ghosh, N, Manna, P, Das, J & Sil, PC (2019) Targeted delivery of quercetin *via* pH-responsive zinc oxide nanoparticles for breast cancer therapy. *Mater Sci Eng C,* 100, 129-40.
[http://dx.doi.org/10.1016/j.msec.2019.02.096] [PMID: 30948047]

Saha, S, Yakati, V, Shankar, G, Jaggarapu, MMCS, Moku, G, Madhusudana, K, Banerjee, R, Ramkrishna, S, Srinivas, R & Chaudhuri, A (2020) Amphetamine decorated cationic lipid nanoparticles cross the blood-brain barrier: therapeutic promise for combating glioblastoma. *J Mater Chem B Mater Biol Med,* 8, 4318-30.
[http://dx.doi.org/10.1039/C9TB02700A] [PMID: 32330214]

Sala, M, Diab, R, Elaissari, A & Fessi, H (2018) Lipid nanocarriers as skin drug delivery systems: Properties, mechanisms of skin interactions and medical applications. *Int J Pharm,* 535, 1-17.
[http://dx.doi.org/10.1016/j.ijpharm.2017.10.046] [PMID: 29111097]

Salatin, S & Yari Khosroushahi, A (2017) Overviews on the cellular uptake mechanism of polysaccharide colloidal nanoparticles. *J Cell Mol Med,* 21, 1668-86.
[http://dx.doi.org/10.1111/jcmm.13110] [PMID: 28244656]

Saleh, T, Soudi, T & Shojaosadati, SA (2019) Aptamer functionalized curcumin-loaded human serum albumin (HSA) nanoparticles for targeted delivery to HER-2 positive breast cancer cells. *Int J Biol Macromol,* 130, 109-16.
[http://dx.doi.org/10.1016/j.ijbiomac.2019.02.129] [PMID: 30802519]

Sánchez-López, E, Guerra, M, Dias-Ferreira, J, Lopez-Machado, A, Ettcheto, M, Cano, A, Espina, M, Camins, A, Garcia, ML & Souto, EB (2019) 'Current applications of nanoemulsions in cancer therapeutics'. *Nanomaterials (Basel),* 9, 821.
[http://dx.doi.org/10.3390/nano9060821] [PMID: 31159219]

Sebak, S, Mirzaei, M, Malhotra, M, Kulamarva, A & Prakash, S (2010) Human serum albumin nanoparticles as an efficient noscapine drug delivery system for potential use in breast cancer: preparation and *in vitro* analysis. *Int J Nanomedicine,* 5, 525-32.
[PMID: 20957217]

Shah, S, Sasmal, PK & Lee, KB (2014) 'Photo-triggerable hydrogel nanoparticle hybrid scaffolds for remotely controlled drug delivery'. *J Mater Chem B Mater Biol Med,* 2, 7685-93.
[http://dx.doi.org/10.1039/C4TB01436G] [PMID: 25580246]

Shargh, VH, Hondermarck, H & Liang, M (2016) Antibody-targeted biodegradable nanoparticles for cancer therapy. *Nanomedicine (Lond),* 11, 63-79.
[http://dx.doi.org/10.2217/nnm.15.186] [PMID: 26654068]

Sharifi, S, Behzadi, S, Laurent, S, Forrest, ML, Stroeve, P & Mahmoudi, M (2012) Toxicity of nanomaterials. *Chem Soc Rev,* 41, 2323-43.
[http://dx.doi.org/10.1039/C1CS15188F] [PMID: 22170510]

Sharma, A, Goyal, AK & Rath, G (2018) Recent advances in metal nanoparticles in cancer therapy. *J Drug Target,* 26, 617-32.
[http://dx.doi.org/10.1080/1061186X.2017.1400553] [PMID: 29095640]

Sharma, A, Kaur, A, Jain, UK, Chandra, R & Madan, J (2017) Stealth recombinant human serum albumin nanoparticles conjugating 5-fluorouracil augmented drug delivery and cytotoxicity in human colon cancer, HT-29 cells. *Colloids Surf B Biointerfaces,* 155, 200-8.
[http://dx.doi.org/10.1016/j.colsurfb.2017.04.020] [PMID: 28431329]

Shen, J, Sun, H, Meng, Q, Yin, Q, Zhang, Z, Yu, H & Li, Y (2014) Simultaneous inhibition of tumor growth and angiogenesis for resistant hepatocellular carcinoma by co-delivery of sorafenib and survivin small hairpin

RNA. *Mol Pharm,* 11, 3342-51.
[http://dx.doi.org/10.1021/mp4006408] [PMID: 24495194]

Smith, T, Affram, K, Nottingham, EL, Han, B, Amissah, F, Krishnan, S, Trevino, J & Agyare, E (2020) 'Application of smart solid lipid nanoparticles to enhance the efficacy of 5-fluorouracil in the treatment of colorectal cancer'. *Sci Rep,* 10, 1-14.
[http://dx.doi.org/10.1038/s41598-020-73218-6] [PMID: 31913322]

Soares, S, Sousa, J, Pais, A & Vitorino, C (2018) 'Nanomedicine: principles, properties, and regulatory issues'. *Front Chem,* 6, 360.
[http://dx.doi.org/10.3389/fchem.2018.00360] [PMID: 30177965]

Soni, N, Soni, N, Pandey, H, Maheshwari, R, Kesharwani, P & Tekade, RK (2016) Augmented delivery of gemcitabine in lung cancer cells exploring mannose anchored solid lipid nanoparticles. *J Colloid Interface Sci,* 481, 107-16.
[http://dx.doi.org/10.1016/j.jcis.2016.07.020] [PMID: 27459173]

Straubinger, RM, Lopez, NG, Debs, RJ, Hong, K & Papahadjopoulos, D (1988) Liposome-based therapy of human ovarian cancer: parameters determining potency of negatively charged and antibody-targeted liposomes. *Cancer Res,* 48, 5237-45.
[PMID: 3409248]

Stylianopoulos, T (2013) EPR-effect: utilizing size-dependent nanoparticle delivery to solid tumors. *Ther Deliv,* 4, 421-3.
[http://dx.doi.org/10.4155/tde.13.8] [PMID: 23557281]

Sukhanova, A, Bozrova, S, Sokolov, P, Berestovoy, M, Karaulov, A & Nabiev, I (2018) 'Dependence of Nanoparticle Toxicity on Their Physical and Chemical Properties', *Nanoscale Research Letters. Nanoscale Res Lett,* •••, 13.

Summerlin, N, Soo, E, Thakur, S, Qu, Z, Jambhrunkar, S & Popat, A (2015) Resveratrol nanoformulations: challenges and opportunities. *Int J Pharm,* 479, 282-90.
[http://dx.doi.org/10.1016/j.ijpharm.2015.01.003] [PMID: 25572692]

Sun, H & Zu, Y (2015) Aptamers and their applications in nanomedicine. *Small,* 11, 2352-64.
[http://dx.doi.org/10.1002/smll.201403073] [PMID: 25677591]

Sun, Y, Zhao, Y, Teng, S, Hao, F, Zhang, H, Meng, F, Zhao, X, Zheng, X, Bi, Y, Yao, Y, Lee, RJ & Teng, L (2018) Folic acid receptor-targeted human serum albumin nanoparticle formulation of cabazitaxel for tumor therapy. *Int J Nanomedicine,* 14, 135-48.
[http://dx.doi.org/10.2147/IJN.S181296] [PMID: 30613142]

Tomuleasa, C, Soritau, O, Orza, A, Dudea, M, Petrushev, B, Mosteanu, O, Susman, S, Florea, A, Pall, E, Aldea, M, Kacso, G, Cristea, V, Berindan-Neagoe, I & Irimie, A (2012) Gold nanoparticles conjugated with cisplatin/doxorubicin/capecitabine lower the chemoresistance of hepatocellular carcinoma-derived cancer cells. *J Gastrointestin Liver Dis,* 21, 187-96.
[PMID: 22720309]

Torchilin, V (2008) Antibody-modified liposomes for cancer chemotherapy. *Expert Opin Drug Deliv,* 5, 1003-25.
[http://dx.doi.org/10.1517/17425247.5.9.1003] [PMID: 18754750]

Torchilin, VP (2005) Recent advances with liposomes as pharmaceutical carriers. *Nat Rev Drug Discov,* 4, 145-60.
[http://dx.doi.org/10.1038/nrd1632] [PMID: 15688077]

Torre, LA, Bray, F, Siegel, RL, Ferlay, J, Lortet-Tieulent, J & Jemal, A (2015) Global cancer statistics, 2012. *CA Cancer J Clin,* 65, 87-108.
[http://dx.doi.org/10.3322/caac.21262] [PMID: 25651787]

Tsuchiya, N, Sawada, Y, Endo, I, Saito, K, Uemura, Y & Nakatsura, T (2015) Biomarkers for the early diagnosis of hepatocellular carcinoma. *World J Gastroenterol,* 21, 10573-83.

[http://dx.doi.org/10.3748/wjg.v21.i37.10573] [PMID: 26457017]

Varshosaz, J & Farzan, M (2015) Nanoparticles for targeted delivery of therapeutics and small interfering RNAs in hepatocellular carcinoma. *World J Gastroenterol,* 21, 12022-41.
[http://dx.doi.org/10.3748/wjg.v21.i42.12022] [PMID: 26576089]

Vivek, R, Nipun Babu, V, Thangam, R, Subramanian, KS & Kannan, S (2013) pH-responsive drug delivery of chitosan nanoparticles as Tamoxifen carriers for effective anti-tumor activity in breast cancer cells. *Colloids Surf B Biointerfaces,* 111, 117-23.
[http://dx.doi.org/10.1016/j.colsurfb.2013.05.018] [PMID: 23787278]

Wais, U, Jackson, AW, He, T & Zhang, H (2016) Nanoformulation and encapsulation approaches for poorly water-soluble drug nanoparticles. *Nanoscale,* 8, 1746-69.
[http://dx.doi.org/10.1039/C5NR07161E] [PMID: 26731460]

Wakaskar, RR (2017) 'Passive and active targeting in tumor microenvironment'. *International Journal of Drug Development and Research,* 9, 37-41.

Wang, W, Zhang, L, Chen, T, Guo, W, Bao, X, Wang, D, Ren, B, Wang, H, Li, Y, Wang, Y & Chen, S (2017) 'Anticancer effects of resveratrol-loaded solid lipid nanoparticles on human breast cancer cells'. *Molecules,* 22, 1814.
[http://dx.doi.org/10.3390/molecules22111814]

Wang, D, Sun, Y, Liu, Y, Meng, F & Lee, RJ (2018) Clinical translation of immunoliposomes for cancer therapy: recent perspectives. *Expert Opin Drug Deliv,* 15, 893-903.
[http://dx.doi.org/10.1080/17425247.2018.1517747] [PMID: 30169978]

Wang, Q, Zhang, P, Li, Z, Feng, X, Lv, C, Zhang, H, Xiao, H, Ding, J & Chen, X (2019) 'Evaluation of polymer nanoformulations in hepatoma therapy by established rodent models'. *Theranostics,* 9, 1426-52.
[http://dx.doi.org/10.7150/thno.31683] [PMID: 30867842]

Wang, Y, Zhao, Q, Han, N, Bai, L, Li, J, Liu, J, Che, E, Hu, L, Zhang, Q, Jiang, T & Wang, S (2015) Mesoporous silica nanoparticles in drug delivery and biomedical applications. *Nanomedicine,* 11, 313-27.
[http://dx.doi.org/10.1016/j.nano.2014.09.014] [PMID: 25461284]

Wang, Yinsong (2013) PH-sensitive pullulan-based nanoparticle carrier of methotrexate and combretastatin A4 for the combination therapy against hepatocellular carcinoma *Biomaterials* Elsevier Ltd 7181-90.

Weiss, GJ, Chao, J, Neidhart, JD, Ramanathan, RK, Bassett, D, Neidhart, JA, Choi, CHJ, Chow, W, Chung, V, Forman, SJ, Garmey, E, Hwang, J, Kalinoski, DL, Koczywas, M, Longmate, J, Melton, RJ, Morgan, R, Oliver, J, Peterkin, JJ, Ryan, JL, Schluep, T, Synold, TW, Twardowski, P, Davis, ME & Yen, Y (2013) First-in-human phase 1/2a trial of CRLX101, a cyclodextrin-containing polymer-camptothecin nanopharmaceutical in patients with advanced solid tumor malignancies. *Invest New Drugs,* 31, 986-1000.
[http://dx.doi.org/10.1007/s10637-012-9921-8] [PMID: 23397498]

Wong, HL, Bendayan, R, Rauth, AM, Li, Y & Wu, XY (2007) Chemotherapy with anticancer drugs encapsulated in solid lipid nanoparticles. *Adv Drug Deliv Rev,* 59, 491-504.
[http://dx.doi.org/10.1016/j.addr.2007.04.008] [PMID: 17532091]

Xu, J, Cheng, X, Tan, L, Fu, C, Ahmed, M, Tian, J, Dou, J, Zhou, Q, Ren, X, Wu, Q, Tang, S, Zhou, H, Meng, X, Yu, J & Liang, P (2019) 'Microwave responsive nanoplatform *via* P-selectin mediated drug delivery for treatment of hepatocellular carcinoma with distant metastasis'. *Nano Lett,* 19, 2914-27.
[http://dx.doi.org/10.1021/acs.nanolett.8b05202] [PMID: 30929452]

Xu, X, Ho, W, Zhang, X, Bertrand, N & Farokhzad, O (2015) Cancer nanomedicine: from targeted delivery to combination therapy. *Trends Mol Med,* 21, 223-32.
[http://dx.doi.org/10.1016/j.molmed.2015.01.001] [PMID: 25656384]

Yadav, AS, Radharani, NNV, Gorain, M, Bulbule, A, Shetti, D, Roy, G, Baby, T & Kundu, GC (2020) RGD functionalized chitosan nanoparticle mediated targeted delivery of raloxifene selectively suppresses angiogenesis and tumor growth in breast cancer. *Nanoscale,* 12, 10664-84.
[http://dx.doi.org/10.1039/C9NR10673A] [PMID: 32374338]

Yallapu, MM, Gupta, BK, Jaggi, M & Chauhan, SC (2010) Fabrication of curcumin encapsulated PLGA nanoparticles for improved therapeutic effects in metastatic cancer cells. *J Colloid Interface Sci,* 351, 19-29. [http://dx.doi.org/10.1016/j.jcis.2010.05.022] [PMID: 20627257]

Yallapu, MM, Nagesh, PKB, Jaggi, M & Chauhan, SC (2015) 'Therapeutic applications of curcumin nanoformulations'. *AAPS J,* 17, 1341-56. [http://dx.doi.org/10.1208/s12248-015-9811-z] [PMID: 26335307]

Yan, B, Gu, Y, Zhao, J, Liu, Y, Wang, L & Wang, Y (2019) 'Self-microemulsion Technology for Water-insoluble Drug Delivery'. *Curr Nanosci,* 15, 576-88. a [http://dx.doi.org/10.2174/1573413715666190112122107]

Yan, H, Xue, Z, Xie, J, Dong, Y, Ma, Z, Sun, X, Kebebe Borga, D, Liu, Z & Li, J (2019) Toxicity of carbon nanotubes as anti-tumor drug carriers. *Int J Nanomedicine,* 14, 10179-94. b [http://dx.doi.org/10.2147/IJN.S220087] [PMID: 32021160]

Yaqoob, SB, Adnan, R, Rameez Khan, RM & Rashid, M (2020) Gold, Silver, and Palladium Nanoparticles: A Chemical Tool for Biomedical Applications. *Front Chem,* 8, 376. [http://dx.doi.org/10.3389/fchem.2020.00376] [PMID: 32582621]

Yetisgin, AA, Cetinel, S, Zuvin, M, Kosar, A & Kutlu, O (2020) Therapeutic Nanoparticles and Their Targeted Delivery Applications. *Molecules,* 25, 2193. [http://dx.doi.org/10.3390/molecules25092193] [PMID: 32397080]

Yingchoncharoen, P, Kalinowski, DS & Richardson, DR (2016) 'Lipid-based drug delivery systems in cancer therapy: what is available and what is yet to come'. *Pharmacol Rev,* 68, 701-87. [http://dx.doi.org/10.1124/pr.115.012070] [PMID: 27363439]

Yousef, S, Alsaab, HO, Sau, S & Iyer, AK (2018) Development of asialoglycoprotein receptor directed nanoparticles for selective delivery of curcumin derivative to hepatocellular carcinoma. *Heliyon,* 4, e01071. [http://dx.doi.org/10.1016/j.heliyon.2018.e01071] [PMID: 30603704]

Yu, Z, Li, Q, Wang, J, Yu, Y, Wang, Y, Zhou, Q & Li, P (2020) Reactive Oxygen Species-Related Nanoparticle Toxicity in the Biomedical Field. *Nanoscale Res Lett,* 15, 115. [http://dx.doi.org/10.1186/s11671-020-03344-7] [PMID: 32436107]

Zhang, H (2016) Onivyde for the therapy of multiple solid tumors. *OncoTargets Ther,* 9, 3001-7. a [http://dx.doi.org/10.2147/OTT.S105587] [PMID: 27284250]

Zhang, J, Chen, Y, Li, X, Liang, X & Luo, X (2016) The influence of different long-circulating materials on the pharmacokinetics of liposomal vincristine sulfate. *Int J Nanomedicine,* 11, 4187-97. b [http://dx.doi.org/10.2147/IJN.S109547] [PMID: 27616886]

Zhang, Z, Tsai, PC, Ramezanli, T & Michniak-Kohn, BB (2013) Polymeric nanoparticles-based topical delivery systems for the treatment of dermatological diseases. *Wiley Interdiscip Rev Nanomed Nanobiotechnol,* 5, 205-18. [http://dx.doi.org/10.1002/wnan.1211] [PMID: 23386536]

Zhang, T, Chen, Y, Ge, Y, Hu, Y, Li, M & Jin, Y (2018) Inhalation treatment of primary lung cancer using liposomal curcumin dry powder inhalers. *Acta Pharm Sin B,* 8, 440-8. [http://dx.doi.org/10.1016/j.apsb.2018.03.004] [PMID: 29881683]

Zhang, X, Wang, Q, Qin, L, Fu, H, Fang, Y, Han, B & Duan, Y (2016) EGF-modified mPEG-PLGA-PLL nanoparticle for delivering doxorubicin combined with Bcl-2 siRNA as a potential treatment strategy for lung cancer. *Drug Deliv,* 23, 2936-45. c [http://dx.doi.org/10.3109/10717544.2015.1126769] [PMID: 26739487]

Zhang, Y, Sriraman, SK, Kenny, HA, Luther, E, Torchilin, V & Lengyel, E (2016) 'Reversal of chemoresistance in ovarian cancer by co-delivery of a P-glycoprotein inhibitor and paclitaxel in a liposomal platform'. *Mol Cancer Ther,* 15, 2282-93. d [http://dx.doi.org/10.1158/1535-7163.MCT-15-0986] [PMID: 27466355]

Zheng, N, Gao, Y, Ji, H, Wu, L, Qi, X, Liu, X & Tang, J (2016) Vitamin E derivative-based multifunctional nanoemulsions for overcoming multidrug resistance in cancer. *J Drug Target,* 24, 663-9.
[http://dx.doi.org/10.3109/1061186X.2015.1135335] [PMID: 26710274]

Zhou, Q, Ching, AKK, Leung, WKC, Szeto, CYY, Ho, SM, Chan, PKS, Yuan, YF, Lai, PBS, Yeo, W & Wong, N (2011) Novel therapeutic potential in targeting microtubules by nanoparticle albumin-bound paclitaxel in hepatocellular carcinoma. *Int J Oncol,* 38, 721-31.
[PMID: 21240457]

Zhou, SK, Rueckert, D, Fichtinger, G (2019). *Handbook of medical image computing and computer assisted intervention.*Academic Press.

Zhu, B, Li, Y, Lin, Z, Zhao, M, Xu, T, Wang, C & Deng, N (2016) 'Silver nanoparticles induce HePG-2 cells apoptosis through ROS-mediated signaling pathways'. *Nanoscale Res Lett,* 11, 1-8.
[http://dx.doi.org/10.1186/s11671-016-1419-4] [PMID: 26729219]

CHAPTER 4

Nanoformulations to Limit Challenges of Conventional Therapy Against Hepatocellular Carcinoma – An Overview

Suresh Ajmeera[1] and **V. Badireenath Konkimalla**[1,*]

[1] *School of Biological Sciences, National Institute of Science Education and Research, HBNI, Khordha, Jatni, Odisha 752050, India*

Abstract: The chapter primarily deals with different nano-drug delivery approaches to overcome current HCC chemotherapy challenges. The objective of organizing the various sections in this chapter is to highlight the different nanoformulations that are currently being explored, benefits of nanoformulations over the free drug, different approaches and molecular blocks utilized for preparation on different nanoformulations and their applications in the context of the development of novel drug delivery approaches in HCC. Conventional chemotherapy and its limitations for HCC, different targeting approaches for HCC, need for nanoparticulate approach in HCC, different strategies for delivery of nanoformulations with different targeting approaches, different nanoformulations (liposomes, micelles, hydrogels, *etc.*) that are currently studied in HCC, different molecular blocks under preparation, the current status of clinical trials of different nanoformulations studied for HCC therapy and perspective for futuristic role of nanoformulations in HCC have been discussed in the present chapter.

Keywords: Active targeting, Albumin, Amphiphilic formulations, Biocompatibility, Clinical trials, Combinational nanoformulations, Emulsomes, Hydrogels, Liposomes, Metallic nanoparticles, Micelles, miRNAs, Multidrug therapy, Multikinase inhibitor, Nanoparticles, Passive targeting, Polysaccharides, Site-specific targeting, Sorafenib, Stimuli-responsive nanoparticles, Targeted delivery.

INTRODUCTION

Hepatocellular carcinoma (HCC) is a liver malignancy and the leading cause of most cancer-related deaths. In the past four decades, liver cancer incidences have more than tripled, with approximately 700,000 new cases diagnosed with liver

* **Corresponding author V. Badireenath Konkimalla:** School of Biological Sciences, National Institute of Science Education and Research, HBNI, Khordha, Jatni, Odisha 752050, India; E-mail: badireenath@niser.ac.in

cancer every year (Dhanasekaran *et al.*, 2012). As per the GLOBOCAN report, a significant number of liver cancer cases are reported from the less developed countries with higher occurrences of HCC reported in males than females (2.4:1) (Balogh *et al.*, 2016). Various risk factors contribute to HCC: inflammation, viral infections (Hepatitis-B and -C), toxicity due to alcohol and aflatoxins, and other diseases such as non-alcoholic fatty liver disease, diabetes, cirrhosis, and autoimmune hepatitis. Despite advances in preventive methods, screening, and state-of-the-art technologies in diagnosis and treatment, incidence and mortality continue to rise. From the total HCC cases, only 25% are detected within the early stages, as HCC lacks specific symptoms, leading to advanced non-curable stages. From studies on different HCC samples and body fluids, various biomarkers have been reported for the prognosis and evaluation of HCC. Of these, the well-investigated HCC biomarkers are (1) the AFP, its isoform lens culinaris agglutinin-reactive fraction of alpha-fetoprotein (AFP-L3); and (2) des-γ-carboxy prothrombin (DCP). Further research investigations are underway to establish a few more potential molecules as specific biomarkers of HCC, which includes glypican-3 (GPC3), fibroblast growth factor 3/4 (FGF3/4), glutamine synthase (GS), squamous cell carcinoma antigen (SCCA), Golgi protein 73 (GP73), midkine, osteopontin (OPN), cytokeratin 19 (CK19), heat shock protein 70 (HSP70), Annexin A2, micro-RNAs (miRNAs), Long non-coding RNAs (lncRNAs), circulating tumors cells (CTCs), cell-free DNA (cfDNA).

In the prognosis of HCC, genetic signatures play a crucial role and are accounted for among possible disease biomarkers (Chaiteerakij *et al.*, 2015). Epigenetic changes with modified DNA methylation and histone modifications perturb the gene expression, although the sequence remains unchanged. Interestingly, by deciphering the mechanism at a molecular level, a few epigenetic regulators such as *P16*, DLC1 RhoA GTPase activating protein, *RASSF1A*, runt-related transcription factor 3, and suppressor of cytokine signaling one were observed to be involved in HCC pathogenesis (Khan *et al.*, 2017; Umeda *et al.*, 2018). While the discovery of biomarkers is confined to HCC diagnosis, they are also used for drug targeting (epigenetic modifiers) or to study a therapeutic response (Dhanak *et al.*, 2014; Di Costanzo *et al.*, 2014). For example, panobinostat and belinostat are histone deacetylase inhibitors that have shown good therapeutic efficiency in HCC (Pathil *et al.*, 2006; Yeo *et al.*, 2012). In another study, Zhu *et al.* utilized alpha-fetoprotein (AFP), a biomarker for HCC, to evaluate the therapeutic response and efficacy of ramucirumab following treatment (Zhu *et al.*, 2018).

From histological studies, different subtypes and markers of HCC have been identified and classified to place and confirm various stages of HCC for possible treatment or prognosis. It has been observed that the disease progression shows different developmental patterns (a) A traditional type where the cancer cells spread tentacle-like growths through the liver (b) a proliferating single tumor can metastasize to other parts of the liver as the disease advances (c) as nodules at several places in the liver are observed in cirrhosis condition, a chronic liver disease (Castaldo *et al.*, 2000). In some cases, the pattern is still non-elucidative as there is no substantial evidence that either correlates with the cause of the disease, cell type being affected, *etc.* Among them, fibrolamellar is a vital indicator that is very uncommon and accumulates up to less than 1% of HCCs, which is most often recognized in younger patients between 10-35 years of age (Lafaro *et al.*, 2015). The alarming growth rate of HCC incidence and survival in the population is a grave concern worldwide and requires more attention. While different treatment options are available depending on the stage of HCC profiles such as surgical resection, transarterial embolization (TACE), liver transplantation, radiotherapy, ablation, and chemotherapy, nevertheless, these conventional therapies suffer challenges due to chemoresistance, untoward effects, and promotion of cancer metastasis following surgical intervention (Daher *et al.*, 2018). Most drugs available for treating HCC are conventionally used drugs that exhibit profound cytotoxicity by acting on the vital pathways involving DNA and/or RNA machinery of the cell, arresting its ways for replication, repair, and proliferation (Marin *et al.*, 2020). Thus, prognosis, diagnosis, and therapy of HCC are still not considered successful, and efforts are to utilize the advantages of nanotechnology to manage the disease better therapeutically. The present chapter will focus on nano-drug delivery systems that could limit conventional cancer therapy challenges.

Anticancer Drugs in HCC and its Limitations

Table **1** summarizes a list of conventional anti-cancer drugs with their cellular targets. While these drugs show significant cytotoxicity towards cancerous cells, nevertheless, these are non-selective. These chemicals significantly kill the normal cells leading to severe side/adverse effects limiting its further usage for cancer therapy. The non-specific activity of these drugs arises primarily due to non-uniform bio-distribution of the drug other than the unintended organ, action on multiple biomolecular targets, or activity on a target that has no causative role (Ul-Islam *et al.*, 2018). Table **2** summarizes the adverse effects observed in clinical trials for chemotherapeutic agents intended to treat HCC conditions.

As HCC therapy involves long-term drug therapy, it is vital to develop modalities that can reduce its distribution to other organs, reduce side effects, and improve efficacy. Understandably, the liver being the largest reticuloendothelial organ, researchers worldwide have been focusing on developing specific inhibitors that target the receptors of the causative pathways.

Table 1. Conventionally used anti-cancer agents and their cellular targets.

Therapeutic Drug	Site of Action	References
5-Flurouracil	Inhibition of thymidylate synthase Mis-incorporation of nucleotide analogues	(Longley *et al.*, 2003)
Cisplatin	DNA damage	(Eastman, 2006)
Gemcitabine	Mis-incorporation of nucleotide analogues	(Burris *et al.*, 1997; Yamada *et al.*, 1997)
Capecitabine	Inhibition of DNA synthesis	(Venook *et al.*, 2000)
Doxorubicin	Production of free radicals, intercalation into DNA	(Wassermann *et al.*, 1990)
Mitoxantrone	Intercalates with DNA and inhibits DNA replication and RNA synthesis	(Zhou *et al.*, 2009)
Etoposide	Suppression of DNA topoisomerase II	(Wang *et al.*, 2013)
Tamoxifen	mTOR, PI3K-Akt, MAPK	(Guo *et al.*, 2009)
Octreotide	IGF-I/IGF-II	(Siveke *et al.*, 2003; Liu *et al.*, 2004)
Thalidomide	IL-6, bFGF, VEGF, TNFα	(Pinter *et al.*, 2008)
Thymophysin and α---Thymosin	IFN/IL-2	(Dollinger *et al.*, 2010)
Interferon	JAK-STAT	(Darnell *et al.*, 1994)

Table 2. Current status of therapeutic agents used in HCC (data obtained from ClinicalTrials.gov on Dec 2020).

Therapeutic Drug	Significant Adverse Events	Status	Clinical Trial
Atezolizumab (Tecentriq) with Bevacizumab	Hypertension, Epistaxis, Decreased Platelet, Lymphocytes, Hemoglobin, Leukocyte, and Neutrophil, Increased Bilirubin	Phase 3, Active, not recruiting	NCT03434379
Cabozantinib-S-Malate	Stomatitis, Dyspepsia, Asthenia, Palmar-plantar erythrodysesthesia, Hypertension, Hypothyroidism, Dysphonia, Dyspnea, Decreased platelets, Neutropenia, Increased hemoglobin, Hypophosphatemia, Hypoalbuminemia, Hypokalemia, Hypomagnesemia, Hypocalcemia	Phase 4, Active not recruiting	NCT03963206
Ramucirumab (Cyramza)	Peripheral edema, Hypertension, Epistaxis, Thrombocytopenia, Neutropenia, Hypoaluminemia, Hyponatremia, Hypocalcemia	Phase 3, recruiting	NCT02435433

(Table 2) cont.....

Therapeutic Drug	Significant Adverse Events	Status	Clinical Trial
Pembrolizumab	Pruritus, Asthenia, Increased aspartate aminotransferase, Myalgia, Hypothyroidism, Increased alanine aminotransferase, Arthralgia, Maculopapular rash, Hyperbilirubinaemia, Dyspnoea, Anaemia, Adrenal insufficiency, Cardiac failure, Diabetic metabolic vein thrombosis, Gastric ulcer, Hyperlipasaemia, Cholestatic jaundice, Lichenoid keratosis, Lung infection, Mucosal inflammation, Type 1 Diabetes Mellitus, Vena cava thrombosis, Ulcerative oesophagitis	Phase 2, not recruiting	NCT02702414
Lenvatinib Mesylate (Lenvima)	Hypothyroidism, Abdominal pain, Constipation, Ascites, Stomatitis, Pyrexia, Peripheral edema, Decreased appetite and weight, Arthralgia/Myalgia, Dysphonia, Palmar-plantar erythrodysesthesia syndrome, Hypertension, Hemorrhagic events, Hyponatremia, Hyperbilirubinemia, Increased AST and ALT, Increased alkaline phosphate and lipase, Hypokalemia, Hyperkalemia, Decreased albumin, Increased creatinine, Thrombocytopenia, Lymphopenia, Neutropenia, Anemia	Phase 4, not yet recruiting	NCT04297254
Sorafenib Tosylate (Nexavar)	Anorexia, Alopecia, Liver dysfunction, Hypoalbuminemia, Lymphopenia, Thrombocytopenia, Hypophosphatemia, Increased Amylase, Hypocalcemia, Hypokalemia,	Phase 3, Terminated	NCT02867280
Nivolumab (Opdivo) with Lpilimumab, Sorafenib, and Cabozantinib	Pruritus, Arthralgia, Ascites, Dyspepsia, Stomatitis, Abdominal distension, Dyspnea, Pneumonitis, Malaise, Influenza-like illness, Hypothyroidism, Adrenal insufficiency, Anemia, Influenza, Upper respiratory tract infection, Hypotension, Lymphopenia, Anemia, Neutropenia, Leukopenia, Thrombocytopenia, Increased AST, ALT, Bilirubin, Hyponatremia, Hypocalcemia, Increased alkaline phosphate, Increase amylase, Hypokalemia, Hyperkalemia, Increased creatinine, Hypomagnesemia	Phase 1 and 2, Active, not recruiting	NCT01658878

HCC Chemotherapy and Molecular Targets

The tumor microenvironment of HCC is heterogeneous. Various factors in the *milieu* (hypoxia, inflammation, and oxidative stress) contribute to the pathogenesis from tumor initiation to metastasis (Aravalli *et al.*, 2008; Marrero *et al.*, 2010). The gradual accumulation of mutations due to chronic inflammation and oxidative stress results in an altered hepatocyte genome. This way, the altered gene expression affects various underlying signaling pathways, thereby causing liver damage and cancer manifestation (Kumar *et al.*, 2011). By understanding the HCC disease pathogenesis, tumor microenvironment, and gene expression patterns at a molecular level, different therapeutic modalities and approaches can be developed to treat HCC. The cancer cells of HCC express different growth factor receptors, and the HCC microenvironment is highly vascularized and populated with different immune cells. Further, the hepatocytes of the liver are the body's detoxification systems that inactivate different classes of drugs entering the systemic circulation. In contrast, a few drugs are poorly absorbed and less bioavailable. These factors shield the cancer cells of HCC from any significant activity by any chemotherapeutic agent.

From HCC progression, it is understood that apart from the heterogeneous cancerous hepatocytes, the immune cells and the vascular endothelial cells present alongside in the tumor microenvironment contribute significantly to tumor survival and metastasis. Therefore, for effective HCC therapy, different receptors and their growth factors that are associated with angiogenesis (VEGFR, VEGF), activation of immune checkpoints (PD-1, PD-L1), growth factors (EGFR, PDGFR, and FGFR) are chosen as suitable targets to treat HCC condition. Moreover, different other receptors whose protein expression is altered at mRNA or protein levels in different stages of tumor progression are reported, such as the over-expression of TGF-alpha, IGF1R, and IGF-II (in cirrhosis), reduced expression of TGF-betaRII (in early HCC), and over-expression of HGF (metastasis) (Siracusano *et al.*, 2020). By profiling these proteins to canonical pathways available in a database like KEGG, a clear idea of various other proteins involved and pathways that would have been deregulated or as a molecular target can be deduced from a network map. Fig. (**1**) illustrates the network map available for hepatocellular carcinoma presenting the various pathways and cellular response.

To date, different therapeutic approaches have been developed against a few molecular targets, either as small molecules, antibody or miRNA that inhibit proliferation, angiogenesis, or inactivate the immune checkpoint. Multidrug therapy is also a much-sought therapy option to negate the HCC progression. (Fig. **2**) illustrates the various treatment approaches with therapeutic agents available for HCC treatment.

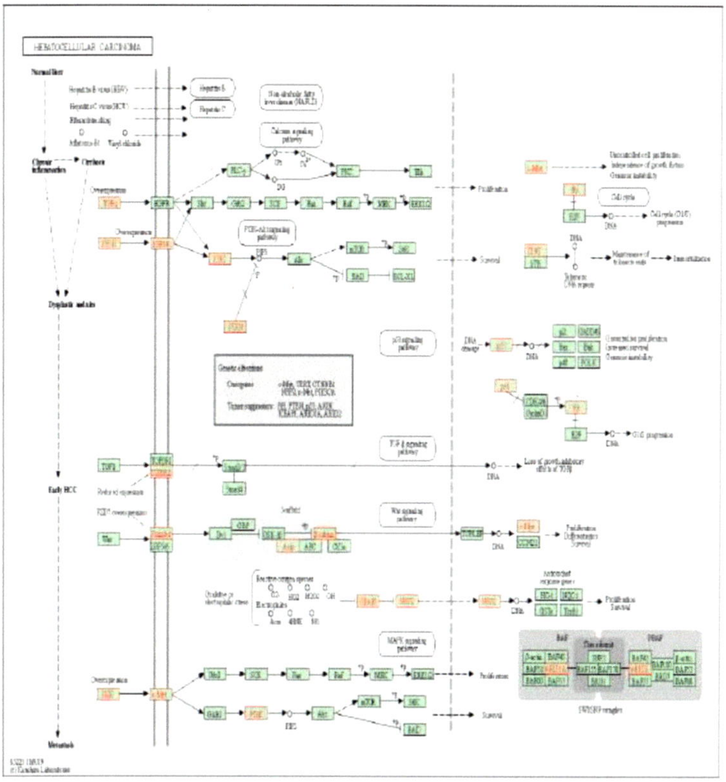

Fig. (1). An illustration of different pathways that are involved in various stages of HCC progression. The receptors highlighted in red are reported to be involved in HCC progression. (KEGG database entry).

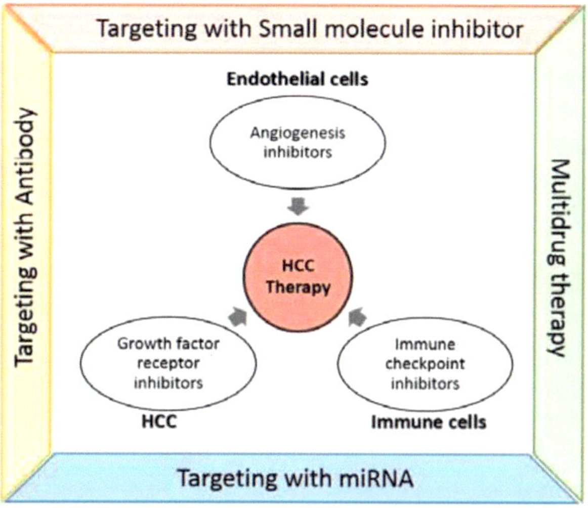

Fig. (2). Different therapeutic agents and their targeting approach for HCC therapy.

Small Molecule and Antibody-Based Inhibitors in HCC

Sorafenib (Nexavar®, Bayer Pharmaceuticals) is the first multi-kinase inhibitor approved as first-line therapy by US-FDA for HCC patients. Sorafenib elicits its potent anti-cancer activity by effectively inhibiting multiple receptors of the tyrosine kinase family [Raf serine/threonine kinases (BRAF), vascular endothelial growth factor receptor (VEGFR-1, -2, -3) and platelet-derived growth factor receptor (PDGFR- β)], thereby blocking tumor growth, cell proliferation and angiogenesis (Wilhelm *et al.*, 2006). For a decade, Sorafenib was the only drug for treating HCC, followed by the successful emergence of regorafenib, lenvatinib, cabozantinib, and ramucirumab (Raoul *et al.*, 2019). Preclinical studies with Bevacizumab (angiogenesis blocker) in HCC have shown significantly reduced microvessel density, minimal off-target mediated toxicity as similarly observed in small molecules in addition to extended progression time in orthotopic human tumors in mice. By critically understanding and correlating the preclinical outcomes to the VEGF pathway, numerous investigations have explored the use of Bevacizumab either as a single agent or in combination with cytotoxic or molecularly targeted agents in patients with advanced HCC (Finn *et al.*, 2009).

Among the different immune checkpoint-related molecules, PD-1 receptor found on the surface of cancer cells and stromal cells, and cytotoxic T lymphocyte-associated protein 4 (CTLA-4) found on T cell surface a vital role in suppressing T-cell activation by cancer cells. Therefore, as part of the immune checkpoint mechanism, the PD-L1/PD-1 pathway is considered a hot target for HCC treatment. This way, as a priority, current efforts are focused on developing antibodies against immune checkpoint inhibitors as monotherapy for HCC. Spartalizumab, Pembrolizumab, Nivolumab, Camrelizumab as anti-PD-1 antibodies, Avelumab, Atezolizumab, and Durvalumab anti-PD-L1 antibodies are developed in the process to target solid tumors, including HCC (Okusaka *et al.*, 2018; Lee *et al.*, 2020).

From intense research in the past decade, researchers have successfully developed specific inhibitors and antibodies that target different receptors expressed in HCC or the receptors that can negate HCC progression (angiogenesis or immune checkpoints). Crystal structures of ligand-binding domain with their inhibitors have been deduced for some receptors in a suitable resolution that can also serve as a template in a virtual screening platform for identifying novel drug candidates. Tables **3** and **4** summarize the drugs and antibodies that bind to the receptors involved in HCC. Figs. (**3**, **4** and **5**) show the ligand-binding site of the inhibitor in the receptor.

Table 3. Therapeutic drugs and reported targeting receptors in HCC.

Drugs	Target Receptors	References
Apatinib	VEGFR2	(Zhao *et al.*, 2020)
Axitinib	VEGFR	(Chan *et al.*, 2017)
Cabozantinib	c-MET	(Shang *et al.*, 2020)
Capmatinib	MET	(Qin *et al.*, 2019)
Epacadostat	IDO1	(Luo *et al.*, 2018)
FGF401 (Roblitinib)	FGFR4	(Fairhurst *et al.*, 2020)
Galunisertib (LY2157299)	TGF-βR1	(Kelley *et al.*, 2019)
Lenvatinib	VEGFR2, VEGFR3	(Matsuki *et al.*, 2018)
Linifanib	PDGFR-B	(Toh *et al.*, 2013)
Ponatinib	FGFR4	(Gao *et al.*, 2017)
Regorafenib	VEGFR, TIE2, C-KIT, RET	(Montironi *et al.*, 2019)
Sorafenib	VEGFR, C-KIT, PDGFR, RAF	(Wilhelm *et al.*, 2008)
Sunitinib	VEGFR (-1, -2, -3), c-KIT, PDGFR, FLT-3, RET	(Morse *et al.*, 2019)
Tivantinib	c-MET	(Weekes *et al.*, 2018)
XL888	Hsp90	(Bussenius *et al.*, 2012)

Table 4. Antibody-based therapeutics and their targeting sites in HCC.

Molecular Target	Therapeutic Antibody	References
PD-L1	Atezolizumab, Avelumab, Durvalumab, Nivolumab	(Okusaka *et al.*, 2018)
PD-1	Spartalizumab, Pembrolizumab, Camrelizumab	(Lee *et al.*, 2020)
VEGF	Bevacizumab	(Finn *et al.*, 2009)
CTLA-4	Tremelimumab, Ipilimumab	(Kudo, 2019)
CCR4	Mogamulizumab	(Doi *et al.*, 2019)
VEGFR2	Ramucirumab	(Turkes *et al.*, 2019)

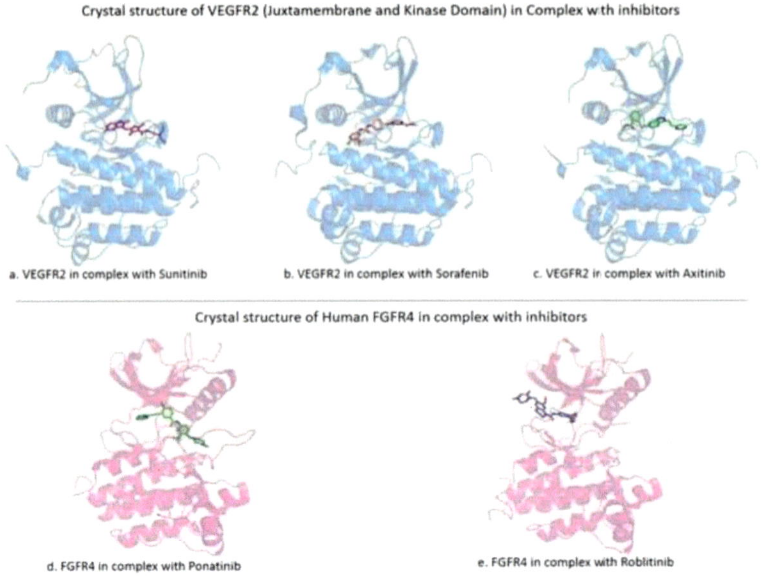

Fig. (3). Crystal structures of various drugs used in HCC therapy in complex with their receptors.
a. VEGFR2 in complex with Sunitinib (PDB: 4AGD, (McTigue *et al.*, 2012)); b. VEGFR2 in complex with Sorafenib (PDB: 4ASD, (McTigue *et al.*, 2012)); c. VEGFR2 in complex with Axitinib (PDB: 4AGC, (McTigue *et al.*, 2012)); d. FGFR4 in complex with Ponatinib (PDB: 4UXQ, (Tucker *et al.*, 2014)); e. FGFR4 in complex with Roblitinib (PDB: 6YI8, (Fairhurst *et al.*, 2020)).

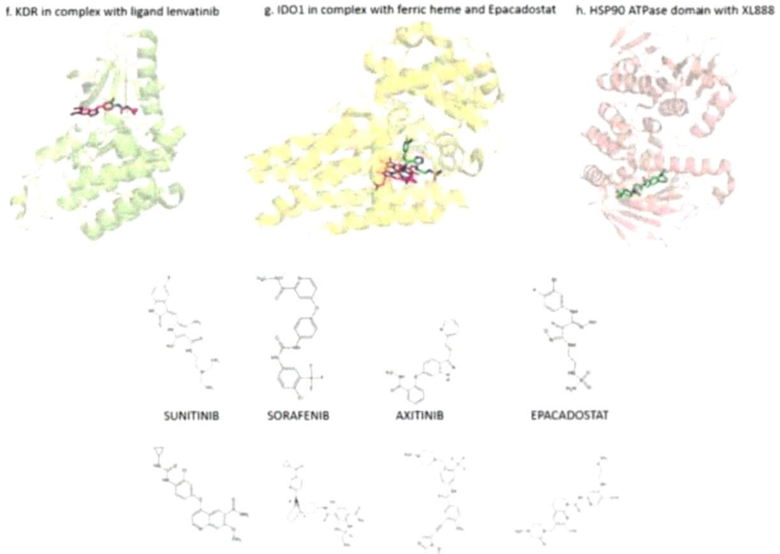

Fig. (4). Crystal structures of various drugs used HCC therapy in complex with their receptors.
f. KDR in complex with ligand lenvatinib (PDB: 3WZD); g. IDO1 in complex with ferric heme and Epacadostat (PDB: 6E40); h. HSP90 ATPase domain with XL888 (PDB: 4AWO). The detailed structure can be accessed from www.rcsb.org using the given PDB code.

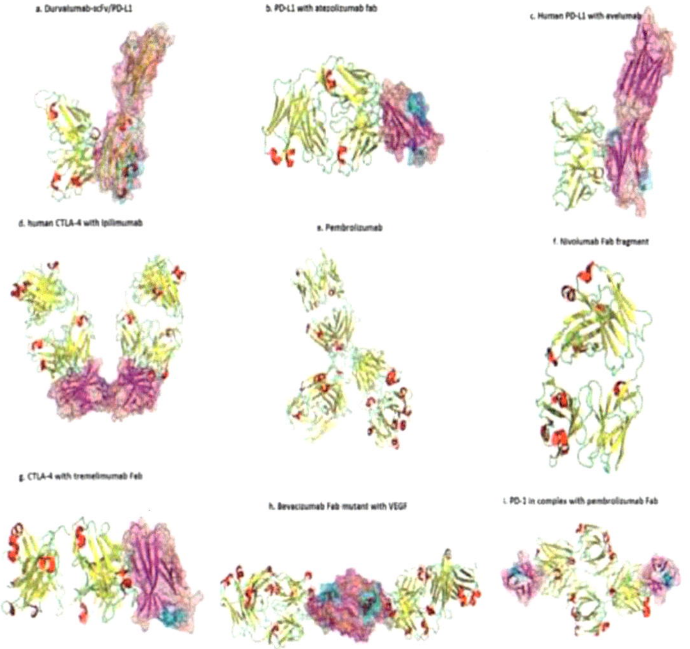

Fig. (5). Crystal structures of different antibody fragments used for HCC therapy.
a. Durvalumab-scFv/PD-L1 (PDB : 5XJ4); b. PD-L1 with atezolizumab fab (PDB: 5XXY); c. Human PD-L1 with avelumab (PDB: 5GRJ); d. human CTLA-4 with Ipilimumab (PDB: 5TRU); e. Pembrolizumab (PDB: 5DK3); f. Nivolumab Fab fragment (PDB: 5GGQ) g. CTLA-4 with tremelimumab Fab (PDB: 5GGV); h. Bevacizumab Fab mutant with VEGF(PDB: 6BFT); i. PD-1 in complex with pembrolizumab Fab (PDB: 5GGS). The detailed structure can be accessed from www.rcsb.org using the given PDB code. The antibodies are rendered in the cartoon. The respective receptors are represented with a *brown* mesh surface using the 3D coordinates obtained from the repository (Burley *et al*., 2021) (www.rcsb.org) the given PDB code. The 3D structures are generated using PyMOL (DeLano *et al*., 2000) (https:// www.pymol.org). The detailed design can be accessed from www.rcsb.org using the given PDB code.

MicroRNAs (or miRNAs) are short (18 25 nucleotides long) non-coding RNA involved in gene expression regulation post-transcriptionally. These miRNAs are evolutionarily conserved and generally located in the intergenic (non-coding) regions of DNA with endogenous expression in the cytoplasm. The miRNAs maintain cellular homeostasis by counteracting insults or stress caused to cells by any extrinsic or intrinsic factor. A miRNA with improper base pairing can bind to the 3`-UTR region of different mRNAs and post-transcriptionally perturb further biosynthesis of proteins involved in different cellular pathways responsible for cell proliferation, survival, and death. Detailed investigations report the role of miRNAs in various stages of disease onset and progression, such as cancer, a neurodegenerative disorder, and cardiovascular diseases. Differential expressions of miRNA observed between the normal and the disease states have resulted in miRNA implication as diagnostic markers or therapeutic targets (Lee *et al.,* 2019).

miRNAs Based Therapeutics in HCC

In the context of HCC, different pathways and processes of HCC development, invasiveness and prognosis are associated with sustained dysregulation of miRNA expression that exerts their function as oncogenes or tumor suppressors depending on their cellular targets. A single miRNA has a broad range of therapeutic targets that regulate multiple gene expression and repression. By studying the differential expression of miRNAs in a tumor microenvironment, the genes or pathways associated with invasion, metastasis, and angiogenesis of HCC can be obtained. As of June 2020, miR-Cancer (a microRNA-cancer association database) has documented 9080 miR-cancer associations from 196 cancer types, of which 46 are reported for HCC (Xie *et al.*, 2013). Fig. (**6**) is a comprehensive list of miRNAs that are up-regulated or down-regulated. The expression of target mRNA is altered, leading to various stages of HCC progression (information is presented as obtained from the KEGG database).

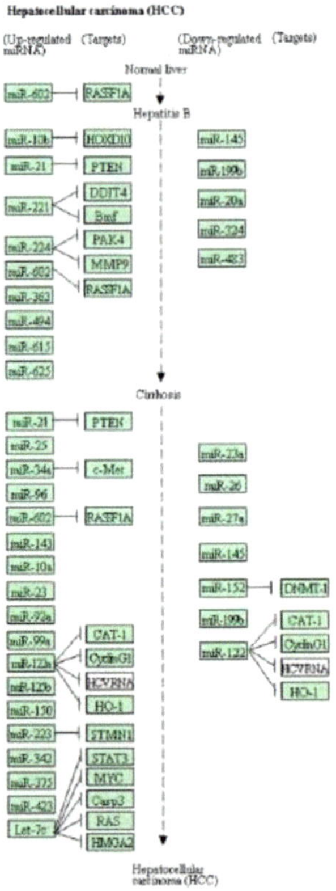

Fig. (6). List of miRNAs reported in various stages of HCC progression (KEGG database entry hsa05206: https://www.genome.jp/kegg-bin/show_pathway?hsa05206). It is adapted with permission from Kanehisa Laboratories (Kanehisa *et al.*, 2000).

The discovery of miRNA and its many targets has immensely contributed to the development of miRNA therapeutics. Anti-miR (miRNA inhibition therapy) or miR-mimics (miRNA reinforcement or replacement therapy) are developed as cancer miRNA therapeutics depending on the expressed target miRNA (Montgomery *et al.*, 2011; Bouchie, 2013). Treatment with miRNA delivery is a promising approach with a unique advantage. However, the naked molecules lack efficacy due to poor targeting, reduced circulation time, and off-target effects. Nevertheless, the small miRNA facilitates encapsulation into NPs, thereby enhancing the efficiency, delivery, circulation, and targeted accumulation (Xie *et al.*, 2017). An effective strategy was developed where nanoformulation encapsulating miRNA and a drug resulted in enhanced cytotoxicity both in *in vitro* and *in vivo* conditions (Santos-Carballal *et al.*, 2015).

The usage of miRNA and miRNA-based nanoformulations as therapeutics in HCC treatment is still in its nascent stages. A countable number of miRNAs are currently investigated in pre-clinical and clinical stages for HCC therapy. In a Flank nude mice model of hepatocellular carcinoma (HCC), lipid-based NPs are prepared by encapsulating miR-122 (liver-specific tumor suppressor) in the aqueous core of PEGylated cationic/neutral liposomes, which showed 50% reduced tumor growth after 30 days of systemic delivery (Hsu *et al.*, 2013). The miR-101 is generally low-expressed in HCC. However, over-expression effectively suppressed liver tumor formation induced by the oncogenes (c-Myc and AKT/Ras). In a study, a miRNA-chemotherapeutic combination of mir-101 and Doxorubicin (DOX) as liposomal formulation was studied for the nano combination's tumor-suppressive effect in an HCC xenograft model of mice. An enhanced tumor inhibitory activity was reported from the results due to a synergistic cytotoxic effect of DOX and simultaneous suppression of miR-10--targeting downstream-related genes both transcriptionally and post-transcriptionally (Xu *et al.*, 2017). The miR-221 overexpression has a poor prognosis in HCC but correlates well to cirrhosis, tumor size, and tumor staging. In a study on HepG2 cells, which overexpressed miR-221, targeted-liposomes loaded with a miR-221 antisense oligonucleotide (anti-miR-221) [loaded into negatively charged liposomes with transferrin (Tf) as liposome-targeting moiety] showed improved transfection efficiency and delivery of miR-221 in TfRs-elevated HepG2 cells. Cell-based studies upon delivery of Tf-R liposomes (Tf-RL) showed significant activation of apoptosis and cell cycle arrest in the G_0-G_1 phase due to inhibition of miR-221 expression correlated with upregulation of PTEN, $P27^{kip1}$, and TIMP3 by the anti-miR-221 encapsulated in the liposomes (Zhang *et al.*, 2015). In a study by Yang *et al.*, a synergistic and improved therapeutic effect with drug-resistant impairment was reported for cisplatin-coated liposomes loaded with miR-375 in HCC. Analysis of the *in vitro* study revealed that the co-delivery showed an efficient escape of miR-375 and increased apoptosis rate and cell cycle arrest in HCC cells (Yang *et al.*, 2016).

Multidrug Therapy in HCC

Multidrug therapy is also a classically adopted approach for various disease conditions such as anti-microbial, anti-viral, cancer, *etc.* Here, different drugs acting on different pathways are combined to achieve an additive or synergistic therapeutic effect. HCC is a deadly disease with fewer therapeutic options available. Adopting multidrug therapy is much needed; however, this has its problems of adverse effects when the combination is rationally selected. This way, combinations of two drugs or antibodies or miRNA or a mix of drugs, antibodies, and miRNA have been studied for HCC therapy. Table **5** below summarizes a few clinical trials of different combinations in various clinical trials (accessed in Jan 2021). A recent update for the same can be accessed from https://clinicaltrials.gov/.

Table 5. Phase trials of multidrug therapy used in HCC.

NCT	Therapeutic Drug	Clinical Stage	Current Status
NCT03434379	Atezolizumab and Bevacizumab	Phase 3	Active, not recruiting
NCT01908426	Cabozantinib	Phase 3	Active, not recruiting
NCT01761266	Lenvatinib and Sorafenib	Phase 3	Active, not recruiting
NCT02528643	Enzalutamide	Phase 2	Active, not recruiting
NCT02702401	Pembrolizumab	Phase 3	Active, not recruiting
NCT03222076	Nivolumab and Ipilimumab	Phase 2	Active, not recruiting
NCT02178358	LY2157299 and Sorafenib	Phase 2	Active, not recruiting
NCT02178722	MK-3475 and INCB024360	Phase 1 and Phase 2	Active, not recruiting
NCT02795429	Spartalizumab and Capmatinib	Phase 1 and Phase 2	Active, not recruiting
NCT03006926	Pembrolizumab and Lenvatinib	Phase 1	Active, not recruiting
NCT03347292	Regorafenib and Pembrolizumab	Phase 1	Active, not recruiting
NCT03299946	Cabozantinib and Nivolumab	Phase 1	Active, not recruiting
NCT02572687	Ramucirumab and Durvalumab	Phase 1	Active, not recruiting
NCT03298451	Durvalumab and Tremelimumab	Phase 3	Recruiting
NCT02942329	Apatinib and SHR-1210	Phase 1 and Phase 2	Recruiting (last updated Feb 26, 2018)
NCT03211416	Pembrolizumab and Sorafenib	Phase 1 and Phase 2	Recruiting
NCT03095781	XL888 and Pembrolizumab	Phase 1	Recruiting

(Table 5) cont.....

NCT	Therapeutic Drug	Clinical Stage	Current Status
NCT02705105	Mogamulizumab and Nivolumab	Phase 1 and Phase 2	Completed
NCT02423343	Galunisertib and Nivolumab	Phase 1 and Phase 2	Completed
NCT02325739	FGF401 and Spartalizumab	Phase 1 and Phase 2	Completed
NCT03289533	Avelumab and Axitinib	Phase 1	Completed
NCT01406574	OPB-31121	Phase 1 and Phase 2	Completed
NCT00790218	CF-102	Phase 1 and Phase 2	Completed

Need for Nanoformulations in HCC

The application of nanotechnology in biomedicine resulting in the emergence of a distinct domain of nanomedicine is indeed a great boon in the area of drug delivery. In recent decades, nanoparticle drug delivery systems have been the most sought and investigated delivery systems for various biomedical and pharmaceutical applications ranging from diagnosis, imaging, therapy, *etc.* When administered to the systemic circulation, a drug in its free form suffers from different pharmacokinetics and pharmacodynamics problems such as solubility, biodegradability, biocompatibility, toxicity, circulation time, premature release, *etc.* (Kumari *et al.,* 2010). These issues can be well-addressed without altering the drug's chemical structure by adopting a nanotechnology approach. An improved therapeutic efficacy can also be achieved by applying a suitable technique that brings an effective solution upon considering the various drug properties (Masood, 2016). In the case of poorly water-soluble drugs, decreasing size to a nanoscale significantly enhances their solubility. At the same time, the efficacy can be improved by developing them as targeted delivery.

Improved efficacy of the drug encapsulated in a nanoformulation compared to its free-form was also reported from various studies making nanoparticle drug delivery a much-desired approach. Sorafenib (SF), a multi-kinase inhibitor, is a drug of choice for treating late-stage HCC patients. However, adverse events of SF as a free-drug were observed later due to paradoxical activation and triggering of mitogen-activated protein kinases (MAPKs) related cellular pathways responsible for cancer advancement (Peluso *et al.,* 2019). In order to minimize such adverse events, Chen and his team prepared lipid-coated PLGA nanoformulations encapsulating SF and MEK suppressor AZD6244 for synergistic effect with high loading efficacy (~70%) (Chen *et al.,* 2017). CTCE-9908, an antagonist peptide ligand, was incorporated on the surface of the nanoformulation to target and bind to CXCR4, a chemokine receptor highly expressed in HCC, thus making this nanoformulation a targeted delivery. Due to the ligand specificity, increased cellular internalization of nanoformulation and synergistic cytotoxic activity against HCC both *in-vitro* and *in-vivo* was observed bypassing the SF-induced activation of MAPKs and its associated side effects when administered in its free-form.

In another study, Zhao *et al.* demonstrated co-delivery of Doxorubicin (DOX) and Curcumin (Cur) loaded lipid nanoformulations in DEN-induced HCC mice model. Here, the combination, when co-delivered, showed a synergistic effect in inducing apoptosis, proliferation, and angiogenesis despite differences in their solubility and pharmacokinetic properties. Further, as a nanoformulation, the adverse effects of DOX were considerably reduced (Zhao *et al.,* 2015).

Site-specific Drug Transporter Systems in HCC

Nanoformulation as a targeted drug transporter system has numerous benefits, including shielding normal cells from the cytotoxic therapeutic agents, reducing dose-related adverse events, and counteracting drug-resistant cancerous cells. The size and shape achieved as NPs are a significant advantage as they facilitate tissue/organ penetration, distribution, targeting specific cellular trafficking pathways, or controlling drug release. Different nanoformulations for the drug (liposomes, micelles, dendrimers, polysaccharides, *etc.*) entrapped in a polymer (lipid or matrix) protect the drug from unfavorable physiological microenvironments. Further, the polymer offers various functional groups that enable surface modification and anchoring of specific targeting agents. Surface alteration of NPs with targeting ligands enhances the efficiency of active targeting (Table **6**). Passive targeting depends on the enhanced permeability and retention (EPR) effect. The NPs internalize at the tumor site due to increased permeability of tumor vasculature and absence of lymphatic drainage (El-Say *et al.,* 2017). In due course, numerous stimuli-responsive factors such as pH reduction, thermal, photodynamic therapy, and photothermal therapy were also incorporated in the delivery systems to enhance the drug deployment based on the conditions of the tumor environment. In recent years, stimuli-responsive linkages have been widely explored in various nanoformulations.

In HCC, Sorafenib was the only FDA-approved drug for treating HCC from 2007 to 2016. Therefore, it was extensively studied in nano-delivery to improve its limitations (low response rate and high toxicity) (Kudo, 2018). Over time, various other chemotherapeutic agents such as small molecules, antibody or miRNA were developed as nanoformulations for active, passive, and stimuli-responsive targeting purposes.

Table 6. Overexpressed receptors and their respective ligands for HCC.

Overexpressed Receptors	Name	Ligands	References
ASGPR	Asialoglycoprotein receptor	Galactose, Cholesterol, Pectin	(Zhang *et al.*, 2012; Anirudhan *et al.*, 2016; Pathak *et al.*, 2016; Varshosaz *et al.*, 2019 a)
PDGFR	Platelet-derived growth factor receptor	Octreotide	(Varshosaz *et al.*, 2019 b)
LDLR	Low-density lipoprotein receptor	ApoE, Cholesterol, AFP-L3	(Okagawa *et al.*, 2016; Monajati *et al.*, 2018; Li *et al.*, 2020)

Active Targeting

Active targeting (AT) is a much-sought approach to traverse the chemotherapeutics to a specific site to avoid interaction with normal tissues/organs that guarantees increased therapeutic efficacy and limited adverse events. By AT, the concentration of the drug transported to the directed cell can be considerably enhanced in contrast to free-drug or passively targeted delivery systems. The liver cells consist of Kupffer cells, endothelial cells, stellate cells, hepatocytes expressing different plasma membrane-bound receptors with specific activator ligand (Mishra *et al.*, 2013). The receptors that are generally overexpressed in the HCC and their ligands are summarized (Table 7). AT is achieved by tagging the drug encapsulated-nanocarrier surfaces with specific ligands of the receptors that are generally overexpressed by the cancer cells of HCC. These ligands are directed to the respective receptor site, and upon recognition by the liver cancer cells, the nanocarrier gains entry in the cells *via* receptor-mediated endocytosis. For example, ASGPR is overexpressed in HCC cells, and upon tagging the nanoformulation with galactose for active targeting, higher accumulation and cell death were observed in the endocytosed cells. To date, many different nanoformulations such as liposomes, micelles, and hydrogel are prepared to target ASGPR with different ligands actively. Similarly, Glypican-3A is an emerging biomarker for HCC that is currently used for AT (Zhou *et al.*, 2018).

Various gene silencing technologies such as antisense technologies are also applied for AT in HCC. Here, the small activating RNAs (saRNAs) that upregulate the enhancer-binding protein-α (CEBPA) are actively targeted to the liver to inhibit HCC. Activating the C/EBP-α pathway is the therapeutic aim for saRNA to suppress liver tumor growth (Voutila *et al.*, 2017). Kim *et al.* demonstrated an advanced therapeutic approach by attaching N-acetylgalactosamine (GalNAc) to antisense oligonucleotides (ASO), which elevated antitumor activity in the HCC tumor model. In another study, Harada *et al.* altered antisense oligonucleotide (ASO) to efficaciously reduce the ADP-ribosylation 4C (ARL4C) expression, which is significantly expressed in HCC (Kim *et al.*, 2019). Fig. (**7**) is an illustration of the various components to be considered for the preparation of a nanoformulation. Table **7** summarizes the nanoformulations prepared using different ligands as molecular units directed towards the intended target (based on the receptor overexpressing in the HCC) (Harada *et al.*, 2019).

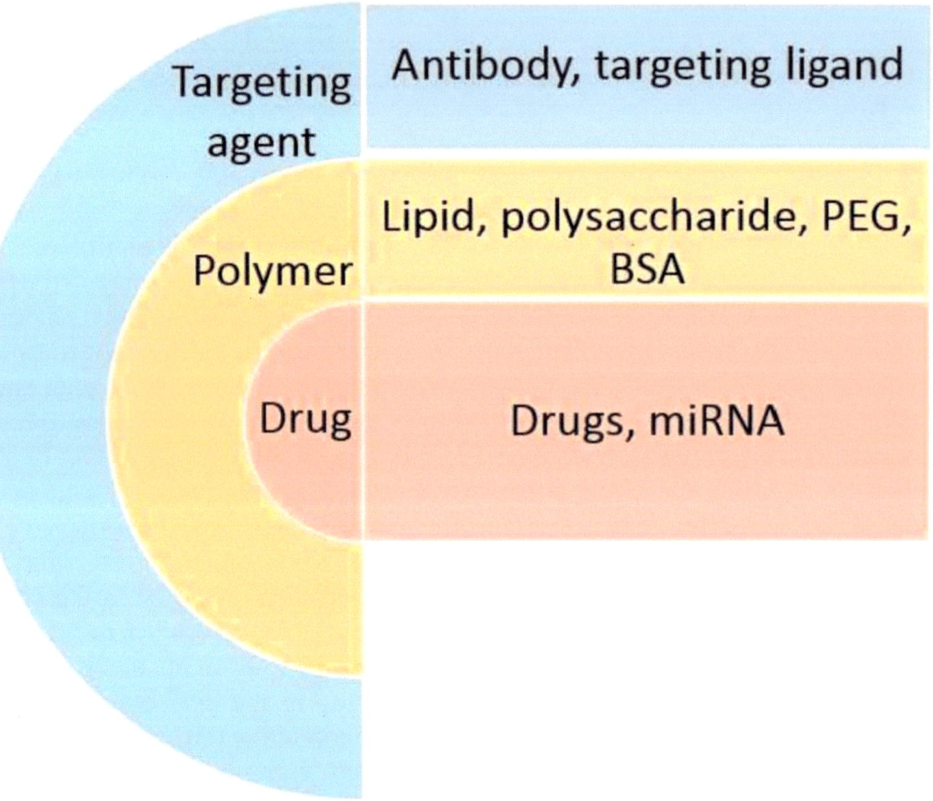

Fig. (7). Different components to be considered for preparation of a nanoformulation.

Table 7. Different nanoformulations investigated for active targeting of HCC.

Molecular Units	**Formulation**	**Ligands**	**Receptors**	**References**
Fuc-Lip-Sf with HDACi	Liposome	AFP-L3	LDLRs	(Baig *et al.*, 2019)
LPG (MX-LPG)	Liposome	Galactose	ASGPR	(Zhang *et al.*, 2012)

(Table 7) cont.....

Molecular Units	Formulation	Ligands	Receptors	References
CHOL-AL-AG and PL90/PL90H/CHOL	Liposome	Cholesterol	ASGPR	(Pathak *et al.*, 2016)
ApoE-PEG-P(CL-DTC)	Micelle	ApoE	LDLRs	(Li *et al.*, 2020)
P-DOCA	Micelle	Pectin	ASGPR	(Varshosaz *et al.*, 2019 a)
PEGylated PEI-CL	Micelle	Cholesterol	LDLRs	(Monajati *et al.*, 2018)
PHEA-EDA-PLA-GAL	Micelle	Galactose	ASGPR	(Craparo *et al.*, 2014)
Gal-PEG-PCL	Micelle	Galactose	ASGPR	(Yang *et al.*, 2011)
PEGylated TMC-EMs	Emulsomes	Octreotide	PDGFR and VEGFR	(Varshosaz *et al.*, 2019 b)
Galactosylated Chitosan Nanoparticles	Polysaccharide	Galactose	ASGPR	(Nair *et al.*, 2019)
GHDx	Polysaccharide	Glycyrrhetinic acid	ASGPR	(Anirudhan *et al.*, 2016)

Passive Targeting

Passive targeting (PT) solely depends on transporter factors such as size, molecular weight, hydrophobicity, hydrophilicity, circulation time, and tumor biologies such as temperature, vascularity, leakiness, and surface charge of tumor cells (Maeda, 2001; Fang *et al.*, 2011; Xiao *et al.*, 2011; Ferreira *et al.*, 2013; Prabhu *et al.*, 2015). Passive targeting of nanotherapeutics to cancerous hepatocytes is achieved by taking advantage of its anatomic and pathophysiological features. The fenestrations present in the liver sinusoid capillaries range between 100 – 200 nm and lack basal lamina. By preferentially controlling the particle size (< 200 nm) or suitable surface modification of NPs, a high accumulation of NPs can be achieved passively at the site of action or tumor site. This way desired pharmacological effect can be achieved, thereby reducing undesirable side effects.

Further, the distinctive features of most tumors, such as leaky and incomplete vasculature and impaired lymphatic drainage, result in enhanced permeability (macromolecule size > 40 kDa) with retention of NPs during transport of oxygen and other nutrients to the tumor tissues (Torchilin, 2011). High tumor interstitial accumulation of NPs can also be obtained due to efficient extravasation through endothelial cell gap junctions (ranging from 400 – 600 nm). This way, the primary benefit of passively targeting nanoformulations would result in prolonged retention in the bloodstream, permitting the drug to accumulate at the diseased site due to EPR. However, this unique characteristic will not apply to small-molecule therapeutic agents, as most have short circulation time and clearance from the tumor site. Therefore, loading small-molecule drugs in nano-sized drug transporters increases its pharmacokinetics, resulting in tumor selectivity and reducing its adverse events. In a study, supramolecular complexes obtained from nonionic amphiphilic cyclodextrin with SF were developed as nanoformulation (Bondì *et al.*, 2015). The strong interaction of SF with nonionic amphiphilic cyclodextrin enabled passive targeting and increased the stability of the drug by a couple of weeks in an aqueous medium. Interestingly, these nanoformulations exhibited very low hemolytic activity. Table **8** summarizes the different PEGylated molecular units in different nanoformulations for passively targeting HCC.

Table 8. Different PEGylated nanoformulations prepared for passive targeting of HCC.

Molecular Units	Nanoformulation	References
DPPC-DSPE-PEG2000-CL	Liposome	(He *et al.*, 2018)
Lipoid E80-DSPE- MPEG2000-CL	Liposome	(Yin *et al.*, 2018)
PEI modified liposome SF-PL/siGPC3	Liposome	(Sun *et al.*, 2017)
PEGylated PLGA	Micelle	(Devulapally *et al.*, 2016)
CPDG/CHS-PEG1500	Micelle	(Du *et al.*, 2016)
PLGA	Micelle	(Ghosh *et al.*, 2012)
PLGA-PEG-PLGA	Hydrogel	(Zheng *et al.*, 2019)

Stimuli-responsive Nanoparticles

Following cellular internalization, selective deployment of the drug either in the cytosol or subcellular target is a significant challenge. Numerous studies have explored the design of stimuli-responsive nanoparticles to achieve sustained drug release at the desired site. The stimuli-responsive NPs can be prepared for either active or passive targeting. For HCC, nanoformulations such as liposomes, micelle, hydrogels, metallic nanoparticles, emulsions, and polysaccharides are utilized with stimuli-responsive linkages such as pH, reduction, thermal, magnetic, PTT, and PDT (Table **9**).

Table 9. Different stimuli-responsive nanoformulations developed for HCC treatment.

Molecular Units	Nanoformulation	Stimuli	References
Lipoid E80-CL modified SF/Gd-liposome	Liposome	PDT	(Xiao *et al.*, 2016)
Lipoid E80-DSPE- MPEG2000-CL	Liposome	pH	(Yin *et al.*, 2018)

(Table 9) cont.....

Molecular Units	Nanoformulation	Stimuli	References
PEI modified liposome SF-PL/siGPC3	Liposome	pH	(Sun *et al.*, 2017)
DPPC-DSPE-PEG2000-CL	Liposome	PTT and PDT	(He *et al.*, 2018)
CMCS-SiSf-CL	Liposome	pH	(Yao *et al.*, 2019)
LPG (MX-LPG)	Liposome	pH	(Zhang *et al.*, 2012)
CHOL-AL-AG, PL90/PL90H/CHOL	Liposome	pH	(Pathak *et al.*, 2016)
ApoE-PEG-P(CL-DTC)	Micelle	Reduction	(Li *et al.*, 2020)
P-DOCA	Micelle	Temperature	(Varshosaz *et al.*, 2019 a)
PEGylated PEI-CL	Micelle	pH and Temperature	(Monajati *et al.*, 2018)
PHEA-EDA-PLA-GAL	Micelle	pH	(Craparo *et al.*, 2014)
Gal-PEG-PCL	Micelle	pH	(Yang *et al.*, 2011)
PEGylated PLGA	Micelle	pH	(Devulapally *et al.*, 2016)
CPDG/CHS-PEG1500	Micelle	pH	(Du *et al.*, 2016)
GOA/miR-122 NPs	Micelle	pH	(Zhang *et al.*, 2019)
PEGylated TMC-Ems	Emulsome	pH	(Varshosaz *et al.*, 2019 b)
PLGA-PEG-PLGA	Hydrogel	Thermo	(Zheng *et al.*, 2019)
Dox-pMNCs	Metallic	Magnetic	(Jeon *et al.*, 2016)
GHDx	Polysaccharide	pH and Temperature	(Anirudhan *et al.*, 2016)
GA-CH-NPs	Polysaccharide	pH	(Nair *et al.*, 2019)

Nanoformulations in HCC – a Detailed Summary

The sections below describe the different nanoformulations (albumin-based, liposomes, micelles, and hydrogels) prepared to treat HCC (Fig. **8**). Each section consists of a table that summarizes various components utilized to prepare a formulation, such as drugs encapsulated, molecular units prepared with the ligand to target a receptor either actively or passively with/without a stimulus.

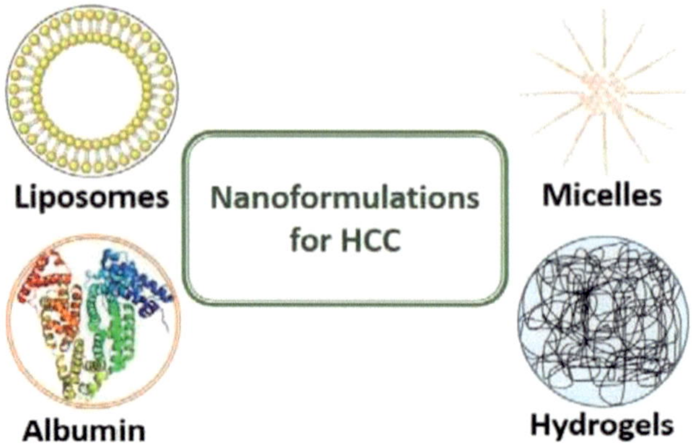

Fig. (8). Nanoformulations studied in HCC condition.

Albumin-Based Nanocarriers

Albumin, a polymer of amino acid, is a natural protein that possesses multiple functional groups present in the side chains of various amino acids. This unique feature makes it a versatile carrier and an ideal candidate for various drug delivery applications. As a blood protein, it is a resourceful transporter in cancer therapeutics. The albumin nanoparticles can traverse to various organs and localize in the inflamed tumor cells releasing its co-loaded therapeutics. In addition, NPs of albumin can be conjugated with different tracking dyes to monitor their entry and localization inside cancerous cells (Kratz, 2008). In a study, albumin-bound paclitaxel showed significantly higher cytotoxicity in HCC xenograft models than other taxane drugs, as evident from the lower IC_{50} values (Zhou *et al.,* 2011).

Liposomes

Liposomes are vesicles containing amphiphilic phospholipids and cholesterol used for encapsulating different types of both lipophilic and hydrophilic chemotherapeutic agents. They are the most preferred nanoformulations for drug delivery purposes as they have several unique features. They contain the aqueous core-shell enclosed within a lipid bilayer to accommodate both water and lipid-soluble drugs. The preparation is easy, and the size of the liposomes can be varied by using a suitable technique such as extrusion, sonication, *etc.* Moreover, the constituents used for preparing liposomes (lipids and cholesterol) are highly biocompatible and mimic the physiological membrane leading to fusion and significant internalization in the cells (Hann *et al.*, 2001; Baig *et al.*, 2019). Liposome nanoparticles are extensively used as therapeutic drug transporters to enhance the efficacy of chemotherapy. Entrapment of DOX within PEGylated liposomes for HCC has been investigated where PEGylated liposomal DOX

(PLD) showed potential to treat HCC clinically (Lombardi *et al.,* 2011). PLD is attributed to enhanced liver uptake and localization to the liver and spleen (Needham *et al.,* 2006).

To date, several PLD nanoformulations have been studied and evaluated in cell lines, rat and mice models, and clinical trials for HCC treatment (Tables **7** and **11**). Xiao *et al.* prepared liposomes co-loaded with Sorafenib (SF) and Gadolinium (Gd) (SF/Gd-liposome) to deliver SF for real-time detection using Magnetic Resonance Imaging. The SF/Gd-liposomes were fabricated with Lipoid-E80, Cholesterol, and SF using thin-film hydration and hydrated with a commercial Gd-DTPA solution. The solubility of SF was noticeably elevated from 0.21 μg/mL to 250 μg/mL in SF/Gd-liposome. Also, the *in-vivo* mice model bearing H22 tumor showed better antitumor effects than the oral SF solution. The *in-vitro* release studies of SF and Gd-DTPA using a dialysis method in phosphate buffer saline (PBS, 0.01, pH 7.4) showed 50% SF release in ~60h in a sustained and controlled manner. On the other hand, the release of Gd-DTPA was relatively fast at about 16% for 4 h and 100% at 12 h following drug administration. Moreover, *in-vitro* cytotoxicity tests in HepG2 cells by MTT assay revealed that the Gd-liposome group exhibited promising biocompatibility, and SF showed a dose-dependent increase in cytotoxicity in cells (Xiao *et al.,* 2016). Okagawa *et al.* prepared Cy5.5-encapsulated L-fucose-liposomes (Fuc-Lip-Cy5.5) to suppress the FUT8 (fucosyltransferase-8) expression in HCC tumor progression. SF-loaded L-fucose decorated uniform micelles were obtained by mixing dipalmitoylphosphati-dylcholine, cholesterol, diacetyl phosphate, ganglioside, and dipalmitoyl phos-phatidylethanolamine with varying molar ratios of cholic acid to facilitate micelle formation followed by solvent evaporation, sonication, and hydrophilization treatment. The cytotoxicity of L-fucose-bound liposome co-loaded with SF (Fuc-Lip-SF) and histone deacetylase inhibitor (HDACi) was assessed *in-vivo* and *in-vitro*. From the studies in AFP-L3 expressing HCC cells, significant uptake of Fuc-Lip-Cy5.5 was reported in a p53- and FUT8- dependent manner. HDACi presence elevated apoptosis and elevated Fuc-Lip-Cy5.5 uptake due to increased FUT8 as a consequence of acetylated -p53 (Okagawa *et al.,* 2016). Yin *et al.* proposed a combinatory approach by preparing SF and Ceramide (CE) co-loaded liposomes (SF/CE-liposomes). CE is an endogenous bioactive sphingolipid that possesses a great potential to suppress numerous tumors. Here, SF/CE-liposomes of particle size of 174 4 nm were prepared with lipoid E80, DSPE-MPEG 2000, cholesterol, SF, and CE by solvent evaporation method followed by thin-film hydration method. The SF and CE showed maximum synergistic antitumor effect by acting on different tumor-suppressing pathways. Further, *in-vitro* cellular uptake studies were performed with free coumarin-6 and coumarin-6/CE-liposomes on HepG2 cells, and *in-vitro* release of SF was characterized by dynamic membrane dialysis under horizontal vibration. The outcomes suggested that the release kinetics of SF from SF-liposomes and SF/CE-liposomes were the same, and CE had no significant impact on the release of SF. Also, the *in-vivo* examination on H22-bearing mice exhibited robust antitumor activity of SF/CE-liposomes in preventing tumor advancement (Yin *et al.*, 2018). Sun *et al.* developed a co-delivery system with SF and siRNA targeting the GPC3 gene using PEI-modified liposomes by a thin-film hydration method. Liposome/siRNA complexes of SF-PL/siGPC3 and SF PEI-liposomes/SCR (SF-PL/SCR) were prepared by adding GPC3 siRNA or scrambled siRNA (SCR) into cationic b-PEI liposomes. AF750 (a NIR fluorescent dye) labeled SCR complexed with PL was utilized to examine nude BALB/c mice bearing human HepG2 hepatoma xenografts. A promising anticancer outcome was obtained from co-delivered therapeutic agents due to suppression of anti-apoptotic GPC3 gene and the proliferative cyclin D1 gene expression in HCC (Sun *et al.*, 2017). He *et al.* 2018 fabricated a NIR fluorescence imaging-guided photothermally responsive nanoliposomes encapsulating SF and Indocyanine Green (ICG) to resolve SF-dependent treatment difficulties in developed HCC. SF-ICG-Liposomes (SILs) containing DPPC, Cholesterol, DSPE-PEG2000, and SF were produced by the thin-film hydration method. The fluorescence intensity from cellular uptake of both free and ICG encapsulated in SILs in Hep3B cells was compared upon NIR laser irradiation. The ROS production and photothermal energy observed upon treatment indicated cellular internalization (He *et al.*, 2018). Yao *et al.* investigated a synergistic effect of co-loaded SF and Cy3-siRNA encapsulated in pH-responsive carboxymethyl chitosan-modified liposomes (CMC-SiSf-CL). The outcomes confirmed co-delivery and penetration into HepG2 cells cultured as 2D, 3D tumor spheroids, and H22 tumor-bearing mice. Also, in contrast with the free siRNA and single sheathed carrier, liposome co-delivery showed increased VEGF downregulation, leading to early cell apoptosis (Yao *et al.*, 2019).

Zhang X *et al.*, with nanomaterial (Gal-P123), designed a dual-functional liposome (LPG) that targets cancerous cells that demonstrated reversal of multidrug resistance in HCC cells. A 97.3% encapsulation efficiency was obtained for mitoxantrone (MX) encapsulated LPG (MX-LPG). From cytotoxicity and cellular internalization studies in Huh-7 cells, MX and MX-LPG exhibited a 2.3-fold increase in cytotoxicity and a 14.9-fold increased cellular accumulation of MX in MDCKII/BCRP cells. Additionally, MX-LPG showed antitumor activity and enhanced specificity in BALB/c mice bearing orthotopic xenograft HCC tumors (Zhang *et al.*, 2012). Wang *et al.* prepared anti-CD44 antibody-mediated liposomal nanoparticle as a theranostic agent for imaging in HCC and as a targeted therapy using a liver tumor model implanted in NOD/SCID mice. Here, an *in situ* model was established by injecting a double fusion reporter gene (firefly luciferase and green fluorescent protein) into HepG2 cells encoded as a reporter system.

Further, the triple fusion gene incorporating the herpes simplex virus truncated thymidine kinase and renilla luciferase. The red fluorescent protein-loaded anti-CD44 antibody-mediated nanoliposome was introduced in the same model. The outcomes of this study showed the benefits of gene therapy and chemotherapy by quantitatively imaging reporter gene expression and tumor volumes by targeting cancer stem cells (Wang *et al.*, 2012). Pathak *et al.* designed cholesterol decorated pH-sensitive DOX-loaded liposomes with palmitoylated arabinogalactan with 90% encapsulation efficacy where ASGPR (+) HepG2 cells revealed a specific ligand-receptor interaction. From bio-distribution studies, liposomal concentration in the liver was reported to be sustained even after 3 h of administration (Pathak *et al.*, 2016).

Table **10** summarizes a list of various drug-loaded nanoliposomal studied in different cell- and animal-based models of HCC.

Table 10. Different nanosize liposomes studied in HCC condition.

Drugs	Molecular Units	Stimuli	Targeting Receptor	Ligand	Active/Passive	Cells/Model Organisms	Reference
Sorafenib	Lipoid E80-CL modified SF/Gd-liposome	PDT	VEGFR, PDGF		Passive	HepG2 and H22 bearing mice	(Xiao *et al.*, 2016)
Sorafenib	Fuc-Lip-Sf with HDACi		LDLRs	AFP-L3	Active	HepG2	(Okagawa *et al.*, 2016)
Sorafenib and Ceramide	Lipoid E80-DSPE-MPEG2000-CL	pH	Ras/Raf/MAPK Kinase and VEGFR	NA	Passive	HepG2 and H22 bearing mice	(Yin *et al.*, 2018)
Sorafenib and GPC3 siRNA	PEI modified liposome SF-PL/siGPC3	pH	GPC3 gene, HSPG	NA	Passive	HepG2 xenograft nude mice	(Sun *et al.*, 2017)
Sorafenib and Indocyanine	DPPC-DSPE-PEG2000-CL	PTT and PDT	VEGFR	NA	Passive	Hep3B bearing mice	(He *et al.*, 2018)
Sorafenib and VEGF-siRNA	CMCS-SiSf-CL	pH	VEGFR	NA	passive	2D-HepG2, 3D-HepG2 Spheroids, and H22 bearing mice	(Yao *et al.*, 2019)
Mitoxantrone	LPG (MX-LPG)	pH	ASGPR	Galactose	Active	Huh-7, MDCKII/BCRP, BALB/c mice	(Zhang *et al.*, 2012)
Anti-CD44 antibody	PcDNA3.1-RFP-Rluc-HSV-ttk and Lipo-CD44-TF	NA	NA	NA	NA	HepG2	(Wang *et al.*, 2012)
Doxorubicin	CHOL-AL-AG and PL90/PL90H/CHOL	pH	ASGPR	Cholesterol	Active	HepG2	(Pathak *et al.*, 2016)

Micelles

Micelles are amphiphilic colloidal particles (5-100 nm) comprising hydrophilic and hydrophobic building blocks that self-assemble to form micelles (Torchilin, 2006; Husseini *et al.*, 2008). The inner hydrophobic core prevents the drug from deteriorating, and the outer hydrophilic shell elevates phagocytic clearance for EPR. Micelles as transporters are particularly effective for transporting lipophilic therapeutic agents by increasing their solubility and enhancing circulation time in the body. Most importantly, the micelles anchor the targeting ligands intact without altering the inherent property of the ligand. There are numerous studies concerning HCC where different micelles were prepared with varying targeting ligands such as Apolipoprotein E peptide, Pectin, Cholesterol, AFP-L3, Octreotide, and Galactose (see Table **6**).

Moreover, a much productive micelle assembly is the application of Pluronics of application in drug delivery. Pluronic micelles are small-sized micelles ranging from 10-100 nm, suitable for injection into the tumor site for enhanced accumulation (Hanahan *et al.*, 2011). In another study, Pluronic-F68 was combined with hematoporphyrin (HP) and doxorubicin (DOX) to design a multifunctional nanosystem that is simple and biocompatible.

Li *et al.* designed an Apolipoprotein-E peptide decorated to micellar SF (ApoE-Ms-SF) for directed therapy using block polymers that are disulfide cross-linked for reduction-triggered intracellular release HCC. With a loading capacity of 7.0 wt% and 37 nm size, the cytotoxicity studies for ApoE-Ms-SF on low-density lipoprotein receptors (LDLRs) overexpressing SMMC- 7721 human liver cancer cells showed ApoE density-dependent antitumor potency in comparison to free SF (Li *et al.,* 2020). Varshosaz*et al.* synthesized co-polymeric SF micelles encapsulated pectin-deoxycholic acid (P-DOCA) to target the ASGPR overexpressed in hepatocytes using pectin. From migration studies in HepG2 cells, SF-loaded micelles showed reduced migration (6.67%) in contrast to free SF (26.67%) (Varshosaz *et al.,* 2019 a). Monajati *et al.* fabricated PEGylated Cholesterol-Polyethyleneimine (PEI) biopolymers to encapsulate SF. PEI-Cholesterol conjugates were responsible for cellular uptake through endocytosis binding with the LDL receptor. Moreover, the investigation on HepG2 cells indicated improved bioavailability upon PEGylation due to shielding the positive surface charges. However, this study was limited to the characterization of biopolymers and *in-vitro*, but *in-vivo* study might proffer interesting outcomes (Monajati *et al.*, 2018). Craparo *et al.* designed a galactosylated α, β- Poly (N---hydroxyethyl) (2-aminoethylcarbamate)-D, L- Aspartamide- Polylactic acid-Galactose (PHEA-EDA-PLA-GAL) copolymer to target the carbohydrate receptor overexpressing hepatocytes, ASGPR. Biodistribution studies on mice, following oral administration of SF, loaded PHEA-EDA-PLA-GAL copolymer demonstrated promising SF accumulation in the liver, indicating a promising approach to treat HCC (Craparo *et al.,* 2014).

Yang *et al.* fabricated novel galactose-decorated covalently cross-linked biodegradable micelles based on photo-cross-linked PEG-PAC-CL and galactose-conjugated PEG-PCL (Gal-PEG-PCL) copolymers for increased hepatoma-directing delivery of paclitaxel (PTX). From cytotoxicity studies in HepG2 cells, high anti-tumor activity was reported for Gal-decorated PTX-encapsulated cross-linked polymers in contrast to the PTX-encapsulated cross-linked polymers without Ga ligands and Gal-decorated PTX-encapsulated non-cross-linked micelles. Moreover, studies in SMMC-7721 human hepatoma-bearing nude mice exhibited the same efficacy as the HepG2 cell lines (Yang *et al.,* 2011). Devulapally *et al.* developed an optimized technique for synthesizing antisense-miRNA-21 and gemcitabine (GEM) co-loaded PEGylated-PLGA nanoparticles. Following treatment in Hep3B and HepG2 cells, cellular accumulation of nanoparticles increased in a time-dependent manner. Also, from flow cytometry analysis, no cellular toxicity was observed in nanoparticles, and antisense-miRNA-21 encapsulated nanoparticles for both the cells, whereas 9% and 15% apoptosis was observed in GEM and GEM-encapsulated nanoparticles, respectively. Overall, this study demonstrated the significance of down-regulation of an endogenous miRNA-21 function using an antisense-miRNA approach to minimize HCC cell viability and proliferation in response to GEM treatment (Devulapally *et al.,* 2016). Du *et al.* synthesized long-circulating nanoassemblies of amphiphilic GEM derivative, cyclic phosphoryl N-dodecanoyl GEM (CPDG)/CHS-PEG-1500 (9:1, mol/mol) to target HCC. CPDG demonstrated much rapid degradation at pH 2.0. In contrast, in weak acidic and neutral pH conditions (pH 5.0- 7.4), the preparations were relatively stable with a degradation half-life ($t_{1/2}$) of about 43 h in the mouse plasma. In HCC tumor-bearing mice for biodistribution studies, the intravenously administered dose of CPDG/CHS- PEG 1500 nanoassemblies displayed a higher anticancer effect than GEM. In conclusion, this study revealed that tumor-targeting nanoassemble-based on the HepDirect prodrug method and self-assembled drug delivery systems concept are potential methods to alter the pharmacologically active nucleosides to treat some liver diseases (Du *et al.,* 2016). Zhang *et al.* fabricated amphiphilic GOA/miR NPs loaded with miR-122 or miR-34a and reported efficient internalization into HepG2 cells that noticeably downregulated the target gene expression levels after lysosome escape and pH-sensitive release. In contrast to GOA micelles, GOA/miR NPs showed higher tumor suppression following an intravenous injection in HCC xenograft-nude mice with rapid clearance from normal liver tissues (Zhang *et al.,* 2019). Ghosh *et al.* synthesized Cur-loaded PLGA nanoparticles (Nano-Cur) against DEN-induced HCC in rats, where an effective formulation to combat oxidative destruction of hepatic cells was observed compared to the ineffective free Cur form (Ghosh *et al.*, 2012). A summary of prepared drug-loaded micellar nanoparticles studied in cell- and animal-based models of HCC is listed in Table **11**.

Table 11. Different micellar nanoparticles developed for HCC treatment.

Drugs	Molecular Units	Stimuli	Targeting Receptor	Ligand	Active/Passive Targeting	Cells	References
Sorafenib	ApoE-PEG-P(CL-DTC)	Reduction	LDLRs	ApoE	Active	SMMC-7721	(Li *et al.*, 2020)
Sorafenib	P-DOCA	Temperature	ASGPR	Pectin	Active	HepG2	(Varshosaz *et al.*, 2019 a)
Sorafenib	PEGylated PEI-CL	pH and Temperature	LDLRs	Cholesterol	Active	HepG2	(Monajati *et al.*, 2018)
Sorafenib	PHEA-EDA-PLA-GAL	pH	ASGPR	Galactose	Active	Hepatic cell	(Craparo *et al.*, 2014)
Paclitaxel	Gal-PEG-PCL	pH	ASGPR	Galactose	Active	HepG2, SMMC-7721	(Yang *et al.*, 2011)
Gemcitabine and antisense-miRNA-21	PEGylated PLGA	pH	NA	NA	Passive	Hep3B, HepG2	(Devulapally *et al.*, 2016)
Gemcitabine	CPDG/CHS-PEG1500	pH	NA	NA	Passive	HCC bearing mice	(Du *et al.*, 2016)
Gemcitabine and miR-122 or miR-34a	GOA/miR-122 NPs	pH	NA	NA	Passive	HepG2, nude mice xenografted with HCC	(Zhang *et al.*, 2019)
Curcumin	PLGA	NA	NA	NA	Passive	DEN induced HCC in rat	(Ghosh *et al.*, 2012)

Emulsomes

Emulsomes are vesicles used as drug carrier systems that comprise a solid fat core entrapped in a phospholipid bilayer stabilized by cholesterol and soy lecithin. These lipoidal vesicular systems possess a dual property of both liposomes and emulsions. With solidified or semi-solidified internal solid fat core, their properties can be tuned by various lipid mixtures for different purposes. This way, emulsomes are highly preferred to sheath lipophilic drugs in high concentrations. Additionally, a regulated release is achieved as they also have the ability to load water-soluble therapeutic agents in aqueous layers of adjoining phospholipid layers. Varshosaz *et al.* prepared an Octreotide decorated PEGylated Trimethyl chitosan (TMC) as emulsome by emulsion evaporation method for directed delivery of SF to PDGFR and VEGFR overexpressed HepG2 cells. This study showed higher cytotoxicity in targeted emulsomes in comparison to free SF. Also, cell cycle studies showed a noticeable accumulation of the drug in the G1 phase for emulsomes treated HepG2 cells compared to the free and non-targeted emulsomes treated cells (Varshosaz *et al.*, 2019 b).

Hydrogels

Hydrogels are a network of cross-linked hydrophilic polymer chains that are occasionally available as a colloidal gel with water as a dispersion medium. Polymeric hydrogels have been extensively used in medical devices, drug delivery, and tissue engineering applications. In recent years, different stimuli-responsive and injectable hydrogels have been prepared from natural and synthetic polymers for biomedical and therapeutic purposes (Shi *et al.*, 2020 and Caló *et al.*, 2015). Of these, stimuli-responsive block copolymer has received substantial importance as a drug carrier system due to its unique biodegradability, biocompatibility, low-toxicity, and high-drug loading site-specificity, persistent, and regulated drug release characteristics.

Zheng *et al.* synthesized a thermosensitive composite of Gel-SF-Lipiodol Ultra fluid- Selenium nanoparticles (Gel-SF-LUF-SeNPs) to obtain a synergistic effect of chemoradiotherapy when the gel is localized at a particular tumor site of HCC. Here, the gel comprising of poly(D, L-lactic acid- co-glycolic acid)-b-Poly (ethylene glycol)-b- Poly (D, L-lactic acid- co-glycolic acid) (PLGA-PEG-PLGA) co-loaded with SF and SeNPs was injected into HepG2 tumor-bearing nude mice. The combined feature of localization and chemoradiotherapy enhanced the apoptosis by suppressing Ki67 and CD34 and activating the caspase-3 signaling pathway. Further investigations on this system demonstrated site-specific and prolonged anticancer effects in mice up to 21 days after a single subcutaneous injection with no significant side effects (Zheng *et al.*, 2019). Fong *et al.* engineered a 3D-macroporous cellulosic sponge system as an *in-vitro* habitat conducive to HCC patient-derived xenograft (HCC-PDX) organoid derived from a panel of 14 separate HCC-PDX lines (Fong *et al.*, 2018). The system was prepared using hydroxypropyl cellulose (HPC) modified based on a previous report on cellulose-based hydrogels (Yue *et al.*, 2010; Nugraha *et al.*, 2011). The *in-vitro* HCC-PDX models were evaluated using whole-exome sequencing and RNA-sequencing. The effect of SF and BGJ-398, a pan fibroblast growth factor receptor (FGFR) inhibitor, was evaluated in this platform, wherein immunoblot analysis demonstrated a dose-dependent decrease in phosphorylated-Erk and phosphorylated-Akt levels, respectively.

Zhao *et al.* 2019 designed an injectable intraperitoneal depot of supramolecular peptide hydrogel for localized and persistent release of triptolide orthotopic in the HCC model. Here, the peptide amphiphile (C_{16}-GNNQQNYKD-OH) based nanofibre acted as a gelator and transporter for triptolide. The *in-vitro* study showed regulated triptolide release from the hydrogel that attained higher accumulation over 14 days. From cytotoxicity studies, increased cell death was observed in HCC Bel-7402 cells compared to L-02 fetal hepatocytes. Also, following intraperitoneal injection, the hydrogel demonstrated persistent retention over 13 days with safe accumulation in the liver (Zhao *et al.*, 2019). Table **12** summarizes different polymeric hydrogels studied in HCC condition.

Table 12. Different polymeric hydrogels studied used in HCC condition.

Drugs	Molecular Units	Stimuli	Targeting Receptor	Ligand	Active/Passive Targeting	Cells	References
Sorafenib	PLGA-PEG-PLGA	Thermo	Ki67, CD34, caspase-3 signaling pathway	NA	Passive	HepG2 bearing mice	(Zheng *et al.*, 2019)
Sorafenib	MA-HPC	NA	NA	NA	Passive	HCC-PDX	(Fong *et al.*, 2018)
Triptolide	C_{16}-GNNQQNYK--OH nanofibre	NA	NA	NA	Passive	Human HCC Bel-7402	(Zhao *et al.*, 2019)

Metallic Nanoparticles

Metallic nanoparticles are distinguished by their distinctive physical and chemical properties in the nanoscale than those in their bulk (Horikoshi *et al.*, 2013). Several metallic nanoparticle investigations have been conducted on gold and silver nanoparticles as potential therapeutic options for cancer chemotherapy (Comfort *et al.*, 2011). Gold nanoparticles have been studied in various biomedical applications due to their ease of fabrication, functionalization, and extraordinary optical and photothermal properties (Huang *et al.*, 2010). Due to the photothermal property, gold nanoparticles cause local hyperthermia due to the absorption and scattering of visible laser light destroying cancerous cells (Salem *et al.*, 2018). On the other hand, silver nanoparticles possess significant antimicrobial activities (Dar *et al.*, 2013). Silver nanoparticles that are biologically fabricated have distinguished properties such as biocompatibility, stability, solubility and can be synthesized in a high yield without aggregation (Gurunathan *et al.*, 2015). Ahmadian *et al.* conducted an *in-vitro* study on HepG2 cells. Silver nanoparticles exhibited cytotoxic effects and up-regulated the pro-apoptotic factor implying it to be an effective nanoparticle to target HCC. Gold nanoparticles comprise submicron colloidal particles of gold dispersed in liquids, preferably aqueous solutions (Ahmadian *et al.*, 2018). Gold nanoparticles possess antiangiogenic characteristics to inhibit heparin interlinked growth factors such as bFGF and VEGF (Cherukuri *et al.*, 2010).

Jeon *et al.(2016)* designed multifunctional drug carriers Dox-pMNCs as an intra-arterial transcatheter infusion for chemoembolization or radioembolization. The porous structure with carboxylic functional groups on the MNCs had higher drug encapsulation, sustained drug release with good magnetic properties resulting in high MRI T2-weighted image contrast. Also, a comparative study was performed to investigate the safety and efficacy of Dox-pMNCs within iodinated oil, Dox-pMNCs, and Dox within iodinated oil, targeting the liver tumors in a rabbit model. Upon administration as an infusion, MRI and the histological study showed sustained drug release and retention of Dox-pMNCs within iodinated oil, enhancing liver cancer cell fatality (Jeon *et al.*, 2016). Zheng *et al.* synthesized ASGPR-targeting mesoporous silica nanocarrier (MSN) for co-delivery of SF and VEGF-targeted siRNA for chemotherapy and gene therapy to treat HCC. The *in vitro* studies in HepG2 and Huh7 cells demonstrated that MSN-LA nanocarrier not only induced S-phase cell cycle arrest, enhanced the cytotoxicity, and improved the tumor targeting of SF and siVEGF, but also enhanced the siVEGF transfection efficacy in ASGPR-overexpressing Huh7 cells (Zheng *et al.*, 2018). Table **13** summarizes different metallic nanoparticles studied in HCC conditions.

Table 13. Different metallic nanoparticles studied in HCC condition.

Drugs	Nanoformulations	Molecular Units	Stimuli	Targeting Receptor	Ligand	Cells	References
Doxorubicin	Magnetic nanoclusters	Dox-pMNCs	Magnetic	NA	NA	Rabbit model	(Jeon *et al.*, 2016)
Sorafenib and siVEGF	Silica nanocarriers	MSN-LA		ASGPR	NA	HepG2, Huh7	(Zheng *et al.*, 2018)

Polysaccharides

Polysaccharides are natural polymers with extraordinary biocompatibility and multifunctionality that permit further structural advancements to entrap different drugs. Dextran is one such naturally occurring polymer with a complex branched polysaccharide that has been vastly implemented in drug delivery. Dextran has been utilized as a nano-sized drug transporter to encapsulate Curcumin (Cur) to increase its biocompatibility and therapeutic potential. Cytotoxicity studies in HepG2 cells showed dose-dependent cytotoxicity of the drug in the dextran nanoparticles compared to treatment with free-form of Cur, thus, making it protective and more potent for treating HCC (Moghimi *et al.*, 2001). Anirudhan *et al.* synthesized dextran-based glycyrrhetinic acid decorated nano-sized drug transporter (GHDx) to deliver Cur. *In vitro* cytotoxicity examination on L929 and HepG2 cells demonstrated that GHDx was a non-toxic transporter, but Cur encapsulated GHDx revealed more significant toxicity with slow drug release towards hepatic cells (Anirudhan *et al.*, 2016). Nair *et al.* fabricated five different galactosylated chitosan nanoparticles (G1-G5) with the varying drug: polymer ratios to deliver GEM in ASGPR-overexpressed hepatocytes. G4 showed higher drug content and release. Biodistribution studies on G4 in rats showed a biphasic release with greater drug concentration favoring pharmacotherapy in the liver. Rapid clearance of GEM from G4 was observed in rats compared to the free-form highlighting the benefits of preparing targeted nanoformulation (Nair *et al.*, 2019). Table **14** summarizes different polysaccharide-based nanoformulation studies used in HCC condition

Table 14. Different polysaccharide-based nanoformulations studied in HCC condition.

Drugs	Nanoformulations	Molecular Units	Stimuli	Targeting Receptor	Ligand	Active/Passive Targeting	Cells	References
Curcumin	Dextran	GHDx	pH and Temperature	ASGPR	Glycyrrhetinic acid	Active	HepG2, L929	(Anirudhan *et al.*, 2016)
Gemcitabine	Chitosan Nanoformulation	Galactosylated Chitosan Nanoparticles	pH	ASGPR	Galactose	Active	HCC bearing rats	(Nair *et al.*, 2019)

Current Status Clinical Trials for different Nanoformulation used in HCC

MRX34 is a liposomal formulation of tumor suppressor miR-34a, an effective miRNA mimic therapy for cancer. Although this study does not compare adverse effects between the liposomal delivery system and free miR-34a but suggests that adverse effects were also observed due to the liposomal carrier, which can be further reduced by dexamethasone premedication (Beg *et al.*, 2017). In contrast, from a phase I study on BCL-2 targeted, single-stranded DNA oligonucleotide, Tolcher *et al.* demonstrated that the liposomal delivery system similar to the MRX34 had no association of the carrier with frequent and adverse infusion-related reactions (Tolcher *et al.*, 2014).

Doxorubicin is an effective therapeutic drug; however, DOX as a free drug is associated with high morbidity in cirrhosis (Lai *et al.*, 1988). The result remained unaltered when combined with SF (Abou-Alfa *et al.*, 2016). DOX-loaded nanoparticles (DOX-NPs) in the liver effectively counteracted chemoresistance by suppressing the efflux pump genes (Barraud *et al.*, 2005). Thus, administration of DOX-NPs diminished adverse events when the drug was injected through the hepatic arterial route. However, acute respiratory distress syndrome was observed in a few patients due to intrahepatic arterial injection of DOX-NPs in the phase I-

II trial, which showed no clinically noticeable pulmonary treatment-related adverse events following 6 h of intravenous perfusion in RELIVE (Merle *et al.*, 2017).

TKM-080301 is a lipid nanoparticle consisting of four lipids and a synthetic, double-stranded siRNA targeted against human polo-like kinase 1 (PLK1) mRNA. Chemically fabricated siRNAs are a duplex of complementary RNA oligonucleotides outlined to attain post-transcriptional gene suppression by the RNA interference mechanism (Dorsett *et al.*, 2004). In general, nanoformulations such as lipid, liposome, and micelle possess a better EPR effect. The lipid constituents of TKM-080301 also protected the siRNA from degradation by tissue nucleases in the plasma, thereby avoiding quick clearance of the siRNA. Moreover, enhanced intracellular uptake of the PLK1-targeting siRNA into hepatic cancer cells was reported (Judge *et al.*, 2009).

Mitoxantrone (Dihydroxyanthracenedione, DHAD) is a therapeutic antineoplastic drug implemented in cancer treatment, and clinical studies also exhibited its potential outcomes in HCC. Polybutylcyanacrylate (PBCA) is a bio-reconcilable and bioavailable polymer used as a medical adhesive for the past few decades. However, PBCA nanoparticles showed a toxic effect on the liver (Fernandezurrusuno *et al.*, 1995). DHAD-PBCA- nanoparticles have shown a therapeutic advantage for patients with unresected HCC in different stages of clinical investigation.

Earlier, Daunorubicin (Liposomal Da) and Doxorubicin were reported to induce lower levels of cardiac toxicity in animals (Fichtner *et al.*, 1984). Generally, the liposomal formulations change drug distribution in organs tissues, thereby reducing the exposure of cardiac tissue to high anthracycline concentrations. However, the change of anthracycline metabolism, specifically the reduction in the formation of the alcohol metabolite, can reduce cardiac toxicity. Therefore, most clinical investigations reported to date had no cardiotoxicity in patients despite acquiring a cumulative high dose of 1 g/m^2. Moreover, a reduction in adverse events such as alopecia was also achieved without losing the potential of anthracyclines (Guaglianone *et al.*, 1994).

From the studies currently available on the nanoformulations, several techniques and methods are established to specifically design and synthesize potential nanoparticles to deliver the drugs/therapeutic agents for HCC. Various *in-vitro* cell-based approaches and *in-vivo* biodistribution examinations on animal models exhibited favorable outcomes when the drugs were encapsulated/cross-linked with targeted nanoparticles compared to the free forms. Currently, different clinical trials comparing single-drug therapy and multi-drug therapy are being pursued.

From detailed investigations, specific drugs, miRNA, and antibodies designed to target HCC are also developed as nanoformulations to improve efficacy. As targeted nanoparticles, many of these chemotherapeutics have shown exciting results and reduced adverse events compared to the respective free therapeutics. Further studies on preparing multi-chemotherapeutics as a nanoformulation would be a promising way ahead for treating HCC effectively.

Table **15** provides a list of drug-loaded nanoformulations at the different phases of clinical trials for HCC treatment.

Table 15. Current status of different nanoformulations in clinical trials in HCC treatment.

Drugs	Formulation	Molecular Units	Clinical Stage	Adverse Events	Remarks	References
Cisplatin	Liposome	Lipoplatin (DPPG, SPC-3, CL, mMPEG2000-DSPE)	Preclinical (4 patients, one with HCC)	NA	Preferentially accumulate in malignant tissue both of primary and metastatic origin.	(Boulikas *et al.*, 2005)
Doxorubicin associated with Capecitabine or Gemcitabine	Liposome	PLD	Preclinical (31 patients)	Neutropenia, Anemia, Thrombocytopenia, Skin rash, Mucositis, Hand-foot syndrome	PEGylated liposomal doxorubicin-based combination chemotherapy with Capecitabine or Gemcitabine was not effective in advanced HCC.	(Poh *et al.*, 2005)
MRX34	Liposome	Liposomal miR-34a (cationic amphoteric lipids) (if necessary)	Phase 1 (47 patients) NCT01829971 Status: Terminated (2016)	Lymphopenia, Neutropenia, Thrombocytopenia, increased bilirubin, AST and ALT, Hyperglycemia, and Hyponatremia.	The miRNA therapy with MRX34 was feasible and tolerable under adequate dexamethasone premedication. Shows preliminary signs of antitumor activity.	(Beg *et al.*, 2017)
TKM-080301	Lipid Nanoparticle	siRNA against PLK1	Phase 1 (43 patients) NCT02191878 Status-Completed (2016)	Thrombocytopenia, Leucocytosis, Cardiac disorder, Ascites, hemorrhage, Gastric ulcer, Peritoneal hemorrhage, Pyrexia, Cholangitis, Non-cardiac chest pain, Hepatic failure,	Antitumor effect was limited for this study.	(El Dika *et al.*, 2019)

(Table 15) cont.....

Drugs	Formulation	Molecular Units	Clinical Stage	Adverse Events	Remarks	References
				Thrombocytopenia, Leucocytosis, Cardiac disorder, Ascites, hemorrhage, Gastric ulcer, Peritoneal hemorrhage, Pyrexia, Cholangitis, Non-cardiac chest pain, Hepatic failure,		
Doxorubicin	Liposome	LTLD	Phase I (22 patients) NCT00617981 Status: Completed (2017)	Hair loss, Leucopenia, decreased neutrophil count, Decreased hemoglobin level, Abdominal pain, Weight loss	RFA with heat target delivery chemotherapy facilitated better tumor coagulation necrosis without additional toxicity.	(Yang *et al.*, 2019)
Gemcitabine and Doxorubicin	Liposome	LD	Phase I (21 patients)	Hematological toxicity, Thrombocytopenia, Stomatitis, and Neutropenia	The combinatory therapy was safe and efficacious in the treatment of HCC.	(Pastorelli *et al.*, 2006)
Doxorubicin and Temsirolimus	Liposome	PLD	Phase I (23 patients)	Mucositis, Stomatitis, Anorexia, Thrombocytopenia, ALT, Dyspnea, Dyspepsia, Desquamation	Combinatory therapy was tolerable and attained a clinical advantage.	(Wang-Gillam *et al.*, 2014)
Doxorubicin and Radiofrequency ablation therapy	Liposome	LD	Phase I (14 patients)	NA	The adjuvant Doxil chemotherapy increased tumor suppression in contrast with radiofrequency ablation therapy alone.	(Goldberg *et al.*, 2002)
Mitoxantrone	Nanoparticle	DHAD-PBCA-NPs	Phase II (108 patients) Sichuan Food and Drug Administration (registration no. 1999-266)	Mucositis, Bilirubin, Aminotransferase, Alkaline phosphate, Serum creatinine, Leukopenia, and Anemia	Increased cytotoxicity and prolonged the median survival period.	(Zhou *et al.*, 2009)

(Table 15) cont.....

Drugs	Formulation	Molecular Units	Clinical Stage	Adverse Events	Remarks	References
Daunorubicin	Liposome	DaunoXome	Phase II (14 patients) Independent Ethics Committee of the Chinese University of Hong Kong 1999	Treatment-related laboratory abnormalities were infrequent and unlikely adverse events.	Further assessment was not warranted.	(Yeo *et al.*, 1999)
Doxorubicin	Liposome	PLD	Phase II (16 patients)	Hypersensitivity, Grade 3 and 4 toxicities were increased liver enzymes, and hematologic toxicity	Not effective for the treatment of advanced HCC.	(Halm *et al.*, 2000)
Gemcitabine and Doxorubicin	Liposome	PLD	Phase II (41 patients)	Hematological toxicity, Neutropenia, anemia, Thrombocytopenia, Stomatitis, HFS, Liver toxicity	Active and safe in advanced HCC.	(Lombardi *et al.*, 2011)
Doxorubicin	Liposome	PLD	Phase II (15 patients)	Palmoplantar erythrodysesthesia, Thrombocytopenia, Leucopenia, Neutropenia, Dyspnoea, severe chronic obstructive lung disease, and Ascites	Further assessment was necessary.	(Lind *et al.*, 2007)
Doxorubicin	Liposome	PLD	Phase II (16 patients)	Lethargy, Cutaneous, Anorexia, Sepsis, Mucositis, Alopecia, Constipation, and Cardiac	PLD has almost no activity in advanced HCC. Further evaluation is needed with better-targeted therapy.	(Valle *et al.*, 2005)
Doxorubicin, 5-Fluorouracil, and Folinic acid	Liposome	PLD	Phase II (31 patients) Institutional review board	Neutropenia, Anemia, Thrombocytopenia, Oral Stomatitis, Hand-foot syndrome, Hepatic dysfunction, and Peripheral neuropathy	Combination appeared to be capable of achieving durable stabilization of HCC.	(Di Lorenzo *et al.*, 2007)

(Table 15) cont.....

Drugs	Formulation	Molecular Units	Clinical Stage	Adverse Events	Remarks	References
Doxorubicin	Liposome	PLD	Phase II (40 patients) Human Investigation Committee	Stomatitis, Alopecia, Skin, Leukopenia, Thrombocytopenia, Anemia, Hepatitis, and Infection	The disposition of PLD in patients with liver dysfunction was not inhibited, but it did not reveal better activity in contrast with free drugs.	(Hong *et al.*, 2003)
Doxorubicin	Liposome	LTLD	Phase III (701 patients)	Alopecia, Neutropenia, Leukopenia, Thrombocytopenia, Aspartate aminotransferase increased, Alanine aminotransferase increased, Pyrexia, Blood bilirubin increased	Adding LTLD to RFA was determined to be safe but did not elevate PFS or OS.	(Tak *et al.*, 2018)
Doxorubicin	Liposome	Doxorubicin loaded nanoparticles	Phase 3 (11 countries, 397 patients) Trial registered number - NCT01655693 Status- Completed (2019)	Asthenia, Peripheral edema, Ascites, Anorexia, Abdominal pain, Dyspnea, Cough, Paraesthesia, Anaemia, Neutropenia, Asthenia, and Thrombocytopenia	This study did not enhance overall survival for patients with HCC in whom earlier Sorafenib treatment had been unsuccessful.	(Merle *et al.*, 2019)

From Table **15** on clinical trials of different nanoformulations studied in HCC patients, it is observed that a chemotherapeutic agent, whether as a small molecule or miRNA or an antibody when administered alone or in combination, suffers severe adverse effects. However, as a nanoformulation, these effects were mitigated to a great extent. By comparing the information listed in Tables **2** and **15**, one may observe reduced adverse events when the drug is delivered in a nanoparticle as a delivery system. However, one cannot exclude adverse events with the nano drug-delivery systems for the lack of targeting moieties or bioavailability of the designed nanosystem polymers or premature drug release caused by stimulus-responsive linkages. However, a successful delivery system may be attained by creating active/passive/stimuli-responsive directed nano-particles.

FUTURE SCOPE

The administration of free-drug and nanoparticle-loaded therapeutic agents has demonstrated different outcomes. The specific cellular internalization and trafficking mechanisms of nanoparticles permit the delivery of chemotherapeutics to their intended target sites in their active form, at required concentration with reduced accumulation in non-specific organs/tissues. However, it is expected that cytosolic internalization of a drug does not imply its interaction with the target organelle. Therefore, organelle-specific targeting would be an approach for better therapeutic outcomes. This can be achieved by tagging therapeutic agents with organelle-specific localization ligands, especially in the case of miRNA or gene-based nanotherapeutics that allow them to even reach inside the nucleus for their site-specific functions.

CONCLUDING REMARKS

The emergence of nanotechnology and its application in medicine as nano-medicine is a boon to humankind. Especially in a situation where there are very few therapeutic options available for HCC treatment, developing nanoformulation has contributed to more sensible therapeutic options, raising HCC patients' hopes for a successful therapy and enhanced survival. It has indeed led to the development and exploration of numerous novel methodologies to target HCC. To obtain a successful treatment for HCC, targeting mRNA of oncogenes through miRNA or targeting the overexpressed receptor using drugs and antibodies are the therapeutic approaches currently followed. However, with conventional therapy obtaining reasonable success without adverse effects remains questionable. The medicines and miRNA now available have potential off-targets and have issues about their bioavailability.

On the other hand, a targeted nanoparticulate approach is a promising approach. It comes in handy as it provides ample options to deliver the chemotherapeutic agent effectively. The application of nanotechnology in drug delivery of HCC is indeed a successful attempt and must be pursued further with a rational approach.

LIST OF ABBREVIATIONS

ApoE-PEG-P (CL-DTC)	Apolipoprotein E peptide decorated poly (ethylene glycol)-b-poly (ε-caprolactone-dithiolane trimethylene carbonate)- mefenamate;
AFP-L3	α-Fetoprotein;
ASGPR	Asialoglycoprotein;
bFGF	basic Fibroblast Growth Factor;
BCRP	Breast Cancer Resistance Protein;
CHOL-AL-AG	Cholesterol-Alanine-Arabinogalactan;
CMCS-SiSf-CL	Carboxymethyl Chitosan Sorafenib and Cy3- siRNA co-loaded Cationic Liposomes;
CPDG/CHS-PEG1500	Cyclic phosphoryl N-dodecanoyl gemcitabine/Cholesterol Hemisuccinate Poly (ethylene glycol) 1500;

DEN	Diethylnitrosamine;
Dox-pMNCs	Doxorubicin loaded magnetic nanoclusters;
DPPC-DSPE-PEG2000-CL	1,2- Dipalmitoyl-sn-glycero-3- Phosphocholine- 1,2- Distearoyl-s- -glyceri- Phosphoethanolamine- N-methoxy (polyethylene glycol) Cholesterol;
Fuc-Lip-Sf with HDACi	L-Fucose-Liposomes-Sorafenib with Histone Deacetylase Inhibitor;
GA-CH-NPs	Galactosylated Chitosan Nanoparticles;
Gd	Gadolinium;
Gal-P123	Galactosyl conjugated Pluronic P123;
Gal-PEG-PCL	Galactose conjugated Poly (ethylene glycol)-b-Poly (ε-caprolactone);
GOA/miR-122 NPs	Gemcitabine- oleic acid prodrugs binding miRNAs nanoparticles;
HSPG	Heparan Sulfate Proteoglycan; IL-6- Interleukin-6;
IFN	Interferons;
JAK-STAT	Janus Kinase-Signal Transducer and Activator of Transcription;
LDLRs	Low-Density Lipoprotein Receptors;
Lipo-CD44-TF	Liposomes-CD44-Triple fusion;
Lipoid E80-DSPE- MPEG2000-CL	Lipoid E80 1,2- Distearoyl-sn-glyceri-3-Phosphoethanolamine- N-methoxy (polyethylene glycol) Cholesterol;
LPG	Dual functional Gal-P123 modified liposome;
MA-HPC	Methacrylic Anhydride- Hydroxypropylcellulose;
MAPK	Mitogen Activated Protein Kinases;
MSN-LA	Mesoporous Silica nanoparticles- Lactobionic acid;
mTOR	mammalian Target of Rapamycin;
IGF	Insulin-like Growth Factor;
MAPK	Mitogen-Activated Protein Kinase;
PcDNA3.1-RFP-Rluc-HSV-ttk	pcDNA- monomeric red fluorescence protein- renilla luciferase-herpes simplex virus truncated thymidine kinase;
PDGFR	Platelet-Derived Growth Factor Receptor;
P-DOCA	Pectin-deoxycholic acid;
PDT	Photo Dynamic Therapy;
PDX	Patient Derived Xenograft;
PEGylated-PLGA	PEGylated Poly (D, L-lactic acid- co-glycolic acid);
PEI-CL	Polyethylenimine Cholesterol;
PHEA-EDA-PLA-GAL	α,β- Poly (N-2-hydroxyethyl) (2-aminoethylcarbamate)-D,L-Aspartamide- Polylactic acid- Galactose;
PI3K-Akt	Phosphatidylinositol 3-Kinase- Protein kinase B;

PL90/PL90H/CHOL	Phospholipon 90G/ Phospholipon 90H/ Cholesterol;
PLGA-PEG-PLGA	Poly (D, L-lactic acid- co-glycolic acid)-b-Poly (ethylene glycol)-b-Poly (D, L-lactic acid- co-glycolic acid);
PTT	Photo Thermal Therapy;
SF	Sorafenib;
SF-PL/siGPC3	Sorafenib PEI modified Liposome/small interfering Glypican-3;
TKI	Tyrosine Kinase Inhibitor;
TMC-Ems	Trimethyl Chitosan Emulsomes;
TNFα	Tumour Necrosis Factor;
VEGF	Vascular Endothelial Growth Factor;
VEGFR	Vascular Endothelial Growth Factor Receptor

CONSENT FOR PUBLICATION

Not applicable

CONFLICT OF INTEREST

The authors declare no conflict of interest, financial or otherwise.

ACKNOWLEDGEMENTS

The authors acknowledge the intramural funding of NISER for the support.

REFERENCES

Abou-Alfa, GK, Niedzwieski, D, Knox, JJ, Kaubisch, A, Posey, J, Tan, BR, Kavan, P, Goel, R, Murray, JJ, Bekaii-Saab, TS, Tam, VC, Rajdev, L, Kelley, RK, Siegel, A, Balletti, J, Harding, JJ, Schwartz, LH, Goldberg, RM & Bertagnolli, MM (2016) Phase III randomized study of sorafenib plus doxorubicin *versus* sorafenib in patients with advanced hepatocellular carcinoma (HCC): CALGB 80802 (Alliance). *J Clin Oncol,* 192-2.
[http://dx.doi.org/10.1200/jco.2016.34.4_suppl.192]

Ahmadian, E, Dizaj, SM, Rahimpour, E, Hasanzadeh, A, Eftekhari, A, Hosain Zadegan, H, Halajzadeh, J & Ahmadian, H (2018) Effect of silver nanoparticles in the induction of apoptosis on human hepatocellular carcinoma (HepG2) cell line. *Mater Sci Eng C,* 93, 465-71.
[http://dx.doi.org/10.1016/j.msec.2018.08.027] [PMID: 30274079]

Anirudhan, TS & Binusreejayan, (2016) Dextran based nanosized carrier for the controlled and targeted delivery of curcumin to liver cancer cells. *Int J Biol Macromol,* 88, 222-35.
[http://dx.doi.org/10.1016/j.ijbiomac.2016.03.040] [PMID: 27012895]

Aravalli, RN, Steer, CJ & Cressman, ENK (2008) Molecular mechanisms of hepatocellular carcinoma. *Hepatology,* 48, 2047-63.
[http://dx.doi.org/10.1002/hep.22580] [PMID: 19003900]

Baig, B, Halim, SA, Farrukh, A, Greish, Y & Amin, A (2019) Current status of nanomaterial-based treatment for hepatocellular carcinoma. *Biomed Pharmacother,* 116, 108852.
[http://dx.doi.org/10.1016/j.biopha.2019.108852] [PMID: 30999152]

Balogh, J, Iii, DV, Gordon, S, Li, X & Ghobrial, RM, Jr (2016) HPM (2016), 'Jhc-3-041' *Journal of Hepatocellular Carcinoma,* 3, 41-53.

Barraud, L, Merle, P, Soma, E, Lefrançois, L, Guerret, S, Chevallier, M, Dubernet, C, Couvreur, P, Trépo, C & Vitvitski, L (2005) Increase of doxorubicin sensitivity by doxorubicin-loading into nanoparticles for hepatocellular carcinoma cells *in vitro* and *in vivo. J Hepatol,* 42, 736-43.
[http://dx.doi.org/10.1016/j.jhep.2004.12.035] [PMID: 15826724]

Beg, MS, Brenner, AJ, Sachdev, J, Borad, M, Kang, YK, Stoudemire, J, Smith, S, Bader, AG, Kim, S & Hong, DS (2017) Phase I study of MRX34, a liposomal miR-34a mimic, administered twice weekly in patients with advanced solid tumors. *Invest New Drugs,* 35, 180-8.
[http://dx.doi.org/10.1007/s10637-016-0407-y] [PMID: 27917453]

Bondì, ML, Scala, A, Sortino, G, Amore, E, Botto, C, Azzolina, A, Balasus, D, Cervello, M & Mazzaglia, A (2015) Nanoassemblies Based on Supramolecular Complexes of Nonionic Amphiphilic Cyclodextrin and Sorafenib as Effective Weapons to Kill Human HCC Cells. *Biomacromolecules,* 16, 3784-91.
[http://dx.doi.org/10.1021/acs.biomac.5b01082] [PMID: 26528591]

Bouchie, A (2013) First microRNA mimic enters clinic. *Nat Biotechnol,* 31, 577.
[http://dx.doi.org/10.1038/nbt0713-577] [PMID: 23839128]

Boulikas, T, Stathopoulos, GP, Volakakis, N & Vougiouka, M (2005) Systemic Lipoplatin infusion results in preferential tumor uptake in human studies. *Anticancer Res,* 25, 3031-9.
[PMID: 16080562]

Burley, SK, Bhikadiya, C, Bi, C, Bittrich, S, Chen, L, Crichlow, GV, Christie, CH, Dalenberg, K, Di Costanzo, L, Duarte, JM, Dutta, S, Feng, Z, Ganesan, S, Goodsell, DS, Ghosh, S, Green, RK, Guranović, V & Guzenko, D (2021) Hudson, BP et al*RCSB Protein Data Bank,* D437-51.

Burris, HA, III, Moore, MJ, Andersen, J, Green, MR, Rothenberg, ML, Modiano, MR, Cripps, MC, Portenoy, RK, Storniolo, AM, Tarassoff, P, Nelson, R, Dorr, FA, Stephens, CD & Von Hoff, DD (1997) Improvements in survival and clinical benefit with gemcitabine as first-line therapy for patients with advanced pancreas cancer: a randomized trial. *J Clin Oncol,* 15, 2403-13.
[http://dx.doi.org/10.1200/JCO.1997.15.6.2403] [PMID: 9196156]

Bussenius, J, Blazey, CM, Aay, N, Anand, NK, Arcalas, A, Baik, T, Bowles, OJ, Buhr, CA, Costanzo, S, Curtis, JK, DeFina, SC, Dubenko, L, Heuer, TS, Huang, P, Jaeger, C, Joshi, A, Kennedy, AR, Kim, AI, Lara, K, Lee, J, Li, J, Lougheed, JC, Ma, S, Malek, S, Manalo, JC, Martini, JF, McGrath, G, Nicoll, M, Nuss, JM, Pack, M, Peto, CJ, Tsang, TH, Wang, L, Womble, SW, Yakes, M, Zhang, W & Rice, KD (2012) Discovery of XL888: a novel tropane-derived small molecule inhibitor of HSP90. *Bioorg Med Chem Lett,* 22, 5396-404.
[http://dx.doi.org/10.1016/j.bmcl.2012.07.052] [PMID: 22877636]

Caló, E & Khutoryanskiy, VV (2015) Biomedical applications of hydrogels: A review of patents and commercial products. *Eur Polym J,* 252-67.
[http://dx.doi.org/10.1016/j.eurpolymj.2014.11.024]

Castaldo, G, Calcagno, G, Sibillo, R, Cuomo, R, Nardone, G, Castellano, L, Del Vecchio Blanco, C, Budillon, G & Salvatore, F (2000) Quantitative analysis of aldolase A mRNA in liver discriminates between hepatocellular carcinoma and cirrhosis. *Clin Chem,* 46, 901-6.
[http://dx.doi.org/10.1093/clinchem/46.7.901] [PMID: 10894831]

Chaiteerakij, R, Zhang, X, Addissie, BD, Mohamed, EA, Harmsen, WS, Theobald, PJ, Peters, BE, Balsanek, JG, Ward, MM, Giama, NH, Moser, CD, Oseini, AM, Umeda, N, Venkatesh, S, Harnois, DM, Charlton, MR, Yamada, H, Satomura, S, Algeciras-Schimnich, A, Snyder, MR, Therneau, TM & Roberts, LR (2015) Combinations of biomarkers and Milan criteria for predicting hepatocellular carcinoma recurrence after liver transplantation. *Liver Transpl,* 21, 599-606.
[http://dx.doi.org/10.1002/lt.24117] [PMID: 25789635]

Chan, SL, Yeo, W, Mo, F, Chan, AWH, Koh, J, Li, L, Hui, EP, Chong, CCN, Lai, PBS, Mok, TSK & Yu, SCH (2017) A phase 2 study of the efficacy and biomarker on the combination of transarterial chemoembolization and axitinib in the treatment of inoperable hepatocellular carcinoma. *Cancer,* 123, 3977-

85.
[http://dx.doi.org/10.1002/cncr.30825] [PMID: 28640364]

Chen, Y, Liu, YC, Sung, YC, Ramjiawan, RR, Lin, TT, Chang, CC, Jeng, KS, Chang, CF, Liu, CH, Gao, DY, Hsu, FF, Duyverman, AM, Kitahara, S, Huang, P, Dima, S, Popescu, I, Flaherty, KT, Zhu, AX, Bardeesy, N, Jain, RK, Benes, CH & Duda, DG (2017) Overcoming sorafenib evasion in hepatocellular carcinoma using CXCR4-targeted nanoparticles to co-deliver MEK-inhibitors. *Sci Rep,* 7, 44123.
[http://dx.doi.org/10.1038/srep44123] [PMID: 28276530]

Cherukuri, P, Glazer, ES & Curley, SA (2010) Targeted hyperthermia using metal nanoparticles. *Adv Drug Deliv Rev,* 62, 339-45.
[http://dx.doi.org/10.1016/j.addr.2009.11.006] [PMID: 19909777]

Comfort, KK, Maurer, EI, Braydich-Stolle, LK & Hussain, SM (2011) Interference of silver, gold, and iron oxide nanoparticles on epidermal growth factor signal transduction in epithelial cells. *ACS Nano,* 5, 10000-8.
[http://dx.doi.org/10.1021/nn203785a] [PMID: 22070748]

Craparo, EF, Sardo, C, Serio, R, Zizzo, MG, Bondì, ML, Giammona, G & Cavallaro, G (2014) Galactosylated polymeric carriers for liver targeting of sorafenib. *Int J Pharm,* 466, 172-80.
[http://dx.doi.org/10.1016/j.ijpharm.2014.02.047] [PMID: 24607205]

Daher, S, Massarwa, M, Benson, AA & Khoury, T (2018) Current and future treatment of hepatocellular carcinoma: An updated comprehensive review. *J Clin Transl Hepatol,* 6, 69-78.
[http://dx.doi.org/10.14218/JCTH.2017.00031] [PMID: 29607307]

Dar, MA, Ingle, A & Rai, M (2013) Enhanced antimicrobial activity of silver nanoparticles synthesized by Cryphonectria sp. evaluated singly and in combination with antibiotics. *Nanomedicine,* 9, 105-10.
[http://dx.doi.org/10.1016/j.nano.2012.04.007] [PMID: 22633901]

Darnell, JE, Jr, Kerr, IM & Stark, GR (1994) Jak-STAT pathways and transcriptional activation in response to IFNs and other extracellular signaling proteins. *Science,* 264, 1415-21.
[http://dx.doi.org/10.1126/science.8197455] [PMID: 8197455]

DeLano, WL, Ultsch, MH, de Vos, AM & Wells, JA (2000) Convergent solutions to binding at a protein-protein interface. *Science,* 287, 1279-83.
[http://dx.doi.org/10.1126/science.287.5456.1279] [PMID: 10678837]

Devulapally, R, Foygel, K, Sekar, TV, Willmann, JK & Paulmurugan, R (2016) Gemcitabine and Antisense-microRNA Co-encapsulated PLGA-PEG Polymer Nanoparticles for Hepatocellular Carcinoma Therapy. *ACS Appl Mater Interfaces,* 8, 33412-22.
[http://dx.doi.org/10.1021/acsami.6b08153] [PMID: 27960411]

Dhanak, D & Jackson, P (2014) Development and classes of epigenetic drugs for cancer. *Biochem Biophys Res Commun,* 455, 58-69.
[http://dx.doi.org/10.1016/j.bbrc.2014.07.006] [PMID: 25016182]

Dhanasekaran, R, Limaye, A & Cabrera, R (2012) Hepatocellular carcinoma: current trends in worldwide epidemiology, risk factors, diagnosis, and therapeutics. *Hepat Med,* 4, 19-37.
[PMID: 24367230]

Di Costanzo, A, Del Gaudio, N, Migliaccio, A & Altucci, L (2014) Epigenetic drugs against cancer: an evolving landscape. *Arch Toxicol,* 88, 1651-68.
[http://dx.doi.org/10.1007/s00204-014-1315-6] [PMID: 25085708]

Di Lorenzo, G, Rea, A, Carlomagno, C, Pepe, S, Palmieri, G, Labianca, R, Chirianni, A, De Stefano, A, Esposito, V, De Placido, S & Montesarchio, V (2007) Activity and safety of pegylated liposomal doxorubicin, 5-fluorouracil and folinic acid in inoperable hepatocellular carcinoma: a phase II study. *World J Gastroenterol,* 13, 6553-7.
[http://dx.doi.org/10.3748/wjg.v13.i48.6553] [PMID: 18161926]

Doi, T, Muro, K, Ishii, H, Kato, T, Tsushima, T, Takenoyama, M, Oizumi, S, Gemmoto, K, Suna, H, Enokitani, K, Kawakami, T, Nishikawa, H & Yamamoto, N (2019) A phase I study of the anti-CC chemokine

receptor 4 antibody, mogamulizumab, in combination with nivolumab in patients with advanced or metastatic solid tumors. *Clin Cancer Res,* 25, 6614-22.
[http://dx.doi.org/10.1158/1078-0432.CCR-19-1090] [PMID: 31455681]

Dollinger, MM, Lautenschlaeger, C, Lesske, J, Tannapfel, A, Wagner, AD, Schoppmeyer, K, Nehls, O, Welker, MW, Wiest, R & Fleig, WE (2010) Thymostimulin *versus* placebo for palliative treatment of locally advanced or metastasised hepatocellular carcinoma: a phase III clinical trial. *BMC Cancer,* 10, 457.
[http://dx.doi.org/10.1186/1471-2407-10-457] [PMID: 20735834]

Dorsett, Y & Tuschl, T (2004) siRNAs: applications in functional genomics and potential as therapeutics. *Nat Rev Drug Discov,* 3, 318-29.
[http://dx.doi.org/10.1038/nrd1345] [PMID: 15060527]

Du, L, Zhang, B, Lei, Y, Wang, S & Jin, Y (2016) Long-circulating and liver-targeted nanoassemblies of cyclic phosphoryl N-dodecanoyl gemcitabine for the treatment of hepatocellular carcinoma. *Biomed Pharmacother,* 79, 208-14.
[http://dx.doi.org/10.1016/j.biopha.2016.02.024] [PMID: 27044830]

Eastman, A (2006) *'The Mechanism of Action of Cisplatin: From Adducts to Apoptosis', Cisplatin: Chemistry and Biochemistry of a Leading Anticancer Drug* Verlag Helvetica Chimica Acta, Zürich 111-34.

El-Say, KM & El-Sawy, HS (2017) Polymeric nanoparticles: Promising platform for drug delivery. *Int J Pharm,* 528, 675-91.
[http://dx.doi.org/10.1016/j.ijpharm.2017.06.052] [PMID: 28629982]

El Dika, I, Lim, HY, Yong, WP, Lin, CC, Yoon, JH, Modiano, M, Freilich, B, Choi, HJ, Chao, TY, Kelley, RK, Brown, J, Knox, J, Ryoo, BY, Yau, T & Abou-Alfa, GK (2019) An Open-Label, Multicenter, Phase I, Dose Escalation Study with Phase II Expansion Cohort to Determine the Safety, Pharmacokinetics, and Preliminary Antitumor Activity of Intravenous TKM-080301 in Subjects with Advanced Hepatocellular Carcinoma. *Oncologist,* 24, 747-e218.
[http://dx.doi.org/10.1634/theoncologist.2018-0838] [PMID: 30598500]

Fairhurst, RA, Knoepfel, T, Buschmann, N, Leblanc, C, Mah, R, Todorov, M, Nimsgern, P, Ripoche, S, Niklaus, M, Warin, N, Luu, VH, Madoerin, M, Wirth, J, Graus-Porta, D, Weiss, A, Kiffe, M, Wartmann, M, Kinyamu-Akunda, J, Sterker, D, Stamm, C, Adler, F, Buhles, A, Schadt, H, Couttet, P, Blank, J, Galuba, I, Trappe, J, Voshol, J, Ostermann, N, Zou, C, Berghausen, J, Del Rio Espinola, A, Jahnke, W & Furet, P (2020) Discovery of Roblitinib (FGF401) as a Reversible-Covalent Inhibitor of the Kinase Activity of Fibroblast Growth Factor Receptor 4. *J Med Chem,* 63, 12542-73.
[http://dx.doi.org/10.1021/acs.jmedchem.0c01019] [PMID: 32930584]

Fang, J, Nakamura, H & Maeda, H (2011) The EPR effect: Unique features of tumor blood vessels for drug delivery, factors involved, and limitations and augmentation of the effect. *Adv Drug Deliv Rev,* 63, 136-51.
[http://dx.doi.org/10.1016/j.addr.2010.04.009] [PMID: 20441782]

Fernandez-Urrusuno, R, Fattal, E, Porquet, D, Feger, J & Couvreur, P (1995) Evaluation of liver toxicological effects induced by polyalkylcyanoacrylate nanoparticles. *Toxicol Appl Pharmacol,* 130, 272-9.
[http://dx.doi.org/10.1006/taap.1995.1032] [PMID: 7871540]

Ferreira, DdosS, Lopes, SCDA, Franco, MS & Oliveira, MC (2013) pH-sensitive liposomes for drug delivery in cancer treatment. *Ther Deliv,* 4, 1099-123.
[http://dx.doi.org/10.4155/tde.13.80] [PMID: 24024511]

Fichtner, I, Arndt, D, Elbe, B & Reszka, R (1984) Cardiotoxicity of free and liposomally encapsulated rubomycin (daunorubicin) in mice. *Oncology,* 41, 363-9.
[http://dx.doi.org/10.1159/000225854] [PMID: 6472773]

Finn, RS & Zhu, AX (2009) Targeting angiogenesis in hepatocellular carcinoma: focus on VEGF and bevacizumab. *Expert Rev Anticancer Ther,* 9, 503-9.
[http://dx.doi.org/10.1586/era.09.6] [PMID: 19374603]

Fong, ELS, Toh, TB, Lin, QXX, Liu, Z, Hooi, L, Mohd Abdul Rashid, MB, Benoukraf, T, Chow, EKH, Huynh, TH & Yu, H (2018) Generation of matched patient-derived xenograft *in vitro-in vivo* models using

3D macroporous hydrogels for the study of liver cancer. *Biomaterials,* 159, 229-40. [http://dx.doi.org/10.1016/j.biomaterials.2017.12.026] [PMID: 29353739]

Gao, L, Wang, X, Tang, Y, Huang, S, Hu, CAA & Teng, Y (2017) FGF19/FGFR4 signaling contributes to the resistance of hepatocellular carcinoma to sorafenib. *J Exp Clin Cancer Res,* 36, 8. [http://dx.doi.org/10.1186/s13046-016-0478-9] [PMID: 28069043]

Ghosh, D, Choudhury, ST, Ghosh, S, Mandal, AK, Sarkar, S, Ghosh, A, Saha, KD & Das, N (2012) Nanocapsulated curcumin: oral chemopreventive formulation against diethylnitrosamine induced hepatocellular carcinoma in rat. *Chem Biol Interact,* 195, 206-14. [http://dx.doi.org/10.1016/j.cbi.2011.12.004] [PMID: 22197969]

Goldberg, SN, Kamel, IR, Kruskal, JB, Reynolds, K, Monsky, WL, Stuart, KE, Ahmed, M & Raptopoulos, V (2002) Radiofrequency ablation of hepatic tumors: increased tumor destruction with adjuvant liposomal doxorubicin therapy. *AJR Am J Roentgenol,* 179, 93-101. [http://dx.doi.org/10.2214/ajr.179.1.1790093] [PMID: 12076912]

Guaglianone, P, Chan, K, DelaFlor-Weiss, E, Hanisch, R, Jeffers, S, Sharma, D & Muggia, F (1994) Phase I and pharmacologic study of liposomal daunorubicin (DaunoXome). *Invest New Drugs,* 12, 103-10. [http://dx.doi.org/10.1007/BF00874439] [PMID: 7860226]

Guo, R, Huang, Z, Shu, Y, Jin, S & Ge, H (2009) Tamoxifen inhibits proliferation and induces apoptosis in human hepatocellular carcinoma cell line HepG2 *via* down-regulation of survivin expression. *Biomed Pharmacother,* 63, 375-9. [http://dx.doi.org/10.1016/j.biopha.2008.09.010] [PMID: 18993026]

Gurunathan, S, Park, JH, Han, JW & Kim, JH (2015) Comparative assessment of the apoptotic potential of silver nanoparticles synthesized by Bacillus tequilensis and Calocybe indica in MDA-MB-231 human breast cancer cells: targeting p53 for anticancer therapy. *Int J Nanomedicine,* 10, 4203-22. [http://dx.doi.org/10.2147/IJN.S83953] [PMID: 26170659]

Halm, U, Etzrodt, G, Schiefke, I, Schmidt, F, Witzigmann, H, Mössner, J & Berr, F (2000) A phase II study of pegylated liposomal doxorubicin for treatment of advanced hepatocellular carcinoma. *Ann Oncol,* 11, 113-4. [http://dx.doi.org/10.1023/A:1008386822906] [PMID: 10690399]

Hanahan, D & Weinberg, RA (2011) Hallmarks of cancer: the next generation. *Cell,* 144, 646-74. [http://dx.doi.org/10.1016/j.cell.2011.02.013] [PMID: 21376230]

Hann, IM & Prentice, HG (2001) Lipid-based amphotericin B: a review of the last 10 years of use. *Int J Antimicrob Agents,* 17, 161-9. [http://dx.doi.org/10.1016/S0924-8579(00)00341-1] [PMID: 11282260]

Harada, T, Matsumoto, S, Hirota, S, Kimura, H, Fujii, S, Kasahara, Y, Gon, H, Yoshida, T, Itoh, T, Haraguchi, N, Mizushima, T, Noda, T, Eguchi, H, Nojima, S, Morii, E, Fukumoto, T, Obika, S & Kikuchi, A (2019) Chemically Modified Antisense Oligonucleotide Against ARL4C Inhibits Primary and Metastatic Liver Tumor Growth. *Mol Cancer Ther,* 18, 602-12. [http://dx.doi.org/10.1158/1535-7163.MCT-18-0824] [PMID: 30647122]

He, Q, He, X, Deng, B, Shi, C, Lin, L, Liu, P, Yang, Z, Yang, S & Xu, Z (2018) Sorafenib and indocyanine green co-loaded in photothermally sensitive liposomes for diagnosis and treatment of advanced hepatocellular carcinoma. *J Mater Chem B Mater Biol Med,* 6, 5823-34. [http://dx.doi.org/10.1039/C8TB01641K] [PMID: 32254989]

Hong, RL & Tseng, YL (2003) A phase II and pharmacokinetic study of pegylated liposomal doxorubicin in patients with advanced hepatocellular carcinoma. *Cancer Chemother Pharmacol,* 51, 433-8. [http://dx.doi.org/10.1007/s00280-003-0583-2] [PMID: 12736762]

Horikoshi, S & Serpone, N *Microwaves in Nanoparticle Synthesis: Fundamentals and Applications.* Wiley-VCH Verlag GmbH & Co. [http://dx.doi.org/10.1002/9783527648122]

S hao, Hsu,, B, Yu,, X, Wang,, Y, Lu,, CR, Schmidt,, RJ, Lee,, LJ, Lee,, ST, Jacob, & K, Ghoshal, (2013) Cationic lipid nanoparticles for therapeutic delivery of siRNA and miRNA to murine liver tumor. *Nanomedicine: Nanotechnology, Biology and Medicine,* 9, 1169-80.

Huang, X & El-Sayed, MA (2010) Gold nanoparticles: Optical properties and implementations in cancer diagnosis and photothermal therapy. *J Adv Res,* 13-28.
[http://dx.doi.org/10.1016/j.jare.2010.02.002]

Husseini, GA & Pitt, WG (2008) Micelles and nanoparticles for ultrasonic drug and gene delivery. *Adv Drug Deliv Rev,* 60, 1137-52.
[http://dx.doi.org/10.1016/j.addr.2008.03.008] [PMID: 18486269]

Jeon, MJ, Gordon, AC, Larson, AC, Chung, JW, Kim, YI & Kim, DH (2016) Transcatheter intra-arterial infusion of doxorubicin loaded porous magnetic nano-clusters with iodinated oil for the treatment of liver cancer. *Biomaterials,* 88, 25-33.
[http://dx.doi.org/10.1016/j.biomaterials.2016.02.021] [PMID: 26938029]

Joshi, MD, Patravale, V & Prabhu, R (2015) Polymeric nanoparticles for targeted treatment in oncology: current insights. *International Journal of Nanomedicine,* 1001.
[PMID: 25678788]

Judge, AD, Robbins, M, Tavakoli, I, Levi, J, Hu, L, Fronda, A, Ambegia, E, McClintock, K & MacLachlan, I (2009) Confirming the RNAi-mediated mechanism of action of siRNA-based cancer therapeutics in mice. *J Clin Invest,* 119, 661-73.
[http://dx.doi.org/10.1172/JCI37515] [PMID: 19229107]

Kanehisa, M & Goto, S (2000) KEGG: kyoto encyclopedia of genes and genomes. *Nucleic Acids Res,* 28, 27-30.
[http://dx.doi.org/10.1093/nar/28.1.27] [PMID: 10592173]

Kelley, RK, Gane, E, Assenat, E, Siebler, J, Galle, PR, Merle, P, Hourmand, IO, Cleverly, A, Zhao, Y, Gueorguieva, I, Lahn, M, Faivre, S, Benhadji, KA & Giannelli, G (2019) A phase 2 study of galunisertib (TGF-b1 Receptor Type i Inhibitor) and sorafenib in patients with advanced hepatocellular carcinoma. *Clin Transl Gastroenterol,* 10, e00056.
[http://dx.doi.org/10.14309/ctg.0000000000000056] [PMID: 31295152]

Khan, FS, Ali, I, Afridi, UK, Ishtiaq, M & Mehmood, R (2017) Epigenetic mechanisms regulating the development of hepatocellular carcinoma and their promise for therapeutics. *Hepatol Int,* 11, 45-53.
[http://dx.doi.org/10.1007/s12072-016-9743-4] [PMID: 27271356]

Kim, Y, Jo, M, Schmidt, J, Luo, X, Prakash, TP, Zhou, T, Klein, S, Xiao, X, Post, N, Yin, Z & MacLeod, AR (2019) Enhanced Potency of GalNAc-Conjugated Antisense Oligonucleotides in Hepatocellular Cancer Models. *Mol Ther,* 27, 1547-57.
[http://dx.doi.org/10.1016/j.ymthe.2019.06.009] [PMID: 31303442]

Kratz, F (2008) Albumin as a drug carrier: design of prodrugs, drug conjugates and nanoparticles. *J Control Release,* 132, 171-83.
[http://dx.doi.org/10.1016/j.jconrel.2008.05.010] [PMID: 18582981]

Kudo, M (2018) Systemic therapy for hepatocellular carcinoma: Latest advances. *Cancers (Basel),* 10, 412.
[http://dx.doi.org/10.3390/cancers10110412] [PMID: 30380773]

Kudo, M (2019) Combination cancer immunotherapy with molecular targeted agents/Anti-CTLA-4 antibody for hepatocellular carcinoma. *Liver Cancer,* 8, 1-11.
[http://dx.doi.org/10.1159/000496277] [PMID: 30815391]

Kumar, M, Zhao, X & Wang, XW (2011) Molecular carcinogenesis of hepatocellular carcinoma and intrahepatic cholangiocarcinoma: one step closer to personalized medicine? *Cell Biosci,* 1, 5.
[http://dx.doi.org/10.1186/2045-3701-1-5] [PMID: 21711594]

Kumari, A, Yadav, SK & Yadav, SC (2010) Biodegradable polymeric nanoparticles based drug delivery systems. *Colloids Surf B Biointerfaces,* 75, 1-18.

[http://dx.doi.org/10.1016/j.colsurfb.2009.09.001] [PMID: 19782542]

Lafaro, KJ & Pawlik, TM (2015) Fibrolamellar hepatocellular carcinoma: current clinical perspectives. *J Hepatocell Carcinoma,* 2, 151-7.
[PMID: 27508204]

Lai, C-L, Wu, P-C, Chan, GC, Lok, AS & Lin, H-J (1988) Doxorubicin *versus* no antitumor therapy in inoperable hepatocellular carcinoma. A prospective randomized trial. *Cancer,* 62, 479-83.
[http://dx.doi.org/10.1002/1097-0142(19880801)62:3<479::AID-CNCR2820620306>3.0.CO;2-L] [PMID: 2839280]

Lee, HW, Cho, KJ & Park, JY (2020) Current status and future direction of immunotherapy in hepatocellular carcinoma: What do the data suggest? *Immune Netw,* 20, e11.
[http://dx.doi.org/10.4110/in.2020.20.e11] [PMID: 32158599]

Lee, JY, Lee, HT, Shin, W, Chae, J, Choi, J, Kim, SH, Lim, H, Won Heo, T, Park, KY, Lee, YJ, Ryu, SE, Son, JY, Lee, JU & Heo, YS (2016) Structural basis of checkpoint blockade by monoclonal antibodies in cancer immunotherapy. *Nat Commun,* 7, 13354.
[http://dx.doi.org/10.1038/ncomms13354] [PMID: 27796306]

Lee, SWL, Paoletti, C, Campisi, M, Osaki, T, Adriani, G, Kamm, RD, Mattu, C & Chiono, V (2019) MicroRNA delivery through nanoparticles. *J Control Release,* 313, 80-95.
[http://dx.doi.org/10.1016/j.jconrel.2019.10.007] [PMID: 31622695]

Li, Y, Wei, J, Wei, Y, Cheng, L, Guo, B, Meng, F, Li, F & Zhong, Z (2020) Apolipoprotein E Peptide-Guided Disulfide-Cross-Linked Micelles for Targeted Delivery of Sorafenib to Hepatocellular Carcinoma. *Biomacromolecules,* 21, 716-24.
[http://dx.doi.org/10.1021/acs.biomac.9b01419] [PMID: 31809037]

Lind, PA, Naucler, G, Holm, A, Gubanski, M & Svensson, C (2007) Efficacy of pegylated liposomal doxorubicin in patients with advanced hepatocellular carcinoma. *Acta Oncol,* 46, 230-3.
[http://dx.doi.org/10.1080/02841860600693473] [PMID: 17453374]

Liu, HL, Huo, L & Wang, L (2004) Octreotide inhibits proliferation and induces apoptosis of hepatocellular carcinoma cells. *Acta Pharmacol Sin,* 25, 1380-6.
[PMID: 15456543]

Liu, K, Tan, S, Chai, Y, Chen, D, Song, H, Zhang, CWH, Shi, Y, Liu, J, Tan, W, Lyu, J, Gao, S, Yan, J, Qi, J & Gao, GF (2017) Structural basis of anti-PD-L1 monoclonal antibody avelumab for tumor therapy. *Cell Res,* 27, 151-3.
[http://dx.doi.org/10.1038/cr.2016.102] [PMID: 27573173]

Lombardi, G, Zustovich, F, Farinati, F, Cillo, U, Vitale, A, Zanus, G, Donach, M, Farina, M, Zovato, S & Pastorelli, D (2011) Pegylated liposomal doxorubicin and gemcitabine in patients with advanced hepatocellular carcinoma: results of a phase 2 study. *Cancer,* 117, 125-33.
[http://dx.doi.org/10.1002/cncr.25578] [PMID: 21058409]

Longley, DB, Latif, T, Boyer, J, Allen, WL, Maxwell, PJ & Johnston, PG (2003) The interaction of thymidylate synthase expression with p53-regulated signaling pathways in tumor cells. *Semin Oncol,* 30 (Suppl. 6), 3-9.
[http://dx.doi.org/10.1016/S0093-7754(03)70019-0] [PMID: 12802789]

Luo, S, Xu, K, Xiang, S, Chen, J, Chen, C, Guo, C, Tong, Y & Tong, L (2018) High-resolution structures of inhibitor complexes of human indoleamine 2,3-dioxygenase 1 in a new crystal form. *Acta Crystallogr F Struct Biol Commun,* 74, 717-24.
[http://dx.doi.org/10.1107/S2053230X18012955] [PMID: 30387777]

Maeda, H (2001) The enhanced permeability and retention (EPR) effect in tumor vasculature: the key role of tumor-selective macromolecular drug targeting. *Adv Enzyme Regul,* 41, 189-207.
[http://dx.doi.org/10.1016/S0065-2571(00)00013-3] [PMID: 11384745]

Marin, JJG, Macias, RIR, Monte, MJ, Romero, MR, Asensio, M, Sanchez-Martin, A, Cives-Losada, C,

Temprano, AG, Espinosa-Escudero, R, Reviejo, M, Bohorquez, LH & Briz, O (2020) Molecular bases of drug resistance in hepatocellular carcinoma. *Cancers (Basel),* 12, 1-26.
[http://dx.doi.org/10.3390/cancers12061663] [PMID: 32585893]

Marrero, JA, Kudo, M & Bronowicki, JP (2010) The challenge of prognosis and staging for hepatocellular carcinoma. *Oncologist,* 15 (Suppl. 4), 23-33.
[http://dx.doi.org/10.1634/theoncologist.2010-S4-23] [PMID: 21115578]

Masood, F (2016) Polymeric nanoparticles for targeted drug delivery system for cancer therapy. *Mater Sci Eng C,* 60, 569-78.
[http://dx.doi.org/10.1016/j.msec.2015.11.067] [PMID: 26706565]

Matsuki, M, Hoshi, T, Yamamoto, Y, Ikemori-Kawada, M, Minoshima, Y, Funahashi, Y & Matsui, J (2018) Lenvatinib inhibits angiogenesis and tumor fibroblast growth factor signaling pathways in human hepatocellular carcinoma models. *Cancer Med,* 7, 2641-53.
[http://dx.doi.org/10.1002/cam4.1517] [PMID: 29733511]

McTigue, M, Murray, BW, Chen, JH, Deng, YL, Solowiej, J & Kania, RS (2012) Molecular conformations, interactions, and properties associated with drug efficiency and clinical performance among VEGFR TK inhibitors. *PNAS,* 109(45), 8281-9.
[http://dx.doi.org/10.1073/pnas.1207759109]

Merle, P, Camus, P, Abergel, A, Pageaux, GP, Masliah, C, Bronowicki, JP, Zarski, JP, Pelletier, G, Bouattour, M, Farloux, L, Dorval, E, Verset, G, Si-Ahmed, SN, Doffoel, M, Couzigou, P, Taieb, J, Vasseur, B & Attali, P (2017) Safety and efficacy of intra-arterial hepatic chemotherapy with doxorubicin-loaded nanoparticles in hepatocellular carcinoma. *ESMO Open,* 2, e000238.
[http://dx.doi.org/10.1136/esmoopen-2017-000238] [PMID: 29104762]

Merle, P, Blanc, JF, Phelip, JM, Pelletier, G, Bronowicki, JP, Touchefeu, Y, Pageaux, G, Gerolami, R, Habersetzer, F, Nguyen-Khac, E, Casadei-Gardini, A, Borbath, I, Tran, A, Wege, H, Saad, AS, Colombo, M, Abergel, A, Richou, C, Waked, I, Yee, NS, Molé, A, Attali, P, Le Boulicaut, J & Vasseur, B (2019) Doxorubicin-loaded nanoparticles for patients with advanced hepatocellular carcinoma after sorafenib treatment failure (RELIVE): a phase 3 randomised controlled trial. *Lancet Gastroenterol Hepatol,* 4, 454-65.
[http://dx.doi.org/10.1016/S2468-1253(19)30040-8] [PMID: 30954567]

Mishra, N, Yadav, NP, Rai, VK, Sinha, P, Yadav, KS, Jain, S & Arora, S (2013) Efficient hepatic delivery of drugs: Novel strategies and their significance *BioMed Research International,* 1-20.
[http://dx.doi.org/10.1155/2013/382184]

Moghimi, SM, Hunter, AC & Murray, JC (2001) Long-circulating and target-specific nanoparticles: theory to practice. *Pharmacol Rev,* 53, 283-318.
[PMID: 11356986]

Monajati, M, Tavakoli, S, Abolmaali, SS, Yousefi, G & Tamaddon, A (2018) Effect of PEGylation on assembly morphology and cellular uptake of poly ethyleneimine-cholesterol conjugates for delivery of sorafenib tosylate in hepatocellular carcinoma. *Bioimpacts,* 8, 241-52.
[http://dx.doi.org/10.15171/bi.2018.27] [PMID: 30397579]

Montgomery, RL, Hullinger, TG, Semus, HM, Dickinson, BA, Seto, AG, Lynch, JM, Stack, C, Latimer, PA, Olson, EN & van Rooij, E (2011) Therapeutic inhibition of miR-208a improves cardiac function and survival during heart failure. *Circulation,* 124, 1537-47.
[http://dx.doi.org/10.1161/CIRCULATIONAHA.111.030932] [PMID: 21900086]

Montironi, C, Montal, R & Llovet, JM (2019) New Drugs Effective in the Systemic Treatment of Hepatocellular Carcinoma. *Clin Liver Dis (Hoboken),* 14, 56-61.
[http://dx.doi.org/10.1002/cld.796] [PMID: 31508221]

Morse, MA, Sun, W, Kim, R, He, AR, Abada, PB, Mynderse, M & Finn, RS (2019) The role of angiogenesis in hepatocellular carcinoma. *Clin Cancer Res,* 25, 912-20.
[http://dx.doi.org/10.1158/1078-0432.CCR-18-1254] [PMID: 30274981]

Nair, AB, Shah, J, Al-Dhubiab, BE, Patel, SS, Morsy, MA, Patel, V, Chavda, V, Jacob, S, Sreeharsha, N,

Shinu, P, Attimarad, M & Venugopala, KN (2019) Development of asialoglycoprotein receptor-targeted nanoparticles for selective delivery of gemcitabine to hepatocellular carcinoma. *Molecules,* 24, 4566. [http://dx.doi.org/10.3390/molecules24244566] [PMID: 31847085]

Needham, D & Ponce, A (2006) Nanoscale Drug Delivery Vehicles for Solid Tumors: A New Paradigm for Localized Drug Delivery Using Temperature Sensitive Liposomes', Nanotechnology for Cancer Therapy. CRC Press 677-719.

Nugraha, B, Hong, X, Mo, X, Tan, L, Zhang, W, Chan, PM, Kang, CH, Wang, Y, Beng, LT, Sun, W, Choudhury, D, Robens, JM, McMillian, M, Silva, J, Dallas, S, Tan, CH, Yue, Z & Yu, H (2011) Galactosylated cellulosic sponge for multi-well drug safety testing. *Biomaterials,* 32, 6982-94. [http://dx.doi.org/10.1016/j.biomaterials.2011.05.087] [PMID: 21741702]

Okagawa, Y, Takada, K, Arihara, Y, Kikuchi, S, Osuga, T, Nakamura, H, Kamihara, Y, Hayasaka, N, Usami, M, Murase, K, Miyanishi, K, Kobune, M & Kato, J (2016) Activated p53 with histone deacetylase inhibitor enhances L-Fucose-mediated drug delivery through induction of fucosyltransferase 8 expression in hepatocellular carcinoma cells. *PLoS One,* 11, e0168355. [http://dx.doi.org/10.1371/journal.pone.0168355] [PMID: 27977808]

Okamoto, K, Ikemori-Kawada, M, Jestel, A, von König, K, Funahashi, Y, Matsushima, T, Tsuruoka, A, Inoue, A & Matsui, J (2014) Distinct binding mode of multikinase inhibitor lenvatinib revealed by biochemical characterization. *ACS Med Chem Lett,* 6, 89-94. [http://dx.doi.org/10.1021/ml500394m] [PMID: 25589937]

Okusaka, T & Ikeda, M (2018) Immunotherapy for hepatocellular carcinoma: current status and future perspectives. *ESMO Open,* 3 (Suppl. 1), e000455. [http://dx.doi.org/10.1136/esmoopen-2018-000455] [PMID: 30622744]

Pastorelli, D, Cartei, G, Zustovich, F, Marchese, F, Artioli, G, Zovato, S, Binato, S, Ceravolo, R, Cingarlini, S, Salmaso, F, Mattiazzi, M, Sanavio, C, Farinati, F, Zanus, G & Cillo, U (2006) Gemcitabine and liposomal doxorubicin in biliary and hepatic carcinoma (HCC) chemotherapy: preliminary results and review of the literature. *Ann Oncol,* 17 (Suppl. 5), v153-7. [http://dx.doi.org/10.1093/annonc/mdj972] [PMID: 16807446]

Pathak, P, Dhawan, V, Magarkar, A, Danne, R, Govindarajan, S, Ghosh, S, Steiniger, F, Chaudhari, P, Gopal, V, Bunker, A, Róg, T, Fahr, A & Nagarsenker, M (2016) Design of cholesterol arabinogalactan anchored liposomes for asialoglycoprotein receptor mediated targeting to hepatocellular carcinoma: *In silico* modeling, *in vitro* and *in vivo* evaluation. *Int J Pharm,* 509, 149-58. [http://dx.doi.org/10.1016/j.ijpharm.2016.05.041] [PMID: 27231122]

Pathil, A, Armeanu, S, Venturelli, S, Mascagni, P, Weiss, TS, Gregor, M, Lauer, UM & Bitzer, M (2006) HDAC inhibitor treatment of hepatoma cells induces both TRAIL-independent apoptosis and restoration of sensitivity to TRAIL. *Hepatology,* 43, 425-34. [http://dx.doi.org/10.1002/hep.21054] [PMID: 16583461]

Peluso, I, Yarla, NS, Ambra, R, Pastore, G & Perry, G (2019) MAPK signalling pathway in cancers: Olive products as cancer preventive and therapeutic agents. *Semin Cancer Biol,* 56, 185-95. [http://dx.doi.org/10.1016/j.semcancer.2017.09.002] [PMID: 28912082]

Pinter, M, Wichlas, M, Schmid, K, Plank, C, Müller, C, Wrba, F & Peck-Radosavljevic, M (2008) Thalidomide in advanced hepatocellular carcinoma as antiangiogenic treatment approach: a phase I/II trial. *Eur J Gastroenterol Hepatol,* 20, 1012-9. [http://dx.doi.org/10.1097/MEG.0b013e3283036740] [PMID: 18787470]

Poh, SB, Bai, LY & Chen, PM (2005) Pegylated liposomal doxorubicin-based combination chemotherapy as salvage treatment in patients with advanced hepatocellular carcinoma. *Am J Clin Oncol,* 28, 540-6. [http://dx.doi.org/10.1097/01.coc.0000177911.36579.3d] [PMID: 16317261]

Qin, S, Chan, SL, Sukeepaisarnjaroen, W, Han, G, Choo, SP, Sriuranpong, V, Pan, H, Yau, T, Guo, Y, Chen, M, Ren, Z, Xu, J, Yen, CJ, Lin, ZZ, Manenti, L, Gu, Y, Sun, Y, Tiedt, R, Hao, L, Song, W & Tanwandee, T (2019) A phase II study of the efficacy and safety of the MET inhibitor capmatinib (INC280) in patients with advanced hepatocellular carcinoma. *Ther Adv Med Oncol,* 11, 1758835919889001. [http://dx.doi.org/10.1177/1758835919889001] [PMID: 31853265]

Ramagopal, UA, Liu, W, Garrett-Thomson, SC, Bonanno, JB, Yan, Q, Srinivasan, M, Wong, SC, Bell, A, Mankikar, S, Rangan, VS, Deshpande, S, Korman, AJ & Almo, SC (2017) Structural basis for cancer immunotherapy by the first-in-class checkpoint inhibitor ipilimumab. *PNAS,* 114, E4223-32. [http://dx.doi.org/10.1073/pnas.1617941114]

Raoul, JL, Frenel, JS, Raimbourg, J & Gilabert, M (2019) Current options and future possibilities for the systemic treatment of hepatocellular carcinoma. *Hepat Oncol,* 6, HEP11. [http://dx.doi.org/10.2217/hep-2019-0001] [PMID: 31244990]

Salem, DS, Sliem, MA, El-Sesy, M, Shouman, SA & Badr, Y (2018) Improved chemo-photothermal therapy of hepatocellular carcinoma using chitosan-coated gold nanoparticles. *J Photochem Photobiol B,* 182, 92-9. [http://dx.doi.org/10.1016/j.jphotobiol.2018.03.024] [PMID: 29653312]

Santos-Carballal, B, Aaldering, LJ, Ritzefeld, M, Pereira, S, Sewald, N, Moerschbacher, BM, Götte, M & Goycoolea, FM (2015) Physicochemical and biological characterization of chitosan-microRNA nanocomplexes for gene delivery to MCF-7 breast cancer cells. *Sci Rep,* 5, 13567. [http://dx.doi.org/10.1038/srep13567] [PMID: 26324407]

Scapin, G, Yang, X, Prosise, WW, McCoy, M, Reichert, P, Johnston, JM, Kashi, RS & Strickland, C (2015) Structure of full-length human anti-PD1 therapeutic IgG4 antibody pembrolizumab. *Nat Struct Mol Biol,* 22, 953-8. [http://dx.doi.org/10.1038/nsmb.3129] [PMID: 26595420]

Shang, R, Song, X, Wang, P, Zhou, Y, Lu, X, Wang, J, Xu, M, Chen, X, Utpatel, K, Che, L, Liang, B, Cigliano, A, Evert, M, Calvisi, DF & Chen, X (2020) Cabozantinib-based combination therapy for the treatment of hepatocellular carcinoma. *Gut,* 1-12. [PMID: 33144318]

Shi, W, Hass, B, Kuss, MA, Zhang, H, Ryu, S, Zhang, D, Li, T, Li, YL & Duan, B (2020) Fabrication of versatile dynamic hyaluronic acid-based hydrogels. *Carbohydr Polym,* 233, 115803. [http://dx.doi.org/10.1016/j.carbpol.2019.115803] [PMID: 32059877]

Siracusano, G, Tagliamonte, M, Buonaguro, L & Lopalco, L (2020) Cell surface proteins in hepatocellular carcinoma: From bench to bedside. *Vaccines (Basel),* 8, 1-23. [http://dx.doi.org/10.3390/vaccines8010041] [PMID: 31991677]

Siveke, JT, Herberhold, C & Folwaczny, C (2003) Complete regression of advanced HCC with long acting octreotide. *Gut,* 52, 1531. [http://dx.doi.org/10.1136/gut.52.10.1531-a] [PMID: 12970151]

Sun, W, Wang, Y, Cai, M, Lin, L, Chen, X, Cao, Z, Zhu, K & Shuai, X (2017) Codelivery of sorafenib and GPC3 siRNA with PEI-modified liposomes for hepatoma therapy. *Biomater Sci,* 5, 2468-79. [http://dx.doi.org/10.1039/C7BM00866J] [PMID: 29106433]

Tak, WY, Lin, SM, Wang, Y, Zheng, J, Vecchione, A, Park, SY, Chen, MH, Wong, S, Xu, R, Peng, CY, Chiou, YY, Huang, GT, Cai, J, Abdullah, BJJ, Lee, JS, Lee, JY, Choi, JY, Gopez-Cervantes, J, Sherman, M, Finn, RS, Omata, M, O'Neal, M, Makris, L, Borys, N, Poon, R & Lencioni, R (2018) Phase III HEAT study adding lyso-thermosensitive liposomal doxorubicin to radiofrequency ablation in patients with unresectable hepatocellular carcinoma lesions. *Clin Cancer Res,* 24, 73-83. [http://dx.doi.org/10.1158/1078-0432.CCR-16-2433] [PMID: 29018051]

Tan, S, Liu, K, Chai, Y, Zhang, CWH, Gao, S, Gao, GF & Qi, J (2018) Distinct PD-L1 binding characteristics of therapeutic monoclonal antibody durvalumab. *Protein Cell,* 9, 135-9. [http://dx.doi.org/10.1007/s13238-017-0412-8] [PMID: 28488247]

Toh, HC, Chen, PJ, Carr, BI, Knox, JJ, Gill, S, Ansell, P, McKeegan, EM, Dowell, B, Pedersen, M, Qin, Q, Qian, J, Scappaticci, FA, Ricker, JL, Carlson, DM & Yong, WP (2013) Phase 2 trial of linifanib (ABT-869) in patients with unresectable or metastatic hepatocellular carcinoma. *Cancer,* 119, 380-7.

[http://dx.doi.org/10.1002/cncr.27758] [PMID: 22833179]

Tolcher, AW, Rodrigueza, WV, Rasco, DW, Patnaik, A, Papadopoulos, KP, Amaya, A, Moore, TD, Gaylor, SK, Bisgaier, CL, Sooch, MP, Woolliscroft, MJ & Messmann, RA (2014) A phase 1 study of the BCL2-targeted deoxyribonucleic acid inhibitor (DNAi) PNT2258 in patients with advanced solid tumors. *Cancer Chemother Pharmacol,* 73, 363-71.
[http://dx.doi.org/10.1007/s00280-013-2361-0] [PMID: 24297683]

Torchilin, V (2011) Tumor delivery of macromolecular drugs based on the EPR effect. *Adv Drug Deliv Rev,* 63, 131-5.
[http://dx.doi.org/10.1016/j.addr.2010.03.011] [PMID: 20304019]

Torchilin, VP (2007) Micellar nanocarriers: pharmaceutical perspectives. *Pharm Res,* 24, 1-16.
[http://dx.doi.org/10.1007/s11095-006-9132-0] [PMID: 17109211]

Tucker, JA, Klein, T, Breed, J, Breeze, AL, Overman, R, Phillips, C & Norman, RA (2014) Structural insights into FGFR kinase isoform selectivity: diverse binding modes of AZD4547 and ponatinib in complex with FGFR1 and FGFR4. *Structure (London, England : 1993),* 22, 1764-74.
[http://dx.doi.org/10.1016/j.str.2014.09.019]

Turkes, F & Chau, I (2019) Ramucirumab and its use in the treatment of hepatocellular carcinoma. *Future Oncol,* 15, 979-88.
[http://dx.doi.org/10.2217/fon-2018-0822] [PMID: 30644314]

Ul-Islam, S, Ahmed, MB, Shehzad, A, Ul-Islam, M & Lee, YS (2018) Failure of Chemotherapy in Hepatocellular Carcinoma Due to Impaired and Dysregulated Primary Liver Drug Metabolizing Enzymes and Drug Transport Proteins: What to Do? *Curr Drug Metab,* 19, 819-29.
[http://dx.doi.org/10.2174/1389200219666180529113818] [PMID: 29807513]

Umeda, S, Kanda, M & Kodera, Y (2018) Emerging evidence of molecular biomarkers in hepatocellular carcinoma. *Histol Histopathol,* 33, 343-55.
[PMID: 28959824]

Valle, JW, Dangoor, A, Beech, J, Sherlock, DJ, Lee, SM, Scarffe, JH, Swindell, R & Ranson, M (2005) Treatment of inoperable hepatocellular carcinoma with pegylated liposomal doxorubicin (PLD): results of a phase II study. *Br J Cancer,* 92, 628-30.
[http://dx.doi.org/10.1038/sj.bjc.6602394] [PMID: 15700038]

Varshosaz, J, Sadri, F, Rostami, M, Mirian, M & Taymouri, S (2019) Synthesis of pectin-deoxycholic acid conjugate for targeted delivery of anticancer drugs in hepatocellular carcinoma. *Int J Biol Macromol,* 139, 665-77.
[http://dx.doi.org/10.1016/j.ijbiomac.2019.07.225] [PMID: 31377298]

Varshosaz, J, Raghami, F, Rostami, M & Jahanian, A (2019) PEGylated trimethylchitosan emulsomes conjugated to octreotide for targeted delivery of sorafenib to hepatocellular carcinoma cells of HepG2. *J Liposome Res,* 29, 383-98.
[http://dx.doi.org/10.1080/08982104.2019.1570250] [PMID: 30668221]

Venook, AP, Egorin, MJ, Rosner, GL, Hollis, D, Mani, S, Hawkins, M, Byrd, J, Hohl, R, Budman, D, Meropol, NJ & Ratain, MJ (2000) Phase I and pharmacokinetic trial of gemcitabine in patients with hepatic or renal dysfunction: Cancer and Leukemia Group B 9565. *J Clin Oncol,* 18, 2780-7.
[http://dx.doi.org/10.1200/JCO.2000.18.14.2780] [PMID: 10894879]

Voutila, J, Reebye, V, Roberts, TC, Protopapa, P, Andrikakou, P, Blakey, DC, Habib, R, Huber, H, Saetrom, P, Rossi, JJ & Habib, NA (2017) Development and mechanism of small activating RNA targeting CEBPA, a novel therapeutic in clinical trials for liver cancer. *Mol Ther,* 25, 2705-14.
[http://dx.doi.org/10.1016/j.ymthe.2017.07.018] [PMID: 28882451]

Wang-Gillam, A, Thakkar, N, Lockhart, AC, Williams, K, Baggstrom, M, Naughton, M, Suresh, R, Ma, C, Tan, B, Lee, W, Jiang, X, Mwandoro, T, Trull, L, Belanger, S, Creekmore, AN, Gao, F, Fracasso, PM & Picus, J (2014) A phase I study of pegylated liposomal doxorubicin and temsirolimus in patients with refractory solid malignancies. *Cancer Chemother Pharmacol,* 74, 419-26.

[http://dx.doi.org/10.1007/s00280-014-2493-x] [PMID: 24916546]

Wang, L, Su, W, Liu, Z, Zhou, M, Chen, S, Chen, Y, Lu, D, Liu, Y, Fan, Y, Zheng, Y, Han, Z, Kong, D, Wu, JC, Xiang, R & Li, Z (2012) CD44 antibody-targeted liposomal nanoparticles for molecular imaging and therapy of hepatocellular carcinoma. *Biomaterials,* 33, 5107-14.
[http://dx.doi.org/10.1016/j.biomaterials.2012.03.067] [PMID: 22494888]

Wang, N, Zhu, M, Tsao, SW, Man, K, Zhang, Z & Feng, Y (2013) MiR-23a-mediated inhibition of topoisomerase 1 expression potentiates cell response to etoposide in human hepatocellular carcinoma. *Mol Cancer,* 12, 119.
[http://dx.doi.org/10.1186/1476-4598-12-119] [PMID: 24103454]

Wassermann, K, Markovits, J, Jaxel, C, Capranico, G, Kohn, KW & Pommier, Y (1990) Effects of morpholinyl doxorubicins, doxorubicin, and actinomycin D on mammalian DNA topoisomerases I and II. *Mol Pharmacol,* 38, 38-45.
[PMID: 2164630]

Weekes, CD, Clark, JW & Zhu, AX (2018) Tivantinib for advanced hepatocellular carcinoma: is MET still a viable target? *Lancet Oncol,* 19, 591-2.
[http://dx.doi.org/10.1016/S1470-2045(18)30249-3] [PMID: 29625880]

Wilhelm, S, Carter, C, Lynch, M, Lowinger, T, Dumas, J, Smith, RA, Schwartz, B, Simantov, R & Kelley, S (2006) Discovery and development of sorafenib: a multikinase inhibitor for treating cancer. *Nat Rev Drug Discov,* 5, 835-44.
[http://dx.doi.org/10.1038/nrd2130] [PMID: 17016424]

Wilhelm, SM, Adnane, L, Newell, P, Villanueva, A, Llovet, JM & Lynch, M (2008) Preclinical overview of sorafenib, a multikinase inhibitor that targets both Raf and VEGF and PDGF receptor tyrosine kinase signaling. *Mol Cancer Ther,* 7, 3129-40.
[http://dx.doi.org/10.1158/1535-7163.MCT-08-0013] [PMID: 18852116]

Xiao, K, Li, Y, Luo, J, Lee, JS, Xiao, W, Gonik, AM, Agarwal, RG & Lam, KS (2011) The effect of surface charge on *in vivo* biodistribution of PEG-oligocholic acid based micellar nanoparticles. *Biomaterials,* 32, 3435-46.
[http://dx.doi.org/10.1016/j.biomaterials.2011.01.021] [PMID: 21295849]

Xiao, Y, Liu, Y, Yang, S, Zhang, B, Wang, T, Jiang, D, Zhang, J, Yu, D & Zhang, N (2016) Sorafenib and gadolinium co-loaded liposomes for drug delivery and MRI-guided HCC treatment. *Colloids Surf B Biointerfaces,* 141, 83-92.
[http://dx.doi.org/10.1016/j.colsurfb.2016.01.016] [PMID: 26844644]

Xie, B, Ding, Q, Han, H & Wu, D (2013) miRCancer: a microRNA-cancer association database constructed by text mining on literature. *Bioinformatics,* 29, 638-44.
[http://dx.doi.org/10.1093/bioinformatics/btt014] [PMID: 23325619]

Xie, Y, Murray-Stewart, T, Wang, Y, Yu, F, Li, J, Marton, LJ, Casero, RA, Jr & Oupický, D (2017) Self-immolative nanoparticles for simultaneous delivery of microRNA and targeting of polyamine metabolism in combination cancer therapy. *J Control Release,* 246, 110-9.
[http://dx.doi.org/10.1016/j.jconrel.2016.12.017] [PMID: 28017891]

Xu, F, Liao, JZ, Xiang, GY, Zhao, PX, Ye, F, Zhao, Q & He, XX (2017) MiR-101 and doxorubicin codelivered by liposomes suppressing malignant properties of hepatocellular carcinoma. *Cancer Med,* 6, 651-61.
[http://dx.doi.org/10.1002/cam4.1016] [PMID: 28135055]

Yamada, M, O'Regan, E, Brown, R & Karran, P (1997) Selective recognition of a cisplatin-DNA adduct by human mismatch repair proteins. *Nucleic Acids Res,* 25, 491-6.
[http://dx.doi.org/10.1093/nar/25.3.491] [PMID: 9016586]

Yang, R, Meng, F, Ma, S, Huang, F, Liu, H & Zhong, Z (2011) Galactose-decorated cross-linked biodegradable poly(ethylene glycol)-b-poly(ε-caprolactone) block copolymer micelles for enhanced hepatoma-targeting delivery of paclitaxel. *Biomacromolecules,* 12, 3047-55.

[http://dx.doi.org/10.1021/bm2006856] [PMID: 21726090]

Yang, T, Zhao, P, Rong, Z, Li, B, Xue, H, You, J, He, C, Li, W, He, X, Lee, RJ, Ma, X & Xiang, G (2016) Anti-tumor efficiency of lipid-coated cisplatin nanoparticles co-loaded with microRNA-375. *Theranostics,* 6, 142-54.
[http://dx.doi.org/10.7150/thno.13130] [PMID: 26722380]

Yang, W, Lee, JC, Chen, MH, Zhang, ZY, Bai, XM, Yin, SS, Cao, K, Wang, S, Wu, W & Yan, K (2019) Thermosensitive liposomal doxorubicin plus radiofrequency ablation increased tumor destruction and improved survival in patients with medium and large hepatocellular carcinoma: A randomized, double-blinded, dummy-controlled clinical trial in a single center. *J Cancer Res Ther,* 15, 773-83.
[http://dx.doi.org/10.4103/jcrt.JCRT_801_18] [PMID: 31436231]

Yao, Y, Wang, T, Liu, Y & Zhang, N (2019) Co-delivery of sorafenib and VEGF-siRNA *via* pH-sensitive liposomes for the synergistic treatment of hepatocellular carcinoma. *Artif Cells Nanomed Biotechnol,* 47, 1374-83.
[http://dx.doi.org/10.1080/21691401.2019.1596943] [PMID: 30977418]

Yeo, W, Chan, KK, Mukwaya, G, Ross, M, Leung, WT, Ho, S, Chan, ATC & Johnson, PJ (1999) Phase II studies with DaunoXome in patients with nonresectable hepatocellular carcinoma: clinical and pharmacokinetic outcomes. *Cancer Chemother Pharmacol,* 44, 124-30.
[http://dx.doi.org/10.1007/s002800050956] [PMID: 10412946]

Yeo, W, Chung, HC, Chan, SL, Wang, LZ, Lim, R, Picus, J, Boyer, M, Mo, FKF, Koh, J, Rha, SY, Hui, EP, Jeung, HC, Roh, JK, Yu, SCH, To, KF, Tao, Q, Ma, BB, Chan, AWH, Tong, JHM, Erlichman, C, Chan, AT & Goh, BC (2012) Epigenetic therapy using belinostat for patients with unresectable hepatocellular carcinoma: a multicenter phase I/II study with biomarker and pharmacokinetic analysis of tumors from patients in the Mayo Phase II Consortium and the Cancer Therapeutics Research Group. *J Clin Oncol,* 30, 3361-7.
[http://dx.doi.org/10.1200/JCO.2011.41.2395] [PMID: 22915658]

Yin, X, Xiao, Y, Han, L, Zhang, B, Wang, T, Su, Z & Zhang, N (2018) Ceramide-Fabricated Co-Loaded Liposomes for the Synergistic Treatment of Hepatocellular Carcinoma. *AAPS PharmSciTech,* 19, 2133-43.
[http://dx.doi.org/10.1208/s12249-018-1005-4] [PMID: 29714002]

Yue, Z, Wen, F, Gao, S, Ang, MY, Pallathadka, PK, Liu, L & Yu, H (2010) Preparation of three-dimensional interconnected macroporous cellulosic hydrogels for soft tissue engineering. *Biomaterials,* 31, 8141-52.
[http://dx.doi.org/10.1016/j.biomaterials.2010.07.059] [PMID: 20691470]

Zhang, F, Qi, X, Wang, X, Wei, D, Wu, J, Feng, L, Cai, H, Wang, Y, Zeng, N, Xu, T, Zhou, A & Zheng, Y (2017) Structural basis of the therapeutic anti-PD-L1 antibody atezolizumab. *Oncotarget,* 8, 90215-24.
[http://dx.doi.org/10.18632/oncotarget.21652] [PMID: 29163822]

Zhang, HT, Sun, J, Yan, Y, Cui, SH, Wang, H, Wang, CH, Qiu, C, Chen, X, Ding, JS, Qian, HG, Wang, JC & Zhang, Q (2019) Encapsulated microRNA by gemcitabine prodrug for cancer treatment. *J Control Release,* 316, 317-30.
[http://dx.doi.org/10.1016/j.jconrel.2019.11.010] [PMID: 31733293]

Zhang, W, Peng, F, Zhou, T, Huang, Y, Zhang, L, Ye, P, Lu, M, Yang, G, Gai, Y, Yang, T, Ma, X & Xiang, G (2015) Targeted delivery of chemically modified anti-miR-221 to hepatocellular carcinoma with negatively charged liposomes. *Int J Nanomedicine,* 10, 4825-36.
[PMID: 26251599]

Zhang, X, Guo, S, Fan, R, Yu, M, Li, F, Zhu, C & Gan, Y (2012) Dual-functional liposome for tumor targeting and overcoming multidrug resistance in hepatocellular carcinoma cells. *Biomaterials,* 33, 7103-14.
[http://dx.doi.org/10.1016/j.biomaterials.2012.06.048] [PMID: 22796159]

Zhao, S, Zhang, T, Dou, W, Wang, E, Wang, M, Wang, C, Du, X & Liu, L (2020) A comparison of transcatheter arterial chemoembolization used with and without apatinib for intermediate- to advanced-stage hepatocellular carcinoma: a systematic review and meta-analysis. *Ann Transl Med,* 8, 542-2.
[http://dx.doi.org/10.21037/atm.2020.02.125] [PMID: 32411765]

Zhao, X, Chen, Q, Li, Y, Tang, H, Liu, W & Yang, X (2015) Doxorubicin and curcumin co-delivery by lipid nanoparticles for enhanced treatment of diethylnitrosamine-induced hepatocellular carcinoma in mice. *Eur J Pharm Biopharm,* 93, 27-36.
[http://dx.doi.org/10.1016/j.ejpb.2015.03.003] [PMID: 25770771]

Zhao, X, Liu, X, Zhang, P, Liu, Y, Ran, W, Cai, Y, Wang, J, Zhai, Y, Wang, G, Ding, Y & Li, Y (2019) Injectable peptide hydrogel as intraperitoneal triptolide depot for the treatment of orthotopic hepatocellular carcinoma. *Acta Pharm Sin B,* 9, 1050-60.
[http://dx.doi.org/10.1016/j.apsb.2019.06.001] [PMID: 31649853]

Zheng, G, Zhao, R, Xu, A, Shen, Z, Chen, X & Shao, J (2018) Co-delivery of sorafenib and siVEGF based on mesoporous silica nanoparticles for ASGPR mediated targeted HCC therapy. *Eur J Pharm Sci,* 111, 492-502.
[http://dx.doi.org/10.1016/j.ejps.2017.10.036] [PMID: 29107835]

Zheng, L, Li, C, Huang, X, Lin, X, Lin, W, Yang, F & Chen, T (2019) Thermosensitive hydrogels for sustained-release of sorafenib and selenium nanoparticles for localized synergistic chemoradiotherapy. *Biomaterials,* 216, 119220.
[http://dx.doi.org/10.1016/j.biomaterials.2019.05.031] [PMID: 31200144]

Zhou, F, Shang, W, Yu, X & Tian, J (2018) Glypican-3: A promising biomarker for hepatocellular carcinoma diagnosis and treatment. *Med Res Rev,* 38, 741-67.
[http://dx.doi.org/10.1002/med.21455] [PMID: 28621802]

Zhou, Q, Sun, X, Zeng, L, Liu, J & Zhang, Z (2009) A randomized multicenter phase II clinical trial of mitoxantrone-loaded nanoparticles in the treatment of 108 patients with unresected hepatocellular carcinoma. *Nanomedicine,* 5, 419-23.
[http://dx.doi.org/10.1016/j.nano.2009.01.009] [PMID: 19523421]

Zhou, Q, Ching, AKK, Leung, WKC, Szeto, CYY, Ho, SM, Chan, PKS, Yuan, YF, Lai, PBS, Yeo, W & Wong, N (2011) Novel therapeutic potential in targeting microtubules by nanoparticle albumin-bound paclitaxel in hepatocellular carcinoma. *Int J Oncol,* 38, 721-31.
[PMID: 21240457]

Zhu, AX, Finn, RS, Edeline, J, Cattan, S, Ogasawara, S, Palmer, D, Verslype, C, Zagonel, V, Fartoux, L, Vogel, A, Sarker, D, Verset, G, Chan, SL, Knox, J, Daniele, B, Webber, AL, Ebbinghaus, SW, Ma, J, Siegel, AB, Cheng, AL & Kudo, M (2018) Pembrolizumab in patients with advanced hepatocellular carcinoma previously treated with sorafenib (KEYNOTE-224): a non-randomised, open-label phase 2 trial. *Lancet Oncol,* 19, 940-52.
[http://dx.doi.org/10.1016/S1470-2045(18)30351-6] [PMID: 29875066]

CHAPTER 5

Nanotherapeutics for the Treatment of Hepatocellular Carcinoma

Kishor Mazumder[1,2,3,4,*], **Md. Emran Hossain**[2] and **Asma Aktar**[2]

[1] *School of Biomedical Sciences, Charles Sturt University, Wagga Wagga, NSW 2650, Australia*

[2] *Department of Pharmacy, Jashore University of Science and Technology, Jashore-7408, Bangladesh*

[3] *School of Optometry and Vision Science, UNSW Medicine*

[4] *University of New South Wales (UNSW), Sydney, NSW, Australia*

Abstract: Currently, hepatocellular carcinoma (HCC) is the third leading cause of mortality among cancerous diseases. It is a primary type of liver cancer possessing unique features like solid malignant tumor type growth, leaky vasculature, and angiogenesis. The success of conventional treatment in the management of HCC is constrained due to unresponsiveness to particular approaches, drug resistance, systemic side effects, and recurrence of malignancy. The development of nanotherapeutics offers an impending key for overcoming these challenges. Nanotherapeutics utilizes nanosized or nanostructured materials to attain particular therapeutic and pharmacokinetic purposes. The diverse targeting strategies and site-specific drug release patterns of this approach enlighten the hope for effective management of HCC. Scientists have developed several nanomaterials like nanoparticles, nanogel, and liposomes to deliver chemotherapeutic agents specifically to HCC sites with improved efficacy, safety, and selectivity. Active targeting has remained most common and effective in HCC management among active, passive, and stimuli-responsive targeting strategies. Hopefully, some nanoformulations for HCC treatment have proved their promising effects in clinical trials. In this chapter, an attempt is made to illustrate the overview of HCC, the impact of nanotherapeutics, along with recent developments, suitability, and challenges of various nanotherapeutic approaches for HCC management.

Keywords: Chemotherapy, Hepatocellular carcinoma, Nanomedicine, Nano-particles, Primary cancer, Nanotheranostic, Selectivity, Targeting.

* **Corresponding author Kishor Mazumder:** School of Biomedical Sciences, Charles Sturt University, Wagga Wagga, NSW 2650, Australia and Department of Pharmacy, Jashore University of Science and Technology, Jashore-7408, Bangladesh; E-mails: kmazumder@csu.edu.au, k.mazumder@unsw.edu.au and kmazumder@just.edu.bd

Biswajit Mukherjee (Ed.)

INTRODUCTION

Hepatocellular carcinoma (HCC), the most predominant form of liver cancer, is recognized as the 5th common cancer and the third leading cause of mortality among all neoplastic diseases worldwide. It is a primary malignant tumor that occurs as a result of oncogenesis in hepatocytes triggered by multiple risk factors, involving hepatitis B and C viral infections, non-alcoholic fatty liver disease, metabolic syndrome triggered steatohepatitis, chronic smoking, and consumptions of alcohol, aflatoxin B_1 and anabolic steroids (Elnaggar *et al.*, 2019).

Several methods, including resection, radiation therapy, thermal ablation, and chemotherapy, are developed for HCC treatment. Yet, the success of the recovery is still a challenge for healthcare professionals as well as patients. Choosing a suitable treatment method for a patient is not easy because of the need to consider the stage of HCC, the magnitude of hepatic damage, the short survival period of patients (usually 1-3 months), and treatment costs. Surgical resection and chemotherapy are the most adopted techniques that have been effective for optimal recovery. Due to the high price, metastatic stage of HCC, and poor liver functionality, more than 80% of patients are unresponsive to surgery. Moreover, the chemotherapeutic agent lacks selectivity and sensitivity to HCC. Thus, it is associated with poor efficacy as well as undesirable toxicities, multidrug resistance, recurrence, and therapeutic failures (Chi *et al.*, 2020).

Cancer nanotherapeutics have been achieving enormous popularity in drug delivery and diagnosis of specific cancerous organs and tissues. This approach allows the delivery of nanostructured or nanosized materials with specific therapeutic and/or targeting purposes to achieve promising objectives, including controlling drug release, enhancing drug stability, accumulating drugs at a specific site, imaging, *etc.* In addition, chemotherapeutic drugs (chemotherapy), DNA or RNA (gene therapy), heat-generating drugs (thermotherapy), radioactive isotopes (radiotherapy), diagnostic chemicals (diagnosis), *etc.*, can be delivered successfully to the cancerous region (Wagner *et al.*, 2006). Nanotherapeutics offer an emerging scope for managing HCC because of its salient features that may cause acidosis or decreased pH, hypoxia or lack of oxygen, lack of nutrition, and leaky vasculature within the solid tumorous mass (Chi *et al.*, 2020). Consequently, scientists have addressed numerous nanotherapeutic approaches aiming at HCC management with promising outcomes in experimental, preclinical, and clinical stages of research.

In this chapter, a substantial overview of nanotherapeutics for effective management of HCC has been discussed with the perspective of associated challenges, recent developmental strategies, and future recommendations.

HEPATOCELLULAR CARCINOMA: AN OVERVIEW

HCC is the deadliest and most predominant (about 80-85%) (Elnaggar *et al.*, 2019). It is unique and clinically characterized as the primary malignancy of liver cells, which results from a series of genetic and/or epigenetic alterations leading to trigger initiation of oncogenesis. Multiple symptoms are observed in HCC patients, such as upper right abdominal pain, hepatomegaly, splenomegaly, swelling and bloating in the stomach, anorexia, pale yellowish color of skin, urine, and eyes (jaundice like symptoms), *etc.* The common risk factors for the progression of this disease include chronic hepatic inflammations due to viral hepatitis, parasitic infection in the liver, metabolic syndrome triggered steatohepatitis, fatty liver disease, chronic smoking, and consumptions of alcohol, and several chemicals (aflatoxin B_1, diethylnitrosamine, and anabolic steroids, carbon-tetrachloride and thioacetamide). Besides, obesity, diabetes, age, gender, and lifestyle also influence the progression of the disease. Among these risk factors, hepatitis B infection has been found to progress HCC in 50% of patients (Usmani and Mishra, 2017).

Pathogenesis of HCC and Molecular Targets

Several molecular events, such as lack of sensitivity to anti-growth factors, overexpression of growth factors and specific receptors, angiogenesis, invasion, and metastasis, are the collective outcomes of genetic mutation, amplifications, and deletions, as well as deactivation of genetic material, arises in the progression of HCC (Usmani *et al.*, 2018). These molecular alterations vary in the HCC stage and etiology. Accountable functional molecules of these pathogenic pathways would be promising targets for developing treatment strategies of HCC.

Considerable alteration of specific tumor suppressor genes is observed predominantly in the pathogenesis of HCC, particularly in an advanced stage, for example, p53 and retinoblastoma. Besides, signal transduction pathways are altered in this disease resulting in the initiation of oncogenesis in hepatocytes. Tyrosine kinase pathway has been observed as the most prominent pathway that comprises RAS/RAF/MEK/ERK, PI_3K/Akt/mTOR, and NF-kB (nuclear factor-kappa B). RAF is a kinase protein responsible for the hepatocellular proliferation, angiogenesis, and apoptosis. Thus, targeting RAF can be an effective strategy to treat HCC. Another signal transduction pathway, namely the WNT/b-catenin pathway, is also altered in this disease, making cancer highly resistant and nonresponsive to conventional therapies. Moreover, there is an overexpression of growth factors like VEGF (vascular endothelial growth factor) and PDGFRβ (platelet-derived growth factor receptor beta) on cell surface resulting angiogenesis by mediating enhancement of vascular permeability (Elnaggar *et al.*,

2019). Hence, these growth factors might be considered promising molecular targets for resisting the angiogenesis of HCC.

However, the expression of surface receptors and proteins in hepatocytes are also altered during the progression of HCC (Elnaggar *et al.*, 2019). For example, (a) malignant hepatocytes overexpress asialoglycoprotein receptor (ASGPR), IgA-receptor, transferrin receptor, and insulin receptors; (b) hepatic stellate cells overexpress mannose-6-phosphate/insulin growth factor II receptor, ferritin receptor, plasminogen receptor, α_2 macroglobulin receptor, and thrombin receptor; (c) endothelial cells overexpress mannose/N-acetyl glucosamine receptor, Fc receptor immune complexes, and hyaluronan fibronectin; and (d) cancerous Kupffer cells overexpress galactose particle receptor, galactose specific receptor, fibronectin, Fc receptor, complement receptor, and macroglobulin receptors.

Current Treatment Approaches for HCC

Numerous treatment options involving radiation therapy, resection or surgery, thermal ablation, and chemotherapy have been developed for HCC. The selection of a suitable approach for HCC treatment is a challenging task for health care professionals. Stages of HCC, the magnitude of liver damage, patient's financial conditions, responsiveness, *etc.*, play a considerable role in choosing appropriate treatment strategies. Resection or surgery is known as the most effective technique for HCC treatment, but hepatic decompensation is observed in this case. The patients with tolerable reimbursed cirrhosis are considered for surgery only when they comply score 'A' in Child-Pugh class (Ascites and encephalopathy: absent; bilirubin: <2.0 mg/dL; albumin: >3.5 g/dL; and prothrombin time: 1-3 s). Besides, the risk of this cancer recurrence is higher after resection. Liver transplantation is a suitable strategy for hepatic decompensated patients who match the Milan criteria: the presence of either one lesion of not less than 5 cm or three lesions of not less than 3 cm each. Besides, it offers a low rate of recurrence in patients with a reasonable survival rate. Radiotherapy is suitable for patients with the intermediate stage of HCC. In this approach, radioactive nanocarriers and drug conjugates are administered directly into the blood vessels formed by angiogenesis with the intention of treating the cancerous lumps. Trans-hepatic artery chemoembolization is the approach of delivering chemotherapeutics in the form of a suspension in iodized oil *via* the hepatic artery. It is selected along with a combination of other therapy for patients unable to respond to curative treatments. This approach is associated with post-embolization syndrome in most cases. Furthermore, hepatic artery injury, biliary tract damage, and variceal hemorrhage are also found, which may lead to acute liver decompensation (Elnaggar *et al.*, 2019).

Barriers for Management of HCC

Molecular environments and salient features of HCC make HCC unique. Several treatment options are available to combat this malignancy, yet desirable effects are out of the reach for scientists. Following challenges need to be addressed for a practical treatment approach:

i. Lack of selectivity of the malignant tumor

ii. Poor specificity and sensitivity of the malignant cells to the drug molecules

iii. Undesirable adverse effects

iv. Poor bioavailability of chemotherapeutic drugs

v. Recurrence of the hepatic malignancy

Most of the therapeutic agents in the market are unable to overcome all of these barriers. Such a novel approach capable of overcoming these barriers is a search of the present era. Fortunately, HCC cells possess special features enlisted below, which can help design a novel delivery system.

a. Leaky vasculature and higher permeability

b. Accumulation of substances having affinity to the specific biochemical of cancer cells

c. Specific criteria of microenvironments (that may function as stimuli of the drug delivery system, such as hypoxia, lower pH, presence of particular enzyme or biochemical, *etc.*).

NANOTHERAPEUTICS: A NOVEL APPROACH

Particles with a size range of 1 to 100 nanometers are considered nanoparticles (Pal *et al.*, 2011). Nanotechnology is the art and science of formulating nanoparticles and applying them for various purposes. It is the ability to work at atomic, molecular, or supra-molecular levels to understand, create, and utilize materials or devices to improve their performance because of their small structure. The significant advantages of the physical and chemical properties of these nanoparticles arise from their decreased size, which causes an increase in the surface area leading to more dominant quantum effects, surface properties, and large surface area to volume ratio. It is a powerful tool for creating 'smart' materials, but the method is challenging, and perfection is still far from being achieved.

Nanotechnology involves novel drug delivery in the treatment of life-threatening diseases like cancer. The growth of nanotechnology has paved the way for different new vistas in medical science, particularly in the drug delivery system. As the novel drug discovery process becomes enriched with each passing year, newer moieties are being discovered for treating disease. However, biotechnology has given us several more recent and more potent drugs, many of them encounter the common problem of poor delivery in the physiological system. The efficiency of drug therapy is significantly halted because of their side effects in the biological system owing to their specific chemical structure. Nanotechnology can substantially increase site-specific delivery and achieve real progress in the fields of drug targeting. However, the pharmaceutical industry faces various challenges, including low bioavailability, low solubility of drugs, instability, adverse effects, non-targeted delivery, low therapeutic outcome, inconsistent plasma drug concentration, and frequent dosing by developing nanotechnology-based therapeutics. The prospect of a nanotechnology-based drug delivery system has the potential to overcome these hurdles along the way.

Method of Preparing Nanoparticles

In a nanoparticulate system, drug(s) to deliver can be dissolved, encapsulated, or entrapped into the matrix based on the method of preparation. The success of nanoparticle formulation relies solely on some of the major considerations, such as average size and size distribution, physicochemical properties, surface morphology, compatibility with a biological system, biodegradability and toxicity, release kinetics of the active drugs from the nanoparticulate system, response of body's immune system to the nanoparticle matrix, *etc.* Various methods have been developed for preparing nanoparticles. The most common methods work with a dispersion of preformed polymer/polymerization of monomers/ionic gelation or coacervation of hydrophilic polymers and salting out.

Dispersion of preformed polymers is the most common method for preparing nanoparticles, especially for biodegradable nanoparticles. Polylactic acid (PLA), poly D,L-glycolide (PLG), ploy D,L-lactide-co-glycolide (PLGA), and ploy cyanoacrylate (PCA) are the most common biodegradable polymers used in this method (Ueda and Kreuter, 1997). This method (Fig. **1 A**) is performed by solvent evaporation and solvent diffusion techniques. In solvent evaporation technique, the hydrophobic polymers (as a matrix) and the active ingredients are dissolved in a suitable organic solvent (acetone, n-hexane, chloroform, ethyl acetate) followed by adding drop by drop to the aqueous solution under continuous stirring. It leads to the formation of oil in water (O/W) emulsion, stabilized by a suitable emulsifying agent stabilizer. The emulsion is then homogenized, and the organic solvent is removed to obtain nanoparticles. The concentration of the organic and aqueous solution, type and concentration of the emulsifying agent used, and homogenizing speed determine the size distribution of the synthesized nanoparticles. Increased homogenizing speed and ultrasonication can be performed to obtain smaller particles. Solvent diffusion or spontaneous emulsification method is a modified version of solvent evaporation method where a water-miscible solvent and a small amount of water-immiscible nonpolar solvent are used. In this technique, nanoparticles are formed by turbulence generation at the interphase between the two phases by spontaneous solvent transfer from one phase to another (Vandervoort and Ludwig, 2002).

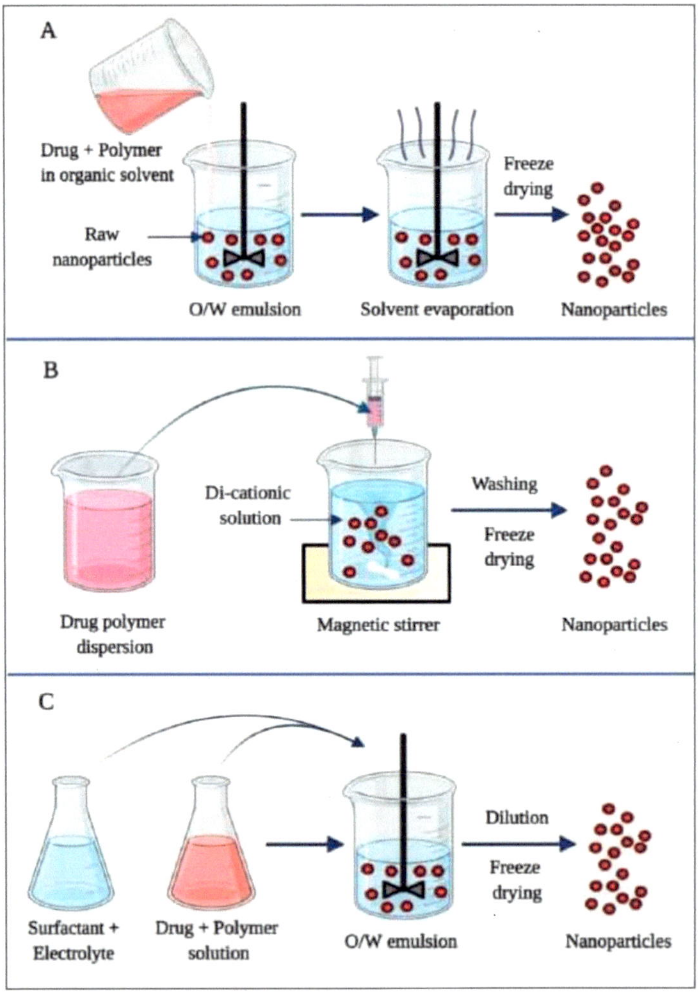

Fig. (1). Most typical methods of preparing nanoparticles; A, B, and C represent dispersion, ionic gelation, and salting-out methods, respectively.

In the polymerization method, nanoparticles are formed during the polymerization process. The active ingredients are incorporated into the nanoparticles either by adsorption of the drug on the surface of the polymeric particle or the addition of the drug in the reaction medium followed by subsequent entrapment into the cross-linked polymer. After the formation of the nanoparticle, they are separated by ultracentrifugation. Separated particles are then resuspended into an isotonic solution in order to remove the surfactant and other reagents used for the polymerization process (Yordanov, 2012). The size of the nanoparticles is dependent on the nature and amount of surfactant and other stabilizing agents. This method is suitable for preparing poly butyl cyanoacrylate and other poly alkyl cyanoacrylate nanoparticles.

The ionic gelation method has been developed to manufacture nanoparticles utilizing biodegradable hydrophilic polymeric compounds such as gelatin, chitosan, sodium alginate, *etc.* In this method (Fig. **1 B**), a biodegradable hydrophilic polymeric compound is solubilized into a diblock copolymer (for example, ethylene oxide or propylene oxide) and reacted to polyanion sodium triphosphate solution containing a positively charged amino group and negatively charged triphosphate. These two opposite charged moieties interact and convert from liquid to gel form at normal temperature, leading to the nanosized coacervate formation (Pedroso-Santana and Fleitas-Salazar, 2020).

Salting out is a process that is based on solubility-mediated separation of the distinct compound. In this method (Fig. **1 C**), the active drug and the polymer are solubilized, followed by emulsification with an aqueous gel containing salting-out agents such as $CaCl_2$, $MgCl_2$, or other electrolytes to induce salting out. A suitable stabilizer such as povidone, hydroxyethylcellulose, or other colloidal substances is added to enhance the stability of the emulsion. Then an adequate amount of aqueous solvent is added, resulting in the organic solvent's diffusion into aqueous solvent and the formation of nanospheres (Pal *et al.*, 2011).

NANOTHERAPEUTIC APPROACHES FOR MANAGEMENT OF HCC

The nanotherapeutic approach involves delivering nanosized therapeutic agents with specific therapeutic goals. Cancer cell-targeted nanoparticulate drug delivery system has recently become a promising and hopeful approach for imaging and diagnosing cancer, delivering chemotherapeutic agents at the cancerous region for treatment, and monitoring treatment outcomes (Fig. **2**). Chemotherapeutic agents entrapped into nanoparticles allow them to accumulate in the liver as a natural process of pharmacokinetics. Besides, designing a site-specific delivery system for chemotherapeutic agents by targeting specific receptors, proteins, or other possible molecular targets of the malignant cell surface also seems to be effective in HCC treatment. Apart from these benefits, some polymers, the delivery matrix or shell, are cytotoxic and capable of synergistic effects with the drug molecules (Chi *et al.*, 2020).

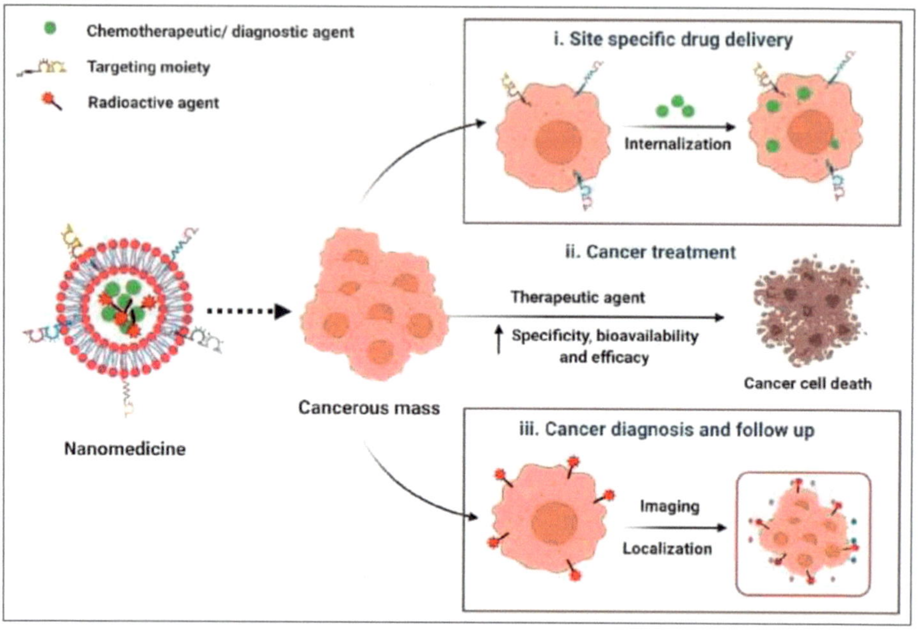

Fig. (2). Divergent roles of nanomedicine in the management of cancer. (i) Specific targeting moiety containing nanomedicine may enhance the selectivity of delivering therapeutic agents. (ii) Nanocarriers may increase the specificity, bioavailability, and efficacy of chemotherapeutic drugs or radioisotopes, leading to effective cancer treatment. (iii) Nanomedicine containing tracing agents may enable localization of cancer and monitoring of treatment outcomes.

Based on origin, various types of advanced inorganic and organic nanoparticles have been developed in the recent advances of nanotherapeutics (Fig. **3**). Gold nanoparticles, iron oxide nanoparticles, nanoshells, silica nanoparticles, carbon nanotubes, and quantum dots are innovative inorganic nanoparticle-specific characteristics and functionalities in pharmaceutical research. Polymer nanoparticles, liposomes, micelles, polymersomes, dendrimers, and solid lipid particles are the most common organic nanoparticle types. For effective treatment, diagnosis, and monitoring of HCC, different types of nanoparticles have been developed, such as liposomal nanoparticles, nanosized micelles, quantum dots, dendrimers, nanoshells, metallic nanoparticles, polymeric nanoparticles, and carbon nanotubes employing nanotherapeutics or nanotheranostics.

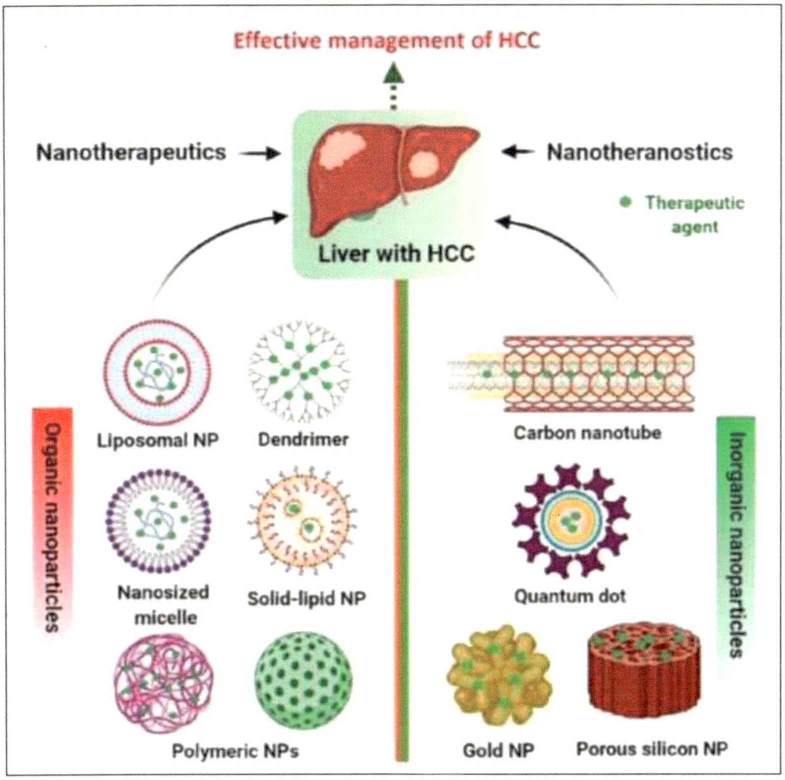

Fig. (3). Different types of nanoparticles for effective treatment, diagnosis, and monitoring of HCC. NP: nanoparticles, small green dot: drug molecules.

The key considerations for the nanotherapeutic approach are the nature of potent drugs, size and type of nanoparticles, and specific targets. The ideal size of this delivery system should be 30-200 nm. The particles with <100 nm sizes are accumulated into the reticuloendothelial system (mainly liver) for metabolism. This facilitates the target-specific delivery for HCC management (Elnaggar *et al.*, 2019). Recent advances in science and research have developed many nanotherapeutic approaches that showed successful outcomes and are under clinical trials (Table **1**).

Table 1. Nanotherapeutic formulations for HCC management under clinical trials.

Product	Company	Delivery System	Therapeutic Agent	Phase	References
ADI-PEG 20	Polaris	PEG protein conjugate	Arginine deaminase	II/III	(Ott *et al.*, 2013)

(Table 1) cont.....

Product	Company	Delivery System	Therapeutic Agent	Phase	References
PK2(PCE28069)	Pfizer	Polymeric conjugate	Doxorubicin	II	(Seymour *et al.*, 2002)
DHAD-PBCA-NP	-	Polymeric NPs	Mitoxantrone	II	(Zhou *et al.*, 2009)
Trans drug BA-003	Bio Alliance	Polymeric NPs	Doxorubicin	III	(Barraud *et al.*, 2005)
Thermodox®	Celsion	Thermo-sensitive lysolipid	Doxorubicin	III	(Hare *et al.*, 2017)

- indicate unknown, NPs indicate nanoparticles

Several chemotherapeutic agents have been delivered successfully to manage HCC (Mohamed *et al.*, 2017). These delivery systems have been designed by implementing varieties of delivery matrices exhibiting distinct targeting principles and/or release strategies with careful consideration of toxic effects of the respective therapeutic agents as well as challenges associated with drug delivery in HCC microenvironments. Many of these delivery systems showed remarkable outcomes in biological assays; for example, nanocurcumin, dextran-based curcumin nanoformulation, doxorubicin-loaded magnetic nanoclusters, folate-conjugated magnetic nanoparticles, docetaxel-loaded polydopamine nanoparticles, SM5-1 conjugated gold nanoparticles, erythrocyte-loaded pravastatin chitosan nanogels, bio-responsive chitin-poly(L-lactic acid) composite nanogels, SMMC-7721 carbon nanotubes, *etc.*, as listed in Table **2**.

Table 2. ***In vitro*** **and** ***in vivo*** **remarks of nanomedicine used in the management of HCC.**

Formulation	Delivery System	Size (nm)	*In vitro* and/or *in vivo* Remarks	References
Bio-responsive chitin-poly (LPA) composite nanogel	Chitin-poly (LPA)	270 ± 20	• HepG2 cell line study showed enhanced cyto-toxicity • Fluorescent micro-scopy study showed improved drug inter-nalization	(Arunraj *et al.*, 2014)

(Table 2) cont.....

Formulation	Delivery System	Size (nm)	*In vitro* and/or *in vivo* Remarks	References
SMMC-7721 carbon nanotubes	Chitosan modified single-walled carbon nanotubes	<500	• SMMC-7721 cell line study showed 68% cell death by 100 mg/mL dose compared to free doxorubicin • *In vivo* SMMC-7721 cell bearing mice model study demonstrated a significant reduction in cell growth	(Ji *et al.*, 2012)
Hematoporphyrin-modified doxorubicin-loaded NPs	Hematoporphyrin	350 ± 15	• Greater accumulation of drug into the tumor site and enhanced phototoxicity in HepG2 • *In vivo* HepG2 tumor-bearing mice model study showed significant improvement in anticancer activity compared to free drug	(Chang *et al.*, 2014)
Gum arabic conjugate curcumin micelles	Highly water-soluble polysaccharide gum arabic	270 ± 5	• *In vitro* studies showed enhanced solubility and stability of curcumin • HepG2 cell line study showed severe cytotoxicity	(Sarika *et al.*, 2015)
SM5-1 (monoclonal antibody) conjugated gold NPs	Gold NPs	~8.5	Orthotropic HCC mice model study showed 39.64 ± 4.87% inhibition of cell proliferation after 31 days of treatment	(Ma *et al.*, 2016)
Erythrocyte-loaded pravastatin chitosan nanogel	Erythrocyte for loading pravastatin and chitosan	129.8 ± 10.5	HepG2cells line study showed a 28% reduction in cells viability compared to unloaded erythrocytes	(Harisa *et al.*, 2016)

(Table 2) cont.....

Formulation	**Delivery System**	**Size (nm)**	***In vitro* and/or *in vivo* Remarks**	**References**
Transferrin-targeted core-shell nanomedicine loaded with doxorubicin (nanocore) and sorafenib (nanoshell)	Poly(vinyl alcohol) nanocore for doxorubicin and albumin nanoshell for sorafenib	~110	• About 92% of cytotoxicity of cancer cells was observed • 3D spheroids studies demonstrated effective penetration all through the tumor site and uniform cell death	(Malarvizhi *et al.*, 2014)
Doxorubicin-intercalated nanohydroxyapatite	Nanosized hydroxyapatite	40 60	*In vivo,* the animal model study showed remarkable suppression of hyperplastic nodules and a minimum num-ber of preneoplastic lesions	(Kundu *et al.*, 2013)
Genistein-loadedNPs	Star-shaped copolymer mannitol-functionalized PLGA TPGS	~250	• Enhanced cellular uptake (1.29-fold high-er nanoparticle concen-trations of 500 µg/mL) • Significant increase of apoptosis • *In vitro* and *in vivo* studies showed higher antitumor efficacy	(Wu *et al.*, 2016)
Epirubicin-loaded CXCR4 targetedpolymericNPs	PLGA/TPGS	138 ± 3.12	HepG2 cell line study showed enhanced cell-ular uptake (3-folded) compared to free and non-targeted drugs and significant tumor cell death	(Di-Wen *et al.*, 2016)
Sorafenib and gadolinium co-loaded liposomes	Liposomes	180 ± 1	• *In vitro* and *in vivo* imaging showed higher signal enhancement a-nd capability of visual-ization of biodistri-bution • *In vivo* antitumor study showed signi-ficant antitumor effi-cacy with reduced toxic effects	(Xiao *et al.*, 2016)

(Table 2) cont.....

Formulation	**Delivery System**	**Size (nm)**	***In vitro* and/or *in vivo* Remarks**	**References**
pHe-triggered charge-reversal and redox-responsive docetaxel NPs	D-α-tocopheryl PEG 1000-poly(β-amino ester) block copolymer with disulfide linkages	103.6 ± 9.2	• Effective suppression of cell proliferation increased the rate of apoptosis and cell cycle arrest in the G2/M phase • HepG2 xenograft tumor-bearing mice model showed significant suppression of tumor growth without side effects	(Chen *et al.*, 2015a)
Folate-conjugated PEGylated PLGA NPs co-encapsulated with sorafenib	Folate-conjugated PEGylated PLGA and magnetic NPs	205 ± 3.12	• BEL7402 cancer cell line study showed enhanced cellular uptake and effective suppression of cell proliferation than that of free drug • MRI properties showed good imaging characteristics and effective inhibition of the colony-forming ability	(Li *et al.*, 2015)
Lactosyl-norcantharidin encapsulated N-trimethyl chitosanNPs	N-trimethyl chitosan	120.6 ± 1.7	• HepG2 cell line study showed an IC_{50} value of this NP was only 24.2% of free drug • Increased *in vitro* cellular uptake • *In vivo* NIR fluorescence real-time imaging showed a higher targeting effi-cacy compared to free drug	(Guan *et al.*, 2012)

(Table 2) cont.....

Formulation	Delivery System	Size (nm)	*In vitro* and/or *in vivo* Remarks	References
Gambogic acidloadedelectrosprayedNPs	Poly D,L-lactide	185.6 ± 33.8	*In vivo,* HCC mice model study showed 82.51% antitumor targeting efficacy, decreased tumor invasion and hepatic cell lesions, recovery of hepatic function after 14 days treatment, and greater survival periods	(Yin *et al.*, 2014)
Galactosylated chitosan/5-FU NPs	Biodegradable galactosylated chitosan	35.19 ± 9.50	• Higher cytotoxicity to cancer cells • *In vivo,* an animal study showed a greater drug accumulation rate in tumor sites compared to free drugs	(Cheng *et al.*, 2012)
pH-sensitive pullulan targetedNPsloaded with methotrexate and combretastatin A4	N-urocanyl pullulan	187.1	• Prolonged circulation time in blood • Increased distributions in liver and tumor • Increased antitumor as well as anti-angiogenic effects	(Wang *et al.*, 2013)
L-aspartate coated gold NPs loaded with doxorubicin, cisplatin, and capecitabine	Gold NPs stabilized with L-aspartate monolayer	-	Reduced cellular proliferation rates and increased susceptibility to doxorubicin, cisplatin, and capecitabine compared to free drug therapy	(Tomuleasa *et al.*, 2012)

HCC TARGETING MECHANISMS BY NANOPARTICLES

In the recent development of nanotherapeutic approaches for HCC management, three types of targeting mechanisms have been utilized for delivering chemotherapeutic agents at the targeted site.

Active Targeting

Active targeting is the most used approach for the management of HCC. In this approach, the delivery system is designed in such a way that it has a specific affinity for a surface marker or targeting moiety (*e.g.*, ligands) of malignant cells, which enables it to bind to specific receptors or proteins, leading to direct delivery of therapeutic agents to the tumorous region by maintaining high specificity, affinity, and efficiency, termed as nanocarrier functionalization. A summarized mechanism of this targeting is illustrated in Fig. (4). Due to the higher surface area of nanoparticles, specialized functionalization has been designed based on the nature of the materials for a better outcome. Various ligands with specific characteristics have been targeted by several types of particular macromolecules and small molecules for active targeting of HCC, which are discussed below.

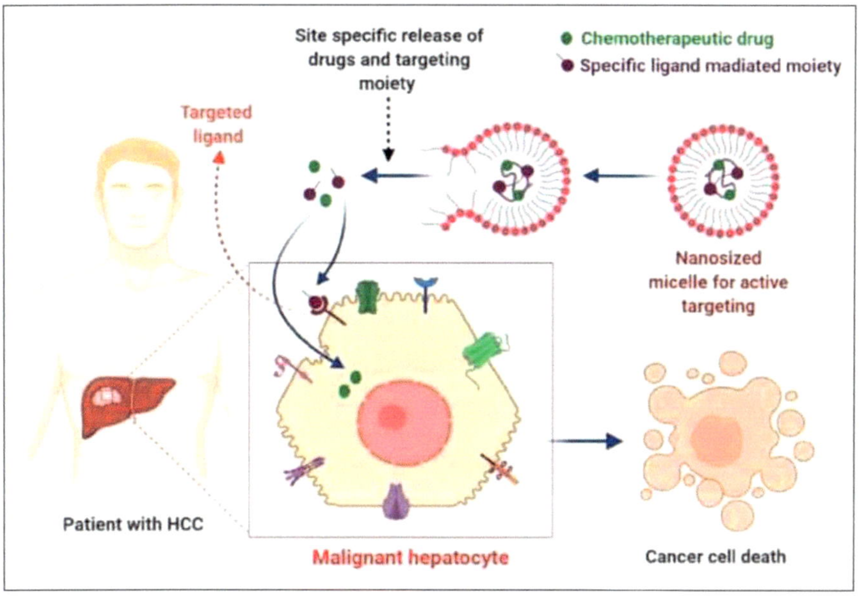

Fig. (4). A summary of the general mechanism of active targeting by using a nanotherapeutic approach, where targeting ligands can be a peptide, antibody, aptamer, or small molecules like saccharide, vitamin specific to a receptor, enzyme, gene, or any bio-molecular chemicals of malignant cells of HCC.

Active Targeting of Ligands by Specific Macromolecules

Active Targeting by Peptide-Mediated Ligands

Specific and characteristic peptides affect distinctive and characteristic macromolecules, such as-Arginine-Glycine-Asparagine (RGD) tripeptides have an affinity for integrin-αvβ3, Gerbich GE11 has an affinity for EGFR, *etc.* Nanoparticles functionalized with these peptides can aid the direct delivery of chemotherapeutic agents to the tumor region. For example, RGD tripeptides have been utilized to functionalize paclitaxel liposome, which has been found to attenuate proliferation with higher efficiency (Chen *et al.*, 2015b) and GE11 incorporation onto doxorubicin-loaded liposomes, leading to increased internalization and cellular uptake of doxorubicin, resulting in efficient antitumor activity (Li *et al.*, 2005).

Active Targeting by Antibody-Mediated Ligands

In HCC, a diversity of specific complementary antigens is found on the cell surface, which can be a promising modality of active targeting. Designing a nanoparticulate system coupled with an antibody targeting complementary antigens can effectively deliver chemotherapeutic agents with higher specificity. This approach helps drug accumulation in a hepatocellular tumor by enhancing cellular uptake and satisfying therapeutic efficacy through a common mechanism of antigen-antibody recognition. Researchers have reported such kinds of tactics for treating HCC. For example, nanoparticles coupled with mAb were designed by targeting SM5-1 binding membrane proteins that overexpress on the cell surface of HCC. These nanoparticles were found to show higher specificity and drug uptake, resulting in desired cytotoxicity (Kou *et al.*, 2008). Other examples of antibody-targeted nanoparticulate systems showing effective therapeutic responses are anti-CD44 antibody-mediated liposomal nanoparticles loaded with doxorubicin (Wang *et al.*, 2012), nanoparticle loaded with 5-fluorouracil and glucose-regulated protein-78mAb-conjugated bovine serum albumin (MATHEW *et al.*, 1996), EGFR mAb-modified polylactic acid-co-L-lysine nanoparticles (Kiss *et al.*, 1997), *etc.*

Active Targeting by Aptamer Mediated Ligands

Oligonucleotides, siRNA (single-stranded RNA), and ssDNA (single-stranded DNA) having binding affinity to other nucleic acids, proteins, and small cellular molecules are known as aptamers. Due to the presence of characteristic genes, proteins, and small cellular molecules (which can be a potential target for aptamer), this approach has achieved enormous HCC therapeutic management popularity. For example, conjugates of salinomycin-loaded poly-(lactic--o-glycolic acid) nanoparticles with aptamers of CD133EGFR termed as A15 (sequence: 5′-NH_2CCCUCCUACAUAGGG-3′) and CL4 (sequence: 5′-GCCUUAGUAACGUGCUUUGAUGUCGAUUCGACAGGAGGC-3′), respectively. This nanoparticle-aptamer conjugate has been designed to target CD133 and EGFR on malignant cells of HCC that have shown enhanced efficacy against HCC (Jiang *et al.*, 2015).

Active Targeting of Small Molecular Ligands

Active Targeting by Saccharide-Mediated Ligands

ASGPR is a calcium-channel receptor that has been shown to overexpress extensively on hepatic cell surfaces. Galactose is a natural ligand for this receptor. N-acetylgalactosamine and N-acetylgalactose are the derivatives of galactose, which have a higher affinity to bind with ASGPR ensuing efficient cellular uptake of drugs *via* receptor-mediated endocytosis. Integration of these small molecules into nanoparticles can be an effective mode of targeting HCC; for example, fluorescence-labeled N-acetylgalactose-modified poly (amidoamine) dendrimers for site-specific delivery and uptake to HCC (Medina *et al.*, 2011), galactose-modified nanocarriers for targeting Huh-7 cells and reversing the multidrug resistance (Yik *et al.*, 2002), and galactosylated cationic dextran for targeting tumor-associated macrophages (Biswas *et al.*, 2006). Likewise, hyaluronic acid, pectin, and pullulan are promising saccharides to be used as actively targeting ligands, which can effectively reduce cell proliferation, migration, and angiogenesis (Li *et al.*, 2016).

Active targeting by Vitamin-Mediated Ligands

Overexpression of certain vitamins, such as folate, biotin, retinoic acid, and dehydroascorbic acid receptors, is observed on the cell surface of HCC. The rapid proliferation of malignant tumors requires an extensive supply of these vitamins. This pathogenicity renders these vitamins as a promising mode of active targeting of these receptors, thus facilitating site-specific delivery of chemotherapeutic agents with higher specificity (Wang *et al.*, 2019). Examples of such approaches are folate conjugated polymeric nanocomposites (D-PCE-FA) (Cao *et al.*, 2011), multifunctional folate-SPIODOX-micelles (Hong *et al.*, 2008), and folate conjugated selenium nanoparticles with therapeutic siRNA (Se–PEI–FA@siRNA) (Xia *et al.*, 2018).

Active Targeting by Transferrin-Mediated Ligands

Transferrin (Tf) is an important small glycoprotein that mediates cellular iron transportation through TFR_1 and TFR_2 receptors. In HCC, TFR_1 is overexpressed, whereas TFR_2 is down-expressed. Nanoparticular systems ligated with Tf can target malignant regions, thus facilitating drug accumulation and the desired therapeutic responses. Such Tf-ligated nanoparticle systems, loaded with sorafenib (loaded into albumin nanoshells) and doxorubicin (loaded into polyvinyl alcohol nanocores), have shown a remarkable increase in cellular uptake of these drugs in HepG2 cells and the resultant cytotoxicity and apoptosis (Malarvizhi *et al.*, 2014).

Passive Targeting

The passive targeting approach is designed on enhanced permeability and retention effect. It results from leaky vasculature of the tumor mass, rapid and flawed angiogenesis, and ineffectual lymphatic flow in the tumor region. Nanoparticles are tiny and distinct in size and shape, thus being internalized and accumulated in tumor cells selectively, facilitating drug delivery (Chi *et al.*, 2020). This targeting technique is shown in Fig. (**5**).

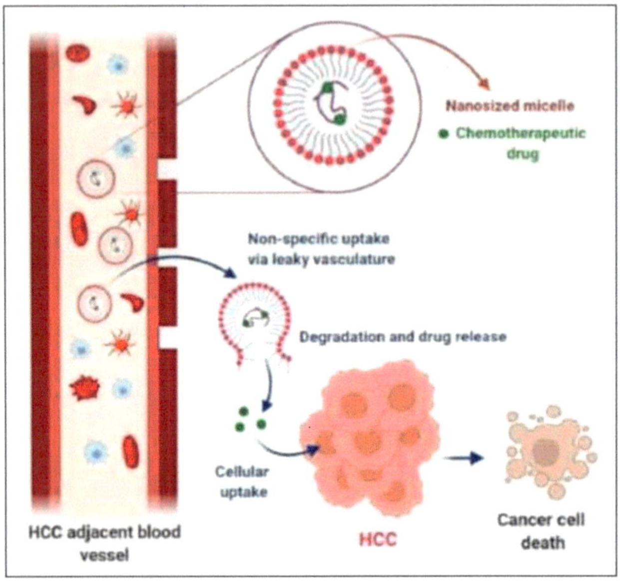

Fig. (5). An illustration of passive targeting of HCC by nanotherapeutic approach.

Usually, by the influence of the enhanced permeability and retention effect, nanoparticles can be accumulated in HCC 3-fold times higher compared to normal healthy tissues. Optimization of physicochemical properties of ligands and nanocarrier may lead to enhance the effect of accumulation. Size, charge, density, and orientation of nanocarrier ligands and hydrophobicity are essential to optimize the nanoparticle system for attaining the most fruitful outcomes. These properties directly affect their blood circulation profiles, distribution, and uptake by cancer cells (Sun *et al.*, 2019). For example, sorafenib cyclodextrin nano-assemblies are passive targeting nano assemblies that are highly stable in the aqueous medium, allowing this drug delivery for two weeks. The approach shows higher efficiency in inhibiting HCC cell proliferation with negligible hemolytic activity.

The passive targeting approach is comparatively less practical than active targeting. Firstly, passive targeting depends on the concentration affected by interstitial pressure, tumor growth, and solid-mass stress. These consequences lower its efficacy. Secondly, passive targeting can hardly meet therapeutic concentration leading to induce multidrug resistance. Finally, the tumors and their differences are hardly recognized by this approach, thus failing selectivity and lack of specificity issues. Conversely, active targeting is dependent on specific molecular targets of tumor cells rather than concentration; therefore, it is free from these complications.

Stimuli-Responsive Nanocarriers Targeting

This targeting system is based on using numerous external (heat, light, radiation, magnetic field, ultrasound, and microwaves) and internal (pH differences, oxygen concentrations, specific enzymes, and cellular chemicals) stimuli for controlling the direction of nanoparticles and allowing drug release to the particular site of the target (Fig. **6**). Numerous approaches regarding this targeting are discussed below.

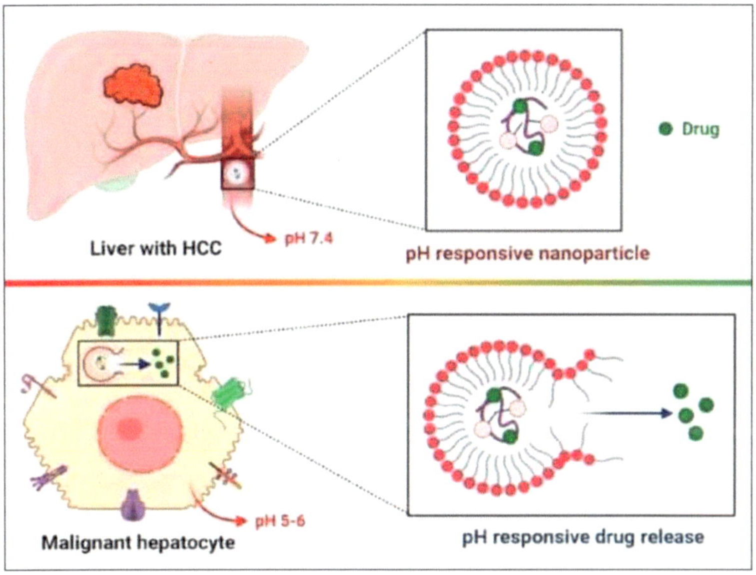

Fig. (6). Drug release from a stimuli-responsive nanoparticle, where specific H^+ concentration functions as a stimulus.

Magnetic Field Responsive Nanoparticles

A nanoparticulate system stimulated by external magnetic fields is an effective drug delivery modality for managing HCC. This approach facilitates the accumulation of drugs in HCC cells selectively, thus increasing therapeutic outcomes and reducing the exposure of healthy tissue to cytotoxic chemotherapeutic agents. Magnetic resonance navigation for endovascular routing of therapeutic magnetic microcarriers enables targeting and monitoring of selective malignant tissues. This strategy enables controlling the biodistribution of chemoembolization agents resulting in the amendment of specificity and deposition of drugs in targeted cancerous regions, thus ensuring minimal toxicity of normal tissues; for example, doxorubicin and magnetic nanoparticles-loaded into biodegradable microcarriers. This system was designed for targeting deep tissue by using vascular magnetic resonance navigation (Pouponneau *et al.*, 2011).

pH-Responsive Nanoparticles

The tumor microenvironment exhibits a comparatively lower pH than normal healthy tissues. A similar pH difference pattern is also found in intracellular endolysosomal compartments of healthy tissues and cancer tissue. This difference may occur due to proton accumulation as the combined effects of the Warburg effect and abnormal vasculature drainage (Chi *et al.*, 2020). This incidence in malignant cells, known as acidosis, is considered a responsive stimulus for controlling drug release. An illustration of this approach is shown in Fig. (**6**). Introducing a pH-responsive linker such as hydrazine or imine to the nanocarriers system is essential for designing this system. It links drugs and nanocarriers. For example, doxorubicin is attached to pH-sensitive mesoporous silica nanoparticles. In this system, drugs and nanoparticles are linked by a hydrazone linker and programmed to release drugs at pH 5.5 rather than at pH 7.4 (Lee *et al.*, 2010).

Moreover, pH-responsive nanocarrier is widely popular. For example, pH-responsive microspheres containing drug-eluting nanocomposites synthesized from sorafenib, iron oxide nanoparticles, biodegradable polymer, and pH-responsive additive released drugs at a higher rate at pH 6.5 compared to pH 7.4 and showed higher cytotoxicity against McA-RH7777 hepatoma cells (Park *et al.*, 2016). Furthermore, silica NPs collapse at low pH; thus, they act as pH-responsive nanocarriers. Arsenite-loaded pH-responsive nanoparticle is an example of this approach, which showed enhanced anticancer efficacy against SMMC-7721cells of HCC (Chi *et al.*, 2019).

Hypoxia-Responsive Nanoparticles

Malignant tumors increase very rapidly and necessitate a significant amount of oxygen. Due to this reason, hypoxia is one of the most common phenomena in cancer cells. Compared to healthy tissues, the partial pressure of oxygen in the tumor region is only 40% (Kim *et al.*, 2009). Utilization of hypoxia in malignant tissues as a stimulus of drug release in the cancerous part is a promising means of treating HCC. Resembling acidosis, hypoxia-responsive linkers such as disulfides are used in synthesizing nanocarriers. This disulfide linker is cleaved by the presence of excess glutathione (GSH), which enables the use of this approach in the treatment of HCC. Organosilica-capped mesoporous silica nanoparticle is a hypoxia-responsive nanocarrier system. When these nanocarriers come to the exposure of excess GSH, the disulfide links get cleaved. It results in the organosilica shell collapsing and releasing doxorubicin. This nanocarrier system showed remarkable cytotoxicity against SMMC-7721 cells of HCC compared to free-drug (Shen *et al.*, 2019).

NANOTHERANOSTIC APPROACH FOR MANAGEMENT OF HCC

The advancement of nanotechnology offers a simplistic approach for imaging and treatment, creating a new modality in biomedical science, known as nanomedicine-based theranostics or nanotheranostics. 'Nanotheranostics' is a multifunctional term arising from 'nano,' 'diagnostics,' and 'therapy,' which states a combination therapy comprising nanomaterials, imaging, and therapeutics. It is a concomitant approach to disease management by single therapy providing imaging, diagnosis, treatment, and follow-up. This approach has received immense acceptance for cancer management because it allows rapid adaptation in cancer therapy, intending to obtain higher therapeutic responses (Kelkar and Reineke, 2011). In HCC management, this approach has been applied efficaciously as well. Integration of nanomedicine with MRI (magnetic resonance imaging) is an effective strategy of nanotheranostics. For example, manganese (II) arsenite nanoparticles-loaded hollow silica nanoparticle system is a pH-responsive nano theranostic approach. This nanomedicine system works by releasing arsenite and Mn^{2+} ions as a response to acidosis H22 tumors in mice. The arsenite works as a therapeutic agent, whereas Mn^{2+} ions permit MRI (contrast-enhanced T_1-weighted), enabling the diagnosis and monitoring of liver cancer (Zhao *et al.*, 2015). Fluorescence imaging integrated with nanomedicine is also a popular strategy of nanotheranostics; for example, cisplatin-containing DSPEmPEG/DCM-S-Pt micelles conjugated with a near-infrared fluorescent dye (DCM-NH_2). About 49% inhibition of liver cancer in the rabbit model was observed by this approach (Chi *et al.*, 2020).

IMPACT OF PHYSICOCHEMICAL FACTORS OF NANOPARTICLES ON HCC MANAGEMENT

The effectiveness of nanomedicine on HCC management depends largely on physicochemical characteristics (Fig. 7) of nanoformulation due to their direct relationship to drug targeting mechanisms and the stability as well as bio-suitability of nanomaterials. Ligand concentration is the first consideration for obtaining desired therapeutic and theranostic effects, especially for active targeting. In this approach, the concentration of ligands on the surface of nanoparticles is directly correlated to the affinity for the molecular targets of HCC. As stated by molecular biology and thermodynamic principles, an increased concentration of ligand may exaggerate the affinity of nanoparticles for targeted moiety, thus intensifying their interactions resulting in the initiation of a biochemical cascade to exert therapeutic response. In contrast, an excessive increase of ligand concentration may negatively impact binding due to steric hindrance, improper orientation, combined effects, and/or competition for the binding moiety of cancer cells; for example, patchy clusters coordination as a negative cooperative effect of ligand-clustered nanoparticles. Therefore, the concentration of a ligand is considered a critical factor that should be optimal for desired outcomes.

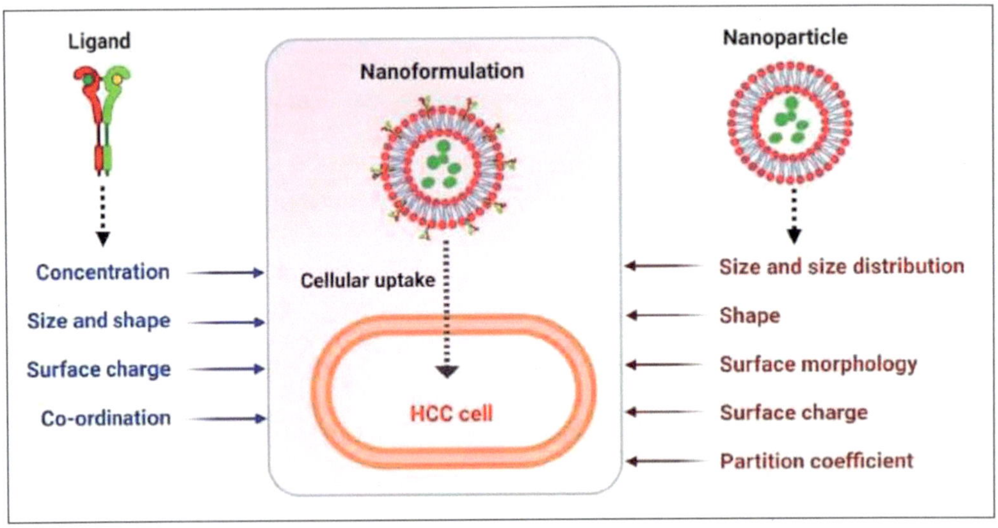

Fig. (7). Physicochemical properties of nanoformulation affecting the therapeutic success of HCC.

In addition, the size, size distribution, shape, surface morphology, surface charge, charge density, partition coefficient, and the nature of the nanocarrier matrix are the factors that affect the outcome of HCC therapy. The size, size distribution, and shape of the nanoformulation must be considered in the formulation stage. In the case of effective HCC therapy, nanoparticles should have sophisticated curvatures and satisfactory ligand functionalization capability after synthesis. Spherical-shaped small-size nanoparticles with a narrow size distribution range represent greater curvatures but are complex in ligand functionalization. Besides, cellular accumulation is dependent on size, while the cellular internalization mechanism depends mostly on the shape of nanoparticles. Spherical-shaped nanoparticles with a range of 2-70 nm size are considered for maximum hepatic accumulation. The hydrophobic core is one of the significant organizational parts of nanoparticles, regardless of the type of nanoparticle. Hydrophobicity affects the self-assembling process, shape, post-synthesis functionalization, and passive targeting mediated non-specific interaction to cancer cells. The surface charge of nanoparticles and ligands perform vital roles in the post-synthesis functionalization process. Opposite charged nanoparticles and ligands can produce a greater conjugation yield and favorable spatial spectacle with optimum particle size because of existing attractive forces. The existing repulsive force causes the complexity of the functionalization process and affects particle size and shape, resulting in poor efficacy (Sun *et al.*, 2019).

CONCLUSION

The nanotherapeutic approach attracts the recent researchers for delivering drugs in a targeted region of the body, especially for neoplastic disease management. Numerous promising outcomes have been observed by nanotherapeutics in the case of HCC management as well. Unfortunately, various challenges are creating hindrances, such as physiochemical characterization variability, toxicity problems, complexity, and costs for formulations. Physiochemical properties, including structure, shape, charge, surface properties, aggregation behavior, solubility to biological fluids, interaction affinity with biological proteins, stability, and others, are alterable after administration. Along with this, significant health and environmental hazards are reported. The commonness of intracellular biomolecules and lack of adequate toxicity assessment methodologies impede research on nano material-related toxicity issues. Moreover, formulation complexity and higher cost of raw materials affect the feasibility of this approach.

CONSENT FOR PUBLICATION

Not applicable.

CONFLICT OF INTEREST

The authors declare no conflict of interest, financial or otherwise.

ACKNOWLEDGEMENT

Declared none.

REFERENCES

Ali, ES, Sharker, SM, Islam, MT, Khan, IN, Shaw, S, Rahman, MA, Uddin, SJ, Shill, MC, Rehman, S, Das, N, Ahmad, S, Shilpi, JA, Tripathi, S, Mishra, SK & Mubarak, MS (2020) Targeting cancer cells with nanotherapeutics and nanodiagnostics: Current status and future perspectives. *Semin Cancer Biol* [PMID: 32014609]

Arunraj, TR, Sanoj Rejinold, N, Ashwin Kumar, N & Jayakumar, R (2014) Bio-responsive chitin-poly(--lactic acid) composite nanogels for liver cancer. *Colloids Surf B Biointerfaces,* 113, 394-402. [http://dx.doi.org/10.1016/j.colsurfb.2013.09.023] [PMID: 24129331]

Barraud, L, Merle, P, Soma, E, Lefrançois, L, Guerret, S, Chevallier, M, Dubernet, C, Couvreur, P, Trépo, C & Vitvitski, L (2005) Increase of doxorubicin sensitivity by doxorubicin-loading into nanoparticles for hepatocellular carcinoma cells *in vitro* and *in vivo*. *J Hepatol,* 42, 736-43. [http://dx.doi.org/10.1016/j.jhep.2004.12.035] [PMID: 15826724]

Biswas, SK, Gangi, L, Paul, S, Schioppa, T, Saccani, A, Sironi, M, Bottazzi, B, Doni, A, Vincenzo, B,

Pasqualini, F, Vago, L, Nebuloni, M, Mantovani, A & Sica, A (2006) A distinct and unique transcriptional program expressed by tumor-associated macrophages (defective NF-kappaB and enhanced IRF-3/STAT1 activation). *Blood,* 107, 2112-22.
[http://dx.doi.org/10.1182/blood-2005-01-0428] [PMID: 16269622]

Cao, N, Cheng, D, Zou, S, Ai, H, Gao, J & Shuai, X (2011) The synergistic effect of hierarchical assemblies of siRNA and chemotherapeutic drugs co-delivered into hepatic cancer cells. *Biomaterials,* 32, 2222-32.
[http://dx.doi.org/10.1016/j.biomaterials.2010.11.061] [PMID: 21186059]

Chang, J-E, Yoon, I-S, Sun, P-L, Yi, E, Jheon, S & Shim, C-K (2014) Anticancer efficacy of photodynamic therapy with hematoporphyrin-modified, doxorubicin-loaded nanoparticles in liver cancer. *J Photochem Photobiol B,* 140, 49-56.
[http://dx.doi.org/10.1016/j.jphotobiol.2014.07.005] [PMID: 25090224]

Chen, F, Zhang, J, Wang, L, Wang, Y & Chen, M (2015) Tumor pH(e)-triggered charge-reversal and redox-responsive nanoparticles for docetaxel delivery in hepatocellular carcinoma treatment. *Nanoscale,* 7, 15763-79. a
[http://dx.doi.org/10.1039/C5NR04612B] [PMID: 26355843]

Chen, L, Liu, Y, Wang, W & Liu, K (2015) Effect of integrin receptor-targeted liposomal paclitaxel for hepatocellular carcinoma targeting and therapy. *Oncol Lett,* 10, 77-84. b
[http://dx.doi.org/10.3892/ol.2015.3242] [PMID: 26170980]

Cheng, M, Han, J, Li, Q, He, B, Zha, B, Wu, J, Zhou, R, Ye, T, Wang, W, Xu, H & Hou, Y (2012) Synthesis of galactosylated chitosan/5-fluorouracil nanoparticles and its characteristics, *in vitro* and *in vivo* release studies. *J Biomed Mater Res B Appl Biomater,* 100, 2035-43.
[http://dx.doi.org/10.1002/jbm.b.32767] [PMID: 22865703]

Chi, X, Liu, K, Luo, X, Yin, Z, Lin, H & Gao, J (2020) Recent advances of nanomedicines for liver cancer therapy. *J Mater Chem B Mater Biol Med,* 8, 3747-71.
[http://dx.doi.org/10.1039/C9TB02871D] [PMID: 32215381]

Chi, X, Zhang, R, Zhao, T, Gong, X, Wei, R, Yin, Z, Lin, H, Li, D, Shan, H & Gao, J (2019) Targeted arsenite-loaded magnetic multifunctional nanoparticles for treatment of hepatocellular carcinoma. *Nanotechnology,* 30, 175101.
[http://dx.doi.org/10.1088/1361-6528/aaff9e] [PMID: 30654348]

Di-Wen, S, Pan, G-Z, Hao, L, Zhang, J, Xue, Q-Z, Wang, P & Yuan, Q-Z (2016) Improved antitumor activity of epirubicin-loaded CXCR4-targeted polymeric nanoparticles in liver cancers. *Int J Pharm,* 500, 54-61.
[http://dx.doi.org/10.1016/j.ijpharm.2015.12.066] [PMID: 26748365]

Elnaggar, MH, Abushouk, AI, Hassan, AHE, Lamloum, HM, Benmelouka, A, Moatamed, SA, Abd-Elmegeed, H, Attia, S, Samir, A, Amr, N, Johar, D & Zaky, S (2019) Nanomedicine as a putative approach for active targeting of hepatocellular carcinoma. *Semin Cancer Biol,* 69, 91-9.
[PMID: 31421265]

Guan, M, Zhou, Y, Zhu, Q-L, Liu, Y, Bei, Y-Y, Zhang, X-N & Zhang, Q (2012) N-trimethyl chitosan nanoparticle-encapsulated lactosyl-norcantharidin for liver cancer therapy with high targeting efficacy. *Nanomedicine,* 8, 1172-81.
[http://dx.doi.org/10.1016/j.nano.2012.01.009] [PMID: 22321383]

Hare, JI, Lammers, T, Ashford, MB, Puri, S, Storm, G & Barry, ST (2017) Challenges and strategies in anti-cancer nanomedicine development: An industry perspective. *Adv Drug Deliv Rev,* 108, 25-38.
[http://dx.doi.org/10.1016/j.addr.2016.04.025] [PMID: 27137110]

Harisa, G I, Badran, M M, Alqahtani, S A, Alanazi, F K & Attia, S M (2016) Pravastatin chitosan nanogels-loaded erythrocytes as a new delivery strategy for targeting liver cancer. *Saudi pharmaceutical journal : SPJ : the official publication of the Saudi Pharmaceutical Society,* 24, 74-81.

Hong, G, Yuan, R, Liang, B, Shen, J, Yang, X & Shuai, X (2008) Folate-functionalized polymeric micelle as hepatic carcinoma-targeted, MRI-ultrasensitive delivery system of antitumor drugs. *Biomed Microdevices,* 10, 693-700.

[http://dx.doi.org/10.1007/s10544-008-9180-9] [PMID: 18350380]

Ji, Z, Lin, G, Lu, Q, Meng, L, Shen, X, Dong, L, Fu, C & Zhang, X (2012) Targeted therapy of SMMC-7721 liver cancer *in vitro* and *in vivo* with carbon nanotubes based drug delivery system. *J Colloid Interface Sci,* 365, 143-9.
[http://dx.doi.org/10.1016/j.jcis.2011.09.013] [PMID: 21974923]

Jiang, J, Chen, H, Yu, C, Zhang, Y, Chen, M, Tian, S & Sun, C (2015) The promotion of salinomycin delivery to hepatocellular carcinoma cells through EGFR and CD133 aptamers conjugation by PLGA nanoparticles. *Nanomedicine (Lond),* 10, 1863-79.
[http://dx.doi.org/10.2217/nnm.15.43] [PMID: 26139123]

Kelkar, SS & Reineke, TM (2011) Theranostics: combining imaging and therapy. *Bioconjug Chem,* 22, 1879-903.
[http://dx.doi.org/10.1021/bc200151q] [PMID: 21830812]

Kim, Y, Lin, Q, Glazer, PM & Yun, Z (2009) Hypoxic tumor microenvironment and cancer cell differentiation. *Curr Mol Med,* 9, 425-34.
[http://dx.doi.org/10.2174/156652409788167113] [PMID: 19519400]

Kiss, A, Wang, N-J, Xie, J-P & Thorgeirsson, SS (1997) Analysis of transforming growth factor (TGF)-alpha/epidermal growth factor receptor, hepatocyte growth Factor/c-met,TGF-beta receptor type II, and p53 expression in human hepatocellular carcinomas. *Clin Cancer Res,* 3, 1059-66.
[PMID: 9815784]

Kou, G, Wang, S, Cheng, C, Gao, J, Li, B, Wang, H, Qian, W, Hou, S, Zhang, D, Dai, J, Gu, H & Guo, Y (2008) Development of SM5-1-conjugated ultrasmall superparamagnetic iron oxide nanoparticles for hepatoma detection. *Biochem Biophys Res Commun,* 374, 192-7.
[http://dx.doi.org/10.1016/j.bbrc.2008.06.126] [PMID: 18621023]

Kundu, B, Ghosh, D, Sinha, MK, Sen, PS, Balla, VK, Das, N & Basu, D (2013) Doxorubicin-intercalated nano-hydroxyapatite drug-delivery system for liver cancer: An animal model. *Ceram Int,* 39, 9557-66.
[http://dx.doi.org/10.1016/j.ceramint.2013.05.074]

Lee, CH, Cheng, SH, Huang, IP, Souris, JS, Yang, CS, Mou, CY & Lo, LW (2010) Intracellular pH-responsive mesoporous silica nanoparticles for the controlled release of anticancer chemotherapeutics. *Angew Chem Int Ed Engl,* 49, 8214-9.
[http://dx.doi.org/10.1002/anie.201002639] [PMID: 20865709]

Li, M, Zhang, W, Wang, B, Gao, Y, Song, Z & Zheng, QC (2016) Ligand-based targeted therapy: a novel strategy for hepatocellular carcinoma. *Int J Nanomedicine,* 11, 5645-69.
[http://dx.doi.org/10.2147/IJN.S115727] [PMID: 27920520]

Li, Y-J, Dong, M, Kong, F-M & Zhou, J-P (2015) Folate-decorated anticancer drug and magnetic nanoparticles encapsulated polymeric carrier for liver cancer therapeutics. *Int J Pharm,* 489, 83-90.
[http://dx.doi.org/10.1016/j.ijpharm.2015.04.028] [PMID: 25888801]

Li, Z, Zhao, R, Wu, X, Sun, Y, Yao, M, Li, J, Xu, Y & Gu, J (2005) Identification and characterization of a novel peptide ligand of epidermal growth factor receptor for targeted delivery of therapeutics. *FASEB J,* 19, 1978-85.
[http://dx.doi.org/10.1096/fj.05-4058com] [PMID: 16319141]

Ma, X, Hui, H, Jin, Y, Dong, D, Liang, X, Yang, X, Tan, K, Dai, Z, Cheng, Z & Tian, J (2016) Enhanced immunotherapy of SM5-1 in hepatocellular carcinoma by conjugating with gold nanoparticles and its *in vivo* bioluminescence tomographic evaluation. *Biomaterials,* 87, 46-56.
[http://dx.doi.org/10.1016/j.biomaterials.2016.02.007] [PMID: 26897539]

Malarvizhi, GL, Retnakumari, AP, Nair, S & Koyakutty, M (2014) Transferrin targeted core-shell nanomedicine for combinatorial delivery of doxorubicin and sorafenib against hepatocellular carcinoma. *Nanomedicine,* 10, 1649-59.
[http://dx.doi.org/10.1016/j.nano.2014.05.011] [PMID: 24905399]

Mathew, J, Hines, JE, Obafunwa, JO, Burr, AW, Toole, K & Burt, AD (1996) CD44 is expressed in hepatocellular carcinomas showing vascular invasion. *J Pathol,* 179, 74-9.
[http://dx.doi.org/10.1002/(SICI)1096-9896(199605)179:1<74::AID-PATH531>3.0.CO;2-E] [PMID: 8691349]

Medina, SH, Tekumalla, V, Chevliakov, MV, Shewach, DS, Ensminger, WD & El-Sayed, ME (2011) N-acetylgalactosamine-functionalized dendrimers as hepatic cancer cell-targeted carriers. *Biomaterials,* 32, 4118-29.
[http://dx.doi.org/10.1016/j.biomaterials.2010.11.068] [PMID: 21429574]

Mohamed, NK, Hamad, MA, Hafez, MZ, Wooley, KL & Elsabahy, M (2017) Nanomedicine in management of hepatocellular carcinoma: Challenges and opportunities. *Int J Cancer,* 140, 1475-84.
[http://dx.doi.org/10.1002/ijc.30517] [PMID: 27861850]

Ott, PA, Carvajal, RD, Pandit-Taskar, N, Jungbluth, AA, Hoffman, EW, Wu, BW, Bomalaski, JS, Venhaus, R, Pan, L, Old, LJ, Pavlick, AC & Wolchok, JD (2013) Phase I/II study of pegylated arginine deiminase (ADI-PEG 20) in patients with advanced melanoma. *Invest New Drugs,* 31, 425-34.
[http://dx.doi.org/10.1007/s10637-012-9862-2] [PMID: 22864522]

Pal, SL, Jana, U, Manna, PK, Mohanta, GP & Manavalan, R (2011) Nanoparticle: An overview of preparation and characterization. *J Appl Pharm Sci,* 1, 228-34.

Park, W, Chen, J, Cho, S, Park, S-J, Larson, AC, Na, K & Kim, D-H (2016) Acidic pH-triggered drug-eluting nanocomposites for magnetic resonance imaging-monitored intra-arterial drug delivery to hepatocellular carcinoma. *ACS Appl Mater Interfaces,* 8, 12711-9.
[http://dx.doi.org/10.1021/acsami.6b03505] [PMID: 27159350]

Pedroso-Santana, S & Fleitas-Salazar, N (2020) Ionotropic gelation method in the synthesis of nanoparticles/microparticles for biomedical purposes. *Polym Int,* 69, 443-7.
[http://dx.doi.org/10.1002/pi.5970]

Pouponneau, P, Leroux, J-C, Soulez, G, Gaboury, L & Martel, S (2011) Co-encapsulation of magnetic nanoparticles and doxorubicin into biodegradable microcarriers for deep tissue targeting by vascular MRI navigation. *Biomaterials,* 32, 3481-6.
[http://dx.doi.org/10.1016/j.biomaterials.2010.12.059] [PMID: 21315445]

Sarika, PR, James, NR, Kumar, PR, Raj, DK & Kumary, TV (2015) Gum arabic-curcumin conjugate micelles with enhanced loading for curcumin delivery to hepatocarcinoma cells. *Carbohydr Polym,* 134, 167-74.
[http://dx.doi.org/10.1016/j.carbpol.2015.07.068] [PMID: 26428113]

Seymour, LW, Ferry, DR, Anderson, D, Hesslewood, S, Julyan, PJ, Poyner, R, Doran, J, Young, AM, Burtles, S & Kerr, DJ (2002) Hepatic drug targeting: phase I evaluation of polymer-bound doxorubicin. *J Clin Oncol,* 20, 1668-76.
[http://dx.doi.org/10.1200/JCO.2002.20.6.1668] [PMID: 11896118]

Shen, L, Pan, S, Niu, D, He, J, Jia, X, Hao, J, Gu, J, Zhao, W, Li, P & Li, Y (2019) Facile synthesis of organosilica-capped mesoporous silica nanocarriers with selective redox-triggered drug release properties for safe tumor chemotherapy. *Biomater Sci,* 7, 1825-32.
[http://dx.doi.org/10.1039/C8BM01669K] [PMID: 30892297]

Sun, Y, Ma, W, Yang, Y, He, M, Li, A, Bai, L, Yu, B & Yu, Z (2019) Cancer nanotechnology: Enhancing tumor cell response to chemotherapy for hepatocellular carcinoma therapy. *Asian journal of pharmaceutical sciences,* 14, 581-94.

Tomuleasa, C, Soritau, O, Orza, A, Dudea, M, Petrushev, B, Mosteanu, O, Susman, S, Florea, A, Pall, E & Aldea, M (2012) Gold nanoparticles conjugated with cisplatin/doxorubicin/capecitabine lower the chemoresistance of hepatocellular carcinoma-derived cancer cells. *Journal of Gastrointestinal & Liver Diseases,* 21

Ueda, M & Kreuter, J (1997) Optimization of the preparation of loperamide-loaded poly (L-lactide) nanoparticles by high pressure emulsification-solvent evaporation. *J Microencapsul,* 14, 593-605.

[http://dx.doi.org/10.3109/02652049709006812] [PMID: 9292435]

Usmani, A & Mishra, A (2017) *Current Updates on Risk Factors of Hepatocellular Carcinoma,* 8, 23-31.

Usmani, A, Mishra, A & Ahmad, M (2018) Nanomedicines: a theranostic approach for hepatocellular carcinoma. *Artif Cells Nanomed Biotechnol,* 46, 680-90.
[http://dx.doi.org/10.1080/21691401.2017.1374282] [PMID: 28884605]

Vandervoort, J & Ludwig, A (2002) Biocompatible stabilizers in the preparation of PLGA nanoparticles: a factorial design study. *Int J Pharm,* 238, 77-92.
[http://dx.doi.org/10.1016/S0378-5173(02)00058-3] [PMID: 11996812]

Wagner, V, Dullaart, A, Bock, AK & Zweck, A (2006) The emerging nanomedicine landscape. *Nat Biotechnol,* 24, 1211-7.
[http://dx.doi.org/10.1038/nbt1006-1211] [PMID: 17033654]

Wang, F, Wang, M, Zhao, L & Li, Q (2019) A new biosafe reactive oxygen species responsive nanoplatform for targeted oral squamous cell carcinoma therapy. *Mater Express,* 9, 1076-81.
[http://dx.doi.org/10.1166/mex.2019.1602]

Wang, JL, Tang, GP, Shen, J, Hu, QL, Xu, FJ, Wang, QQ, Li, ZH & Yang, WT (2012) A gene nanocomplex conjugated with monoclonal antibodies for targeted therapy of hepatocellular carcinoma. *Biomaterials,* 33, 4597-607.
[http://dx.doi.org/10.1016/j.biomaterials.2012.02.045] [PMID: 22469295]

Wang, Y, Chen, H, Liu, Y, Wu, J, Zhou, P, Wang, Y, Li, R, Yang, X & Zhang, N (2013) pH-sensitive pullulan-based nanoparticle carrier of methotrexate and combretastatin A4 for the combination therapy against hepatocellular carcinoma. *Biomaterials,* 34, 7181-90.
[http://dx.doi.org/10.1016/j.biomaterials.2013.05.081] [PMID: 23791500]

Wu, B, Liang, Y, Tan, Y, Xie, C, Shen, J, Zhang, M, Liu, X, Yang, L, Zhang, F, Liu, L, Cai, S, Huai, D, Zheng, D, Zhang, R, Zhang, C, Chen, K, Tang, X & Sui, X (2016) Genistein-loaded nanoparticles of star-shaped diblock copolymer mannitol-core PLGA-TPGS for the treatment of liver cancer. *Mater Sci Eng C,* 59, 792-800.
[http://dx.doi.org/10.1016/j.msec.2015.10.087] [PMID: 26652434]

Xia, Y, Zhao, M, Chen, Y, Hua, L, Xu, T, Wang, C, Li, Y & Zhu, B (2018) Folate-targeted selenium nanoparticles deliver therapeutic siRNA to improve hepatocellular carcinoma therapy. *RSC Advances,* 8, 25932-40.
[http://dx.doi.org/10.1039/C8RA04204G]

Xiao, Y, Liu, Y, Yang, S, Zhang, B, Wang, T, Jiang, D, Zhang, J, Yu, D & Zhang, N (2016) Sorafenib and gadolinium co-loaded liposomes for drug delivery and MRI-guided HCC treatment. *Colloids Surf B Biointerfaces,* 141, 83-92.
[http://dx.doi.org/10.1016/j.colsurfb.2016.01.016] [PMID: 26844644]

Yik, JH, Saxena, A & Weigel, PH (2002) The minor subunit splice variants, H2b and H2c, of the human asialoglycoprotein receptor are present with the major subunit H1 in different hetero-oligomeric receptor complexes. *J Biol Chem,* 277, 23076-83.
[http://dx.doi.org/10.1074/jbc.M202748200] [PMID: 11943787]

Yin, D, Yang, Y, Cai, H, Wang, F, Peng, D & He, L (2014) Gambogic acid-loaded electrosprayed particles for site-specific treatment of hepatocellular carcinoma. *Mol Pharm,* 11, 4107-17.
[http://dx.doi.org/10.1021/mp500214a] [PMID: 25290462]

Yordanov, G (2012) Poly (alkyl cyanoacrylate) nanoparticles as drug carriers: 33 years later. *Bulg J Chem,* 1, 61-72.

Zhao, Z, Wang, X, Zhang, Z, Zhang, H, Liu, H, Zhu, X, Li, H, Chi, X, Yin, Z & Gao, J (2015) Real-time monitoring of arsenic trioxide release and delivery by activatable T(1) imaging. *ACS Nano,* 9, 2749-59.

[http://dx.doi.org/10.1021/nn506640h] [PMID: 25688714]

Zhou, Q, Sun, X, Zeng, L, Liu, J & Zhang, Z (2009) A randomized multicenter phase II clinical trial of mitoxantrone-loaded nanoparticles in the treatment of 108 patients with unresected hepatocellular carcinoma. *Nanomedicine,* 5, 419-23.
[http://dx.doi.org/10.1016/j.nano.2009.01.009] [PMID: 19523421]

CHAPTER 6

A Summarized View of Lipid, Polyplex, Inorganic, and Carbon-Based Nanotherapeutics for Hepatocellular Carcinoma Treatment

Riddhi Trivedi[1], **Sanjay Arora**[1], **Richard N. L. Lamptey**[1], **Bivek Chaulagain**[1], **Jagdish Singh**[1,*] and **Buddhadev Layek**[1,*]

[1] *Department of Pharmaceutical Sciences, North Dakota State University, Fargo, North Dakota 58105, USA*

Abstract: Liver cancer is one of the primary causes of global cancer deaths after lung cancer and colorectal cancer. In 2021, an estimated 42,230 new liver cancer cases will be diagnosed, and approximately 30 thousand people will die of these cancers in the United States alone. Hepatocellular carcinoma (HCC) alone accounts for nearly 75% of all liver cancers. Early detection of HCC enables multiple treatment choices resulting in improved therapeutic outcomes. Unfortunately, most HCC cases are typically diagnosed at advanced stages, resulting in poor survival. Among various treatment modalities, chemotherapy remains the mainstay, particularly for treating advanced patients. However, the major drawback of conventional chemotherapeutics is the lack of cancer cell selectivity, leading to significant damage to healthy tissues. These challenges can be circumvented with the help of targeted nanotherapeutics containing anticancer drugs. These nanotherapeutics are increasingly favored over their conventional counterparts due to their specific cancer cell targeting with low off-target effects. Therefore, in this book chapter, we focus on different types of nanocarriers to treat hepatocellular carcinoma. Furthermore, current nanotherapeutics in clinical trials and the future perspective of nanomedicine in liver cancer are discussed.

Keywords: Cancer, Carbon nanotubes, Chemotherapeutics, Chronic hepatitis, Cirrhosis, Drug resistance, Enhanced permeability and retention effect, Fullerenes, Hepatocellular carcinoma, Hepatocytes, Inorganic nanoparticles, Liposomes, Metastases, Micelles, Nanoparticles, Nanostructured lipid carriers, Polyplex, Quantum dots, Solid lipid nanoparticles, Targeted drug delivery.

* **Corresponding authors Buddhadev Layek and Jagdish Singh:** Department of Pharmaceutical Sciences, North Dakota State University, Fargo, North Dakota 58105 USA; Tel: +1(701) 231-7906 (B.L.), +1(701) 231-7943 (J.S.); Fax: +1(701) 231-8333; E-mails: buddhadev.layek@ndsu.edu, Jagdish.Singh@ndsu.edu

INTRODUCTION

Liver cancer is the third leading cause of global cancer death (8.3% of the total cancer deaths) after lung cancer (18.0%) and colorectal cancer (9.4%) (Ferlay J 2020). Liver cancer is much more predominant in Southeast Asia and sub-Saharan Africa than in the USA. In many of these countries, it is the most prevalent cancer type. More than 840,000 people are diagnosed with liver cancer each year globally, in addition to 781,000 annual deaths (Bray *et al.*, 2018). In 2021, an estimated 42,230 new liver cancer cases will be diagnosed, and approximately 30,230 people will die of these cancers in the United States, according to the American Cancer Society (Siegel *et al.*, 2021). More notably, the liver cancer incidence rate has increased more than three times since 1980, while the death rate has more than doubled during this time.

Hepatocellular carcinoma (HCC) alone accounts for nearly 75% of all liver cancers. However, most of these cases are avoidable since majority of the liver cancer risk factors are modifiable. In addition to cirrhosis and chronic liver diseases, excessive alcohol consumption, cigarette smoking, and viral hepatitis (both hepatitis B and hepatitis C) are also the top risk factors of HCC (Crissien and Frenette 2014, Turati *et al.* 2014, Islami *et al.* 2018). Chronic hepatitis C infection is the most critical risk factor and accounts for 1 in 4 liver cancer cases in the USA (Edlin *et al.*, 2015). Cirrhosis can also be developed due to hepatitis, resulting in regenerative nodules due to increased hepatocyte proliferation (Balogh *et al.*, 2016). Therefore, it is believed that improved treatment and vaccination against hepatitis can prevent almost 50% of all HCC worldwide.

Early detection of HCC enables multiple treatment choices resulting in improved outcomes (van Meer *et al.* 2015). Numerous modalities are available for the detection of HCC, like ultrasound, computed tomography (CT) imaging, and magnetic resonance imaging (MRI) (Gish 2014). Biological markers such as serum α-fetoprotein (AFP) and des-γ-carboxy prothrombin (DCP) levels are also used in diagnosing HCC (Balogh *et al.* 2016, Gish 2014). Unfortunately, most HCC cases are typically diagnosed at advanced stages, resulting in poor survival (median survival varies between 6-20 months) (Golabi *et al.*, 2017). Surgical and non-surgical approaches are available to treat HCC. The patients with liver diseases other than cirrhosis undergo surgical resection, which offers the best chances of 5-year survival at 41–74% (Allemann *et al.*, 2013). The surgical removal of the tumor is dependent on its location, size, and remaining liver volume post-surgery. Only patients with confined tumors are suitable for surgical resection (Wong and Frenette 2011). Therefore, candidate selection is a vital part of preventing mortality after surgical procedures. Liver transplantation is also another option for these patients with cirrhosis (Mazzaferro *et al.*, 1996).

Among various treatment modalities, chemotherapy remains the mainstay, particularly for treating advanced cases. For unresectable HCC, sorafenib has been used as the first-line treatment ("EASL Clinical Practice Guidelines: Management of hepatocellular carcinoma," 2018). Various other therapies were evaluated; however, no superior efficacy to sorafenib was found. The major drawback of conventional chemotherapeutics is the lack of cancer cell selectivity, leading to significant damage to healthy tissues. Therefore, it is vital to develop novel approaches that enable the targeted delivery of chemotherapeutics to the tumor tissues while sparing the healthy tissue (Brannon-Peppas and Blanchette 2004). Furthermore, most chemotherapeutic drugs lack adequate aqueous solubility and desired pharmacokinetic profiles, causing poor drug distribution at the tumor sites (Danhier *et al.*, 2010).

These challenges can be circumvented with the help of targeted nanotherapeutics containing anticancer drugs. These nanotherapeutics are increasingly favored over their conventional counterparts due to their specific cancer cell targeting with low off-target effects (Fig. **1**). However, the true potential of these nanotherapeutics can be realized if they can circumvent various biological barriers and deliver therapeutics to the tumor microenvironment (Sriraman *et al.*, 2014, Brigger *et al.*, 2012, Sanna *et al.*, 2014).

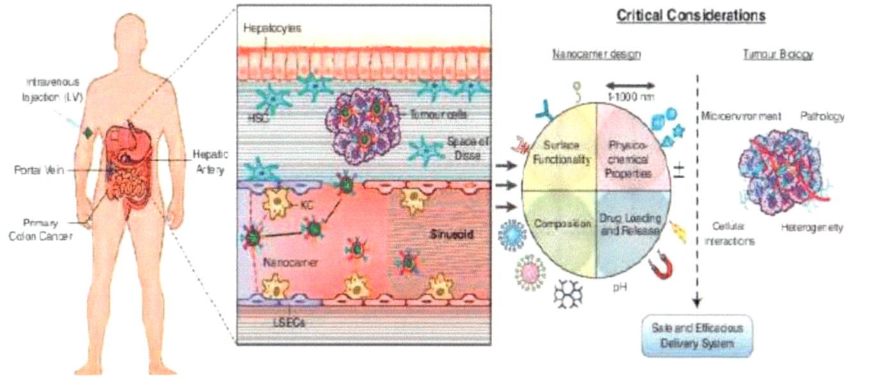

Fig. (1). Schematic representation of nanotherapeutics designed for liver cancer (From Arshad, U, Sutton, PA, Ashford, MB, *et al.* Critical considerations for targeting colorectal liver metastases with nanotechnology. WIREs Nanomed Nanobiotechnol. 2020; 12:e1588, under an open access Creative Commons CC BY license).

The tumor microenvironment contains tumor cells and noncancerous stromal cells, supporting tumor cells in various processes such as proliferation and escaping the immune system (Bissell and Hines 2011). Therefore, for effective treatment, tumor microenvironment modification can be performed by targeting therapeutics to this site (Thakkar *et al.* 2020, Bailey *et al.* 2012). Monumental evidence shows that nanoparticle targeting has led to dose reduction with reduced toxicity. However, there are numerous barriers *in vivo,* resulting in attenuating the effect of these nanotherapeutics at the target site, leading to an increase in drug resistance chances (Tekade and Chougule 2013). This limitation of nanotherapeutics can be worsened if it develops against an entire group of drugs resulting in multidrug resistance.

After the entry of nanoparticles into the systemic circulation, the immune system gets activated, leading to their bloodstream withdrawal. The remaining nanoparticles have to extravasate from the capillaries to the tumor site. Although tumor interstitium also presents a significant barrier, nanoparticles with appropriate physicochemical characteristics can overcome this layer and deliver the therapeutic to the intended site (Thakkar *et al.* 2020). Nanoparticles of various sizes and shapes can be fabricated using diverse materials and their combinations. Different materials are used in preparing these nanoparticles, such as lipids, polymers, inorganic or carbon-based materials (Aghebati-Maleki *et al.* 2020). Based on the material, structure, and surface modifications, these nanoparticles can be modified to achieve the desired characteristics. These properties can include controlled release, protection of therapeutic, small size, targeting, and biocompatibility. Over the last several decades, there has been an exponential advancement in chemistry, biology, polymer science, and physics, resulting in improved nanocarriers for therapeutic delivery (Aghebati-Maleki *et al.* 2020).

In recent years, various nanotherapeutics have been developed for targeting HCC. These nanoparticles have shown promising effects in their preclinical assessment. Therefore, we have discussed various nanotherapeutics investigated for the management of HCC further in detail.

Nanotherapeutics for Hepatocellular Carcinoma (HCC)

Lipid-based Nanotherapeutics

Lipid-based nanotherapeutics have been widely used to enhance the efficacy of chemotherapeutics (Layek *et al.*, 2020). Further, these nanotherapeutics also show the potential to boost the pharmacokinetic profile and stability of the therapeutic agents. Lipid-based nanotherapeutics majorly comprise liposomes, solid lipid nanoparticles (SLNs), and nanostructured lipid carriers (NLCs). The major advantage of employing lipid-based delivery systems is the lipophilicity of several chemotherapeutic agents. Hydrophobic drugs lack dissolution in the aqueous biological environment, leading to low oral bioavailability and poor absorption (Subramaniam *et al.*, 2020). Therefore, lipid-based nanotherapeutics help drug and gene targeting, cellular internalization, and deliver the chemotherapeutics to the site of action.

Nanocarriers can either passively target tumour or actively target it using targeting ligands. The passive tumor targeting is primarily based on the enhanced permeability and retention (EPR) effect (Fig. **2**). In contrast to small-molecule drugs, nanotherapeutics are unable to penetrate through the tight endothelial junctions of healthy blood vessels. Nevertheless, most solid tumors usually have leaky vasculature, enabling nanoparticle extravasation to the tumor tissue (Wu *et al.*, 2018, Iyer *et al.*, 2006, Chow and Ho, 2013). Tumors also lack a fully functional lymphatic drainage system that facilitates nanoparticle accumulation in the tumor tissues (Maeda, 2001, Matsumura and Maeda, 1986, Greish *et al.*, 2003). Therefore, intratumoral nanoparticle concentration is increased by several folds as compared to the healthy tissues. The physicochemical and biological properties of nanotherapeutics can be further improved by altering their composition, morphology, size, or surface functionalization. Active targeting is a promising tool for cancer treatment because of its ability to increase therapeutic effectiveness and minimize potential side effects. These nanocarriers have the ability to incorporate therapeutic agents for secondary or tertiary levels of drug targeting (Mukherjee *et al.*, 2009).

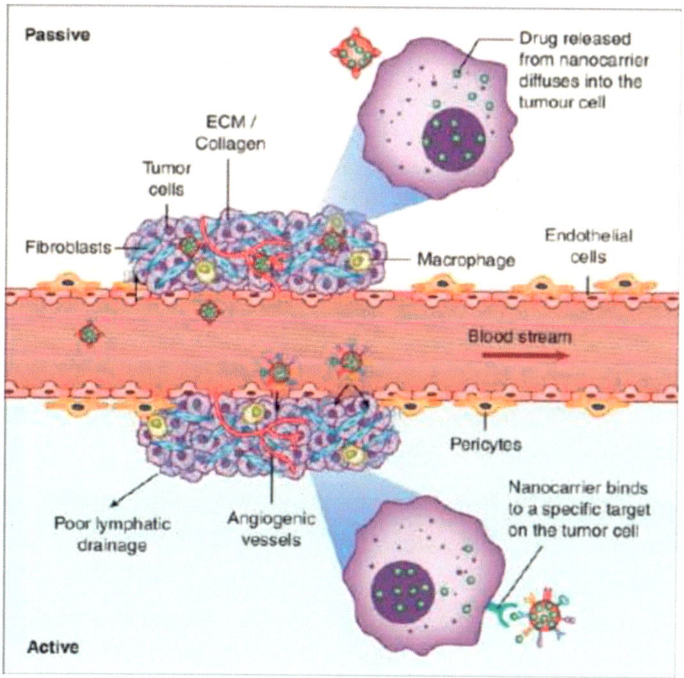

Fig. (2). Schematic representation of passively and actively targeted nanoparticle (NP) delivery systems. (From Arshad, U, Sutton, PA, Ashford, MB *et al.* Critical considerations for targeting colorectal liver metastases with nanotechnology. WIREs Nanomed Nanobiotechnol. 2020; 12:e1588, under an open access Creative Commons CC BY license).

Liposomes

Liposomes are spherical amphiphilic bilayered vesicles that contain an internal aqueous cavity. They are capable of entrapping both hydrophilic and hydrophobic drugs. The hydrophobic drugs are retained on the bilayered lipid membrane, while the hydrophilic drugs can be encapsulated in the central aqueous cavity. When used as a nanocarrier, they offer numerous benefits, including controlled release kinetics, tunable surface modification, which make them "targeted" to the site of action and help minimize toxic effects of the therapeutic agent (Iwasaki *et al.* 2007, Deepak *et al.* 2020). A variety of lipids can be used to formulate liposomes. Cationic lipids are generally preferred for gene delivery as the positive charge enables cationic liposomes to entrap and deliver the genetic materials efficiently. In association with the cationic lipids, neutral lipids have also been employed in gene delivery formulations to circumvent the side effects seen with cationic lipids (Deepak *et al.* 2020). Besides gene delivery, liposomes have been extensively studied as drug carriers. A liposomal formulation containing chemotherapeutic drug doxorubicin, anchored with a 19-amino acid peptide, demonstrated effective targeting in HCC. This peptide chain was used to target hepatic heparan sulfate glycosaminoglycan on the liver cells (Longmuir *et al.*, 2006). These liposomes majorly accumulated in the liver compared to the trace amounts detected in the lung, kidney, and heart (Longmuir *et al.*, 2009).

Efforts have also been made to enhance the targeting efficiencies of liposomes to HCC. The doxorubicin-loaded thermoresponsive liposomal formulation was developed to release encapsulated drugs under mild hyperthermic temperatures for treating HCC (Ponce *et al.* 2006). The liposomal system was formulated using a variety of lipids and a lysolipid. These liposomes demonstrated complete drug release within ~10–20 s at 40–42°C (*i.e.*, main phase transition temperature). The same formulation retained all the encapsulated drugs above or below the main phase transition temperature. This system demonstrated increased drug concentration at the tumor site and improved cytotoxicity of doxorubicin.

Another liposomal formulation was developed to aim at the co-delivery of a vascular endothelial growth factor siRNA (VEGF-siRNA) and hydrophobic chemotherapeutic agent sorafenib for the treatment of HCC (Yao *et al.* 2019). VEGF and its receptor (VEGFR) have a vital role in angiogenesis and cancer cell proliferation. The VEGF-siRNA suppressed tumor growth and angiogenesis, while the chemotherapeutic led to significant cell killing when the formulation was tested on a 2D monolayer and 3D spheroid tumor model.

Apart from developing targeted liposomal drug delivery, the focus has also been shifted to developing theranostics to monitor or diagnose tumors while actively targeting treatment. Liposomes containing CD44 antibodies were developed for molecular imaging and HCC therapy (Wang *et al.*, 2012). An HCC model was developed by an in-situ injection of green fluorescence protein (GFP)-tagged HepG2 cells in mice to monitor tumor progression. The liposomes bearing antibody CD44 were marked with a red fluorescent protein, making it easier to monitor both the tumor and the treatment throughout the therapy with their respective fluorescence.

Liposomal formulations have also been used to prevent multidrug resistance (MDR) of chemotherapeutics. Mitoxantrone encapsulated liposomes were prepared and surface-modified using synthetic polymeric nano-biomaterial (Gal-P123) (Zhang *et al.*, 2012). The polymeric nano-biomaterial was responsible for reversing or preventing MDR. This system demonstrated a significant increase in cytotoxicity and bypassed efflux transporters, responsible for the development of the MDR.

Solid Lipid Nanoparticles (SLNs)

Solid lipid nanoparticles (SLNs) are spherical and formulated using biocompatible and biodegradable lipids. These nanocarriers have a solid lipid core that is stabilized by surfactants. There are several advantages of selecting SLNs as a nanocarrier over other colloidal carriers, such as high and enhanced drug loading, the ability to incorporate hydrophilic and hydrophobic agents, making SLNs a versatile formulation (Layek *et al.* 2020, Mukherjee *et al.* 2009). Apart from these, SLNs are formulated through a water-based technology and avoid organic solvents, and this confers a huge advantage over other nanocarriers. SLNs are also known to be easy to sterilize and scale up. Due to all these advantages, SLNs have been well explored for drug delivery in HCC.

A cationic SLN formulation of resveratrol was formulated for targeting HCC due to the beneficial properties such as increased affinity towards cell membrane and serum proteins, enhanced cellular uptake, and stimulation of cellular receptor interaction (M. Rahman *et al.* 2020). The antitumor and biodistribution study indicated that the cationic SLNs accumulated significantly with higher concentrations resulting in a remarkable reduction in tumor volume compared to the non-ionic SLN and free drug. Similar to resveratrol, other naturally occurring compounds have also shown promising effects on HCC. It is commonly known that such types of agents require a carrier due to their rapid enzymatic degradation in the body. SLN entrapped ganoderic acid, an active constituent extracted from the medicinal mushroom *Ganoderma lucidum*, was formulated to treat HCC (Mahfoozur Rahman *et al.* 2020). The *in vitro* data indicated that the formulation demonstrated a lowered IC_{50} than the free drug. SLNs showed a marked reduction in the size of hepatic nodules and change in the oxidative stress levels in male Wistar rats in a dose-dependent manner.

Considering that the stability of the delivery vehicle is crucial while encapsulating a drug, efforts have been made to develop SLNs that target HCC and are comparatively more stable. Keeping the stability and antitumor efficacy in mind, a nucleoside lipid-based SLN encapsulating sorafenib was developed to target HCC (Benizri *et al.* 2018). Interestingly, the formulated SLNs possessed a parallel-piped structure due to the shape of the nucleolipid used. The stability studies at both 4 and 37 °C demonstrated that even after 30 days, the SLNs retained their initial size. The reason behind the stability reported was π-π stacking, hydrogen bonds, and charge/charge interaction between the nucleolipid and the drug. Enhanced anticancer activity was also seen on liver tumor cells as compared to the free drug.

SLNs have also shown their ability to be compatible with other delivery systems, such as layered double hydroxides (LHD). Co-delivery of drugs without a protected delivery system often results in low bioavailability due to rapid metabolism. Zhu and his co-workers formulated SLNs encapsulating curcumin and LHD modified 5-fluorouracil (5-FU) and evaluated their synergistic anticancer effect (Zhu *et al.*, 2013). Furthermore, LDH-5-FU and SLN-curcumin demonstrated marked synergetic toxicity on SMMC-7721 cells, more significant than that seen with the combination of free drugs. The percentage of apoptosis observed in the cells treated using these formulations was 1.7 times greater compared to the sum of the two carriers used alone.

Nanostructured Lipid Carriers (NLCs)

Nanostructured lipid carriers (NLCs) are said to be an enhanced version of SLNs. NLCs are generally composed of both solid and liquid lipids. Thus, this delivery system has a better drug loading capacity with a lower burst release (Subramaniam *et al.*, 2020). They are also considered superior to other traditional lipid-based nanocarriers due to their improved stability, enhanced drug loading, and better biocompatibility. NLC has been previously administered orally for inflammatory bowel disorders because of their long residence time in the gastrointestinal tract (Liu *et al.*, 2014). Besides, NLCs have also been widely explored for delivering chemotherapeutics such as doxorubicin and paclitaxel through the pulmonary route (Subramaniam *et al.*, 2020). Their versatile compositions make them a good candidate for tailoring them to target drugs to specific sites.

The main problem with the chemotherapeutic agents is their toxic effects on healthy cells. This problem mainly occurs due to the uncontrolled release pattern of the entrapped drug. To address the following problem, Bondì and co-workers developed two different kinds of NLCs comprising tripalmitin solid lipid and a liquid-lipid Captex 355 EP/NF (termed as NLC-A) or Miglyol 812 (termed as NLC-B) (Bondì *et al.* 2015). The drug release profile from NLC-B was similar to the dissolution profile of the free drug. In contrast, NLC-A demonstrated a prolonged release of the drug, reaching a higher concentration of sorafenib at 24 h compared to NLC-B and the free drug. *In vitro* studies on HCC cell lines also demonstrated that both types of NLC had enhanced cytotoxicity compared to the free drug.

The same research group had also tried NLC to deliver epidermal growth factor receptor (EGFR) inhibitor to modulate the regulation of EGFR in HCC (Bondì *et al.*, 2014). The primary reason for choosing NLC as the delivery system was to improve the drug solubility and anticancer activity of this inhibitor. Different types of NLCs were prepared using PEGylated or non-PEGylated solid lipids with or without different liquid lipids. It was seen that the entrapment efficiency was higher for NLC composed of solid and liquid lipids compared with NLCs composed of only solid lipids. The release studies indicated that the non-PEGylated NLCs released the encapsulated drug slower than the PEGylated ones. Apart from having efficient delivery characteristics, these NLCs also demonstrated enhanced inhibition of EGFR and colony formation property of HCC cells compared to the free drug. Table **1** represents a non-exhaustive list of lipid-based formulations investigated for HCC.

Table 1. List of representative lipid-based formulations investigated for hepatocellular carcinoma.

Nanocarriers	Therapeutic Agent	Cell lines/Animal Model	Key Points	References
Liposomes	Cisplatin and curcumin	*In vitro*: HepG2 cells *In vivo*: Mouse hepatoma H22 and human HCC HepG2 xenograft models	• The co-loaded liposomes showed enhanced antitumor efficacy in both mouse hepatoma H22 and human HCC HepG2 xenograft models compared to free drugs or encapsulated mono-drug therapy • Reduced toxicity	(Cheng *et al.* 2018)

(Table 1) cont.....

Nanocarriers	Therapeutic Agent	Cell lines/Animal Model	Key Points	References
Glycyrrhetinic acid (G.A.) and peanut agglutinin (PNA) dual-ligand-modified liposomes	Doxorubicin	*In vitro*: HepG2, MCF-7, and SMMC-7721cells *In vivo*: BALB/c nude mice bearing SMMC-7721 tumors	• The dual-functionalized liposomes demonstrated an excellent antitumor effect *in vitro* and *In vivo* • G.A. and PNA modification led to attractive tumor targeting and attenuated toxic side effects of doxorubicin	(X. Li *et al.* 2020)
Glypican-3 (GPC3)-targeted liposomes	Sorafenib and IR780 iodide (photothermal and near-infrared fluorescence imaging agent)	*In vitro*: HepG2 cells *In vivo*: H22tumor-bearing female K.M. mice	• Facilitate early detection and precise treatment • GPC3-targeted liposomes exhibited better tumor control than folic acid-conjugated liposomes	(Mu *et al.* 2019)
CD147 antibody-conjugated immunoliposomes	Doxorubicin	*In vitro*: Huh-7, HepG2, and HCC3736 cells *In vivo*: BALB/c nude mice bearing Huh-7 xenograft and BALB/c nude mice bearing patient-derived HCC xenograft	• Anti-CD147 immunoliposomes encapsulated doxorubicin demonstrated longer circulation half-life and efficient accumulation in tumors • The immunoliposomal doxorubicin showed superior *in vitro* and *In vivo* antitumor effect	(Wang *et al.* 2018)

(Table 1) cont.....

Nanocarriers	Therapeutic Agent	Cell lines/Animal Model	Key Points	References
Galactosyl conjugated pluronic P123(Gal-P123) modified liposomes	Mitoxantrone	*In vitro*: Huh-7 cells *In vivo*: BALB/c nude mice bearing orthotopic Huh-7 tumors	• Gal-P123 modified mitoxantrone loaded liposomes showed 2.3 times greater cytotoxicity than free mitoxantrone in Huh-7 cells • The liposomal formulation showed prolonged circulation and improved bioavailability of mitoxantrone • Tumor-targeted liposomal formulation of mitoxantrone displayed improved tumor selectivity and enhanced antitumor activity	(Zhang *et al.* 2012)
Cationic SLNs	Resveratrol	*In vitro*: HepG2 cells *In vivo*: Diethyl nitrosamine induced HCC in albino Wister rats	• Resveratrol SLNs demonstrated higher cytotoxicity than resveratrol solution in HepG2 cells • The cationic SLN formulation exhibited significantly ($p < 0.01$) higher tumor accumulation and lower tumor volume than resveratrol solution and resveratrol SLNs	(M. Rahman *et al.* 2020)
SLNs	Ganoderic acid	*In vitro*: HepG2 cells *In vivo*: Diethyl nitrosamine induced HCC in albino Wister rats	• Ganoderic acid SLNs demonstrated higher cytotoxicity than ganoderic solution in HepG2 cells • SLN encapsulated ganoderic acid exhibited a better chemoprotective effect over the free drug	(Mahfoozur Rahman *et al.* 2020)

(Table 1) cont.....

Nanocarriers	Therapeutic Agent	Cell lines/Animal Model	Key Points	References
SLNs	Sorafenib	*In vitro*: Huh-7 and HepG2 cells	• SLN encapsulated sorafenib displayed superior cytotoxicity than the free drug • SLNs encapsulated sorafenib (> 80 μM) exhibited complete cell death	(Benizri *et al.* 2018)
SLNs	Curcumin	*In vitro*: SMMC-7721 cells	• LDH-5-FU and SLN-curcumin combination prompted ~80% apoptosis in SMMC-7721 cells • LDH-5-FU and SLN-curcumin displayed substantial cytotoxicity against SMMC-7721 cell than free drug combination	(Zhu *et al.* 2013)
Galactosylated SLNs	Docetaxel	*In vitro*: BEL7402 cells *In vivo*: Female nude mice bearing hepatoma	• Galactosylated SLNs showed superior *in vitro* cytotoxicity compared to Taxotere® and non-targeted SLNs • Targeted SLNs also demonstrated superior antitumor efficacy and tolerance than Taxotere® or non-targeted SLNs	(Xu *et al.* 2009)
NLCs	Sorafenib	*In vitro*: Hep3B, Huh-7, and PLC/PRF/5 cells	• Lipid nanoparticles demonstrated good hemocompatibility under chosen experimental conditions • Sorafenib loaded NLCs showed superior *in vitro* toxicity than free drug	(Bondì *et al.* 2015)
NLCs	Tyrphostin AG-1478 (EGFR inhibitor)	*In vitro*: HA22T/VGH cells	• NLC-loaded tyrphostin AG-1478 exhibited improved antitumor activity compared to the free drug *in vitro*	(Bondì *et al.* 2014)

(Table 1) cont.....

Nanocarriers	Therapeutic Agent	Cell lines/Animal Model	Key Points	References
Lipid nanoparticles (LNPs)	N-acetylgalactosamine (NAcGal) modified doxorubicin and sorafenib	*In vitro*: HepG2 cells *In vivo*: BALB/c nude mice bearing HepG2 xenograft	• NAcGal functionalized LNPs showed considerably higher cellular uptake than unmodified LNPs. • NAcGal modified and pH-sensitive LNPs system displayed the highest tumor growth inhibition and the lowest systemic toxicity	(Duan and Liu 2018)
LNPs	Interleukin-12 mRNA	*In vivo*: MYC-induced HCC transgenic mice	• Treatment with LNP-loaded IL-12 mRNA significantly reduced liver tumor burden and increased survival in comparison to control mice • Prevented tumor growth without damaging surrounding healthy cells	(Lai *et al.* 2018)

Polymer-Based Nanotherapeutics

Among various delivery systems, polymeric nanocarriers offer several advantages, such as tunable size, transformable surface, prolonged blood circulation time, and higher accumulation at the target site (Yao *et al.*, 2020, Agarwal *et al.*, 2019). Thus, polymeric nanoparticles have been widely used to deliver numerous drugs, genes, biomolecules, and vaccines to the desired site of action (Wang *et al.*, 2019, Layek *et al.*, 2015, Layek and Singh, 2019, Yao *et al.*, 2020). Polymer-based nanocarriers include polymeric micelles, polyplexes, polymeric nanoparticles, and polymer-drug conjugates. Both natural and synthetic polymers can be used to formulate these nanocarriers. The selection of polymers mostly depends on the size of the desired nanocarrier, properties of the therapeutic agent to be administered, surface modifications for targeted delivery, the desired drug release profile, and the final product's antigenicity (Kumar *et al.*, 2012, Ferrari *et al.*, 2018). Polymeric nanocarriers have also been widely explored in delivering chemotherapeutics in various cancers, including HCC.

Polymeric Micelles

Amphiphilic polymers are self-assembled in an aqueous milieu to form polymeric micelles. Above the critical micellar concentration (CMC), these polymers self-assemble into micelles. Micelles are spherical-shaped colloidal particles in the nanoscale range and can effectively deliver drugs and genes to treat various diseases. Polymeric micelles offer several benefits, including increased drug solubility, improved physiological stability, higher bioavailability, better cellular uptake, lower cytotoxicity, and enhanced targeting ability (Majumder *et al.*, 2020). Despite these advantages, as mentioned earlier, the development of drug or gene-loaded micelles has faced some challenges. The significant problems of polymeric micelles are low loading efficiency and difficulty translocating across cell membranes. Several attempts have been made with micellar systems to enhance their payload capacity, controlled release profile, and genetic material encapsulation (Majumder *et al.* 2020, Layek *et al.* 2014, Layek and Singh 2013b, Chen *et al.* 2018).

Amongst various drug delivery systems, polymeric micelles have shown promising results for tumor-targeted delivery of chemotherapeutics. They are primarily chosen due to their quick and straightforward preparation method and thermodynamic stability under physiological conditions (Prabhu *et al.*, 2015). One such system consisting of block copolymer polyphosphoester and poly(ε-caprolactone) was formulated for receptor-mediated drug delivery in HCC (Wang *et al.*, 2008). This micellar formulation was used for targeting asialoglycoprotein receptors on liver cells utilizing its ligand galactosamine, which was surface conjugated on these micelles. This modification resulted in enhanced cell surface binding and internalization, as demonstrated using flow cytometry. Drug-loaded surface-modified micelles also showed improved cytotoxicity on liver tumor cells in comparison with drug-containing unmodified micelles.

Self-assembling polymeric micelles have also been used to deliver natural agents to treat HCC. The hydrophobic core of these micellar systems allows entrapment of hydrophobic agents resulting in enhanced bioavailability of chemotherapeutic agents. The clinical application of ursolic acid, found in many dietary plants, was limited due to its hydrophobic nature. Zhou and his co-workers developed the ursolic acid-loaded polymer micelles (UA-PMs) for enhancing its antitumor effect against HCC (Zhou *et al.* 2019). *In vitro* data demonstrated tumor cell proliferation inhibition without affecting the proliferation of normal liver cells when treated with these polymeric micelles. *In vivo* study also revealed that these nano micelles could significantly retard H22 xenograft tumor growth, leading to the prolonged survival time of tumor-bearing mice.

Apart from the self-assembling polymeric micelles, the focus has been shifted to formulate micelles using more biocompatible and biodegradable components. An effort was made to develop glycyrrhetinicacid (GA) modified doxorubicin micelles to treat HCC (Fan *et al.*, 2018). Gelatin was chosen to formulate micelles due to its biocompatible and biodegradable nature. It is also a substrate of matrix metalloproteinase-2 (MMP-2), thus quickly releasing the encapsulated drug *via* its degradation at the tumor sites. These micelles were also surface modified with GA to bind GA-receptor on hepatic cells for HCC targeting. The efficient liver-targeting activity of these micelles was demonstrated *via in vivo* imaging analysis, indicating their major distribution to the liver and H22 orthotopic tumor site. Also, doxorubicin-loaded micelles exhibited better antitumor activity against H22 orthotopic tumors compared to the free drug.

Polyplex

The complexes between genetic materials and polymers are known as polyplexes. These polyplexes are formed due to electrostatic interactions between the cationic polymer and the negatively charged nucleic acids. The primary role of polyplexes is to protect the nucleic acids from DNase degradation and release the therapeutic agent at the target site (Layek and Singh 2013a, Layek and Singh 2017, Diamantopoulou *et al.* 2017, Kandasamy *et al.* 2020). Polyplexes, being a non-viral gene delivery system, have several advantages over viral vectors, such as better cell or tissue targeting, ease of production, and low immune response. The only setback of using non-viral vectors is their low transfection efficiency. However, polyplexes can be optimized, and their physicochemical properties can be tuned to achieve better results (Prabhu *et al.*, 2015). Due to the cationic nature of these polyplexes, they demonstrate a better association with negatively charged cell surfaces resulting in enhanced cell uptake.

Additionally, PEGylation of the polyplexes can help reduce their interactions with plasma proteins and erythrocytes to achieve a longer circulation time. However, the significant limiting steps for gene transfer through polyplexes are cell surface binding, endosomal escape, translocation to the nucleus, and intracellular unpacking of the polyplexes. A better understanding of these steps could help optimize this delivery system to overcome the barriers and achieve better transfection yields.

siRNAs suppress the expression of the gene through the degradation of mRNA in the cytosol. However, one of the significant challenges of siRNA is their intracellular delivery at active form. Several groups have tried to improve this shortfall by delivering siRNA with the help of polyplexes. Gossart *et al.* modified pyridylthiourea-polyethyleneimine polymer, having the ability to rupture/disassemble in the endosomal acidic environment (Gossart *et al.* 2017). Specifically, pyridylthiourea polymer was responsible for enhancing the hydrophobicity of the polyplex and increased interaction with siRNA. These pH-responsive polyplexes considerably improved the siRNA delivery efficiency to monolayer cells as well as in the spheroid model, demonstrating 90% and 60% cell death, respectively.

The asialoglycoprotein receptor (ASGPR) is overexpressed in HCC cells as compared to normal and healthy hepatocytes. Taking this into consideration, Perrone *et al.* developed a polyplex for targeted siRNA delivery to hepatocytes using the synthetic polymer α,β-poly- (N-2-hydroxyethyl)-D, L-aspartam- -(PHEA) derivatized with diethylenetriamine (DETA) (Perrone *et al.* 2020). As galactose residue can be used to target the ASGPR on the HCC cells, they linked galactose (GAL) to the side chain bearing polyethylene glycol (PEG) to obtain PHEA-DETA-PEG-GAL, PDPG copolymer. This polymeric system demonstrated siRNA protection against degradation by forming a complex and effectively targeting the cancer cells. Due to its efficient targeting property, the off-target effects of this system were found to be minimal.

Apart from gene delivery, polyplexes have also been explored for the co-delivery of drugs and genes for increasing the efficacy of the treatment. One such example is the co-delivery of liver-specific miRNA-122 and chemotherapeutic drug 5-FU in galactosylated chitosan polyplex (Ning *et al.* 2019). The miR-122 was selected due to its abundance and specificity for liver tissue. Additionally, miR-122 can target crucial mediators like ADAM 10 and 17, Bcl-2, and Wnt1, responsible for inhibiting angiogenesis, hepatocarcinogenesis, and epithelial-mesenchymal transition. These are also involved in hepatocytes regulation and differentiation. Therefore, the formulated system displayed enhanced stability, efficient proliferation inhibition, apoptosis of HCC cells, and downregulated expression of Bcl-2 and ADAM17.

Polymeric Nanoparticles

Polymeric nanoparticles are ubiquitous nanocarriers used in cancer therapy, especially those that are made using biodegradable polymers such as poly(lactic-co-glycolic acid) (PLGA), chitosan, alginates, *etc.* (Lu *et al.*, 2018, Karlsson *et al.*, 2018). Among different polymeric nanomaterials, PLGA nanoparticles have been widely used to encapsulate both hydrophilic and hydrophobic drugs (Español *et al.*, 2016). Furthermore, the presence of active functional groups on PLGA allows for easy ligand attachment for tumor targeting.

Similarly, chitosan and its derivatives are frequently used in formulating nanoparticles due to their biocompatibility, biodegradability, nontoxicity, and low immunogenicity. Chitosan-based nanoparticles are also easy to synthesize, exhibit good mucoadhesion and tissue permeation properties, and offer sustained drug release. Moreover, abundant primary amine and hydroxyl groups on the chitosan backbone make it amenable for easy chemical modifications to accomplish desired functional characteristics (Bonferoni *et al.*, 2020, Fu *et al.*, 2016). Chitosan alone or a combination of chitosan-PLGA have been employed in encapsulating various anticancer drugs like hydroxycamptothecin (Han *et al.*, 2015), doxorubicin (Ye *et al.*, 2018), piceatannol (Dhanapal and Balaraman Ravindrran, 2018), and conjugated with CD147 antibody (Zhu *et al.*, 2015) for the targeting and treatment of HCC. Another promising HCC targeted formulation was NP-TPGS-SFB, which included sorafenib (SFB) encapsulated within the biodegradable polymers poly(amidoamine)-poly(γ-benzyl-L-Glutamate--b-D-α-tocopheryl polyethylene glycol 1000 succinate (PAM-PBLG-*b*-TPGS). These nanoparticles exhibited acid-responsive drug release and excellent stability. Compared to the free drug and PEG-coated nanoparticles (NP-PEG-SFB), NP-TPGS-SFB exhibited higher cellular uptake and significantly inhibited tumor growth in HepG2 xenograft mice models (Zihuang Li *et al.*, 2020). Polymeric nanoparticles have been widely exploited due to their tunability and targeting efficiency while being stable, biodegradable, and biocompatible, making them an ideal delivery system for targeting HCC.

Polymer Drug Conjugates

Polymer therapeutics has become an effective and efficient approach for drug delivery, where the therapeutic moiety is linked covalently to the polymer instead of being encapsulated within. The concept of polymer-anticancer conjugates was first proposed in 1975, and their rationale for design and mechanism of action was documented later on in 1992 and 2003 (Duncan 2003). Tumor-specific targeting through the EPR effect can be achieved using polymer-drug conjugates, leading to significant tumor-targeting more than 10-100 fold compared to the free drug (Matsumura Y Fau - Maeda and Maeda). Doxorubicin conjugated with a water-soluble polymer N-(2-hydroxypropyl) methacrylamide (HPMA) has been an effective delivery system to target hepatocellular carcinoma and has completed Phase I clinical trials (*i.e.*, PK1) (Luo *et al.*, 2002, Ekladious *et al.*, 2019, Elnaggar *et al.*, 2021).

Synthesizing polymer conjugates with ligands can lead to more efficient targeting. One such ligand, folic acid, is commonly used in targeted drug delivery due to the overexpression of folate receptors on cancerous cells. PEG was conjugated with two units of folic acid and fluorescein isothiocyanate (ASGPR) through a chemo-enzymatic synthetic process to target HCC in rats. Increased specific uptake of this delivery system was seen in the liver tumor region, evidenced by strong signals of FITC. The PEG polymer enhanced the water solubility and provided flexibility to this system to allow better interaction with folate receptors on cell surfaces (Koirala *et al.*, 2019). Another polymer-drug conjugate, galactosylated pullulan–curcumin (LANH2-Pu Ald-Cur SA) system, was formulated to target HCC. This system exhibited higher specificity and internationalization in HepG2 cells, which indicated uptake *via* ASGPR mediated endocytosis. Although less common than the other polymeric delivery systems mentioned above, polymer-drug conjugates have proven to effectively target the liver for HCC treatment (Sarika *et al.*, 2015).

Inorganic Nanoparticles

Inorganic nanoparticles are an emerging and promising area of cancer nanomedicine due to their potential benefits over the traditional carrier systems comprising polymeric or lipid carriers. High surface area to volume ratio, long-term stability, passive accumulation at the tumor sites because of the EPR effect, easy functionalization, and presence of optical, electrical, or magnetic properties make them an attractive option for drug targeting and delivery in cancer (Luther *et al.*, 2020). Additionally, inorganic nanoparticles are also increasingly finding their foothold in diagnostics and imaging apart from therapeutic interventions. Gold, silica, platinum, iron oxide are commonly used materials for the fabrication of inorganic nanoparticles. Hensify®, a Hafnium oxide-based nanoparticle, is an example of a recently approved inorganic nanoparticle-based therapy (approved by the European Medicines Agency in 2019). It is used for radiotherapy of locally advanced soft tissue sarcoma. It has also been in multiple clinical trials for other cancer types such as prostate cancer, rectal cancer, or liver cancer (Huang *et al.*, 2020). We present some notable studies performed in the area of inorganic nanoparticles specifically focused on the therapeutic management of HCC.

Gold nanoparticles are the most frequently used class of inorganic nanomaterials against liver cancer due to their flexibility. They can be employed either as diagnostic agents due to their potential in imaging or as therapeutic agents in photothermal, radiotherapy, or targeted therapy (Taghizadeh *et al.*, 2019). Radiotherapy and photothermal therapies provide tangible benefits when used in conjunction with chemotherapy. Gao *et al.* fabricated paclitaxel encapsulated gold nanoparticles using galactose as targeting moiety against ASGPR, predominantly expressed in liver tumors (Gao *et al.*, 2017). The targeted nanoparticle uptake was six times higher than that of non-targeted gold nanoparticles in the HepG2 cell line, and drug localization in the liver was increased by 15.7 times compared to non-targeted controls. The tumor reduction was observed in both heterotopic and orthotopic mouse models, where the tumor sizes after 10 days of treatment were 0.75 and 0.37 times, respectively, compared to non-targeted controls. Gold nanoparticles also find their application as a gene delivery agent to treat liver cancer. Share *et al.* used PEI-modified gold nanoparticles to conjugate siRNA against oncogene c-Myc in liver cancer (Shaat *et al.*, 2016). This carrier system efficiently silenced the gene and diminished the protein levels coded by the c-Myc gene in Huh7 cells.

Silica is also another frequently used inorganic material for anticancer drug delivery. Li *et al.* synthesized mesoporous silica nanorattles using anticancer drug docetaxel and found its efficacy in both *in vitro* and *in vivo* hepatic cancer models (Li *et al.*, 2010). The IC_{50} values of the silica nanorattles were 7% of the free drug in HepG2 cells, and they achieved 15% greater tumor growth inhibition compared to the marketed formulation of docetaxel on the subcutaneous hepatocarcinoma model. Tyrosine kinase inhibitors (TKI), sorafenib and sunitinib, are the first-line drug regimen for advanced end-stage liver cancer. However, they come with the shortcomings of low bioavailability and low aqueous solubility. Sedighi *et al.* formulated mesoporous silica nanoparticles to improve the bioavailability of TKIs (Sedighi *et al.*, 2020). Mesoporous silica nanoparticles preserved the drugs in their amorphous form within their core to improve bioavailability but faced challenges like burst release, aggregation, and low cellular internalization to prevent its therapeutic translation. The researchers fabricated a dual system comprising amine-functionalized mesoporous silica nanoparticles capped by cerium oxide nanoparticles (CNPs) to solve these challenges associated with silica nanoparticles. Sorafenib and sunitinib-loaded systems showed increased cytotoxic profiles and enhanced apoptotic activity than the free drug studied in HepG2, Huh7, and Hep3b cell lines.

Shoshan *et al.* recently reported a promising finding against hepatic carcinoma using another inorganic material, platinum (Shoshan *et al.*, 2019). They found that platinum nanoparticles in a size range of 2.5 nm stabilized by the peptide coating were preferentially distributed in the hepatic carcinoma cell lines and found to be more toxic than cisplatin. Platinum employed in these nanoparticles was in the form of inert Pt^0 atoms. Liver cancer cells, where reactive oxygen species are abundant, convert the Pt^0 to more cytotoxic form Pt^{II} to precipitate its anticancer activity. Cisplatin or other platinum-based drugs are notorious for their non-selectivity and extreme side effects. However, the peptide-coated platinum nanoparticles were free of such problems and opened doors to platinum-based therapeutics in liver cancer, with more *in vivo* studies warranted in the future.

Lunov *et al.* reported the use of superparamagnetic iron oxide nanoparticles (SPIONs) to induce apoptosis non-invasively in liver cancer using magnetic force (Lunov *et al.* 2019). They synthesized carboxydextran coated SPIONs averaging 60 nm in diameter and tested their efficacy against three liver cancer cell lines HepG2, Huh7, and Alexander. After the lysosomal uptake of SPIONs, the cells were exposed to a pulsed magnetic field (PMF), generating a 700pN or higher magnetic force to disrupt the lysosomes. It resulted in lysosomal membrane permeabilization (LMP), culminating in a cascade of events leading to cell apoptosis. The system was efficacious in the three-dimensional cell culture model as well but remains to be tested *in vivo* animal models yet.

Quantum dots, also referred to as nanocrystals of semiconducting material, are another class of inorganic particles that exhibit the properties between atoms or bulk semiconductor materials due to their size ranging from 1–10 nm and are increasingly being used in nanomedicine for therapeutic and diagnostic applications. Ahmad *et al.* fabricated the quantum dots of zinc oxide at a size range of 5 ± 2 nm and studied its anticancer effect on HepG2 cells (Ahmad *et al.*, 2015). The ZnO quantum dots resulted in enhanced cytotoxicity and an alteration in the cellular level of mRNA of apoptotic markers (Bcl2, p53, Bax, Caspase-3), the cumulative effect of which led to increased apoptosis. Similarly, Li *et al.* synthesized cadmium tellurium (CDTe) quantum dots and tested their efficacy against liver cancer cell lines (Li *et al.*, 2017). Quantum dots produced higher amounts of ROS inside the hepatocarcinoma cell lines suggesting the enhanced cytotoxicity of quantum dots against liver cancer cell lines. Further, efficacy studies are required in animal models for broader application in the future.

Inorganic nanoparticles have evolved as a promising armament in the arsenal of anticancer agents in the fight against HCC. Numerous studies have shown positive benefits in various liver cancer models *in vitro*. However, there remains a lack of comprehensive *in vivo* studies to support the claim observed so far. The paucity of *in vivo* studies is due to the difficulties in replicating the outcomes observed during *in vitro* animal models. With the advent of more studies in the coming future, we can expect inorganic nanoparticles to create a potential mark in the fight against liver cancer.

Carbon-Based Nanotherapeutics

The efficient use of carbon-based nanoparticles in modern medicine is a research focus that has attracted much interest, both in medicine and engineering. This interest is attributable to the desired physical and chemical properties of these carbon-based nanoparticles. Pristine carbon-based nanoparticles are mostly hydrophobic and present as small-sized molecules. These nanoparticles are routinely functionalized to produce formulations with desired properties. This malleability makes them favorable as a therapeutic tool. Carbon-based nanoparticles are used both in diagnosis and drug delivery. Two primary carboncarbon-based nanoparticles with much interest in drug delivery are the fullerenes and the carbon nanotubes (CNTs).

Fullerenes

Fullerenes, also known as buckyballs, are of exceptional interest in drug delivery due to their unique carbon cage structure (R. Bakry *et al.*, 2007). Fullerenes are simple conjoined carbon molecules that assume a hollow, ring-like, spherical, or ellipsoidal shape. In addition to their cage-like property, fullerenes are hydrophobic, small in size, have a three-dimensional structure and electronic configuration, which allow their conjugation with diverse therapeutics. The most studied fullerenes are the C60 and C70 molecules. Furthermore, the possible functionalization of fullerene surface to yield derivatives with desirable pharmacokinetic properties inspires more interest in their studies.

In HCC, excessive reactive species production is associated with disease pathology. This makes the use of pristine and functionalized fullerenes suitable in HCC due to their antioxidant properties. Kuznietsova *et al.* observed the effect of water-soluble pristine C60 fullerene in a rat HCC model (H. Kuznietsova *et al.*, 2020). The study revealed that C60 fullerene was capable of inhibiting the HepG2 cell growth, along with apoptosis induction, downregulation of glucose--phosphate dehydrogenase, and upregulation of vimentin and p53 expression, and ultimately, altered redox state. *In vivo* studies with HCC at the liver cirrhosis stage also showed that exposure to 0.25mg/kg/day of C60 fullerene and 5-FU treatment resulted in comparable post-treatment survival. Overall, the study concluded that C60 fullerene could inhibit HCC tumor growth and metastasis, thereby improving animal survival.

In a separate study, Sosnowska *et al.* observed that the mechano-signaling induced by fullerene C60 nanofilms arrested the cell cycle in the G2/M phase and decreased hepatocyte cancer proliferation (Sosnowska *et al.*, 2019). In this study, the nanofilms were used to mimic the extracellular matrix and aid in maintaining physicochemical properties. HepG2 and C3A cancer cells were cultured on fullerene nanofilm, and cell viability and proliferation were measured. The experiment revealed the desirable biocompatibility of fullerenes nanofilm and the suitability of fullerene nanofilms as a substitute component for the niche of cancer cells.

The use of C60 has been studied in other related conditions, including cholangitis, where C60 fullerene nanoparticles were shown to inhibit liver inflammation and fibrogenesis (H. M. Kuznietsova *et al.*, 2020). However, the difficult processability of fullerenes prevents their widespread applications in medicine (Rania Bakry *et al.*, 2007, Rašović, 2017). Several studies also report their various toxicities (Chen *et al.*, 2012). Water-soluble fullerene derivatives appeared as less cytotoxic than pristine fullerenes. Also, $C_{60}(OH)_{24}$ derivatives showed no cytotoxicity within their solubility limit, suggesting the importance of functionalization to minimize toxicity (Chen *et al.* 2012, Yamawaki and Iwai, 2006).

Carbon Nanotubes (CNTs)

CNTs are cylinder-shaped macromolecules with a radius in the nanometer scale (Kostarelos *et al.*, 2009). They have a high surface-to-weight ratio, excellent chemical stability, and a rich electronic polyaromatic structure, which gives them desirable electrochemical properties and mechanical strength (Kamedulski *et al.* 2020). These features have inspired interest in the use of carbon nanotubes in diverse medical applications.

CNTs are proposed as excellent drug delivery tools because of their ability to deliver drugs directly into cells without metabolism by the body (He *et al.*, 2013). The most critical property of CNTs is their ability to adsorb or conjugate multifunctional therapeutics, such as small molecules, antibodies, genes, peptides, enzymes, DNA, *etc.*, making them excellent carriers (He *et al.*, 2013). With the rising interest in controlled drug delivery, CNTs have been proposed as a suitable candidate to provide anticipated effect (Newland *et al.*, 2015).

In a study by Elsayed *et al.*, the multikinase inhibitor sorafenib was physically adsorbed on functionalized CNTs, and the therapeutic efficacy was compared with free sorafenib (Elsayed *et al.*, 2019). Their study showed that cancer suppression of CNT conjugated sorafenib was superior to free sorafenib in HepG2 cells and the DENA-induced HCC rat model.

A drawback of the extensive use of pristine CNTs in biomedicine is their hydrophobic surfaces, which renders them insoluble in aqueous solutions. Nonetheless, several surface-functionalized nanotubes have been synthesized to produce desirable properties for medicinal use while maintaining biocompatibility and low toxicity (He *et al.*, 2013). The functionalization of CNTs largely influences their pharmacokinetic and pharmacodynamic profiles.

Nanotherapeutics Under Clinical Trials

Although several FDA-approved nanomedicines are available for treating various cancers, there is still no nanomedicine approved for liver cancer (Layek *et al.*, 2020). However, many nanotherapeutics are currently undergoing different clinical development phases or awaiting approval (Table **2**).

Table 2. List of nanotherapeutics currently under different phases of clinical trials to treat HCC.

Product Name (Development Phase)	Formulation/treatment	Indication	Route of Administration	Sponsor	Current Status	ClinicalTrials.gov Identifiers
PLM60 (Phase I)	Liposome-entrapped mitoxantrone hydrochloride	Advanced hepatocellular carcinoma	Intravenous infusion	CSPC ZhongQi Pharmaceutical Technology Co., Ltd.	Not yet recruiting	NCT04331743
NBTXR3 (Phase I/II)	Hafnium oxide nanoparticles (radio enhancer) activated by stereotactic body radiation therapy	Liver cancer	Intralesional or intraarterial injection	Nanobiotix	Active, not recruiting	NCT02721056
MTL-CEBPA (Phase I)	SMARTICLES• liposomal nanoparticle encapsulating CEBPA-51	Advanced liver cancer	Intravenous injection	Mina Alpha Limited	Unknown	NCT02716012
Lyso-thermosensitive liposomal doxorubicin (Phase I)	Lyso-thermosensitive liposomal doxorubicin and MR-HIFU	Pediatric cancer, Solid tumors, Rhabdomyosarcoma, Ewing sarcoma, Soft tissue sarcomas, Osteosarcoma, Neuroblastoma, Wilms tumor, Hepatic tumor, Germ cell tumors	Intravenous injection	AeRang Kim	Recruiting	NCT02536183
DCR-MYC (Phase I/II)	EnCore™ lipid nanoparticle encapsulating DsiRNA targeting MYC mRNA	Hepatocellular carcinoma	Intravenous infusion	Dicerna Pharmaceuticals, Inc.	Terminated (sponsor decision)	NCT02314052
TKM-080301 (Phase I/II)	Lipid nanoparticles encapsulating siRNA against PLK 1	Hepatocellular carcinoma	Intravenous infusion	Arbutus Biopharma Corporation	Completed	NCT02191878
TARDOX (Phase I)	Lyso-thermosensitive liposomal doxorubicin (ThermoDox•) activated by focused ultrasound-mediated hyperthermia	Liver tumor	Intravenous infusion	University of Oxford	Completed	NCT02181075
MRX34 (Phase I)	Double-stranded RNA mimic of miR-34 encapsulated in liposomes	Primary liver cancer, Lymphoma, Melanoma, SCLC, Renal cell carcinoma, Multiple myeloma, NSCLC	Intravenous injection	Mirna Therapeutics, Inc.	Terminated (five immune-related serious adverse events)	NCT01829971
ThermoDox (Phase III)	Thermally sensitive liposomal doxorubicin with radiofrequency ablation	Hepatocellular carcinoma	Intravenous infusion	Celsion	Completed	NCT00617981
Lipodox (Phase I)	Doxorubicin HCl liposome	Childhood soft tissue sarcoma and liver cancer, Bone cancer, Kidney tumor, Brain tumor	Intravenous infusion	National Cancer Institute (NCI)	Completed	NCT00019630

CEBPA: CCAAT/enhancer-binding protein alpha; DsiRNA: Dicer substrate small interfering RNA; PLK 1: polo-like-kinase 1

CONCLUSION

Over the last few decades, there has been tremendous progress in nanotechnology that resulted in the development of several marketed cancer nanotherapeutics. Still, nanomedicines are in their infancy, and there is enormous scope for improvement. Appropriately designed nanomedicines have the potential to overcome challenges associated with conventional chemotherapeutics by improving their tumor accumulation either by passive or active targeting while sparing the healthy tissues. Moreover, current chemotherapeutics used in liver cancer treatment can be formulated in nanomedicines to enhance their pharmacokinetic profile, improve tumor selectivity, and minimize adverse side effects.

CONSENT FOR PUBLICATION

Not applicable.

CONFLICT OF INTEREST

The authors declare no conflict of interest, financial or otherwise.

ACKNOWLEDGMENTS

This work was supported by the National Institutes of Health Grant R01AG051574 and RF1 AG068034. Buddhadev Layek also acknowledges support from the NIGMS COBRE award 1P20 GM109024 and DaCCoTA CTR pilot feasibility grant U54GM128729.

REFERENCES

Agarwal, S, Dominic, A & Wasnik, S (2019) An overview of polymeric nanoparticles as potential cancer therapeutics. In: Kesharwani, P., Paknikar, K.M., Gajbhiye, V., (Eds.), *Polymeric Nanoparticles as a Promising Tool for Anti-cancer Therapeutics* Academic Press 21-34. [http://dx.doi.org/10.1016/B978-0-12-816963-6.00002-9]

Aghebati-Maleki, A, Dolati, S, Ahmadi, M, Baghbanzhadeh, A, Asadi, M, Fotouhi, A, Yousefi, M & Aghebati-Maleki, L (2020) Nanoparticles and cancer therapy: Perspectives for application of nanoparticles in the treatment of cancers 235, 1962-72. [http://dx.doi.org/10.1002/jcp.29126]

Ahmad, J, Wahab, R, Siddiqui, MA, Musarrat, J & Al-Khedhairy, AA (2015) Zinc oxide quantum dots: a potential candidate to detain liver cancer cells. *Bioprocess Biosyst Eng,* 38, 155-63. [http://dx.doi.org/10.1007/s00449-014-1254-x] [PMID: 25073692]

Allemann, P, Demartines, N, Bouzourene, H, Tempia, A & Halkic, N (2013) Long-term outcome after liver resection for hepatocellular carcinoma larger than 10 cm. *World J Surg,* 37, 452-8. [http://dx.doi.org/10.1007/s00268-012-1840-5] [PMID: 23188527]

Bailey, KM, Wojtkowiak, JW, Hashim, AI & Gillies, RJ (2012) Targeting the metabolic microenvironment of tumors. *Adv Pharmacol,* 65, 63-107.

[http://dx.doi.org/10.1016/B978-0-12-397927-8.00004-X] [PMID: 22959024]

Bakry, R, Vallant, RM, Najam-ul-Haq, M, Rainer, M, Szabo, Z, Huck, CW & Bonn, GK (2007) Medicinal applications of fullerenes. *Int J Nanomedicine,* 2, 639-49.
[PMID: 18203430]

Balogh, J, Victor, D, III, Asham, EH, Burroughs, SG, Boktour, M, Saharia, A, Li, X, Ghobrial, RM & Monsour, HP, Jr (2016) Hepatocellular carcinoma: a review. *J Hepatocell Carcinoma,* 3, 41-53.
[http://dx.doi.org/10.2147/JHC.S61146] [PMID: 27785449]

Benizri, S, Ferey, L, Alies, B, Mebarek, N, Vacher, G, Appavoo, A, Staedel, C, Gaudin, K & Barthélémy, P (2018) Nucleoside-Lipid-Based Nanocarriers for Sorafenib Delivery. *Nanoscale Res Lett,* 13, 17-7.
[http://dx.doi.org/10.1186/s11671-017-2420-2] [PMID: 29327307]

Bissell, MJ & Hines, WC (2011) Why don't we get more cancer? A proposed role of the microenvironment in restraining cancer progression. *Nat Med,* 17, 320-9.
[http://dx.doi.org/10.1038/nm.2328] [PMID: 21383745]

Bondì, ML, Azzolina, A, Craparo, EF, Botto, C, Amore, E, Giammona, G & Cervello, M (2014) Entrapment of an EGFR inhibitor into nanostructured lipid carriers (NLC) improves its antitumor activity against human hepatocarcinoma cells. *J Nanobiotechnology,* 12, 21-1.
[http://dx.doi.org/10.1186/1477-3155-12-21] [PMID: 24886097]

Bondì, ML, Botto, C, Amore, E, Emma, MR, Augello, G, Craparo, EF & Cervello, M (2015) Lipid nanocarriers containing sorafenib inhibit colonies formation in human hepatocarcinoma cells. *Int J Pharm,* 493, 75-85.
[http://dx.doi.org/10.1016/j.ijpharm.2015.07.055] [PMID: 26211902]

Bonferoni, MC, Gavini, E, Rassu, G, Maestri, M & Giunchedi, P (2020) Chitosan Nanoparticles for Therapy and Theranostics of Hepatocellular Carcinoma (HCC) and Liver-Targeting. *Nanomaterials (Basel),* 10, 870.
[http://dx.doi.org/10.3390/nano10050870] [PMID: 32365938]

Brannon-Peppas, L & Blanchette, JO (2004) Nanoparticle and targeted systems for cancer therapy. *Adv Drug Deliv Rev,* 56, 1649-59.
[http://dx.doi.org/10.1016/j.addr.2004.02.014] [PMID: 15350294]

Bray, F, Ferlay, J, Soerjomataram, I, Siegel, RL, Torre, LA & Jemal, A (2018) Global cancer statistics 2018: GLOBOCAN estimates of incidence and mortality worldwide for 36 cancers in 185 countries. *CA Cancer J Clin,* 68, 394-424.
[http://dx.doi.org/10.3322/caac.21492] [PMID: 30207593]

Brigger, I, Dubernet, C & Couvreur, P (2012) Nanoparticles in cancer therapy and diagnosis. *Adv Drug Deliv Rev,* 64, 24-36.
[http://dx.doi.org/10.1016/j.addr.2012.09.006] [PMID: 12204596]

Chen, Q, Zheng, J, Yuan, X, Wang, J & Zhang, L (2018) Folic acid grafted and tertiary amino based pH-responsive pentablock polymeric micelles for targeting anticancer drug delivery. *Mater Sci Eng C,* 82, 1-9.
[http://dx.doi.org/10.1016/j.msec.2017.08.026] [PMID: 29025636]

Chen, Z, Ma, L, Liu, Y & Chen, C (2012) Applications of functionalized fullerenes in tumor theranostics. *Theranostics,* 2, 238-50.
[http://dx.doi.org/10.7150/thno.3509] [PMID: 22509193]

Cheng, Y, Zhao, P, Wu, S, Yang, T, Chen, Y, Zhang, X, He, C, Zheng, C, Li, K, Ma, X & Xiang, G (2018) Cisplatin and curcumin co-loaded nano-liposomes for the treatment of hepatocellular carcinoma. *Int J Pharm,* 545, 261-73.
[http://dx.doi.org/10.1016/j.ijpharm.2018.05.007] [PMID: 29730175]

Chow, EK & Ho, D (2013) Cancer nanomedicine: from drug delivery to imaging. *Sci Transl Med,* 5, 216rv4.
[http://dx.doi.org/10.1126/scitranslmed.3005872] [PMID: 24353161]

Crissien, AM & Frenette, C (2014) Current management of hepatocellular carcinoma. *Gastroenterol Hepatol (N Y),* 10, 153-61.

[PMID: 24829542]

Danhier, F, Feron, O & Préat, V (2010) To exploit the tumor microenvironment: Passive and active tumor targeting of nanocarriers for anti-cancer drug delivery. *Journal of controlled release : official journal of the Controlled Release Society,* 148, 135-46.
[http://dx.doi.org/10.1016/j.jconrel.2010.08.027]

Deepak, P, Siddalingam, R, Kumar, P, Anand, S, Thakur, S, Jagdish, B & Jaiswal, S (2020) Gene based nanocarrier delivery for the treatment of hepatocellular carcinoma. *J Drug Deliv Sci Technol,* 59, 101837.
[http://dx.doi.org/10.1016/j.jddst.2020.101837]

Dhanapal, J & Balaraman Ravindrran, M (2018) Chitosan/poly (lactic acid)-coated piceatannol nanoparticles exert an *in vitro* apoptosis activity on liver, lung and breast cancer cell lines, *Artificial cells, nanomedicine, and biotechnology,* 46, 274-82.
[http://dx.doi.org/10.1080/21691401.2017.1422130]

Diamantopoulou, Z, Gilles, ME, Sader, M, Cossutta, M, Vallée, B, Houppe, C, Habert, D, Brissault, B, Leroy, E, Maione, F, Giraudo, E, Destouches, D, Penelle, J, Courty, J & Cascone, I (2017) Multivalent cationic pseudopeptide polyplexes as a tool for cancer therapy. *Oncotarget,* 8, 90108-22.
[http://dx.doi.org/10.18632/oncotarget.21441] [PMID: 29163814]

Duan, W & Liu, Y (2018) Targeted and synergistic therapy for hepatocellular carcinoma: monosaccharide modified lipid nanoparticles for the co-delivery of doxorubicin and sorafenib. *Drug Des Devel Ther,* 12, 2149-61.
[http://dx.doi.org/10.2147/DDDT.S166402] [PMID: 30034219]

Duncan, R (2003) The dawning era of polymer therapeutics. *Nat Rev Drug Discov,* 2, 347-60.
[http://dx.doi.org/10.1038/nrd1088] [PMID: 12750738]

EASL Clinical Practice Guidelines: Management of hepatocellular carcinoma, *J Hepatol,* 69, 182-236.

Edlin, BR, Eckhardt, BJ, Shu, MA, Holmberg, SD & Swan, T (2015) Toward a more accurate estimate of the prevalence of hepatitis C in the United States. *Hepatology,* 62, 1353-63.
[http://dx.doi.org/10.1002/hep.27978] [PMID: 26171595]

Ekladious, I, Colson, YL & Grinstaff, MW (2019) Polymer-drug conjugate therapeutics: advances, insights and prospects. *Nat Rev Drug Discov,* 18, 273-94.
[http://dx.doi.org/10.1038/s41573-018-0005-0] [PMID: 30542076]

Elnaggar, MH, Abushouk, AI, Hassan, AHE, Lamloum, HM, Benmelouka, A, Moatamed, SA, Abd-Elmegeed, H, Attia, S, Samir, A, Amr, N, Johar, D & Zaky, S (2021) Nanomedicine as a putative approach for active targeting of hepatocellular carcinoma. *Semin Cancer Biol,* 69, 91-9.
[http://dx.doi.org/10.1016/j.semcancer.2019.08.016] [PMID: 31421265]

Elsayed, MM, Mostafa, ME, Alaaeldin, E, Sarhan, HA, Shaykoon, MS, Allam, S, Ahmed, AR & Elsadek, BE (2019) Design And Characterisation Of Novel Sorafenib-Loaded Carbon Nanotubes With Distinct Tumour-Suppressive Activity In Hepatocellular Carcinoma. *Int J Nanomedicine,* 14, 8445-67.
[http://dx.doi.org/10.2147/IJN.S223920] [PMID: 31754301]

Español, L, Larrea, A, Andreu, V, Mendoza, G, Arruebo, M, Sebastian, V, Aurora-Prado, MS, Kedor-Hackmann, ERM, Santoro, MIRM & Santamaria, J (2016) Dual encapsulation of hydrophobic and hydrophilic drugs in PLGA nanoparticles by a single-step method: drug delivery and cytotoxicity assays. *RSC Advances,* 6, 111060-9.
[http://dx.doi.org/10.1039/C6RA23620K]

Fan, D, Yu, J, Yan, R, Xu, X, Wang, Y, Xie, X, Liu, C, Liu, Y & Huang, H (2018) Preparation and Evaluation of Doxorubicin-Loaded Micelles Based on Glycyrrhetinic Acid Modified Gelatin Conjugates for Targeting Hepatocellular Carcinoma. *J Nanomater,* 2018, 8467169.
[http://dx.doi.org/10.1155/2018/8467169]

Ferlay, J, E M, Lam, F, Colombet, M, Mery, L, Piñeros, M, Znaor, A, Soerjomataram, I & Bray, F (2020) Global Cancer Observatory: Cancer Today [online], available: [Accessed 16/01/2021 2021]

Ferrari, R, Sponchioni, M, Morbidelli, M & Moscatelli, D (2018) Polymer nanoparticles for the intravenous delivery of anticancer drugs: the checkpoints on the road from the synthesis to clinical translation. *Nanoscale,* 10, 22701-19.
[http://dx.doi.org/10.1039/C8NR05933K] [PMID: 30512025]

Fu, S, Xia, J & Wu, J (2016) Functional Chitosan Nanoparticles in Cancer Treatment. *J Biomed Nanotechnol,* 12, 1585-603.
[http://dx.doi.org/10.1166/jbn.2016.2228] [PMID: 29341581]

Gao, Y-Y, Chen, H, Zhou, Y-Y, Wang, L-T, Hou, Y, Xia, X-H & Ding, Y (2017) Intraorgan Targeting of Gold Conjugates for Precise Liver Cancer Treatment. *ACS Appl Mater Interfaces,* 9, 31458-68.
[http://dx.doi.org/10.1021/acsami.7b08969] [PMID: 28838233]

Gish, RG (2014) Early detection of hepatocellular carcinoma through surveillance using biomarkers. *Gastroenterol Hepatol (N Y),* 10, 121-3.
[PMID: 24803876]

Golabi, P, Fazel, S, Otgonsuren, M, Sayiner, M, Locklear, CT & Younossi, ZM (2017) Mortality assessment of patients with hepatocellular carcinoma according to underlying disease and treatment modalities. *Medicine (Baltimore),* 96, e5904-4.
[http://dx.doi.org/10.1097/MD.0000000000005904] [PMID: 28248853]

Gossart, JB, Pascal, E, Meyer, F, Heuillard, E, Gonçalves, M, Gossé, F, Robinet, E, Frisch, B, Seguin, C & Zuber, G (2017) Performance of Pyridylthiourea-Polyethylenimine Polyplex for siRNA-Mediated Liver Cancer Therapy in Cell Monolayer, Spheroid, and Tumor Xenograft Models. *Glob Chall,* 1, 1700013.
[http://dx.doi.org/10.1002/gch2.201700013] [PMID: 31565271]

Greish, K, Fang, J, Inutsuka, T, Nagamitsu, A & Maeda, H (2003) Macromolecular therapeutics: advantages and prospects with special emphasis on solid tumour targeting. *Clin Pharmacokinet,* 42, 1089-105.
[http://dx.doi.org/10.2165/00003088-200342130-00002] [PMID: 14531722]

Han, J, Hou, ZQ, Wang, YG & Guo, X (2015) Synthesis and evaluation of hydroxycamptothecin-encapsulated chitosan nanospheres for the treatment of liver cancer. *Technol Cancer Res Treat,* 14, 111-7.
[http://dx.doi.org/10.7785/tcrt.2012.500404] [PMID: 24593290]

He, H, Pham-Huy, LA, Dramou, P, Xiao, D, Zuo, P & Pham-Huy, C (2013) Carbon nanotubes: applications in pharmacy and medicine. *BioMed Res Int,* 2013, 578290.
[http://dx.doi.org/10.1155/2013/578290] [PMID: 24195076]

Huang, H, Feng, W, Chen, Y & Shi, J (2020) Inorganic nanoparticles in clinical trials and translations. *Nano Today,* 35, 100972.
[http://dx.doi.org/10.1016/j.nantod.2020.100972]

Islami, F, Goding Sauer, A, Miller, K D, Siegel, R L, Fedewa, S A, Jacobs, E J, McCullough, M L, Patel, A V, Ma, J, Soerjomataram, I, Flanders, W D, Brawley, O W, Gapstur, S M & Jemal, A (2018) Proportion and number of cancer cases and deaths attributable to potentially modifiable risk factors in the United States 68, 31-54.
[http://dx.doi.org/10.3322/caac.21440]

Iwasaki, Y, Ueda, M, Yamada, T, Kondo, A, Seno, M, Tanizawa, K, Kuroda, S, Sakamoto, M & Kitajima, M (2007) Gene therapy of liver tumors with human liver-specific nanoparticles. *Cancer Gene Ther,* 14, 74-81.
[http://dx.doi.org/10.1038/sj.cgt.7700990] [PMID: 16990844]

Iyer, AK, Khaled, G, Fang, J & Maeda, H (2006) Exploiting the enhanced permeability and retention effect for tumor targeting. *Drug Discov Today,* 11, 812-8.
[http://dx.doi.org/10.1016/j.drudis.2006.07.005] [PMID: 16935749]

Kamedulski, P, Zielinski, W, Nowak, P, Lukaszewicz, JP & Ilnicka, A (2020) 3D hierarchical porous hybrid nanostructure of carbon nanotubes and N-doped activated carbon. *Sci Rep,* 10, 18793.
[http://dx.doi.org/10.1038/s41598-020-75831-x] [PMID: 33139816]

Kandasamy, G, Danilovtseva, EN, Annenkov, VV & Krishnan, UM (2020) Poly(1-vinylimidazole) polyplexes as novel therapeutic gene carriers for lung cancer therapy. *Beilstein J Nanotechnol,* 11, 354-69. [http://dx.doi.org/10.3762/bjnano.11.26] [PMID: 32190532]

Karlsson, J, Vaughan, HJ & Green, JJ (2018) Biodegradable Polymeric Nanoparticles for Therapeutic Cancer Treatments. *Annu Rev Chem Biomol Eng,* 9, 105-27. [http://dx.doi.org/10.1146/annurev-chembioeng-060817-084055] [PMID: 29579402]

Koirala, N, Das, D, Fayazzadeh, E, Sen, S, McClain, A, Puskas, JE, Drazba, JA & McLennan, G (2019) Folic acid conjugated polymeric drug delivery vehicle for targeted cancer detection in hepatocellular carcinoma. *J Biomed Mater Res A,* 107, 2522-35. [http://dx.doi.org/10.1002/jbm.a.36758] [PMID: 31334591]

Kostarelos, K, Bianco, A & Prato, M (2009) Promises, facts and challenges for carbon nanotubes in imaging and therapeutics. *Nat Nanotechnol,* 4, 627-33. [http://dx.doi.org/10.1038/nnano.2009.241] [PMID: 19809452]

Kumar, S, Dilbaghi, N, Saharan, R & Bhanjana, G (2012) Nanotechnology as Emerging Tool for Enhancing Solubility of Poorly Water-Soluble Drugs. *Bionanoscience,* 2, 227-50. [http://dx.doi.org/10.1007/s12668-012-0060-7]

Kuznietsova, H, Dziubenko, N, Herheliuk, T, Prylutskyy, Y, Tauscher, E, Ritter, U & Scharff, P (2020) Water-Soluble Pristine C_{60} Fullerene Inhibits Liver Alterations Associated with Hepatocellular Carcinoma in Rat. *Pharmaceutics,* 12, E794. [http://dx.doi.org/10.3390/pharmaceutics12090794] [PMID: 32842595]

Kuznietsova, HM, Dziubenko, NV, Lynchak, OV, Herheliuk, TS, Zavalny, DK, Remeniak, OV, Prylutskyy, YI & Ritter, U (2020) Effects of Pristine C_{60} Fullerenes on Liver and Pancreas in α-Naphthylisothiocyanat- -Induced Cholangitis. *Dig Dis Sci,* 65, 215-24. [http://dx.doi.org/10.1007/s10620-019-05730-3] [PMID: 31312992]

Lai, I, Swaminathan, S, Baylot, V, Mosley, A, Dhanasekaran, R, Gabay, M & Felsher, DW (2018) Lipid nanoparticles that deliver IL-12 messenger RNA suppress tumorigenesis in MYC oncogene-driven hepatocellular carcinoma. *J Immunother Cancer,* 6, 125. [http://dx.doi.org/10.1186/s40425-018-0431-x] [PMID: 30458889]

Layek, B, Gidwani, B, Tiwari, S, Joshi, V, Jain, V & Vyas, A (2020) Recent Advances in Lipid-based Nanodrug Delivery Systems in Cancer Therapy. *Curr Pharm Des,* 26, 3218-33. [http://dx.doi.org/10.2174/1381612826666200622133407] [PMID: 32568015]

Layek, B, Haldar, MK, Sharma, G, Lipp, L, Mallik, S & Singh, J (2014) Hexanoic acid and polyethylene glycol double grafted amphiphilic chitosan for enhanced gene delivery: influence of hydrophobic and hydrophilic substitution degree. *Mol Pharm,* 11, 982-94. [http://dx.doi.org/10.1021/mp400633r] [PMID: 24499512]

Layek, B, Lipp, L & Singh, J (2015) APC targeted micelle for enhanced intradermal delivery of hepatitis B DNA vaccine *Journal of controlled release: official journal of the Controlled Release Society,* 207, 143-53. [http://dx.doi.org/10.1016/j.jconrel.2015.04.014]

Layek, B & Singh, J (2013) Amino acid grafted chitosan for high performance gene delivery: comparison of amino acid hydrophobicity on vector and polyplex characteristics. *Biomacromolecules,* 14, 485-94. a [http://dx.doi.org/10.1021/bm301720g] [PMID: 23301560]

Layek, B & Singh, J (2013) Cell penetrating peptide conjugated polymeric micelles as a high performance versatile nonviral gene carrier. *Biomacromolecules,* 14, 4071-81. b [http://dx.doi.org/10.1021/bm401204n] [PMID: 24083483]

Layek, B & Singh, J (2017) 8 - Chitosan for DNA and gene therapy.*Chitosan Based Biomaterials* Woodhead Publishing 209-44. [http://dx.doi.org/10.1016/B978-0-08-100228-5.00008-0]

Layek, B & Singh, J (2019) Editorial of Special Issue "Surface-Functionalized Nanoparticles as Drug Carriers". *Int J Mol Sci,* 20, 6352.

[http://dx.doi.org/10.3390/ijms20246352] [PMID: 31861113]

Li, K, Xia, C, Wang, B, Chen, H, Wang, T, He, Q, Cao, H & Wang, Y (2017) Effects of quantum dots on the ROS amount of liver cancer stem cells. *Colloids Surf B Biointerfaces,* 155, 193-9. [http://dx.doi.org/10.1016/j.colsurfb.2017.04.019] [PMID: 28431328]

Li, L, Tang, F, Liu, H, Liu, T, Hao, N, Chen, D, Teng, X & He, J (2010) *In vivo* delivery of silica nanorattle encapsulated docetaxel for liver cancer therapy with low toxicity and high efficacy. *ACS Nano,* 4, 6874-82. [http://dx.doi.org/10.1021/nn100918a] [PMID: 20973487]

Li, X, Diao, W, Xue, H, Wu, F, Wang, W, Jiang, B, Bai, J, Lian, B, Feng, W, Sun, T, Yu, W, Wu, J, Qu, M, Wang, Y & Gao, Z (2020) Improved efficacy of doxorubicin delivery by a novel dual-ligand-modified liposome in hepatocellular carcinoma. *Cancer Lett,* 489, 163-73. [http://dx.doi.org/10.1016/j.canlet.2020.06.017] [PMID: 32592729]

Li, Z, Ye, L, Liu, J, Lian, D & Li, X (2020) Sorafenib-Loaded Nanoparticles Based on Biodegradable Dendritic Polymers for Enhanced Therapy of Hepatocellular Carcinoma. *Int J Nanomedicine,* 15, 1469-80. [http://dx.doi.org/10.2147/IJN.S237335] [PMID: 32184599]

Liu, Y, Wang, L, Zhao, Y, He, M, Zhang, X, Niu, M & Feng, N (2014) Nanostructured lipid carriers *versus* microemulsions for delivery of the poorly water-soluble drug luteolin. *Int J Pharm,* 476, 169-77. [http://dx.doi.org/10.1016/j.ijpharm.2014.09.052] [PMID: 25280882]

Longmuir, KJ, Haynes, SM, Baratta, JL, Kasabwalla, N & Robertson, RT (2009) Liposomal delivery of doxorubicin to hepatocytes *in vivo* by targeting heparan sulfate. *Int J Pharm,* 382, 222-33. [http://dx.doi.org/10.1016/j.ijpharm.2009.07.030] [PMID: 19664697]

Longmuir, KJ, Robertson, RT, Haynes, SM, Baratta, JL & Waring, AJ (2006) Effective targeting of liposomes to liver and hepatocytes *in vivo* by incorporation of a Plasmodium amino acid sequence. *Pharm Res,* 23, 759-69. [http://dx.doi.org/10.1007/s11095-006-9609-x] [PMID: 16550476]

Lu, J, Wang, J & Ling, D (2018) Surface Engineering of Nanoparticles for Targeted Delivery to Hepatocellular Carcinoma. *Small,* 14, 1702037. [http://dx.doi.org/10.1002/smll.201702037] [PMID: 29251419]

Lunov, O, Uzhytchak, M, Smolková, B, Lunova, M, Jirsa, M, Dempsey, N M, Dias, A L, Bonfim, M, Hof, M, Jurkiewicz, P, Petrenko, Y, Kubinová, Š & Dejneka, A (2019) Remote Actuation of Apoptosis in Liver Cancer Cells *via* Magneto-Mechanical Modulation of Iron Oxide Nanoparticles 11, 1873. [http://dx.doi.org/10.3390/cancers11121873]

Luo, Y, Bernshaw, NJ, Lu, ZR, Kopecek, J & Prestwich, GD (2002) Targeted delivery of doxorubicin by HPMA copolymer-hyaluronan bioconjugates. *Pharm Res,* 19, 396-402. [http://dx.doi.org/10.1023/A:1015170907274] [PMID: 12033370]

Luther, DC, Huang, R, Jeon, T, Zhang, X, Lee, YW, Nagaraj, H & Rotello, VM (2020) Delivery of drugs, proteins, and nucleic acids using inorganic nanoparticles. *Adv Drug Deliv Rev,* 156, 188-213. [http://dx.doi.org/10.1016/j.addr.2020.06.020] [PMID: 32610061]

Maeda, H (2001) SMANCS and polymer-conjugated macromolecular drugs: advantages in cancer chemotherapy. *Adv Drug Deliv Rev,* 46, 169-85. [http://dx.doi.org/10.1016/S0169-409X(00)00134-4] [PMID: 11259839]

Majumder, N, G, Das, N & Das, S K (2020) Polymeric micelles for anticancer drug delivery 11, 613-35. [http://dx.doi.org/10.4155/tde-2020-0008]

Matsumura, Y Fau, Maeda, H & Maeda, H A new concept for macromolecular therapeutics in cancer chemotherapy: mechanism of tumoritropic accumulation of proteins and the antitumor agent smancs (0008-5472 (Print))

Matsumura, Y & Maeda, H (1986) A new concept for macromolecular therapeutics in cancer chemotherapy: mechanism of tumoritropic accumulation of proteins and the antitumor agent smancs. *Cancer Res,* 46, 6387-92.

[PMID: 2946403]

Mazzaferro, V, Regalia, E, Doci, R, Andreola, S, Pulvirenti, A, Bozzetti, F, Montalto, F, Ammatuna, M, Morabito, A & Gennari, L (1996) Liver transplantation for the treatment of small hepatocellular carcinomas in patients with cirrhosis. *N Engl J Med,* 334, 693-9.
[http://dx.doi.org/10.1056/NEJM199603143341104] [PMID: 8594428]

Mu, W, Jiang, D, Mu, S, Liang, S, Liu, Y & Zhang, N (2019) Promoting Early Diagnosis and Precise Therapy of Hepatocellular Carcinoma by Glypican-3-Targeted Synergistic Chemo-Photothermal Theranostics. *ACS Appl Mater Interfaces,* 11, 23591-604.
[http://dx.doi.org/10.1021/acsami.9b05526] [PMID: 31179679]

Mukherjee, S, Ray, S & Thakur, RS (2009) Solid lipid nanoparticles: a modern formulation approach in drug delivery system. *Indian J Pharm Sci,* 71, 349-58.
[http://dx.doi.org/10.4103/0250-474X.57282] [PMID: 20502539]

Newland, B, Leupelt, D, Zheng, Y, Thomas, LSV, Werner, C, Steinhart, M & Wang, W (2015) Magnetically Controllable Polymer Nanotubes from a Cyclized Crosslinker for Site-Specific Delivery of Doxorubicin. *Sci Rep,* 5, 17478.
[http://dx.doi.org/10.1038/srep17478] [PMID: 26619814]

Ning, Q, Liu, Y-F, Ye, P-J, Gao, P, Li, Z-P, Tang, S-Y, He, D-X, Tang, S-S, Wei, H & Yu, C-Y (2019) Delivery of Liver-Specific miRNA-122 Using a Targeted Macromolecular Prodrug toward Synergistic Therapy for Hepatocellular Carcinoma. *ACS Appl Mater Interfaces,* 11, 10578-88.
[http://dx.doi.org/10.1021/acsami.9b00634] [PMID: 30802029]

Perrone, F, Craparo, EF, Cemazar, M, Kamensek, U, Drago, SE, Dapas, B, Scaggiante, B, Zanconati, F, Bonazza, D, Grassi, M, Truong, N, Pozzato, G, Farra, R, Cavallaro, G & Grassi, G (2020) Targeted delivery of siRNAs against hepatocellular carcinoma-related genes by a galactosylated polyaspartamide copolymer. *J Control Release.*
[PMID: 33212117]

Ponce, AM, Vujaskovic, Z, Yuan, F, Needham, D & Dewhirst, MW (2006) Hyperthermia mediated liposomal drug delivery. *Int J Hyperthermia,* 22, 205-13.
[http://dx.doi.org/10.1080/02656730600582956] [PMID: 16754340]

Prabhu, RH, Patravale, VB & Joshi, MD (2015) Polymeric nanoparticles for targeted treatment in oncology: current insights. *Int J Nanomedicine,* 10, 1001-18.
[PMID: 25678788]

Rahman, M, Almalki, WH, Afzal, O, Alfawaz Altamimi, AS, Kazmi, I, Al-Abbasi, FA, Choudhry, H, Alenezi, SK, Barkat, MA, Beg, S, Kumar, V & Alhalmi, A (2020) Cationic Solid Lipid Nanoparticles of Resveratrol for Hepatocellular Carcinoma Treatment: Systematic Optimization, *in vitro* Characterization and Preclinical Investigation. *Int J Nanomedicine,* 15, 9283-99.
[http://dx.doi.org/10.2147/IJN.S277545] [PMID: 33262588]

Rahman, M, Beg, S, Alharbi, KS, Alruwaili, NK, Alotaibi, NH, Alzarea, AI, Almalki, WH, Alenezi, SK, Altowayan, WM, Alshammari, MS, Afzal, M, Saleem, S & Kumar, V (2020) Implications of Solid Lipid Nanoparticles of Ganoderic Acid for the Treatment and Management of Hepatocellular Carcinoma. *J Pharm Innov*

Rašović, I (2017) Water-soluble fullerenes for medical applications. *Mater Sci Technol,* 33, 777-94.
[http://dx.doi.org/10.1080/02670836.2016.1198114]

Sanna, V, Pala, N & Sechi, M (2014) Targeted therapy using nanotechnology: focus on cancer. *Int J Nanomedicine,* 9, 467-83.
[PMID: 24531078]

Sarika, PR, James, NR, Nishna, N, Anil Kumar, PR & Raj, DK (2015) Galactosylated pullulan-curcumin conjugate micelles for site specific anticancer activity to hepatocarcinoma cells. *Colloids Surf B Biointerfaces,* 133, 347-55.

[http://dx.doi.org/10.1016/j.colsurfb.2015.06.020] [PMID: 26133239]

Sedighi, M, Rahimi, F, Shahbazi, M-A, Rezayan, AH, Kettiger, H, Einfalt, T, Huwyler, J & Witzigmann, D (2020) Controlled Tyrosine Kinase Inhibitor Delivery to Liver Cancer Cells by Gate-Capped Mesoporous Silica Nanoparticles. *ACS Appl Bio Mater,* 3, 239-51.
[http://dx.doi.org/10.1021/acsabm.9b00772]

Shaat, H, Mostafa, A, Moustafa, M, Gamal-Eldeen, A, Emam, A, El-Hussieny, E & Elhefnawi, M (2016) Modified gold nanoparticles for intracellular delivery of anti-liver cancer siRNA. *Int J Pharm,* 504, 125-33.
[http://dx.doi.org/10.1016/j.ijpharm.2016.03.051] [PMID: 27036397]

Shoshan, MS, Vonderach, T, Hattendorf, B & Wennemers, H (2019) Peptide-Coated Platinum Nanoparticles with Selective Toxicity against Liver Cancer Cells. *Angew Chem Int Ed Engl,* 58, 4901-5.
[http://dx.doi.org/10.1002/anie.201813149] [PMID: 30561882]

Siegel, RL, Miller, KD, Fuchs, HE & Jemal, A (2021) Cancer Statistics, 2021. *CA Cancer J Clin,* 71, 7-33.
[http://dx.doi.org/10.3322/caac.21654] [PMID: 33433946]

Sosnowska, M, Kutwin, M, Jaworski, S, Strojny, B, Wierzbicki, M, Szczepaniak, J, Łojkowski, M, Święszkowski, W, Bałaban, J, Chwalibog, A & Sawosz, E (2019) Mechano-signalling, induced by fullerene C_{60} nanofilms, arrests the cell cycle in the G2/M phase and decreases proliferation of liver cancer cells. *Int J Nanomedicine,* 14, 6197-215.
[http://dx.doi.org/10.2147/IJN.S206934] [PMID: 31496681]

Sriraman, SK, Aryasomayajula, B & Torchilin, VP (2014) Barriers to drug delivery in solid tumors. *Tissue Barriers,* 2, e29528-8.
[http://dx.doi.org/10.4161/tisb.29528] [PMID: 25068098]

Subramaniam, B, Siddik, ZH & Nagoor, NH (2020) Optimization of nanostructured lipid carriers: understanding the types, designs, and parameters in the process of formulations. *J Nanopart Res,* 22, 141.
[http://dx.doi.org/10.1007/s11051-020-04848-0]

Taghizadeh, S, Alimardani, V, Roudbali, PL, Ghasemi, Y & Kaviani, E (2019) Gold nanoparticles application in liver cancer. *Photodiagn Photodyn Ther,* 25, 389-400.
[http://dx.doi.org/10.1016/j.pdpdt.2019.01.027] [PMID: 30684673]

Tekade, RK & Chougule, MB (2013) Formulation development and evaluation of hybrid nanocarrier for cancer therapy: Taguchi orthogonal array based design. *BioMed Res Int,* 2013, 712678.
[http://dx.doi.org/10.1155/2013/712678] [PMID: 24106715]

Thakkar, S, Sharma, D, Kalia, K & Tekade, RK (2020) Tumor microenvironment targeted nanotherapeutics for cancer therapy and diagnosis: A review. *Acta Biomater,* 101, 43-68.
[http://dx.doi.org/10.1016/j.actbio.2019.09.009] [PMID: 31518706]

Turati, F, Galeone, C, Rota, M, Pelucchi, C, Negri, E, Bagnardi, V, Corrao, G, Boffetta, P & La Vecchia, C (2014) Alcohol and liver cancer: a systematic review and meta-analysis of prospective studies. *Ann Oncol,* 25, 1526-35.
[http://dx.doi.org/10.1093/annonc/mdu020] [PMID: 24631946]

van Meer, S, de Man, RA, Coenraad, MJ, Sprengers, D, van Nieuwkerk, KM, Klümpen, HJ, Jansen, PL, IJzermans, JN, van Oijen, MG, Siersema, PD & van Erpecum, KJ (2015) Surveillance for hepatocellular carcinoma is associated with increased survival: Results from a large cohort in the Netherlands. *J Hepatol,* 63, 1156-63.
[http://dx.doi.org/10.1016/j.jhep.2015.06.012] [PMID: 26100498]

Wang, J, Wu, Z, Pan, G, Ni, J, Xie, F, Jiang, B, Wei, L, Gao, J & Zhou, W (2018) Enhanced doxorubicin delivery to hepatocellular carcinoma cells *via* CD147 antibody-conjugated immunoliposomes. *Nanomedicine,* 14, 1949-61.
[http://dx.doi.org/10.1016/j.nano.2017.09.012] [PMID: 29045824]

Wang, L, Su, W, Liu, Z, Zhou, M, Chen, S, Chen, Y, Lu, D, Liu, Y, Fan, Y, Zheng, Y, Han, Z, Kong, D, Wu, JC, Xiang, R & Li, Z (2012) CD44 antibody-targeted liposomal nanoparticles for molecular imaging and

therapy of hepatocellular carcinoma. *Biomaterials,* 33, 5107-14.
[http://dx.doi.org/10.1016/j.biomaterials.2012.03.067] [PMID: 22494888]

Wang, Q, Zhang, P, Li, Z, Feng, X, Lv, C, Zhang, H, Xiao, H, Ding, J & Chen, X (2019) Evaluation of Polymer Nanoformulations in Hepatoma Therapy by Established Rodent Models. *Theranostics,* 9, 1426-52.
[http://dx.doi.org/10.7150/thno.31683] [PMID: 30867842]

Wang, Y-C, Liu, X-Q, Sun, T-M, Xiong, M-H & Wang, J (2008) Functionalized micelles from block copolymer of polyphosphoester and poly(epsilon-caprolactone) for receptor-mediated drug delivery. *J Control Release,* 128, 32-40.
[http://dx.doi.org/10.1016/j.jconrel.2008.01.021] [PMID: 18395283]

Wong, R & Frenette, C (2011) Updates in the management of hepatocellular carcinoma. *Gastroenterol Hepatol (N Y),* 7, 16-24.
[PMID: 21346848]

Wu, CH, Lan, CH, Wu, KL, Wu, YM, Jane, WN, Hsiao, M & Wu, HC (2018) Hepatocellular carcinoma-targeted nanoparticles for cancer therapy. *Int J Oncol,* 52, 389-401.
[PMID: 29207071]

Xu, Z, Chen, L, Gu, W, Gao, Y, Lin, L, Zhang, Z, Xi, Y & Li, Y (2009) The performance of docetaxel-loaded solid lipid nanoparticles targeted to hepatocellular carcinoma. *Biomaterials,* 30, 226-32.
[http://dx.doi.org/10.1016/j.biomaterials.2008.09.014] [PMID: 18851881]

Yamawaki, H & Iwai, N (2006) Cytotoxicity of water-soluble fullerene in vascular endothelial cells. *Am J Physiol Cell Physiol,* 290, C1495-502.
[http://dx.doi.org/10.1152/ajpcell.00481.2005] [PMID: 16407415]

Yao, Y, Wang, T, Liu, Y & Zhang, N (2019) Co-delivery of sorafenib and VEGF-siRNA *via* pH-sensitive liposomes for the synergistic treatment of hepatocellular carcinoma. *Artif Cells Nanomed Biotechnol,* 47, 1374-83.
[http://dx.doi.org/10.1080/21691401.2019.1596943] [PMID: 30977418]

Yao, Y, Zhou, Y, Liu, L, Xu, Y, Chen, Q, Wang, Y, Wu, S, Deng, Y, Zhang, J & Shao, A (2020) Nanoparticle-Based Drug Delivery in Cancer Therapy and Its Role in Overcoming Drug Resistance 7
[http://dx.doi.org/10.3389/fmolb.2020.00193]

Ye, BL, Zheng, R, Ruan, XJ, Zheng, ZH & Cai, HJ (2018) Chitosan-coated doxorubicin nano-particles drug delivery system inhibits cell growth of liver cancer *via* p53/PRC1 pathway. *Biochem Biophys Res Commun,* 495, 414-20.
[http://dx.doi.org/10.1016/j.bbrc.2017.10.156] [PMID: 29097204]

Zhang, X, Guo, S, Fan, R, Yu, M, Li, F, Zhu, C & Gan, Y (2012) Dual-functional liposome for tumor targeting and overcoming multidrug resistance in hepatocellular carcinoma cells. *Biomaterials,* 33, 7103-14.
[http://dx.doi.org/10.1016/j.biomaterials.2012.06.048] [PMID: 22796159]

Zhou, M, Yi, Y, Liu, L, Lin, Y, Li, J, Ruan, J & Zhong, Z (2019) Polymeric micelles loading with ursolic acid enhancing anti-tumor effect on hepatocellular carcinoma. *J Cancer,* 10, 5820-31.
[http://dx.doi.org/10.7150/jca.30865] [PMID: 31737119]

Zhu, R, Wu, X, Xiao, Y, Gao, B, Xie, Q, Liu, H & Wang, S (2013) Synergetic effect of SLN-curcumin and LDH-5-Fu on SMMC-7721 liver cancer cell line. *Cancer Biother Radiopharm,* 28, 579-87.
[http://dx.doi.org/10.1089/cbr.2012.1445] [PMID: 23808828]

Zhu, R, Zhang, CG, Liu, Y, Yuan, ZQ, Chen, WL, Yang, SD, Li, JZ, Zhu, WJ, Zhou, XF, You, BG & Zhang, XN (2015) CD147 monoclonal antibody mediated by chitosan nanoparticles loaded with α-hederin enhances antineoplastic activity and cellular uptake in liver cancer cells. *Sci Rep,* 5, 17904.
[http://dx.doi.org/10.1038/srep17904] [PMID: 26639052]

CHAPTER 7

Aptamers and Their Potential in Site-Specific Nanotherapy Against Hepatocellular Carcinoma

Debasmita Dutta[1,2], **Samrat Chakraborty**[2,3], **Biswajit Mukherjee**[2], **Moumita Dhara**[2] and **Laboni Das**[4]

[1] *Department of Molecular and Human Genetics, Baylor College of Medicine, Houston, Texas 77030, United States*

[2] *Department of Pharmaceutical Technology, Jadavpur University, Kolkata-700032, West Bengal, India*

[3] *Gupta College of Technological Sciences, Asansol-713301, West Bengal, India*

[4] *School of Pharmacy, Techno India University, EM-4, Sector-V, Salt Lake, Kolkata, WB, India*

Abstract: Globally, hepatocellular carcinoma (HCC) is one of the most devastating neoplasia and has a remarkably high mortality rate. Furthermore, the long latent period associated with HCC lends the diagnosis at the intermediate or advanced stages where the chemotherapy is the solitary therapeutic intervention. The responsiveness of HCC towards conventional chemotherapeutic agents is notably poor due to multiple factors. Among them, multiple drug resistance, reduced drug concentration at the tumor site, quicker clearance, and non-specific distribution are the prime causes leading to remarkably high off-target toxicity and mortality. More importantly, the approval of several multikinase inhibitors (MKIs) by the United States Food and Drug Administration (FDA) for the treatment of HCC as targeted therapeutics has been found to be inadequate to make a notable impact on survival. Therefore, ligand-based targeted therapeutics capable of delivering the therapeutic modality specifically into neoplastic hepatocytes have been explored extensively by researchers worldwide. Among the plethora of HCC-targeting ligands, aptamer-based targeted therapeutics in HCC have gained significant momentum compared to others due to some signature characteristics of aptamer, namely non-immunogenicity, low cost, non-toxicity, thermostability, simpler manufacturing, and high suitability for chemical modification. Despite their enormous potential, aptamer-based targeted therapeutics are still in infancy and require smarter thinking and quick translation from e-clinical to clinical application. Thus, the fundamental focus of the book chapter is to highlight promising features of aptamers, their production, chemical modification, mechanism of action, and finally, detailed emphasis has been given on the overall scenario of aptamer-based targeted therapeutics in HCC.

* **Corresponding author Debasmita Dutta:** Department of Molecular and Human Genetics, Baylor College of Medicine, Houston, Texas 77030, United States and Department of Pharmaceutical Technology, Jadavpur University, Kolkata 700032, India; Tel +1-7014046719; Emails: debasmita.dutta@bcm.edu, debasmita.biochem@gmail.com

Keywords: Aptamers, Diagnosis, Hepatocellular carcinoma, Nanoencapsulated drug delivery, Targeted therapy, Theranostic treatment.

INTRODUCTION

The term ‘cancer’ can be defined simply as the uncontrolled growth in abnormal cells present in any part of our body. Several types of carcinogens and genetic alterations are considered the primary factors responsible for cancer development (Maitra *et al.*, 2013). The causative agents that can develop normal cells into abnormally behaving cancer cells may include exposure to different chemicals or toxic compounds, pathogenic factors, ionizing radiation, and inherited or acquired mutations in the human genome. Classification of cancer depends on its location in the body and the kind of originating tissue or fluid, although some cancers may be of mixed type. Carcinoma, sarcoma, lymphoma, leukemia, and myeloma are five broad categories of cancer (https://stanfordhealthcare.org/medical-conditions/cancer/cancer/cancertypes.html).

Hepatocellular carcinoma (HCC), commonly characterized as the initial development of malignancy in hepatocytes, is one of the most frequently diagnosed cancer globally but is extraordinarily heterogeneous in nature. Generally, the heterogeneity in HCC is described by rapid dysregulation of cellular signal transduction pathways and the highly unpredictable tumor microenvironment in the neoplastic hepatocytes. Again, these abnormal alterations in the cellular pathophysiological environment are developed through some genetic and epigenetic changes in hepatocytes, and they are very comprehensively associated with multiple metabolic syndromes such as diabetes, obesity or alcohol abuse, non-alcoholic steatohepatitis (NASH) with altered sex, aging, and various environmental factors, including hepatitis B and hepatitis C along with other viral infections and immunogenic disorders (Dagogo-Jack *et al.*, 2018). Thus, the therapeutic strategies of HCC are extremely challenging, along with minimum off-target cytotoxicity. Depending on the type and extent of cancer spreading, chemotherapy is chosen to treat cancer. For many years in the past, chemotherapy and radiation were options to save or at least prolong the life span of cancer patients. Radiation delays cancer growth, and on the other hand, chemotherapy helps manage different symptoms caused by cancer. However, the medical community is now aware of the extent of damage the chemotherapy and radiation therapy cause during treatment and the consequent health hazards that follow in the future (https://www.ctoam.com/precision-oncology/why-we-exist/standardtreatment/treatment/chemotherapy/). The need for more sophisticated tools for the treatment of cancer will provide selective cell-specific accumulation of chemotherapeutics with reduced side effects to normal cells.

Although chemotherapy has importance in treatment for cancer patients, the toxic effects (*e.g.*, hair loss, nausea, and vomiting, *etc.*) of this conventional cancer therapy that occur due to the inability of chemotherapy to differentiate between cancerous and healthy cells, tendency to develop resistance to the chemical agents, and the necessity of using other treatment forms along with it limit its use (http://www1.udel.edu/chem/C465/senior/fall98/Cancer2/methods.html). Surgery, chemotherapy, and radiation are the mainstream therapeutic approaches for cancer (Padma, 2015; Xu *et al.*, 2001; Dutta *et al.*, 2015; Dutta *et al.*, 2016). The main strategy of targeted therapy is to deliver a drug at the cancer-promoting specific tissue environment or to specific cancerous cells to target a particular protein or genes. The success of the therapy solely depends on targeted drug action in specific cancer cells, thus reducing toxic side effects in normal healthy cells (Gerber *et al.*, 2008; Padma, 2015). By utilizing the "enhanced permeability and retention effects" (EPR) effect, passive targeting to the tumor can be attributed to various macromolecules (Dutta *et al.*, 2019; Kale *et al.*, 2020, Hazra *et al.*, 2021).

On the other hand, direct targeting to a particular target antigen can be achieved through specific monoclonal antibodies or by small molecule drugs that act by altering their signaling. Under indirect approaches, some proteins express specifically on the tumor cell surface and serve as special targeting devices. These can be actively targeted by conjugating the antigen-specific ligand molecules to the drug carrier (Wu *et al.*, 2006).

Different newer technologies have got rapid and huge expansion for the molecular level diagnostics and tumor targeting strategies which made it essential to develop more specific targeting ligands to target definite cell surface molecules expressed uniquely in tumor tissues or cells (Kim *et al.*, 2018). Extensive research is on the pipeline, involving the active targeting to cancer cells utilizing different ligands such as proteins, peptides, monoclonal antibodies, small molecules, and last but not least, the nucleotide sequence-based targeting molecule, aptamers (Ray *et al.*, 2021; Mondal *et al.*, 2019; Mukherjee *et al.*, 2020; Mukherjee *et al.*, 2021). They can recognize cancer cell-specific and unique receptors and bind with them (Sivashankari *et al.*, 2016). The use of aptamer has been widely investigated for its role in targeted therapy, the discovery of biomarkers, *in vivo* imaging, and *in vitro* diagnosis (Sun *et al.*, 2014; Dutta *et al.*, 2018). Aptamers are small, structured oligonucleotides, *i.e.*, RNA or single-stranded DNA ligands that are selective and have a high affinity towards the target molecules.

In this chapter, our main objective is to explore aptamer-mediated targeted therapy, its diagnostic and theranostic use, target receptor-specific designing procedures, modifications, characterizations, mechanism of actions, and valuable applications for the treatment of HCC.

Therapeutic Approach for HCC: Active *vs.* Passive Targeting and Aptamer.

Apart from developing newer systemic chemotherapeutics and immunogenic drugs, the establishment of a novel drug delivery system through active or passive targeting has been in trend for the last two decades. The invention of nanotechnology has embarked on a novel platform to manage malignancy or cancers considerably better and intrigued scientists worldwide for its characteristic versatility. The foremost advantages are accumulating therapeutics at the tumor site through enhancing permeability and EPR effect with its unique nanosize and physio-chemical properties, thus overcoming systemic adverse effects (Adiseshaiah *et al.*, 2016). This process, described as passive targeting, relies upon the availability of these tiny nanoparticles besides the leaky or damaged vasculatures of the impaired lymphatic system, one of the distended features of tumorous tissues (Kalyane *et al.*, 2019). However, the dependability of EPR-based passive targeting has always been under doubt. In recent times, it was reported that the uptake of nanoparticles in tumor tissues was limited to 0.7% of the injected therapeutics (Wilhelm *et al.*, 2016). Researchers are obligated to design a smart nanocarrier system that can proactively reach the target tumor and steadily improvise exclusive neoplastic cellular uptakes. Thus, active targeting has been instigated through conjugating of various tumor-specific ligands such as peptides, aptamers, antibodies, small molecules, *etc.*, with the nanocarriers to recognize and attach with their complementary receptor partners or surface membrane proteins generally overexpressed on target tumor cells (Bazak *et al.*, 2015). Many impediments such as by-passing systemic toxicity, blood-brain barrier, and overcoming multi-drug resistance in tumors seem to be sensibly resolved with active targeting in curing cancer.

Some bio-conjugates such as asialofetuin or their synthetically modified analogues could be applied as conjugating ligands with nanocarriers to reach fibrotic liver efficiently through targeting tumor-specific ASGPR (Asialoglycoprotein receptor is commonly found overexpressed in mammalian liver cells). The site-specific biodistribution of an Alexa647-labeled polyvalent drug carrier to the neoplastic hepatocytes rather than normal parenchymal tissues in rodents was effectively explored depending on ASGPR-directed hepatocellular accumulation of the therapeutics, while prolonged retention time of the formulation was confirmed through GalNAc attached pegylated polymers (Sanhueza *et al.*, 2017). PES (Polyehelenesebacate) -Gantrez®AN- 119 encapsulated Doxorubicin nanoparticles have been formulated for restoring safety and efficacy in hepatocellular carcinoma following this asialoglycoprotein-mediated active targeting (Pranatharthiharan *et al.*, 2017). Another smart bioconjugate has established the potential of ligand-fitted biodegradable micelles (Gal-CLMs) in HCC. Gal-CLMS, a cross-linked copolymer attached with galactose (targeting ligand), efficiently delivers paclitaxel to the tumor-bearing tissues of some nude mice and maintains controlled drug release patterns in a specified physiological pH *in vitro* (Zou *et al.*, 2014). Again, therapeutic superiority of doxorubicin encapsulated liposomes (CHOL-Al-AG) when conjugated with arabinogalactan (a modified galactose with high affinity towards liver tumor tissues) is demonstrated by Pathak *et al.*, compared to basic liposomes *in vitro* (Pathak *et al.*, 2015). Peptide sequence RGD performs as a labeling moiety for collagen VI and is popularly used to target integrin (overexpressed in fibrotic hepatocyte) (Bartneck *et al.*, 2014). Integrin- αv $\beta 3$ targeted nanoliposomal paclitaxel (PTX) was developed by Chen *et al.* to improve solubility and bioavailability of paclitaxel (PTX) for effective drug delivery in HCC (Chen *et al.*, 2015). Both *in vitro* and *in vivo* studies confirmed that encapsulated and conjugated drugs to DSPE-PEG with RGD-motif (RGD-L--PTX) had successfully improved the drug accumulation and enhanced the antitumor activity than the unconjugated or free form of PTX. Another effective amalgamation of doxorubicin and sorafenib with iRGD is fabricated, entrapping these in smart lipid-based hybrid NPs for their efficacious delivery to the target neoplastic hepatocyte both *in vivo* and *in vitro* for boosting anticancer activity (Zhang *et al.*, 2016). Wang *et al.*, 2016 demonstrated that CD44 antibody-triggered nanoliposomal anticancer drug delivery for molecular imaging and therapy in HCC. In a comprehensive review, Ravichandran and Rengan described various therapeutic uses of aptamers as active drugs targeting moiety through attaching with nanocarriers or acting as labeled biosensors (Ravichandran and Rengan, 2020). Dual aptamer (A15 and CL4) factionalized pegylated nanoparticles were successfully developed to target both CD133 and EGFR of HCC to potentiate the cytotoxicity of salinomycin towards HCC stem cells (Jiang *et al.*, 2015). In another comparative study, Chakraborty *et al.* described the affinity of different types of aptamers towards different liver cancer cell lines (Chakraborty *et al.*, 2020).

Aptamer as a Targeting Molecule and its Modifications for *In Vivo* Stability

Single-stranded nucleic acid oligonucleotides combine with their complementary strand and can fold into 3D scaffold conformation to interact with specific target protein receptors overexpressed on the surface of the diseased organ. Small single-stranded DNA or RNA sequences within the size range of 15 to 50 base pairs designed to target several types of receptor molecules are called chemical antibodies or aptamers (Pang *et al.*, 2018, Tabarzad and Jafari, 2016). The term 'Aptamer' originates from the Latin word, 'Aptus', which denotes 'to fit', and the

Greek word 'Meros', which means 'part'. The aptamer is synthesized by systematic evolution of ligands by exponential enrichment (SELEX) method generating a random single-stranded oligonucleotide library for a particular protein receptor family (Tuerk and Gold, 1990). The receptor affinity and selectivity are regulated by conditional modifications such as ionic strength, pH, and temperature of SELEX technology. The chemically synthesized target-specific oligonucleotides are developed according to the 3D conformational shape of the receptor of interest. There are several types of SELEX methodology named Capillary Electrophoresis SELEX (CE-SELEX), Crossover-SELEX, Conditional-SELEX, Tissue slide-based SELEX, Subtractive-SELEX, High-Throughput Sequencing SELEX (HTS-SELEX), Conditional-SELEX, Microfluidic SELEX (M-SELEX), apart from the conventional technology for the modifications of aptamers (Cerchia and de Franciscis, 2010; Hung *et al.*, 2014; Zou *et al.*, 2018). Many advantageous applications are available for aptamer as a targeting moiety over other targeting ligands, primarily antibodies. Aptamers can form into different defined secondary structures such as loop, stem, bugle, hairpin, G-quadruplex, pseudoknot, which are followed by the development of unique form 3D structures that can bind specific receptor molecules by hydrogen bonding, hydrophobic and electrostatic interactions, and van der Waals forces interactions (Camorani *et al.*, 2017). The aptamer and receptor-binding interaction are similar to the antigen-antibody interaction. However, the small size of the aptamer is favorable for deep tissue penetration, especially the desmoplastic stromal barrier developed in different types of tumors with a wide range of targeting possibilities and long shelf-live. The aptamer can be easily conjugated chemically with a variety of nano formulations for targeting purposes to overcome off-target cytotoxicity to the normal tissues. The short production time and low cost have made it a preferable choice of targeting ligand. Apart from targeting specificity, an aptamer can be considered as a therapeutic molecule capable of hindering protein-protein interactions by receptor-ligand binding; therefore, it can function as an antagonist. Thus, some aptamers have agonist-like activities for extracellular receptor domains followed by inhibition of receptor-mediated activation of the downstream signaling pathway. Furthermore, there are various other aptamer applications in the biomedical field, including biosensors, diagnostic, aptasensors, and imaging systems.

Despite its wide range of biological applications, the long-time *in vivo* stability of aptamer is a matter of concern due to the presence of nuclease in the bloodstream. Chemical modifications in the oligonucleotide sequence of aptamers can introduce the nuclease stability in blood circulation sequences. Among several types of aptamer modifications, the most common chemical modifications are the phosphate backbone modification such as oxygen replacement with sulfur in ribose unit or inside the phosphodiester linkage, locked nucleic acids, and circular, multivalent, and dimerization of aptamers, end-capping at the terminal end. The 3′ to 5′ exonuclease attack can be blocked by capping the 3′-end of the aptamer. Another strategy to protect the aptamer from exonuclease activity is the capping of the 3′ end with inverted deoxy-thymidine modification. Cholesterol can be conjugated at the oligonucleotide end by a spacer, resulting in many fold increase in plasma half-life. A major drawback of the small-sized aptamer is the high clearance rate that the conjugation of large PEG molecules can control at the 5′ end of aptamer sequences. The 2′ position of the sugar modifications can improve the half-life of the aptamer sequence. The 2′ -Fluoro (2′ -F), 2′ -amino (2′ -NH2) and 2′ -O-methyl (2′ -OMe)2′ -substitute modifications are the most common 2′ position substitution on ribose unit (Camorani *et al.*, 2017; Esposito *et al.*, 2011; Chen *et al.*, 2019, Mallikaratchy, 2017). The phosphorothioate backbone modification is another aptamer stability procedure that can ensure the long-term stability of the aptamer in plasma. The phosphorothioate backbone modified aptamer conjugated nanoparticle was reported to target EpCAM receptor overexpressed on the surface of colorectal carcinoma (Dutta *et al.*, 2018).

Aptamer and HCC

The steep rise in HCC cases along with poor prognosis acts as a driving force that directs the researchers around the globe to develop strategies that lead to substantially superior and well-organized management of HCC, resulting in distinctively superior outcomes in the present scenario (Zhang *et al.*, 2016b; Li *et al.*, 2016; Mohamed *et al.*, 2017; Sun *et al.*, 2014; Zhou and Rossi 2014). The efficient management should address two key issues: (a) identification of highly efficient biomarkers which will help diagnose the diseases at the early stages; (b) development of substantially effective and safer targeted therapeutics based on the biomarker proteins or receptors having remarkably improved penetration and retention in HCC tissues and significantly lowered off-target toxicity (Zhang *et al.*, 2019). The multiple promising features of aptamers enable them to successfully utilize both the aspects of effective management of HCC (Zhang *et al.*,2016b; Li *et al.*,2016; Mohamed *et al.*,2017; Fu and Xiang 2020; Zhou and Rossi 2014; Ladju *et al.*,2018). For example, TLS11a, one of the most-studied aptamers, was utilized to develop an electrochemical biosensor (aptasensor) which enables straightforward, selective, highly sensitive, and label-free diagnosis of neoplastic hepatocytes (Shangguan *et al.*, 2008; Kashefi-Kheyrabadi *et al.*, 2014). Further, they revealed that the developed aptasensor had the ability to detect the liver cancer cells within a very low concentration (2 cells/ml) and at a wide linear dynamic range. A microcantilever biosensor based on TLS11a that worked on a similar principle as that of aptasensor for the analysis of neoplastic hepatocytes was developed. However, its responsiveness was found to be less as compared to aptasensor (Chen *et al.*,2016). TLS11a was conjugated with gold nanoparticles and horse reddish peroxidase enzyme (HRP), leading to the development of cytosensor, which allows simple and sensitive (30cells/ml) detection of neoplastic hepatocytes (Jo and Ban 2016). In a sequential advancement in the development of diagnostic tools, a combination of TLS11a, indium tin oxide electrode assay, and multifunctional nanoprobes had been used, which showed a much-improved detection limit (Sun *et al.*, 2017). Xu *et al.* (2015) synthesized a series of aptamers capable of distinguishing HCC cells from normal liver cells and had K_D (dissociation constant) values within the range of 64-349 nM, indicating their high affinity. Further, treatment with trypsin substantially decreased the binding of aptamer with HCC cells, signifying that target proteins for aptamer binding were present at the surface of neoplastic hepatocytes. From the outcomes of the study, they concluded that the aptamers developed by them could be successfully explored to develop a tool for early detection, targeted therapeutics, and imaging agents. Santra *et al.* (2010) highlighted the successful implication of fluorescent silica nanoparticles in the imaging of malignant tissue owing to their photostability, brightness, and high emission. Hu *et al.* (2017) labeled the HCC cells with biotinylated TLS11a aptamer (Bio-TLS11a) followed by co-incubation with fluorescent silica nanoparticles functionalized with streptavidin (Sa-FSNPs). The interaction between streptavidin and biotin enabled *in vitro* assessment of HepG2 cells. Further, they claimed that Sa-FSNPs had the ability to specifically detect HepG2 cells with satisfactory sensitivity and were devoid of any notable off-target toxicity. Wang *et al.* (2016) developed an aptamer-based innovative strategy that enabled the detection of circulating tumor cells (CTCs) in HCC. The surface of nanofilm made up of a hydroxyapatite/chitosan (HA/CTS) was functionalized with carbohydrate sialic acid Lewis X (SLex), leading to the formation of the CTC-^{BioT}Chip platform, which exhibited efficient capture and identification of HCC CTCs. HCC can develop upon exposure to a small number of aflatoxin B_1(AFB_1). Joo *et al.* (2017) developed graphene oxide (GO) and fluorescein imide functionalized AFB_1-specific aptamer-based rapid and efficient detection method for AFB_1. The binding of the aptamer to AFB_1 resulted in a conformational change, which enabled the aptamer to interact with GO leading to a decrease or quenching of fluorescence. The published reports in the literature (Watany *et al.*, 2017; Mohammed *et al.*, 2016; Fezza *et al.*, 2019) pointed out the substantial potential of Dickkopf-1 (DKK1), secretory protein (an inhibitor of Wnt signaling transduction pathway) in early detection of HCC. Zhou *et al.* (2019) developed two DKK1-targeting aptamers, such as slow-acting and fast-acting. Experimental evidence showed that slow-acting aptamer was suitable for aptamer-based enzyme-linked immunosorbent assay (ELISA), whereas fast-acting variety was found to be useful in flow cytometry and spot-blot. The latest advancement in the arena of HCC detection based on TLS11a aptamer has involved its conjugation with a fluorescent probe that can differentiate between malignant and normal hepatocytes. Findings of *in vitro* study in liver cancer cells and analysis of frozen HCC tissue section revealed that aptamer-functionalized fluorescent probe emitted fluorescent signal upon binding to targeted cancer cells.

Aptamers and *In Vivo* Imaging in HCC

In vivo imaging plays a pivotal role in the clinical diagnosis of tumors, and it utilizes different techniques such as magnetic resonance imaging (MRI), ultrasound molecular imaging, computed tomography (CT), and fluorescence molecular tomography (Zhang *et al.*, 2019). For remarkable improvement in the efficiency of different *in vivo* imaging techniques, the applications of various aptamer-based contrast agents, probes, and fluorescent groups have been explored. The findings have shown a highly promising outcome. For example, magnetic resonance imaging (MRI) has gained a substantial preference for *in vivo* imaging in HCC to detect tumors because of its exceptional spatial resolution for soft tissues. However, short circulation half-life and a deficiency in tumor-targeting specificity of commercially available MRI-contrast agent, gadolinium-DTPA (diethylenetriamine penta-acetic acid) (Gd^{3+}-DTPA), leads to the feeble outcome of MRI-based imaging in HCC (Bayat *et al.*, 2019; Bouvier-Muller and Duconge 2018; Zhang *et al.*, 2019). To overcome drawbacks along with remarkable improvement of imaging efficiency, Yan *et al.* (2018) synthesized an aptamer by SELEX capable of targeting Endoglin (CD105), type I membrane glycoprotein overexpressed in neoplastic hepatic cells and in the neovasculature of the endothelial cells. The abundant expression of CD105 has been observed in the tumor periphery. The aptamer showed high affinity (K_D 98pmol/L) for the target protein. They successfully developed an HCC-targeting nanoprobe upon conjugating aptamer and imaging reporter, and the prepared nanoprobe allowed successful visualization of orthotopic HCC xenografts with diameters as small as 1-4 mm. Upon successfully completing the study, they concluded that the multimodal nanoprobe has the potential of non-invasive imaging of tiny HCC by pre-operative MRI leading to successful tumor removal *via* intraoperative near-infrared (NIR) fluorescence imaging. Zhao *et al.* (2018) developed ultrasmall superparamagnetic iron oxide (USPIO)-based magnetic resonance probe which was functionalized with AP613-1, capable of targeting glypican-3 (GPC3), a heparan sulfate proteoglycan highly expressed in the plasma membrane of most HCC cells, but not in normal liver tissue or benign hepatocellular nodules, with high affinity and specificity. They synthesized oleic acid-coated USPIO nanoparticles whose surfaces were tailored with amino polyethylene glycol. AP613-1 functionalized USPIO nanoprobes were prepared by the reaction of a 5′-carboxyl group of aptamer with an amino group of USPIO. Findings of *in vitro* investigations in malignant hepatocytes and *in vivo* studies in GPC3-expressing

HCCs in xenograft mice revealed high specificity of the aptamer-functionalized magnetic probe for GPC3 cells leading to targeted imaging effect exclusively in malignant hepatic tissues.

Aptamers and Targeted Delivery in HCC

The significantly high mortality rate in HCC is due to the multiple potential drawbacks of currently available chemotherapeutics in HCC. Among them, certain potential drawbacks that result in greatly compromised therapeutic outcomes in HCC include faster clearance, low drug concentration in HCC cells (only 5-10% of dose accumulated in neoplastic hepatocytes as compared to dose accumulated in the normal liver), resulting in sub-optimal effect and multi-drug resistance (MDR) and non-specific biodistribution, and therefore, severe toxicity in healthy tissues (Zhang *et al.,* 2016). Thus, the rapid development and availability of targeted therapeutics capable of specifically delivering therapeutic payloads into neoplastic hepatocytes and the massive reduction in toxicity in healthy hepatocytes are badly needed at the clinical level for remarkable improvement in therapeutic outcomes. The plenty of evidence in the literature has revealed significant superiority of aptamer over the other targeting ligands in the development of targeted therapeutics in HCC (Sun and Zu 2014; Zhang *et al.,* 2016; Li *et al.,* 2016; Mohammed *et al.,* 2017; Elnaggar *et al.,* 2019; Chen *et al.,* 2019; Li *et al.,* 2016; Ladju *et al.,* 2017). Despite the fact that significant research on targeted chemotherapeutics involving conjugation of aptamer with antitumor drugs, oligonucleotides, or nanocarriers has been undertaken (Shangguan *et al.,* 2008; Trinh *et al.,* 2015; Dong *et al.,* 2017; Weigum *et al.,* 2016), successful targeted therapeutics in HCC is still in infancy. Chakraborty *et al.* (2020) explored the potential of phosphorothioate backbone-modified TLS 9a (designated as L5) selective delivery of therapeutics in HCC cells for the induction of target-specific apoptosis in them. Further, they compared the targeting potential L5 with previously reported HCC-targeting aptamers (TLS-11a, AS-1411, APS 613-1) and non-aptamer ligands (galactosamine/transferrin) by conjugating them with polymeric nanoparticles which were prepared from US Food and Drug Administration (USFDA)-approved polymer, poly(lactic-co-glycolic) acid (PLGA) and evaluated through a series of well-defined *in vitro* and *in vivo* investigations. Findings of the study revealed that L5-functionalized drug-nanocarrier (PTX-NPL5) showed maximum potency to induce apoptosis preferentially in neoplastic hepatocytes among the different types of investigated formulations used in this study. Further, it showed no appreciable toxicity against healthy hepatocytes both *in vitro* and *in vivo,* unveiling a new avenue in the arena of targeted therapeutic against HCC. They highlighted that chain-length and affinity (denoted by K_D value) are equally crucial in selecting aptamers to develop aptamer-functionalized targeted therapeutics by comparing the characteristics of

L5 and TLS 11a (designated as L2). Computational modeling showed L5 specifically targeted surface biomarker proteins, TAG-72 and HSP70, which are the surface biomarkers specifically present on the surface of neoplastic hepatocytes. The examples of aptamer-mediated targeted delivery systems capable of directing therapeutic payloads preferentially in neoplastic hepatocytes have been summarized in Table **1**.

Table 1. Summary of aptamer-functionalized nanocarriers for targeted delivery of therapeutics.

Name of Aptamer	Characteristics of Aptamer	Target	Brief Outcome	References
A15 to target CD133 cells and CL4 to target to target EGFR	A15 and CL4 both were DNA aptamers and their sequences are given below A15- (5′-NH2 -CCCUCCUACAUAGGG-3′) CL4- (5′-NH2- GCCUUAGUAACGUGCUUUGAUGUCGAUUCGACAGGAGGC-3′)	CD133 cells and EGFR receptor	Salinomycin-loaded PLGA nanoparticles (SN) were prepared by multiple emulsion solvent evaporation techniques. Aptamers were conjugated on the surface of SN by using the N-(3-Dimethylamino propyl)-N'-ethyl carbodiimide hydrochloride (EDC) and N-Hydroxysuccinimide (NHS). A15 functionalized, CL4-functionalized, A-15, and CL4-functionalized nanoparticles were designated as CSN, ESN and CESN, respectively. The cytotoxicity study revealed that the cytotoxic potential of CESN in HCC cells and CD133+ HCC cells (MDR cancer cells) was remarkably superior as compared to CSN and ESN nanoparticles. Further, *in vivo* studies in HCC tumor bearing xenograft mice supported the findings of *in vitro* study. Thus, they concluded that substantially superior antitumor activity of CESN might be due to the efficient targeting by dual aptamers leading to much improved preferential delivery of salinomycin to HCC cells.	Jiang *et al.*, 2015

(Table 1) cont.....

Name of Aptamer	Characteristics of Aptamer	Target	Brief Outcome	References
EpDT3	RNA aptamer. The sequences of unmodified and modified EpDT3 are given below. (5'GCGACUGGUUACCCGGUCG-3') -unmodified 5′-FAM-GCGACUGGUUACCCGGUCG-$(CH2)_6$-NH_2-3′- modified aptamer	EGFR receptor	Despite the fact that tumor suppressor gene PTEN (Ad5-PTEN) has enormous potential as an antitumor agent in HCC, several factors such as auto-immunogenicity, non-specific toxicity to normal tissues, and inferior stability in the blood stream because of neutralizing antibody restrict its widespread application. The linker molecule PEG was used to conjugate EpCAM-targeting EpDT3 aptamer with Ad5-PTEN to form EpDT3-PE--Ad5-PTEN conjugate (EPAP) by adopting the chemical synthesis method. Results showed that EPAP was found to 16-times more stable as compared to naked Ad5-PTEN. It significantly elevated gene expression and cellular internalization of EPAP by HepG2 cells, inhibited cell proliferation and migration, and decreased the toxicity in normal liver cells, L02. *In vivo* study in HepG2 xenograft in nude mice showed the substantial antitumor potential of EPAP. In short, EpDT3 had the potential to bind with overexpressed EpCAM receptors with high affinity and specificity, leading to preferential delivery of Ad5-PTEN in HCC cells resulting in remarkably superior therapeutic outcomes.	Liu *et al.*, 2018

(Table 1) cont.....

Name of Aptamer	Characteristics of Aptamer	Target	Brief Outcome	References
TLS11a	DNA aptamer, 63 bp long, the sequence of aptamer was given below 5′-ACA GCA TCC CCA TGT GAA CAA TCG CAT TGT GAT TGT TAC GGT TTC CGC CTC ATG GAC GTG CTG TTTTTTTTTT-SH-3′	Hepatoma cells	Bi-specific T-cell engagers (BiTE) have evolved as an innovative therapeutic approach because of their excellent therapeutic potential in HCC. However, several drawbacks have hindered their successful clinical applications. An aptamer/antibody bispecific system (AAbs) was developed by conjugating TLS11a aptamer and anti-CD3 antibody through a crosslinker, sulfosuccinimidyl 4-(- -maleimidomethyl) cyclohexane-1-carboxylate (sulfo-SMCC) leading to the formation of bi-specific system, TLS11a/CD3. Findings of the study showed that TLS11a/CD3 showed preferential binding with hepatoma cells (H22) and T-cells, leading to the T-cell mediated antigen-specific lysis of hepatoma cells. Further, it promoted significant inhibition of implanted H22 tumors and elongated the survival of mice. In conclusion, simultaneous targeting of H22 and T-cell directed the T-cells to kill the tumor cells effectively, leading to substantial improvement in antitumor activities both *In vitro* and *in vivo*.	Hu *et al.*, 2018

(Table 1) cont.....

Name of Aptamer	Characteristics of Aptamer	Target	Brief Outcome	References
ST21	Peptide aptamer (SFSIIHTPILPL-TAT-SFSIIHTPILPL	HCC cells	A cationic peptide, disulfide cross-linked stearylated poly arginine peptide modified with histidine (H_3R_5) was modified with peptide aptamer S21 which was composed of SP94 and cell-penetrating peptide TAT. SP94 directed the specific binding to HCC cells, whereas the job of the cell-penetrating peptide was to facilitate the movement across the plasma membrane. miRNA-195 (miR195) and fasudil were simultaneously loaded into peptide carriers by condensation through electrostatic interaction and ammonium sulfate-induced transmembrane electrochemical gradient, respectively. Findings revealed that the therapeutic potential of aptamer-functionalized peptide nanoparticles was significantly superior as compared to unmodified counterparts. Thus, aptamer-functionalized peptides possessed the ability of preferential delivery of therapeutic payloads simultaneously into HCC cells.	Liu *et al.*, 2016
TLS1c	DNA aptamer, 5'-ACAGGAGTGATGGTTGTT ATCTGGCCTCAGAGGTTCTCGGGTGTGGTCACTCCT G-3'	BNL 1ME A.7R.1 (MEAR) cells	TLS1c-functionalized cabazitaxel (Cab)-loaded liposome was prepared. Findings revealed that TLS1c resulted in preferential delivery of aptamer-functionalized liposome into neoplastic MEAR cells, leading to remarkably enhanced therapeutic potential and significant reduction in off-target toxicity	Cheng *et al.*, 2019

(Table 1) cont.....

Name of Aptamer	Characteristics of Aptamer	Target	Brief Outcome	References
AS-1411	DNA aptamer, 5′-d(GGTGGTGGTGGTTGTGGTGGTGGTGG)-3′	Nucleolin receptor	Thiol-modified AS-1411 was tailored at the surface of biocompatible and redox-responsive mesoporous silica nanoparticles containing cytochrome c as sealing agent and DOX as therapeutic payload to achieve tumor-targeted triplex therapy. Cytochrome c was immobilized mesoporous silica nanoparticles (MSNs) *via* disulfide linkage resulting in redox-responsive intracellular delivery. Extensive investigations revealed that AS-1411 directed target specific delivery in HCC cells and reluctant, glutathione resulted in release of DOX into cellular microenvironment leading to apoptosis of malignant hepatocytes. Thus, they highlighted that the triplex therapy consisting of DOX, cytochrome c, and AS-1411 possessed a remarkable potential for successfully combating HCC as evidenced from the change of tumor size, TUNEL staining, and HE staining assays.	Zhang *et al.*, 2014

(Table 1) cont.....

Name of Aptamer	Characteristics of Aptamer	Target	Brief Outcome	References
GT-75	A DNA aptamer 5′-TGTTTGTTTGTTTGTTTGTTTGTTTGTTTGTTTGTTTGTTTGTTTGTTTGT TTGTTTGTTTGTTTGTTTGTTTGT-3′	Elongation factor 1A (eEF1A), protein involved in the elongation step of protein synthesis	GT-75 aptamer containing GT repetition was tested in three types of HCC cells, such as HepG2, HuH7, and JHH6. The delivery of G-75 by liposome resulted in time and dose-dependent cytotoxicity. The apoptotic potential was found to be highest in JHH6 cells, however no notable effect on cell cycle was observed. They highlighted that G-75 showed its therapeutic potential upon interaction with eEF1A; as no distinct changes in mRNA or protein level were observed. Upon completion of the successful study, they concluded that liposome-mediated delivery was far superior in reducing the cell viability in panel of HCC cells compared to cholesterol-mediated delivery.	Scaggiante *et al.*, 2016

(Table 1) cont.....

Name of Aptamer	Characteristics of Aptamer	Target	Brief Outcome	References
AP273	RNA aptamer, TCAGGTGCAGTTCTCGACTCGGTCTTGATGTGGGT	α-fetoprotein (AFP)	High expression of AFP has been observed in HCC whereas minimal expression is seen in adult healthy liver tissue. It is one of the key and widely used serum biomarker for the diagnosis of HCC. SELEX technology was employed to synthesize and characterize an RNA aptamer that showed significantly high affinity (K_D ~33nM). Results showed that aptamer exhibited dose-dependent significant inhibition on proliferation of HCC cells by substantially downregulated AFP-dependent oncogenes. Thus, they concluded that AFP had the potential to be acted as an efficient therapeutic and diagnostic agent to achieve significantly improved therapeutic outcome in AFP-related HCC. Later, the study by Dong *et al.*, further supported the outcome of previous study as they pointed out the ability of AP273 to specifically target the HCC cells.	Dong *et al.*, 2015

Aptamer-Functionalized Theranostic in HCC

A theranostic system comprising diagnostic agent and therapeutic modalities may have enormous potential in HCC therapy due to the simultaneous ability of detection or diagnosis and therapy, which could help overcome the problem associated with the diagnosis of HCC and therapy. Further, their functionalization with aptamer boosts the combined outcome of theranostic because of highly preferential and superior delivery to HCC tumors (Usmani *et al.*, 2018). Pilapong *et al.* (2014) developed a smart magnetic–aptamer probe by functionalizing carboxymethyl cellulose modified MNPs (CMC-MNPs) with EpCAM aptamer to target overexpressed EGFR receptor at the surface of malignant hepatocytes. The delivery capability of nontoxic cellulose derivatives to deliver therapeutic payload DOX, targeting potential of EpCAM aptamer, and imaging quality of magnetic nanoparticles have made them popular. Detailed findings of the study revealed that developed aptamer-based magnetic nanoprobe possessed the satisfactory potential of magnetic resonance (MR) imaging *in vitro*, enhanced target-specific delivery potential to deliver DOX into HCC cells, leading to significantly superior cancer diagnosis and treatment. Babei *et al.* (2017) developed 5-fluorouracil (5-FU)-loaded PEGylated mesoporous silica nanoparticles (NPs), which were hybridized with gold nanoparticles as gate keeper leading to the formation of (PEG-Au@Si-5-FU) for theranostic application in HCC. Finally, the developed theranostic system was functionalized with an EGFR-targeting aptamer to make it target-specific for neoplastic hepatocytes due to the ability of aptamer to bind with overexpressed EGFR receptors on the surface of HCC cells. Findings of the study revealed that cytotoxic potential and cellular internalization of aptamer-functionalized theranostic nanoparticles were significantly superior compared to the unmodified counterpart. Thus, they concluded that their research had provided proof-of-concept that reveals the potential application of hybrid nanoparticles as multimodal nanoparticles. Two well-suited HCC cells, HCCLM9 with superior metastatic potential and MHCC97-L with inferior metastatic potential, were explored to identify a potent aptamer capable of detecting the HCC metastasis. The whole SELEX technology was employed by using HCCLM9 as the target cell population and MHCC97-L as the subtractive cell population. Outcomes of the study revealed that out of six different aptamers, LY-1 showed substantially superior binding affinity and specificity for metastatic cell populations' *in vitro* study, a preclinical study in a metastatic animal model, and clinical HCC specimens. Further, LY-1 functionalized magnetic nanoparticles possessed an excellent ability to pick up the HCC cells from whole blood, indicating a promising role of LY-1 as a molecular probe to identify metastatic HCC cells.

Mechanisms of Aptamer Internalization

Aptamers have been developed to target overexpressed proteins or receptors, leading to targeted delivery of therapeutic payload into neoplastic cells and significant reduction of off-target toxicity. Multiple well-defined pathways, namely clathrin- and caveolae-mediated endocytosis, macropinocytosis, and phagocytosis are responsible for the internalization of the aptamer. However, a growing number of published reports has demonstrated that mechanisms of internalization of aptamers are broadly of two types; clathrin-and caveolae-mediated endocytosis, also known as receptor-mediated endocytosis (general mechanism of aptamer internalization) and macropinocytosis (mechanism of internalization of nucleolin-targeting aptamer, AS-1411) (Yoon and Rossi 2018).

The mechanism of aptamer internalization by clathrin-mediated pathway was confirmed by a colocalization study using fluorescently-labeled transferrin. Clathrin-mediated endocytosis (CME) takes place *via* a series of steps which include: (a) selection of cargo and formation of clathrin-coated pits; (b) induction of cargo followed by membrane-invagination; (c) fractionalization of vesicles and uncoating and (d) sorting by endosomes. Caveolae-mediated endocytosis has the following characteristics (a) (CvME) is triggered upon binding of ligand to receptor followed by separation of caveolae vesicles from the plasma membrane by dynamin, (b) the lipid rafts of the caveolae are composed of mainly cholesterol and sphingolipids and (c) the regulator of a caveolin protein family (caveolin-1/2) includes kinases [Src family protein tyrosine kinases, PTKs] and phosphatase (alkaline phosphatase); and the proteins responsible for caveolae-mediated sorting include caveolin-2, cavin, actin, integrin, and Rab family proteins (Yoon and Rossi 2018; Bareford and Swan 2007; Oh and Park 2014).

The 41-mer sgc8 aptamer has a high binding affinity as K_D value is in the picomolar range for human protein tyrosine kinase-7 (PTK7), which is one of the important biomarker proteins present at the surface of leukemic cells and solid tumors. The aptamer is internalized by receptor-mediated endocytosis (RME), which includes invagination of the plasma membrane to form new intracellular vesicles that enclose the composite of sgc8 and PTK7, resulting in the protection of the complex before it reaches the endosomes (Shangguan *et al.,* 2008a). The internalization of other aptamers, such as aptamers against PSMA-targeting, EGFR-targeting, *etc.*, takes place through RME. Plenty of studies have highlighted that RME is considered a standard mechanism for the internalization of aptamers (Soundararajan *et al.,* 2009; Wang *et al.,* 2016; Yoon and Rossi, 2018).

Macropinocytosis, an actin-dependent mechanism, is the process of formation of waving sheet-like extensions of the plasma membrane, which ultimately leads to the generation of large (>200 nm) organelles called macropinosomes upon the closure of the extensions, and unlike other endocytic mechanisms, macropinocytosis is not directly activated by drug or their associated receptors. The polymerization of cytosolic actin is the key for the formation of protrusions in macropinocytosis and is driven by the coordinated action of small family Rho guanosine triphosphatases (GTPases) and phosphoinositide 4,5-bisphosphate (PI(4,5)P2). It is worth mentioning that very few protrusions lead to the formation of macropinosomes, while the rest are pulled back to the plasma membrane. Nucleolin-targeting AS-1411, the sole member in the aptamer family, is internalized by the process of macropinocytosis. Overexpression of nucleolin receptor has been reported in various types of malignancy such as breast cancer, glioma, ovarian cancer, HCC, *etc.* It can shuttle between cytoplasm and nucleus. The half-lives of cytoplasmic and cell-surface nucleolin are 45 minutes, whereas nuclear nucleolin has a half-life of more than 8 h. Evidence in the literature pointed out that the translocation of nucleolin is a temperature-dependent process, and endoplasmic reticulum (ER)-trans-golgi network transport does not play any significant role in the translocation process (Kotula *et al.,* 2012).

The Aptamer-receptor complex RME is fused with endosomes, leading to their sorting for recycling back to the plasma membrane or delivery to late endosomes and lysosomes for degradation. The subcellular distribution of aptamers has been studied using confocal microscopy and transmission electron microscopy (TEM) to gather information regarding the intracellular fate of aptamers (Yoon and Rossi 2018). For example, colocalization of cell-type-specific DNA aptamers with lysosomal-associated membrane protein 1 (LAMP-1) was authenticated by *in situ* fluorescence hybridization in renal proximal tubule RPTEC/TRT1 cells. The fluorescence of PrP^c–functionalized fluorescent QDs provided distinctive clues regarding the intracellular dynamics of aptamer through fluorescent imaging. The findings of the immunofluorescent assay revealed that PrP^c-QD complexes were colocalized in the lysosome, endoplasmic reticulum, and golgi apparatus (Chen *et al.,* 2012; Cesur *et al.,* 2015). Tailoring of aptamers on the surface of the nanoparticles has been done to detect the subcellular localization by optical microscopy or TEM devoid of any fluorescence tag. For example, subcellular localization of nucleolin-targeting AS-1411 was analyzed by TEM upon conjugating them at the surface of nanoparticles in C6 brain glial tumor cells and brain endothelial cells, bEnd.3. It was observed that AS-1411 aptamer-nanoparticle complex was primarily colocalized in endosomes of bEnd3 cells and mitochondria. In contrast, the complex was colocalized in the lysosome and golgi apparatus of C6 cells, indicating varied subcellular localization of aptamer depending on the cell types. The DNA aptamer (5ECdsAP1) targeting transcription factor activating protein 1 (AP-1) was functionalized at the surface of iron oxide or gold nanoparticles, and the TEM study showed localization of aptamer in ER only. Thus, based on the published reports, it has been observed that aptamers are first internalized into endocytic vehicles followed by their redistribution into other subcellular compartments depending on the physiology of the host cells (Liu *et al.,* 2014; Gao *et al.,* 2014).

Factors Affecting *In Vivo* Therapeutic Potency of Aptamer

The development of aptamer having a high binding affinity for the target by *In vitro* SELELX is relatively simple. Translation of their potential for a therapeutic application requires an extensive investigation of their behavior *in vivo*. The following factors need to be adequately addressed to explore the potential of aptamers to a maximum extent for a better therapeutic outcome (Keefe *et al.,* 2010; Morita *et al.,* 2018).

Resistant to Nuclease Enzyme

Aptamers made up of unmodified nucleotides have extremely short serum half-lives which range from several minutes to several tens of minutes due to the abundance of nuclease enzymes in the physiological fluid. The average time for the decay of aptamers in the blood depends on their structure. Increasing evidences in the literature suggest that chemical modification in nucleotide sugars or internucleotide phosphodiester linkages increases serum half-life.

Substitution of 2′-OH in ribose sugar of pyrimidine ring with 2′-fluro (2′-F), 2′-NH_2 (2′-NH_2) and 2′-O-methyl (2′-OMe) imparts resistance to nuclease degradation leading to an elevation of serum half-life. Incorporation of locked nucleic acids (LNAs), which are the analogs of ribonucleotide having a methylene linkage between 2′-O and 4′-C of the sugar ring, results in strengthening of resistance to nucleases and thermostability, leading to the formation of most stable pairs. In contrast to LNA (which is a structurally rigid modification, flexible structural modification), unlocked nucleic acid (UNA), which lacks the bond between C2′- C3′ of sugar, has also been explored to increase the resistance to nucleases. Several modifications in the phosphodiester backbone have also been explored for predominant improvement in resistance to nucleases. Replacement of phosphodiester linkage of aptamers with methyl phosphonate or phosphorothioate analog has been attempted widely. Incorporation of phosphorodithioate linkage (PS2) formed by substituting non-bridging oxygen atoms with sulphur atoms results in a dramatic increase in target-binding affinity. Further, the replacement of phosphodiester linkages with triazole linkage is highly advantageous. Triazole linkage can be established by automated phosphoramidite synthesis using modified dinucleoside blocks or by performing click reactions between azide- and alkyne-bearing nucleosides (Sun *et al.*, 2014; Morita *et al.*, 2018; Keefe *et al.*, 2010).

A chiral transition of the D-form of natural DNA has resulted in the formation of L-DNA, the mirror image of the former, which exhibits significantly better resistance to nuclease as compared to D-form without any notable change in binding affinity. Application of chiral transition in aptamers has resulted in the generation of L-enantiomeric aptamers, known as Spiegelmers, by chemical synthesis. Among the series of chemicals as described above, 2′ -fluoro, 2′-O-methyl-substitutions, 3′-end capping with inverted thymidine and phosphorothioate backbone modifications have been investigated much extensively to develop aptamers highly resistant to nuclease degradation (Keefe *et al.*, 2010; Zhou and Rossi 2014; Sun *et al.*, 2014; Sun and Zu 2015; Zhu and Chen 2018; Lakhin *et al.*, 2013).

Renal Filtration

The molecular masses of most of the aptamers (15-50 nucleotides long) range between 5-15 kDa, which is significantly lower than the molecular mass cut-off for renal glomerulus as it ranges between 30-50 kDa. Therefore, aptamers, irrespective of sensitivity/resistance to nucleases, are susceptible to renal filtration. The most widely used strategy to prevent renal excretion of aptamers is to increase the molecular weight of aptamers by functionalizing them with high molecular weight entities such as polyethylene glycol (PEG), cholesterol, protein, multimerization, and nanomaterials. Cholesterol can be conjugated at the 5′-end of an aptamer to form cholesterol-aptamer conjugate (cholODN) (Keefe *et al.*, 2010; Lakhin *et al.*, 2013; Morita *et al.*, 2018). A study conducted by Lee *et al.* (2013) showed that 2′-F pyrimidine modified RNA aptamer containing 29 nucleotides inhibits the replication of Hepatitis C virus. The aptamer was conjugated with cholesterol to form a cholesterol-conjugated aptamer. Results showed that cholesterol conjugation resulted in a longer half-life and significantly reduced clearance rate, which was approximately nine times lower than that of the non-conjugated aptamer. Conjugation with PEG is a widely used strategy and probably more extensively investigated than cholesterol conjugation to augment the circulating half-life. For example, conjugation of 40 kDa (PEG) to 2′-F or 2′-O-methyl aptamers increased circulating half-life from 0.5 to 12 h when administered to Sprague-Dawley rats (Soutschek *et al.*, 2004). Due to its high molecular weight, the functional hindrance of aptamer binding to its target can be created upon conjugation to PEG. Thus, a case-by-case determination regarding the effect of different parameters such as size, type of PEG, and length of PEG linked to the aptamer on the binding interaction of aptamer to its target should be performed (Morita *et al.*, 2018).

Safety of Aptamers

Majorly, aptamers lack the toxicology class effects associated with antisense oligonucleotides as reported in the literature (Keefe *et al.*, 2010; Morita *et al.*, 2018; Lakhin *et al.*, 2013). Visible accumulation of mononuclear phagocytes as determined histologically is the principal finding in the toxicity study of therapeutic aptamers. This finding does not come under adverse events. A good safety margin between a pharmacologically effective dose and a good safety margin between a toxicologically established no-adverse-effect level has been shown by therapeutic aptamers (Geary *et al.*, 2003; Keefe *et al.*, 2010; Morita *et al.*, 2018). Thus, very restricted information is available regarding the toxicological aspect of aptamers. In some literature, it has been reported that polyanionic effects, unnatural tissue accumulation, extensive chemical modification or conjugation, and non-specific immune activation, especially after continuous or repeated administration of aptamer therapeutics, may be the principal factors that contribute to the potential toxicities associated with aptamers. High negative charges associated with aptamers are responsible for non-specific binding of them with blood proteins, probably leading to their internalization in non-target tissues resulting in unwanted side effects and reduction in therapeutic efficacy. Pieces of evidence in the literature have revealed that accumulation of aptamers primarily occurs in the kidney, liver, and spleen upon intravenous administration (Morita *et al*., 2018), and different techniques, namely immunohistochemistry, *in situ* hybridization, and histopathology, have been employed for qualitative determination of oligonucleotides in various tissues. Although chemical modification is badly needed to impart resistance to nuclease enzymes, sometimes chemically modified aptamer may give rise to toxic chemical effects or become immunogenic. For example, a 2-fold increase in plasma C3a level in mice was reported upon i.v. administration of E-selectin thioaptamer at a dose of 128 μg as compared to that of mice treated with normal saline.

Interestingly, the elevated level was too low to initiate the symptomatic hypersensitive reaction (Kang *et al*., 2015). LNA-modified nucleic acids resulted in severe hepatotoxicity. Thus, it is recommended that chemical modifications be used judiciously, depending on the desired therapeutic effects by using aptamers. Apart from the chemical modification, formulations of therapeutic aptamers, especially PEGylation, can give rise to the adverse response. Pre-existing antibodies to the PEG group are responsible for a severe allergic reaction, as evidenced from a phase-III study of PEGylated RNA aptamer against clotting factor IXa (Morita *et al*., 2018).

SELEX Technology for the Identification and Selection of Aptamers

Systemic evolution of ligand by exponential enrichment (SELEX) is the process that is widely used for the generation of aptamers. Briefly, the SELEX process is composed of five steps (Sun *et al.,* 2014; Morita *et al.,* 2018) as follows: (i) at first, the target of interest is mixed with random oligonucleotide library; (ii) separation of bound sequences from unbound sequences; (iii) generation of the enriched library by the amplification of target-bound sequences; (iv) an initiation of next round of enrichment by blending the target of interest with newly amplified library; and lastly, several repetitions of a round of selection followed by sequencing of enriched aptamer sequences. Several modifications of the conventional SELEX process have been attempted to improve the outcomes of this procedure. The objectives of these modifications are as follows: The exploration of different techniques such as bead-based aptamer selection (Yang *et al.,* 2002; Yang *et al.,* 2003), slow off-rate modified aptamer (SOMAmer) (Kraemer 2011, Huang *et al.,* 2021), magnetic-assisted rapid aptamer selection (MARAS) (Lai and Hong 2014), monoclonal surface display SELEX (MSD-SELEX) (Zhu *et al.,* 2014); inclusion of additional properties in selected aptamers such as X-Aptamers (He *et al.,* 2012) and Cell-SELEX; selection of aptamers which can recognize target at their native conformational state under physiological conditions such as Cell-SELEX, hybrid-SELEX, *in vivo*-SELEX, tissue-based SELEX, *etc*. (Wilner *et al.*, 2012; Ren *et al.*, 2020). Two classical methods, namely traditional purified membrane protein-based SELEX and live cell-based SELEX, have been implemented to develop nucleic acid aptamers, which are used as targeted delivery agents.

Purified Membrane Protein-Based SELEX

This technique develops aptamers against cell-surface biomarker proteins and consists of different steps (Mallikaratchy *et al.*, 2006; Gopinath, 2007; Martin *et al.*, 2013; Zhou and Rossi, 2014). Initially, a random ssDNA library consists of chemically synthesized ssDNA oligonucleotides having 10^{14} - 10^{15} random sequences flanked by conserved primer binding sites, generally, 5′-sense primer sequence-(random primer sequence), antisense primer sequence-3′ composed of 18 to 22 bases in primer sequence and 20-40 nucleic acids in random sequence. The 5′-sense primer sequence is labeled with a fluorochrome reporter to monitor aptamer selection while affinity molecule such as biotin is tagged at 3′-antisense primer to separate single-stranded oligonucleotides, which are generated at each amplification round. The initial pool of DNA aptamers can be selected from a random ssDNA library. In the case of the generation of RNA aptamers, two additional steps are required. These are: (i) addition of T7 RNA polymerase promoter to the 5′-sense primer after the generation of ssDNA library; (ii) Transcription is initiated in 5′-3′ direction using DNA as a template. The second step of SELX includes denaturation and rapid cooling of oligonucleotides to initiate the formation of 3D structures, followed by mixing with the required target for specific binding enrichment. The third step of SELEX involves eliminating unbound nucleotide sequences by using membranes, columns, magnetic beads, and capillary electrophoresis. Later, conventional PCR (DNA aptamers) or RT-PCR (RNA aptamers) is performed to amplify the enriched sequences for the generation of new sequences, which will be used in the next steps of SELEX. Finally, 4-20 rounds of amplification and enrichment are performed for the selection of aptamers. The correct determination of the number of amplification and selection steps depends on the nature of the target, whether a purified protein or a living cell is used on the evolution of aptamer sequence library, which is established by gel electrophoresis, flow cytometry (for target binding), classical cloning and sequencing method and high throughput Next-Generation Sequencing (NGS). The purified recombinant proteins or peptides which express in prokaryotic or eukaryotic cells can serve as a target for the selection of aptamers by SELEX. Certain proteins, especially highly glycosylated proteins, require post-translational modifications, which can only happen under the physiological condition to become active. In that case, newly synthesized aptamers by the SELEX method may not have the ability of selective recognition and interaction with the target proteins, highlighting their demerit for successful biomedical application. To overcome the limitation, SELEX technology based on whole living cells known as Cell-based SELEX has been explored to develop aptamers capable of identifying the target proteins under native conditions.

Live Cell-Based SELEX

This technique provides significant promise for generating aptamers capable of recognizing particular membrane protein under native conditions, signifying the potential of live cell-based SELEX to overcome the drawbacks associated with purified membrane protein-based SELEX. Information such as native conformation, biological function, and identities of cell-surface proteins is not required. All the steps of SELEX described above are also performed in cell-based SELEX (Zhou and Rossi, 2014). The principal objective of live cell-based SELEX is to differentiate between the target cell population (cells express the protein of interest) and the control cell population (cells do not express the protein of interest). Therefore, two selection processes, namely counter selection and positive selection, have been performed in cell-based SELEX (Hicke *et al.*, 2001; Zhou and Rossi, 2014). Incubation of nucleic acid library with the control cells (also known as negative cells) is known as counter selection resulting in the removal of non-specific binding agents. In the positive selection, the target cell population (known as positive cells) is incubated with the nucleic acid library to recover the target-bound sequences.

Some Prospective Use of Aptamers in HCC Therapy

We have already discussed different types of aptamers, their chemical properties, synthesis, isolation procedures, and their advantages during miscellaneous applications in HCC, as an imaging probe or biosensor for diagnosis and as therapeutic agents or therapeutic targeting moiety to recognize respective biomarkers of malignant hepatocytes. Thus, they improve the therapeutic efficacy of presently available chemotherapeutics, whether in a single or a combination form. Here, in Table **2**, we have mentioned some of the very promising aptamers that have been successfully developed and applied against HCC for diagnostic and therapeutic purposes.

Table 2. Aptamers under scientific investigation with promising results for HCC.

Aptamer	Targeting Receptor/Proteins/Cells	Development	Application	Current Status	References
AP613-1-DNA aptamer	Glypican-3 or GPC-3 overexpressed in HCC	Through C-SELEX evolution	Imaging Probe	Under scientific research	Zhao *et al.*, 2018
LNC-2,4 DNA aptamer	Lipocalin-2 in HCC	Through C-SELEX evolution	Diagnosis	Under scientific research	Lee *et al.*, 2015
Aptamer-07S	HepG2	Through C-SELEX evolution	Detection	Under scientific research	Yu *et al.*, 2020
C-2, DNA Aptamer	HepG2	Through C-SELEX evolution	Detection	Under scientific research	Ninomiya *et al.*, 2013
TLS11a, DNA Aptamer	HepG2	Through C-SELEX evolution/ signal Amplification/ Voltametric method	Detection/cell signaling sensors	Under scientific research	Shangguan *et al.*, 2008/ Sun *et al.*, 2015/ Sun *et al.*, 2017.
TLS11a-GC, DNA aptamer	LH86	Through C-SELEX evolution	Drug Delivery	Under scientific research	Meng *et al.*, 2012.
G12msi, a modified DNA aptamer	GPC-3 overexpressed in HCC	Through C-SELEX evolution	Therapeutic targeting	Under scientific research	Park *et al.*, 2020.
TLS11a, DNA Aptamer	HCC cell surface receptors	Through C-SELEX evolution and conjugated with polymeric nanoparticle	Drug delivery	Under scientific research	Weigum *et al.*, 2016
AS1411, DNA Aptamer	Nucleolin, Cancer cell surface receptors	AS1411-Dox adduct/ AS1411-conjugated gold nanoparticles	Drug delivery and therapy	Phase 2 clinical trials.	Trinh *et al.*, 2015 & Kabirian-Dehkordi *et al.*, 2019.
EPAP, RNA Aptamer	EpCAM, cancer stem cell biomarkers	Aptamer- Gene chemical ligation	Therapy	Under scientific research	Xiao *et al.*, 2017
OPN-R3, RNA aptamer	Osteopontin, unique cell growth factor in HCC	Through C-SELEX evolution	Therapy	Under scientific research	Bhattacharya *et al.*, 2012.
GT75, DNA aptamer	(eEF1A), Elongation of cellular growth factor 1A in HCC	Liposome-aptamer ligation	Drug delivery	Under scientific research	Scaggiante *et al.*, 2016.

(Table 2) cont.....

Aptamer	Targeting Receptor/Proteins/Cells	Development	Application	Current Status	References
TLS 9a, DNA aptamer	HCC	Aptamer guided polymeric nanoparticle	Targeted therapy	Under scientific research	Chakraborty *et al.*, 2020.
AFP, RNA Aptamer	AFP, Alpha-fetoprotein	Through C-SELEX evolution	Detection and treatment	Under scientific research	Lee *et al.*, 2012.
Ep-MNPs,DNA Aptamer	EpCAM	Magnetic nanoparticle-aptamer	Imaging and treatment	Under scientific research	Pilapong *et al.*, 2014.
AP273, DNA Aptamer	Alpha-fetoprotein	Through C-SELEX evolution	Imaging and treatment	Under scientific research	Dong *et al.*, 2015
SLeX-AP, DNA Aptamer	moving tumour cells	Biocompatible nanoparticles	managing personalized therapy	Under scientific research	Wang *et al.*, 2016.

CONCLUSION

The molecular environment of HCC can be considered to understand the targeting mechanism through aptamers. The aptamers are generated based on biomarkers specific to HCC. This chapter highlighted the active targeting potential of different possible aptamers for the target-mediated drug delivery in HCC. Streamline research about this particular area of aptamer-mediated targeting in HCC has a significant impact along with different existing patented works and formulations under clinical and preclinical testing in this field.

Compared to other targeting ligands such as antibodies, the aptamers show lesser toxicity due to their high specificity and low immunogenicity. Aptamers resemble antibodies in terms of recognition and target binding capability to the targeting molecule. They provide some advantages over antibodies: shorter generation time, higher range of modifiability, no variability between the batches, improved thermal stability, higher target potential, and low-cost manufacturing. Several useful applications and specifically minimizing off-target cytotoxicity of anticancer drugs make aptamers an extraordinary targeting moiety in the therapeutic and diagnostic tool for HCC treatment. Thus, aptamer-mediated targeted drug delivery can be translated from bench to bedside to combat HCC successfully.

CONSENT FOR PUBLICATION

Not applicable.

CONFLICT OF INTEREST

The authors declare no conflict of interest, financial or otherwise.

ACKNOWLEDGEMENT

Declared none.

REFERENCES

Adiseshaiah, PP, Crist, RM, Hook, SS & McNeil, SE (2016) Nanomedicine strategies to overcome the pathophysiological barriers of pancreatic cancer. *Nat Rev Clin Oncol,* 13, 750-65. [http://dx.doi.org/10.1038/nrclinonc.2016.119] [PMID: 27531700]

Bareford, LM & Swaan, PW (2007) Endocytic mechanisms for targeted drug delivery *Adv Drug Deliv Rev,* 59, 748-5. [http://dx.doi.org/10.1016/j.addr.2007.06.008]

Bartneck, M, Warzecha, KT & Tacke, F (2014) Therapeutic targeting of liver inflammation and fibrosis by nanomedicine. *Hepatobil Surg Nutr,* 3, 364-76.

Bayat, P, Taghdisi, SM, Rafatpanah, H, Abnous, K & Ramezani, M (2019) *In vitro* selection of CD70 binding aptamer and its application in a biosensor design for sensitive detection of SKOV-3 ovarian cells. *Talanta,* 194, 399-405. [http://dx.doi.org/10.1016/j.talanta.2018.10.063] [PMID: 30609550]

Bazak, R, Houri, M, El Achy, S, Kamel, S & Refaat, T (2015) Cancer active targeting by nanoparticles: a comprehensive review of literature. *J Cancer Res Clin Oncol,* 141, 769-84. [http://dx.doi.org/10.1007/s00432-014-1767-3] [PMID: 25005786]

Bhattacharya, SD, Mi, Z, Kim, VM, Guo, H, Talbot, LJ & Kuo, PC (2012) Osteopontin regulates epithelial mesenchymal transition-associated growth of hepatocellular cancer in a mouse xenograft model. *Ann Surg,* 255, 319-25. [http://dx.doi.org/10.1097/SLA.0b013e31823e3a1c] [PMID: 22241292]

Bray, F, Ferlay, J, Soerjomataram, I, Siegel, RL, Torre, LA & Jemal, A (2018) Global cancer statistics 2018: GLOBOCAN estimates of incidence and mortality worldwide for 36 cancers in 185 countries. *Ca - Cancer J Clin,* 68, 394-424. [http://dx.doi.org/10.3322/caac.21492]

Camorani, S, Crescenzi, E, Gramanzini, M, Fedele, M, Zannetti, A & Cerchia, L (2017) Aptamer-mediated impairment of EGFR-integrin αvβ3 complex inhibits vasculogenic mimicry and growth of triple-negative breast cancers. *Sci Rep,* 7, 46659. [http://dx.doi.org/10.1038/srep46659] [PMID: 28425453]

Cerchia, L & de Franciscis, V (2010) Targeting cancer cells with nucleic acid aptamers. *Trends Biotechnol,* 28, 517-25. [http://dx.doi.org/10.1016/j.tibtech.2010.07.005] [PMID: 20719399]

Cesur, O, Nicol, C, Groves, H, Mankouri, J, Blair, GE & Stonehouse, NJ (2015) The subcellular localisation of the human papillomavirus (HPV) 16 E7 protein in cervical cancer cells and its perturbation by RNA aptamers *Viruses,* 7, 3443-61. [http://dx.doi.org/10.3390/v7072780]

Chakraborty, S, Dlie, ZY & Chakraborty, S (2020) Aptamer-functionalized drug nanocarrier improves hepatocellular carcinoma toward normal by targeting neoplastic hepatocytes *Mol Ther Nucleic Acids,* 5, 34-49. [http://dx.doi.org/10.1016/j.omtn.2020.01.034]

Chakraborty, S, Dlie, ZL & Mukherjee, B (2020) Comparative investigation of the ability of various aptamer-functionalized drug nanocarriers to induce selective apoptosis in neoplastic hepatocytes: *in vitro* and *in vivo* outcome *AAPS PharmSciTech,* 21, 1-1.

Chen, L, He, W, Jiang, H, Wu, L, Xiong, W, Li, B, Zhou, Z & Qian, Y (2018) *In vivo* SELEX of bone targeting aptamer in prostate cancer bone metastasis model. *Int J Nanomedicine,* 14, 149-59. [http://dx.doi.org/10.2147/IJN.S188003] [PMID: 30613143]

Chen, LQ, Xiao, SJ, Hu, PP, Peng, L, Ma, J, Luo, LF, Li, YF & Huang, CZ (2012) Aptamer-mediated nanoparticle-based protein labeling platform for intracellular imaging and tracking endocytosis dynamics. *Analytical Chem,* 84, 3099-110. [http://dx.doi.org/10.1021/ac202810b]

Chen, LY, Liu, YB, Wang, WY & Liu, K (2015) Effect of integrin receptor-targeted liposomal paclitaxel for hepatocellular carcinoma targeting and therapy. *Oncol Lett,* 10, 77-84. [http://dx.doi.org/10.3892/ol.2015.3242]

Chen, W, Dong, J, Haiech, J, Kilhoffer, MC & Zeniou, M (2016) Cancer stem cell quiescence and plasticity as major challenges in cancer therapy. *Stem Cells Int* 1740936. [http://dx.doi.org/10.1155/2016/1740936]

Cheng, C, Zhanlun, O, Li, Q, Yang, J, Hu, M, Zhou, Y, Zhuang, X, Zhang, ZL & Guan, S (2019) Cabazitaxel liposomes with aptamer modification enhance tumour targeting efficacy in nude mice. *Mol Med Rep,* 19, 490-8.

Dagogo-Jack, I & Shaw, AT (2018) Tumour heterogeneity and resistance to cancer therapies. *Nat Rev Clin Oncol,* 15, 81-94. [http://dx.doi.org/10.1038/nrclinonc.2017.166]

Dutta, D, Sarkar, A, Chakraborty, B, Chowdhury, C & Das, P (2015) Induction of apoptosis by a potent Betulinic acid derivative in Human colon carcinoma HT-29 cells. *International Journal of Scientific and Research Publications,* 5, 1-7.

Dutta, D, Chakraborty, B, Sarkar, A, Chowdhury, C & Das, P (2016) A novel betulinic acid analogue ascertains an antagonistic mechanism between autophagy and proteosomal degradation pathway in human colon carcinoma cells (HT29). *BMC Cancer,* 16, 1-19.

Dutta, D & Chakraborty, A (2018) Aptamer-conjugated apigenin nanoparticles to target colorectal carcinoma: A promising safe alternative of colorectal cancer chemotherapy *ACS Appl Bio Mater,* 1, 1538-56. [http://dx.doi.org/10.1021/acsabm.8b00441]

Dutta, D, Brahamacharry, P, Mukherjee, B, Mondal, L, Sen, S, Chowdhury, C & Chatterjee, MD (2019) Nanoencapsulated betulinic acid analogue distinctively improves colorectal carcinoma *in vitro* and *in vivo*. *Sci Rep,* 9, 1-20. [http://dx.doi.org/10.1038/s41598-019-47743-y]

Dong, L, Tan, Q, Ye, W, Liu, D, Chen, H, Hu, H, Wen, D, Liu, Y, Cao, Y, Kang, J, Fan, J, Guo, W & Wu, W (2015) Screening and identifying a novel ssDNA aptamer against alphafetoprotein using CE-SELEX. *Sci Rep,* 26, 15552.

Dong, L, Zhou, H, Zhao, M, Gao, X, Liu, Y, Liu, D, Guo, W, Hu, H, Xie, Q, Fan, J, Lin, J & Wu, W (2018) Phosphorothioate-modified AP613-1 specifically targets GPC3 when used for hepatocellular carcinoma cell imaging. *Mol Ther Nucleic Acids,* 13, 376-86. [http://dx.doi.org/10.1016/j.omtn.2018.09.013] [PMID: 30347351]

Elnaggar, MH, Abushouk, AI, Hassan, AHE, Lamloum, HM, Benmelouka, A, Moatamed, SA, Abd-Elmegeed, H, Attia, S, Samir, A, Amr, N, Johar, D & Zaky, S (2021) Nanomedicine as a putative approach for active targeting of hepatocellular carcinoma. *Semin Cancer Biol,* 69, 91-9. [http://dx.doi.org/10.1016/j.semcancer.2019.08.016] [PMID: 31421265]

Esposito, CL, Passaro, D, Longobardo, I, Condorelli, G, Marotta, P, Affuso, A, de Franciscis, V & Cerchia, L (2011) A neutralizing RNA aptamer against EGFR causes selective apoptotic cell death. *PloS One,* 6, e24071.

[http://dx.doi.org/10.1371/journal.pone.0024071]

Fezza, M, Moussa, M, Aoun, R, Haber, R & Hilal, G (2019) DKK1 promotes hepatocellular carcinoma inflammation, migration and invasion: Implication of TGF-β1. *PLoS ONE,* 14, e0223252. [http://dx.doi.org/10.1371/journal.pone.0223252]

Fu, Z & Xiang, J (2020) Aptamers, the nucleic acid antibodies, in cancer therapy *Int J Mol Sci,* 21, 2793. [http://dx.doi.org/10.3390/ijms21082793] [PMID: 32316469]

Gao, H, Yang, Z, Zhang, S, Pang, Z & Jiang, X (2014) Internalization and subcellular fate of aptamer and peptide dual-functioned nanoparticles. *J Drug Target,* 22, 450-9. [http://dx.doi.org/10.3109/1061186X.2014.886038] [PMID: 24512500]

Geary, RS, Yu, RZ, Watanabe, T, Henry, SP, Hardee, GE, Chappell, A, Matson, J, Sasmor, H, Cummins, L & Levin, AA (2003) Pharmacokinetics of a tumor necrosis factor-alpha phosphorothioate 2′-O--2-methoxyethyl) modified antisense oligonucleotide: Comparison across species. *Drug Metabol Disposition,* 31, 1419-28.

Gerber, DE (2008) Targeted therapies: a new generation of cancer treatments.*Am Fam Physician,* 77, 311-9.

Gopinath, SCB (2007) Methods developed for SELEX. *Anal Bioanal Chem,* 387, 171-82.

Hazra, R & Dutta, D (2021) Polymeric composite matrix with high biobased content as pharmaceutically relevant molec-ular encapsulation and release platform *ACS Appl Mater Interfaces,* 13, 40229-48.

He, W, Elizondo-RiGoojas, MA, Li, X, Lokesh, GL, Somasundera, A, Thiviyanathan, V, Volk, DE, Durland, RH, Englehardt, J, Cavasotto, CN & Gorenstein, DG (2012) X-aptamers: a bead-based selection method for random incorporation of druglike moieties onto next-generation aptamers for enhanced binding. *Biochem,* 51, 8321-3.

Hicke, BJ, Marion, C, Chang, YF, Gould, T, Lynott, CK, Parma, D, Schmidt, PG & Warren, S (2001) Tenascin-C aptamers are generated using tumor cells and purified protein. *J Biol Chem,* 276, 48644-54. [http://dx.doi.org/10.1074/jbc.M104651200] [PMID: 11590140]

http://www1.udel.edu/chem/C465/senior/fall98/Cancer2/methods.html

https://stanfordhealthcare.org/medical-conditions/cancer/cancer/cancer-types.html

https://www.ctoam.com/precision-oncology/why-we-exist/standard treatment/treatment/chemotherapy/

Hu, Z, He, J, Gong, W, Zhou, N, Zhou, S, Lai, Z, Zheng, R, Wang, W, Yang, X & Yang, W (2018) TLS11a Aptamer/CD3 antibody antitumor system for liver cancer. *J Biomed Nanotech,* 14, 1645-53.

Hu, Z, Tan, J, Lai, Z, Zheng, R, Zhong, J, Wang, Y, Li, X, Yang, N, Li, J, Yang, W, Huang, Y, Zhao, Y & Lu, X (2017) 'Aptamer combined with fluorescent silica nanoparticles for detection of hepatoma cells'. *Nanoscale Res Lett,* 12, 96. [http://dx.doi.org/10.1186/s11671-017-1890-6] [PMID: 28176286]

Huang, J, Chen, X, Fu, X, Li, Z, Huang, Y & Liang, C (2021) Advances in Aptamer-Based Biomarker Discovery. *Front Cell Dev Biol,* 9, 659760. [http://dx.doi.org/10.3389/fcell.2021.659760] [PMID: 33796540]

Hung, LY, Wang, CH, Hsu, KF, Chou, CY & Lee, GB (2014) An on-chip Cell-SELEX process for automatic selection of high-affinity aptamers specific to different histologically classified ovarian cancer cells. *Lab Chip,* 14, 4017-28.

India Project Team of the International Cancer Genome Consortium (2013) Mutational landscape of gingivo-buccal oral squamous cell carcinoma reveals new recurrently-mutated genes and molecular subgroups. *Nat Commun,* 4, 2873.

Jiang, J, Chen, H, Yu, C, Zhang, Y, Chen, M, Tian, S & Sun, C (2015) The promotion of salinomycin delivery to hepatocellular carcinoma cells through EGFR and CD133 aptam¬ers conjugation by PLGA nanoparticles. *Nanomed (London),* 10, 1863-79.

Jo, H & Ban, C (2016) Aptamer-nanoparticle complexes as powerful diagnostic and therapeutic tools. *Exp*

Mol Med, 48, e230.
[http://dx.doi.org/10.1038/emm.2016.44] [PMID: 27151454]

Joo, M, Baek, SH, Cheon, SA, Chun, HS, Choi, S-W & Park, TJ (2017) Development of aflatoxin B_1 aptasensor based on wide-range fluorescence detection using graphene oxide quencher. *Colloids Surf B Biointerfaces,* 154, 27-32.
[http://dx.doi.org/10.1016/j.colsurfb.2017.03.010] [PMID: 28285035]

Kabirian-Dehkordi, S, Chalabi-Dchar, M, Mertani, HC, Le Guellec, D, Verrier, B, Diaz, J-J, Mehrgardi, MA & Bouvet, P (2019) AS1411-conjugated gold nanoparticles affect cell proliferation through a mechanism that seems independent of nucleolin. *Nanomedicine,* 21, 102060.
[http://dx.doi.org/10.1016/j.nano.2019.102060] [PMID: 31336175]

Kale, NR & Dutta, D (2020) Functional applications of polyargininehyaluronic acid-based electrostatic complexes. *Bioelectricity,* 2, 158-66.

Kalyane, D, Raval, N, Maheshwari, R, Tambe, V, Kalia, K & Tekade, RK (2019) Employment of enhanced permeability and retention effect (EPR): Nanoparticle-based precision tools for targeting of therapeutic and diagnostic agent in cancer. *Mater Sci Eng C,* 98, 1252-76.
[http://dx.doi.org/10.1016/j.msec.2019.01.066] [PMID: 30813007]

Kang, SA, Tsolmon, B, Mann, AP, Zheng, W, Zhao, L, Zhao, YD, Volk, DE, Lokesh, GL, Morris, L, Gupta, V, Razzaq, W, Rui, H, Suh, KS, Gorenstein, DG & Tanaka, T (2015) Safety evaluation of intravenously administered mono-thioated aptamer against e-selectin in mice. *Toxicol Appl Pharmacol,* 287, 86-92.

Kashefi-Kheyrabadi, L, Mehrgardi, MA, Wiechec, E, Turner, AP & Tiwari, A (2014) Ultrasensitive detection of human liver hepatocellular carcinoma cells using a label-free aptasensor. *Anal Chem,* 86, 4956-60.
[http://dx.doi.org/10.1021/ac500375p] [PMID: 24754473]

Keefe, AD, Pai, S & Ellington, A (2010) Aptamers as therapeutics. *Nat Rev Drug Discov,* 9, 537-50.
[http://dx.doi.org/10.1038/nrd3141] [PMID: 20592747]

Kim, M, Kim, D-M, Kim, K-S, Jung, W & Kim, D-E (2018) Applications of cancer cell-specific aptamers in targeted delivery of anticancer therapeutic agents. *Molecules,* 23, 830.

Kotula, JW, Pratico, ED, Ming, X, Nakagawa, O, Juliano, RL & Sullenger, BA (2012) Aptamer-mediated delivery of splice-switching oligonucleotides to the nuclei of cancer cells. *Nucleic Acid Ther,* 22, 187-95.

Kraemer, S, Vaught, JD, Bock, C, Gold, L, Katilius, E, Keeney, TR, Kim, N, Saccomano, NA, Wilcox, SK, Zichi, D & Sanders, GM (2011) From SOMAmer-based biomarker discovery to diagnostic and clinical applications: a SOMAmer-based, streamlined multiplex proteomic assay. *PLoS One,* 6, e26332.
[http://dx.doi.org/10.1371/journal.pone.0026332] [PMID: 22022604]

Ladju, RB, Pascut, D, Massi, MN, Tiribelli, C & Sukowati, CHC (2018) Aptamer: A potential oligonucleotide nanomedicine in the diagnosis and treatment of hepatocellular carcinoma. *Oncotarget,* 9, 2951-61.

Lai, JC & Hong, CY (2014) Magnetic-assisted rapid aptamer selection (MARAS) for generating high-affinity DNA aptamer using rotating magnetic fields. *ACS Comb Sci,* 16, 321-7.
[http://dx.doi.org/10.1021/co5000272] [PMID: 24814701]

Lakhin, AV, Tarantul, VZ & Gening, LV (2013) Aptamers: problems, solutions and prospects. *Acta naturae,* 5, 34-43.

Lee, CH, Lee, YJ, Kim, JY, Lim, JH, Kim, J-H, Han, W, Lee, S-H, Noh, G-H & Lee, SW (2013) Inhibition of hepatitis C virus (HCV) replication by specific RNA aptamers against HCV NS5B R.N.A. Replicase. *J Virol,* 87, 7064-74.

Lee, KA, Ahn, JY, Lee, SH, Singh Sekhon, S, Kim, DG, Min, J & Kim, YH (2015) Aptamer-based sandwich assay and its clinical outlooks for detecting lipocalin-2 in Hepatocellular Carcinoma (HCC). *Sci Rep,* 5, 10897.
[http://dx.doi.org/10.1038/srep10897] [PMID: 26039737]

Lee, YJ & Lee, SW (2012) Regression of hepatocarcinoma cells using RNA aptamer specific to alpha-fetoprotein. *Biochem Biophys Res Commun,* 417, 521-7.
[http://dx.doi.org/10.1016/j.bbrc.2011.11.153] [PMID: 22166203]

Li, M, Zhang, W, Wang, B, Gao, Y, Song, Z & Zheng, QC (2016) Ligand-based targeted therapy: a novel strategy for hepatocellular carcinoma. *Int J Nanomedicine,* 11, 5645-69.
[http://dx.doi.org/10.2147/IJN.S115727] [PMID: 27920520]

Li, L & Wang, H (2016) Heterogeneity of liver cancer and personalized therapy. *Cancer Lett,* 379, 191-7.
[http://dx.doi.org/10.1016/j.canlet.2015.07.018] [PMID: 26213370]

Liu, CH, Ren, J, Liu, CM & Liu, PK (2014) Intracellular gene transcription factor protein guided MRI by DNA aptamers *in vivo*. *FASEB Journal,* 28, 464-73.

Liu, Y, Wu, X, Gao, Y, Zhang, J, Zhang, D, Gu, S, Zhu, G, Liu, G & Li, X (2016) Aptamer-functionalized peptide H3CR5C as a novel nanovehicle for codelivery of fasudil and miRNA-195 targeting hepatocellular carcinoma. *Int J Nanomedicine,* 11, 3891-905.
[http://dx.doi.org/10.2147/IJN.S108128] [PMID: 27574422]

Liu, Z, Sun, X, Xiao, S, Lin, Y, Li, C, Hao, N, Zhou, M, Deng, R, Ke, S & Zhong, Z (2018) Characterization of aptamer-mediated gene delivery system for liver cancer therapy. *Oncotarget,* 9, 6830-40.

Mallikaratchy, P (2017) Evolution of complex target SELEX to identify aptamers against mammalian cell-surface antigens. *Molecules,* 22, 215.

Mallikaratchy, P, Stahelin, RV, Cao, Z, Cho, W & Tan, W (2006) Selection of DNA ligands for protein kinase C-delta. *Chem Comm,* 30, 3229-31.

Martin, JA, Parekh, P, Kim, Y, Morey, TE, Sefah, K, Gravenstein, N, Dennis, DM & Tan, W (2013) Selection of an aptamer antidote to the anticoagulant drug bivalirudin. *PLoS One,* 8, e57341.
[http://dx.doi.org/10.1371/journal.pone.0057341] [PMID: 23483901]

Meng, L, Yang, L, Zhao, X, Zhang, L, Zhu, H, Liu, C & Tan, W (2012) Targeted delivery of chemotherapy agents using a liver cancer-specific aptamer. *PLoS One,* 7, e33434.
[http://dx.doi.org/10.1371/journal.pone.0033434] [PMID: 22558072]

Mohamed, NK, Hamad, MA, Hafez, MZE, Wooley, KL & Elsabahy, M (2017) Nanomedicine in management of hepatocellular carcinoma: challenges and opportunities. *Int J Cancer,* 140, 1475-84.

Mohammed, MK, Shao, C, Wang, J, Wei, Q, Wang, X, Collier, Z, Tang, S, Liu, H, Zhang, F, Huang, J, Guo, D, Lu, M, Liu, F, Liu, J, Ma, C, Shi, LL, Athiviraham, A, He, TC & Lee, MJ (2016) Wnt/-catenin signaling plays an ever-expanding role in stem cell self-renewal, tumorigenesis and cancer chemoresistance. *Genes Dis,* 3, 11-40.

Mondal, L, Mukherjee, B, Das, K, Bhattacharya, S, Dutta, D, Chakraborty, S, Pal, MM, Gaonkar, RH & Debnath, MC (2019) CD-340 functionalized doxorubicin-loaded nanoparticle induces apoptosis and reduces tumor volume along with drug-related cardiotoxicity in mice. *Int J Nanomedicine,* 14, 8073-94.
[http://dx.doi.org/10.2147/IJN.S220740] [PMID: 31632019]

Morita, Y, Leslie, M, Kameyama, H, Volk, DE & Tanaka, T (2018) Aptamer therapeutics in cancer: current and future. *Cancers (Basel),* 10, 80.
[http://dx.doi.org/10.3390/cancers10030080] [PMID: 29562664]

Mukherjee, B (2020) Nanoformulated drug delivery of potential betulinic acid derivatives: A promising approach toward cancer therapy. *In Nanomedicine for Bioactives* Springer: New York, NY, USA 127-53.

Mukherjee, B, Dhara, M, Dutta, D, Chakraborty, A, Chakraborty, S, Sengupta, S, Mondal, L, Dutta, L & Pal, K (2021) Biopolymer-based materials in nanomedicine: Synthesis and characterization. *In Biopolymer-Based Nanomaterials in Drug Delivery and Biomedical Applications.*Elsevier, Academic Press, Cambridge, MA, USA.

Ninomiya, K, Kaneda, K, Kawashima, S, Miyachi, Y, Ogino, C & Shimizu, N (2013) Cell-SELEX based selection and characterization of DNA aptamer recognizing human hepatocarcinoma. *Bioorg Med Chem Lett,*

23, 1797-802.
[http://dx.doi.org/10.1016/j.bmcl.2013.01.040] [PMID: 23403083]

Oh, N & Park, J-H (2014) Endocytosis and exocytosis of nanoparticles in mammalian cells. *Int J Nanomed,* Suppl 1, 51-63.

Padma, VV (2015) An overview of targeted cancer therapy. *BioMed,* 5, 1-6.

Pang, X, Cui, C, Wan, S, Jiang, Y, Zhang, L, Xia, L, Li, L, Li, X & Tan, W (2018) Bioapplications of Cell-SELEX-generated aptamers in cancer diagnostics, therapeutics, theranostics and biomarker discovery: A comprehensive review. *Cancers (Basel),* 10, 47.

Park, JY & Chae, JR (2020) Targeted therapy of hepatocellular carcinoma using gemcitabine-incorporated GPC3 aptamer. *Pharmaceutics,* 12, 985.

Pathak, PO, Nagarsenker, MS, Barhate, CR, Padhye, SG, Dhawan, VV, Bhattacharyya, D, Viswanathan, CL, Steiniger, F & Fahr, A (2015) Cholesterol anchored arabinogalactan for asialoglycoprotein receptor targeting: synthesis, characterization, and proof of concept of hepatospecific delivery. *Carbohydr Res,* 408, 33-43.
[http://dx.doi.org/10.1016/j.carres.2015.03.003] [PMID: 25841057]

Pilapong, C, Sitthichai, S, Thongtem, S & Thongtem, T (2014) Smart magnetic nanoparticle-aptamer probe for targeted imaging and treatment of hepatocellular carcinoma. *Int J Pharm,* 473, 469-74.
[http://dx.doi.org/10.1016/j.ijpharm.2014.07.036] [PMID: 25089503]

Pranatharthiharan, S, Patel, MD & Malshe, VC (2017) Asialoglycoprotein receptor targeted delivery of doxorubicin nanoparticles for hepatocellular carcinoma. *Drug Deliv,* 24, 20-9.

Ravichandran, G (2020) Aptamer-mediated nanotheranostics for cancer treatment: A review *ACS Appl Nano Mater,* 3, 9542-59.

Ray, P & Dutta, D (2021) pH-Sensitive nanodrug carriers for codelivery of ERK inhibitor and gemcitabine enhance the inhibition of tumor growth in pancreatic cancer. *Mol Pharm,* 18, 87-100.

Ren, Q, Ga, L, Lu, Z, Ai, J & Wang, T (2020) Aptamer-functionalized nanomaterials for biological applications. *Mater Chem Front,* 1569.
[http://dx.doi.org/10.1039/C9QM00779B]

Dullea, R, Ammirati, M, Liu, S, Gebhard, D, Finley, JE, Salatto, CT, King-Ahmad, A, Stock, I, Atkinson, K, Reidich, B, Lin, W, Kumar, R, Tu, M, Menhaji-Klotz, E, Price, DA, Liras, S, Finn, MG & Mascitti, V (2017) Efficient liver targeting by polyvalent display of a compact ligand for the asialoglycoprotein receptor. *J Am Chem Soc,* 139, 3528-6.

Santra, S (2010) Fluorescent silica nanoparticles for cancer imaging. *Methods Mol Biol,* 624, 151-62.
[http://dx.doi.org/10.1007/978-1-60761-609-2_10] [PMID: 20217594]

Scaggiante, B, Farra, R, Dapas, B, Baj, G, Pozzato, G, Grassi, M, Zanconati, F & Grassi, G (2016) Aptamer targeting of the elongation factor 1A impairs hepatocarcinoma cells viability and potentiates bortezomib and idarubicin effects. *Int J Pharm,* 506, 268-79.
[http://dx.doi.org/10.1016/j.ijpharm.2016.04.031] [PMID: 27094354]

Shangguan, D, Meng, L, Cao, ZC, Xiao, Z, Fang, X, Li, Y, Cardona, D, Witek, RP, Liu, C & Tan, W (2008) Identification of liver cancer-specific aptamers using whole live cells. *Analytical Chem,* 80, 721-8.

Sivashankari, R & Prabahara, M (2016) Peptides to target tumor vasculature and lymphatics for improved anti-angiogenesis therapy. *Curr Cancer Drug Targets,* 16, 522-35.

Soundararajan, S, Wang, L, Sridharan, V, Chen, W, Courtenay-Luck, N, Jones, D, Spicer, EK & Fernandes, DJ (2009) Plasma membrane nucleolin is a receptor for the anticancer aptamer AS1411 in MV4-11 leukemia cells. *Mol Pharmacol,* 76, 984-91.
[http://dx.doi.org/10.1124/mol.109.055947] [PMID: 19657047]

Soutschek, J, Akinc, A, Bramlage, B, Charisse, K, Constein, R, Donoghue, M, Elbashir, S, Geick, A, Hadwigger, P & Harborth, J (2004) Therapeutic silencing of anendogenous gene by systemic administration of modified siRNAs. *Nature,* 432, 173-8.

Sun, D, Lu, J, Chen, Z, Yu, Y & Mo, M (2015) A repeatable assembling and disassembling electrochemical aptamer cytosensor for ultrasensitive and highly selective detection of human liver cancer cells. *Anal Chim Acta,* 885, 166-73.
[http://dx.doi.org/10.1016/j.aca.2015.05.027] [PMID: 26231902]

Sun, D, Lu, J, Wang, X, Zhang, Y & Chen, Z (2017) Voltametric aptamer-based detection of HepG2 tumor cells by using an indium tin oxide electrode array and multifunctional nanoprobes. *Mikrochim Acta,* 3487-96.
[http://dx.doi.org/10.1007/s00604-017-2376-z]

Sun, H, Zhu, X, Lu, PY, Rosato, RR, Tan, W & Zu, Y (2014) Oligonucleotide aptamers: new tools for targeted cancer therapy. *Mol Ther Nucleic Acids,* 3, e182.

Sun, H & Zu, Y (2015) Aptamers and their applications in nanomedicine. *Small,* 11, 2352-64.

Sun, Y, Ma, W, Yang, Y, He, M, Li, A, Bai, L, Yu, B & Yu, Z (2019) Cancer nanotechnology: Enhancing tumor cell response to chemotherapy for hepatocellular carcinoma therapy. *Asian J Pharm Sci,* 14, 581-94.
[http://dx.doi.org/10.1016/j.ajps.2019.04.005] [PMID: 32104485]

Tabarzad, M & Jafari, M (2016) Trends in the Design and development of specific aptamers against peptides and proteins. *Protein J,* 35, 81-99.

Trinh, TL, Zhu, G, Xiao, X, Puszyk, W, Sefah, K, Wu, Q, Tan, W & Liu, C (2015) A synthetic aptamer-drug adduct for targeted liver cancer therapy. *PLoS One,* 10, e0136673.
[http://dx.doi.org/10.1371/journal.pone.0136673] [PMID: 26523833]

Tuerk, C & Gold, L (2018) Systematic evolution of ligands by exponential enrichment: RNA ligands to bacteriophage T4 DNA polymerase. *Science,* 249, 505-10.

Usmani, A, Mishra, A & Ahmad, M Nanomedicines: a theranostic approach for hepatocellular carcinoma. *Artif Cells Nanomed Biotechnol,* 46, 680-90.

Wang, L, Su, W, Liu, Z, Zhou, M, Chen, S, Chen, Y, Lu, D, Liu, Y, Fan, Y, Zheng, Y, Han, Z, Kong, D, Wu, JC, Xiang, R & Li, Z (2012) CD44 antibody-targeted liposomal nanoparticles for molecular imaging and therapy of hepatocellular carcinoma. *Biomaterials,* 33, 5107-14.
[http://dx.doi.org/10.1016/j.biomaterials.2012.03.067] [PMID: 22494888]

Wang, S, Zhang, C, Wang, G, Cheng, B, Wang, Y, Chen, F, Chen, Y, Feng, M & Xiong, B (2016) Aptamer-mediated transparentbiocompatible nanostructured surfaces for hepotocellular circulating tumor cells enrichment. *Theranostics,* 6, 1877-86.
[http://dx.doi.org/10.7150/thno.15284] [PMID: 27570557]

Wang, Z, Li, Z, Ye, Y, Xie, L & Li, W (2016) Oxidative stress and liver cancer: etiology and therapeutic targets. *Oxid Med Cell Longev* 7891574.

Watany, M, Badawi, R & Eikhalawany, W (2017) Study of Dickkopf-1 (DKK-1) gene expression in hepatocellular carcinoma patients. *J Clin Diagnostic Res,* 11, OC32-4.

Weigum, S, McIvor, E, Munoz, C, Feng, R, Cantu, T, Walsh, K & Betancourt, T (2016) Targeted therapy of hepatocellular carcinoma with aptamer-functionalized biodegradable nanoparticles. *J Nanopart Res,* 341.
[http://dx.doi.org/10.1007/s11051-016-3633-5]

Wilhelm, S, Tavares, AJ, Dai, Q, Ohta, S, Audet, J, Dvorak, HF & Chan, WCW (2016) Analysis of nanoparticle delivery to tumours. *Nat Rev Mater,* 16014.
[http://dx.doi.org/10.1038/natrevmats.2016.14]

Wilner, SE, Wengerter, B, Maier, K, de Lourdes Borba Magalhães, M, Del Amo, DS, Pai, S, Opazo, F, Rizzoli, SO, Yan, A, Levy, M & Levy, M (2012) An RNA alternative to human transferrin: a new tool for targeting human cells. *Mol Ther Nucleic Acids,* 1, e21.
[http://dx.doi.org/10.1038/mtna.2012.14] [PMID: 23344001]

Wu, H-C, Chang, D-K & Huang, C-T (2006) Targeted therapy for cancer. *J Cancer Mol,* 2, 57-66.

Xiao, S, Liu, Z, Deng, R, Li, C, Fu, S, Chen, G, Zhang, X, Ke, F, Ke, S, Yu, X, Wang, S & Zhong, Z (2017)

Aptamer-mediated gene therapy enhanced antitumor activity against human hepatocellular carcinoma *in vitro* and *in vivo*. *J Control Release,* 258, 130-45.
[http://dx.doi.org/10.1016/j.jconrel.2017.05.017] [PMID: 28522194]

Xu, G & McLeod, HL (2001) Strategies for enzyme/prodrug cancer therapy. *Clin Cancer Res,* 7, 3314-24.

Xu, J, Teng, I-T, Zhang, L, Delgado, S, Champanhac, C, Cansiz, S, Wu, C, Shan, H & Tan, W (2015) Molecular recognition of human liver cancer cells using DNA aptamers generated *via* Cell-SELEX. *PLoS One,* 10, e012586.

Yan, H, Gao, X, Zhang, Y, Chang, W, Li, J, Li, X, Du, Q & Li, C (2018) Imaging tiny hepatic tumor xenografts *via* endoglin-targeted paramagnetic/optical nanoprobe. *ACS Appl Mater Interfaces,* 10, 17047-57.
[http://dx.doi.org/10.1021/acsami.8b02648] [PMID: 29708329]

Yoon, S & Rossi, JJ (2018) Aptamers: uptake mechanisms and intracellular applications. *Adv Drug Deliv Rev,* 134, 22-35.

Yu, XX, Ge, KL, Liu, N, Zhang, JY, Xue, ML & Ge, YL (2020) Selection and characterization of a novel DNA Aptamer, Apt-07S specific to hepatocellular carcinoma Cells. *Drug Des Devel Ther,* 14, 1535-45.
[http://dx.doi.org/10.2147/DDDT.S244149] [PMID: 32368012]

Zhang, B, Luo, Z, Liu, J, Ding, X, Li, J & Cai, K (2014) Cytochrome c end-capped mesoporous silica nanoparticles as redox-responsive drug delivery vehicles for liver tumor-targeted triplex therapy *in vitro* and *in vivo*. *J Control Release,* 192, 192-201.
[http://dx.doi.org/10.1016/j.jconrel.2014.06.037] [PMID: 25034575]

Zhang, J, Hu, J, Chan, HF, Skibba, M, Liang, G & Chen, M (2016) iRGD decorated lipid-polymer hybrid nanoparticles for targeted co-delivery of doxorubicin and sorafenib to enhance anti-hepatocellular carcinoma efficacy. *Nanomedicine,* 12, 1303-11.
[http://dx.doi.org/10.1016/j.nano.2016.01.017] [PMID: 26964482]

Zhang, W, Hu, X, Shen, Q & Xing, D (2019) Mitochondria-specific drug release and reactive oxygen species burst induced by polyprodrug nanoreactors can enhance chemotherapy. *Nat Commun,* 10, 1704.
[http://dx.doi.org/10.1038/s41467-019-09566-3] [PMID: 30979885]

Zhang, X, Ng, HLH, Lu, A, Lin, C, Zhou, L, Lin, G, Zhang, Y, Yang, Z & Zhang, H (2016) Drug delivery system targeting advanced hepatocellular carcinoma: current and future. *Nanomed: Nanotechnol Biol Med,* 12, 853-69.

Zhang, Y, Lai, BS & Juhas, M (2019) Recent advances in aptamer discovery and applications. *Molecules,* 24, 941.
[http://dx.doi.org/10.3390/molecules24050941] [PMID: 30866536]

Zhang, YN, Poon, W, Tavares, AJ, McGilvray, ID & Chan, WCW (2016) Nanoparticle-liver interactions: Cellular uptake and hepatobiliary elimination. *J Control Release,* 240, 332-48.
[http://dx.doi.org/10.1016/j.jconrel.2016.01.020] [PMID: 26774224]

Zhao, M, Dong, L, Liu, Z, Yang, S, Wu, W & Lin, J (2018) *In vivo* fluorescence imaging of hepatocellular carcinoma using a novel GPC3-specific aptamer probe. *Quant Imaging Med Surg,* 8, 151-60.

Zhou, J & Rossi, JJ (2014) Cell-type-specific, aptamer-functionalized agents for targeted disease therapy. *Mol Ther Nucleic Acids,* 3, e169.
[http://dx.doi.org/10.1038/mtna.2014.21] [PMID: 24936916]

Zhou, Y, Li, W, Tseng, Y, Zhang, J & Liu, J (2019) Developing slow-off dickkopf-1 aptamers for early-diagnosis of hepatocellular carcinoma. *Talanta,* 194, 422-9.
[http://dx.doi.org/10.1016/j.talanta.2018.10.014] [PMID: 30609553]

Zhu, G & Chen, X (2018) Aptamer-based targeted therapy. *Adv Drug Deliv Rev,* 134, 65-78.
[http://dx.doi.org/10.1016/j.addr.2018.08.005] [PMID: 30125604]

Zhu, Z, Song, Y, Li, C, Zou, Y, Zhu, L, An, Y & Yang, CJ (2014) ?Microfluidic approaches to rapid and efficient aptamer selection. *Anal Chem,* 86, 6572.

Zou, Y, Song, Y, Yang, W, Meng, F, Liu, H & Zhong, Z (2014) Galactose-installed photo-crosslinked pH-sensitive degradable micelles for active targeting chemotherapy of hepatocellular carcinoma in mice. *J Control Release,* 193, 154-61.
[http://dx.doi.org/10.1016/j.jconrel.2014.05.016] [PMID: 24852094]

Zou, Y, Duan, N, Wu, S, Shen, M & Wang, Z (2018) Selection, identification, and binding mechanism studies of an ssDNA aptamer targeted to different stages. *J Agric Food Chem,* 66, 5677-82.

CHAPTER 8

Preclinical Studies on Nanocarrier-Mediated Delivery of Radiosensitizing Agents to Brain and Pancreatic Cancer with a Future Projection to Liver Cancer

Peter Sminia[1,*], **Pei Pei Che**[1,2], **Ben J. Slotman**[1] and **Elisa Giovannetti**[2,3]

[1] *Amsterdam UMC, Vrije Universiteit Amsterdam, Department of Radiation Oncology, Cancer Center Amsterdam, The Netherlands*

[2] *Amsterdam UMC, Vrije Universiteit Amsterdam, Department of Medical Oncology, Cancer Center Amsterdam, The Netherlands*

[3] *Fondazione Pisana per la Scienza, Pisa, Italy*

Abstract: Radiotherapy is one of the primary treatment modalities in oncology. The therapeutic effectiveness of irradiation is dependent on the balance between the tumor control probability (TCP) and the normal tissue complication probability (NTCP), *i.e.*, the induction of side effects. Combination treatment of irradiation with chemotherapy targeted to a tumor or using immune-modulating agents could significantly benefit from nanotechnology strategies, allowing localized delivery of therapeutic compounds to the irradiated tumor volume. When used in combination with irradiation, drugs should be selected on their interaction with the 6 R's, the six Hallmarks of Radiobiology, to sensitize the radiation effect on the molecular, cellular, and tissue level, and in addition to that, positively impact the TCP/NTCP balance. This chapter presents and discusses preclinical data on the combination of irradiation and nanocarrier-mediated delivery of drugs in the brain, pancreatic, and liver cancer. Before implementation into the clinical practice, nanotechnology demands further technical and biological studies on drug loading efficacy, drug release, cellular and tissue uptake, biodistribution, tumor-targeting methods, and administration routes to the patient. Notwithstanding those challenges, the combination of local radiotherapy with tumor-targeted nanocarrier-delivered radiosensitizers, as well as the use of radiosensitizing nanoparticles, are exciting developments with a great clinical prospect.

Keywords: Blood-brain barrier, Binimetinib, Brain tumour, Curcumin, GBM, Hallmarks of radiobiology, Hepatocellular carcinoma, Immune-modulating agents, Nanocarriers, Oncology, Pancreatic cancer, Radiosensitization, Radiotherapy, Six R 's, Therapeutic agents.

* **Corresponding author Peter Sminia:** Amsterdam UMC, Vrije Universiteit Amsterdam, Department of Radiation Oncology, Cancer Center Amsterdam, The Netherlands; Tel: +31204441574; E-mail: p.sminia@amsterdamumc.nl

Biswajit Mukherjee (Ed.)

INTRODUCTION

Radiotherapy is one of the most effective treatment modalities in cancer therapy. However, despite modern precision radiotherapy, it is generally unavoidable to deposit ionizing radiation to the tumor volume without risk of radiation injury to the surrounding healthy normal tissues or organs. Hence, the therapeutic effects of radiation are dependent on the balance between tumor control and normal tissue adverse effects. In fact, the tolerance dose of the normal tissues or organs at risk determines the dose which can be applied safely to the tumor volume. For almost all normal tissues and organs, dose-volume constraints are well documented in the literature, the QUANTEC (Quantitative Analyses of Normal Tissue Effects in the Clinic) data, as guidance in the clinical practice (Marks *et al.*, 2010). The so-called 'therapeutic window,' the window of opportunity between the tumor control probability (TCP) and normal tissue complication probability (NTCP), is large for some tumor types such as lymphoma but small for other tumor types such as the brain and pancreatic cancer. The main strategy to augment the therapeutic window is to enhance the tumor response *via* combination treatment of irradiation with molecular targeting- or immune-modulating drugs (Begg *et al.*, 2011; Bristow *et al.*, 2018; Krause *et al.*, 2020). Although potential drugs for combination studies should be selected based on their interaction with irradiation, this is still an underexplored field in cancer research (Morris and Harari, 2014). Optimally, drugs should be carefully chosen on their ability to exploit the biological effects of irradiation on cells and tissues, considering the 6R's or Hallmarks of Radiobiology (Fig. **1**) (Section I) (Good and Harrington, 2013; Morris and Harari, 2014).

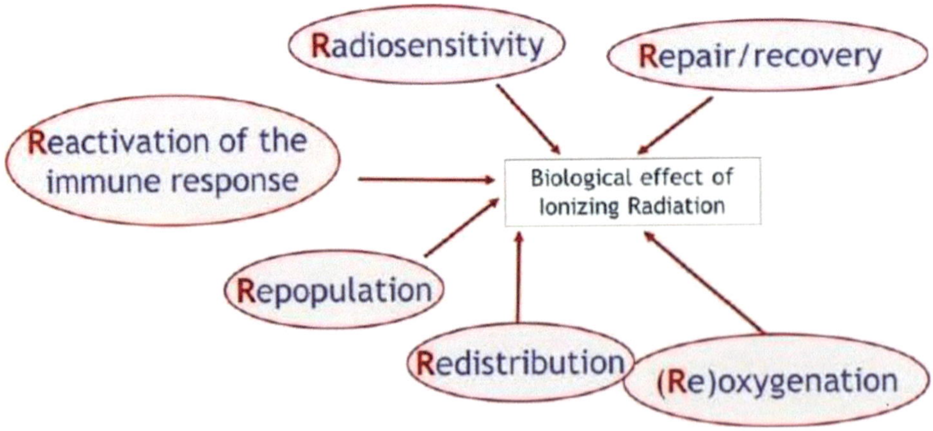

Fig. (1). The Hallmarks of Radiobiology, the 6R's. Six biological phenomena that determine the outcome of radiotherapy in the clinic: *i.e.* the complication rate (side effects due to normal tissue injury) and the tumor control rate (palliation or curation due to tumor sterilization). Details are given in the text.

Section I

Options for modulation of the radiation response should consider these basic principles or Hallmarks of Radiobiology, which has been evolved from Withers' 4R's - 'Recovery/repair, Redistribution, Repopulation and Reoxygenation' - (Withers, 1975), *via* Steels' 5R's - the addition of 'intrinsic cellular Radiosensitivity' - (Steel *et al.*, 1989) to 6R's by including 'Reactivation of the immune response' (Boustani *et al.*, 2019).

The six Hallmarks of Radiobiology (Fig. **1**) include in brief:

• **Radiosensitivity:** Intrinsic and acquired radioresistance of normal tissue cells and tumour cells, in particular, cancer (stem) cells/the heterogenic cancer cell population.

• **Repair:** Capacity, efficiency, and mechanisms of sublethal DNA damage repair and sensitivity to fractionated irradiation.

• **Redistribution:** The redistribution of cells in the cell cycle affects their radioresistance. Cells in mitosis are most sensitive to radiation, while cells in the S phase are radioresistant. Redistribution following irradiation pushes radioresistant S-phase cells toward a radiosensitive cell cycle phase.

• **Repopulation:** Cell repopulation (not by radiation eradicated cancer cells) is involved in the (accelerated) repopulation of the tumour, as well as repopulation of normal tissue cells to recover from injury.

• **Reoxygenation:** Cells in hypoxic niches within the tumor are radioresistant. Reoxygenation between radiation fractions is an important phenomenon to increase the oxygenation status and therewith tumor cell radiosensitivity.

• **Reactivation of the immune response:** Local irradiation induces systemic immune activation to attack distant tumor cell niches.

Preclinical drug research should, therefore, cautiously identify *radiosensitizing* compounds that enhance the effect of irradiation. In general, the drug dose for radiosensitization is in the lower, non-cytotoxic dose range when given as monotherapy, with the benefit of reduced, if any, systemic toxicity. To be noticed is the close link between the Hallmarks of Radiobiology and the Hallmarks of Cancer and therewith related therapeutic options, which have been discussed in detail (Harrington *et al.*, 2007; Bristow *et al.*, 2018).

Considering that conventional radiotherapy is generally applied in a scheme with multiple small-sized dose fractions, typically daily fractions of 1.8-2 Gy, five fractions per week in six to seven weeks, another crucial point is the scheduling of the administration of radiosensitizing drugs during the course of radiotherapy (Sminia and Westerman, 2016). The drug-radiation scheduling issue also applies to hypofractionated irradiation schemes, which are often used nowadays, in which patients are treated with a smaller number of high-dose radiation fractions in a shorter overall treatment duration than the conventional ones. Furthermore, irradiation is locally applied, focused on the tumor location with margins, *i.e.*, the planning target volume (PTV). The PTV includes the gross demonstrable extent of malignant growth and subclinical microscopic lesions and margins for variations in tumor position and shape and patient position, encompassing a small volume of immediate surrounding healthy tissue. In contrast, drugs are administered systemically and might cause side effects in tissues located distant from the primary tumor location. In the case of brain malignancies, drug delivery is further complicated by the presence of the blood-brain barrier (BBB) (Van Tellingen *et al.*, 2015). A significant challenge to current cancer drug treatment is the mode of delivery. Pharmacologically active concentrations of anticancer drugs in the tumors are often reached at the expense of a clinically-relevant exposure to other tissues. This poor specificity creates a toxicological problem that constitutes a major obstacle to effective antitumor therapy. Local drug administration would be preferential because of limited toxicity to healthy tissues. For several reasons, which have been recently reviewed by Reda and colleagues (2020), the nanotechnology strategy is a highly promising approach for imaging and site-specific drug delivery. Apart from the use of nanocarriers for transporting radiosensitizing drugs, nanoparticles composed of high-atomic number metals show radiosensitizing potential by themselves. Indeed, the use of nanosystems in radio oncology is a great mission and challenge, which has been discussed by Kunz-Schughart *et al.* (2017).

In the current chapter, an overview is given on preclinical studies using nanocarriers for drug delivery in the brain and pancreatic cancer. Own laboratory data are presented and discussed on the application of nanocarriers in 3D brain tumor (section II) and pancreatic cancer (section III) *in vitro* models. Finally, a future prospect is given regarding the use of nanocarriers for drug delivery and radiosensitizing nanoparticles in the therapy of hepatocellular carcinoma (section IV).

Section II

Nanocarrier-Mediated Drug Delivery to Brain Tumours

Glioblastoma multiforme (GBM) is the most malignant and common human brain tumor type (Louis *et al.*, 2016). Despite aggressive multimodality therapy with surgery, postoperative radiotherapy, and chemotherapy with the alkylating drug temozolomide, the median survival of GBM patients 5 years after diagnosis is low (Stupp *et al.*, 2009; Siegel *et al.*, 2020). The inadequate treatment response of GBMs has been ascribed to tumor heterogeneity, including the presence of radioresistant glioma stem cells. The space for radiation dose escalation to the tumor location is limited by the radiation sensitivity of neighboring healthy brain tissue. Furthermore, the delivery of most therapeutic agents to the tumor location is abrogated by the presence of the BBB. Thus, the heterogeneous nature of GBMs and related resistance to (radio)therapy, the narrow therapeutic window for escalation of the radiation dose, the presence of the BBB preventing drugs reaching the tumor site, and inadequate clinical treatment response bid for breakthrough strategies and methods to combat this lethal malignancy.

For many years, studies have been performed to facilitate the BBB passaging of drugs. In brief, methods include: (1) non-invasive techniques, such as radiotherapy, ultrasound, as well as several biological approaches, *e.g.*, viral vectors and cell-penetrating peptides; (2) invasive techniques, *e.g.*, convection-enhanced delivery; (3) alternative routes aimed to bypass the cardiovascular system such as intranasal drug application.

Nanomedicine is a sophisticated drug delivery method to brain tumors (Krishnamoorthy *et al.*, 2014; Patra *et al.*, 2018). Different nanotechnology-based structures such as micelles, liposomes, polymeric nanocarriers (polymersomes), dendrimers, and solid lipid nanoparticles have been investigated in the treatment of GBMs. In the present section II, we focus on two drugs that are studied in preclinical brain tumor models: the MAPK inhibitor binimetinib and the natural herb curcumin. We discuss their nanotechnology delivery strategy, uptake, anticancer efficacy, and, in particular, their interaction with irradiation.

Nanocarrier Delivery of the Targeted MAPK Inhibitor Binimetinib

An ingenious method to facilitate the transport of therapeutic agents across the BBB is the application of surface-functionalized nanocarriers. Polymersomes are very attractive since they can be loaded with mixtures of therapeutics *via* encapsulation of water-soluble compounds (*e.g.*, radionuclides) in the closed core together with water-insoluble substances (most drugs) in the hydrophobic outer bilayer. It was for that reason that we investigated the efficacy of polymersomes loaded with a targeted drug *in vitro* GBM models. The polymersomes were developed and loaded with binimetinib by the Radiation Science and Technology research group of the Delft University of Technology in the Netherlands (Wang *et al.*, 2014; De Kruijff *et al.*, 2018; Bikhezar *et al.*, 2020). First of all, they showed that FITC-labeled polymersomes were efficiently taken up in the cytoplasm of

U87 human glioma cells within a few minutes. Confocal microscope imaging was used to visualize the cellular localization of the polymersomes, showing that these nanocarriers, at least in part, were taken up through endocytosis and accumulated in lysosomes (De Kruijff *et al.*, 2018). Next, we studied the biodistribution of the polymersomes in U87MG brain tumor cell spheroids. The 3D spheroid model has a number of advantages compared with cells growing as a monolayer (*e.g.*, Narayan *et al.*, 2017). Spheroids are characterized by cell-cell contact as well as by metabolic and physiological gradients, and therewith representative for brain tumor micrometastases in the patient (Weiswald *et al.*, 2015). To investigate the migration of the nanocarriers from the spheroid-periphery to the center, the spheroids were exposed to PKH26 fluorescently labeled polymersomes. After about 4 days, the polymersomes diffused almost throughout the spheroid volume, and on day 7, the distribution was completely homogeneous (De Kruijff *et al.*, 2018). Next, we tested the therapeutic efficacy of polymersomes-loaded with the allosteric MAPK inhibitor binimetinib (MEK162) on the growth of multicellular U87 human glioma spheroids (Bikhezar *et al.*, 2020). Data presented in Fig. (**2**) demonstrate that binimetinib-loaded polymersomes inhibited spheroid growth and showed interaction with fractionated irradiation and temozolomide.

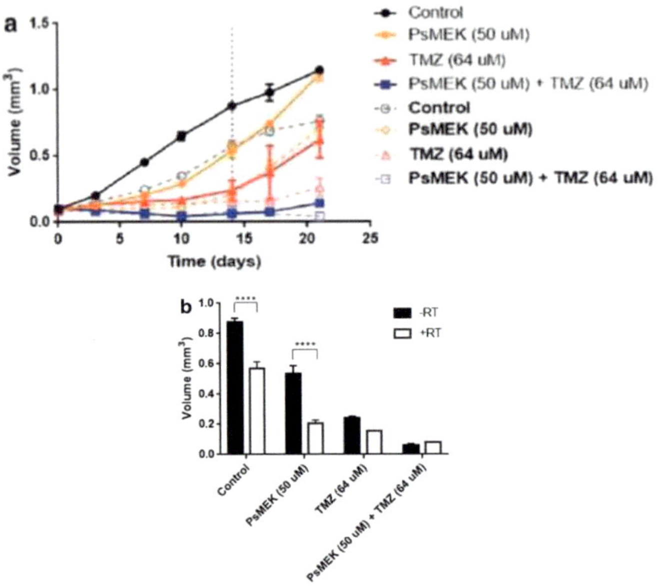

Fig. (2). Combination of 50 μM MEK162 loaded polymersomes (PsMEK), irradiation (RT, 5 daily fractions of 2 Gy), and 64 μM temozolomide (TMZ). (**a**) Growth curve of multicellular U87 human glioma spheroids treated with different conditions (insert) without (straight line) or with (broken line) RT. (**b**) Spheroid volume at day 14 (vertical broken line in Fig.a) after treatment with and without RT. Statistics *via* two-way ANOVA (****p < 0,0001) [Fig. reproduced from Bikhezar *et al.* (2020), licensed under http://creativecommons.org/licenses/by/4.0/.]

Through western blot analysis at 24 hours, binimetinib was found to prevent phosphorylation of its p-ERK target protein in the MAPK pathway. Also, the DNA damage marker γH2AX was found to be upregulated following exposure to binimetinib and irradiation, indicating an increase in radiation-induced DNA double-strand breaks. Next, we tested the transport of the 80 nm diameter-sized polymersomes over the BBB using an *in vitro* transwell BBB model. The data showed passaging of the fluorescent-labeled nanocarriers through the layer of human cerebral microvascular endothelial cells. Overall, our data demonstrated uptake of binimetinib-loaded polymersomes into 3D glioma spheroids, inhibition of the molecular target, and therewith reduced their growth (Bikhezar *et al*., 2020). Using spheroid volume as an endpoint, binimetinib acted as a radiosensitizer, while temozolomide was additive. Our first BBB data demonstrated the passaging of the nanocarriers across the BBB in the '*in vitro* model.'

Nanotechnology offers exciting possibilities in oncology for the directed transport of therapeutic agents within the human body. Application of ligand-conjugated nanocarriers that facilitate BBB crossing for delivery either of radiosensitizing agents and/or radionuclides to brain tumors is the next hurdle. Indeed, the most challenging in developing nanocarriers with BBB crossing potential is their feasibility of joining together with specific proteins. In particular, if selectivity towards the tumor, but not to the normal brain cells, could be obtained, their cargo can be delivered to the desired therapeutic interaction site, increasing the probability of tumor control. In contrast, the likelihood of adverse effects on the normal tissues could be limited. Both glutathione and transferrin are the most promising candidates for conjugation to nanocarriers.

Glutathione interacts with proteins located in the brain that are involved in the transport of molecules across the BBB. Grover *et al.* (2016) studied glutathione-coated nanoparticles loaded with docetaxel in an *in vitro* BBB permeation model. They demonstrated that the nanoparticles that passed the BBB remained cytotoxic for rat glioma cells and produced better effects than with free docetaxel. Targeting of nanoparticles with transferrin has also been reported by Mapanao *et al.* (2018) in a preclinical pancreatic cancer model (see section III).

Nanocarrier Delivery of the Natural Compound Curcumin

The natural compound and dietary spice curcumin has been reported to exert anticancer effects (Hatcher *et al*., 2008). The compound was found to inhibit cell proliferation, and it was cytotoxic for several tumor cell types. Moreover, it was found to interfere with the cellular oxidant status. Recently, we reviewed experimental and clinical data on the interaction between radiotherapy and curcumin in human glioma (Sminia *et al.*, 2020). In addition, we studied the radiosensitizing potential of curcumin on U251 human glioma cells *in vitro*. With clonogenic cell survival as the endpoint, we did not find an interaction between irradiation and curcumin at clinically achievable curcumin concentration. In our review, we concluded that, on the basis of own and preclinical *in vitro* and *in vivo* data from the literature together with clinical bioavailability data, there is no evidence for curcumin to interact synergistically with radiation (Sminia *et al.*, 2020). A crucial problem is the uptake of curcumin in the tumor to reach therapeutic levels. Dutzmann and colleagues (2016) investigated the bioavailability, intra-tumoural concentrations, and efficacy of orally administered micellar curcuminoids in 10 GBM patients (NCT01712542). The mean serum concentration of curcumin they found was 253 ng/ml (range 129-364), *i.e.*, ~0.7 μM. Intratumoral curcumin concentrations ranged between 9 and 151 pg/mg of tissue (mean 56, *i.e.*, ~ 0.15 μM) (Dutzmann *et al.*, 2016). Despite micellar administration, therapeutic levels could not be reached at the tumour site. At present, no clinical trials are ongoing regarding the use of curcumin in the therapy of GBM patients (US Government database, 2020).

Apart from physiological aspects, we face the fact that the compound cannot cross the BBB. In this respect, nanotechnology-based drug delivery approaches aiming to reach high intratumoral curcumin concentrations are challenging (Patra *et al.*, 2018). Curcumin-loaded nanoparticles were demonstrated to enhance blood plasm levels of the compound in humans (Kanai *et al.*, 2012). In another study, improved curcumin oral bioavailability was found *via* liquid micelles (Schiborr *et al.*, 2014). Functionalized, *i.e.*, chemically modified, nanoparticles are currently studied in the laboratory to improve their specificity, bioavailability, and efficacy for localized drug delivery. Curcumin-loaded functionalized nanoliposomes modified by a brain-targeting peptide RDP were investigated in both glioma cells *in vitro* and murine intracranial gliomas *in vivo* (Zhao *et al.*, 2018). The uptake was enhanced, and the nanoliposomes were internalized, which caused a cell cycle arrest at the S-phase and induced apoptosis. Repeated administrations of the curcumin nanoliposomes significantly increased the survival time of the tumor-bearing mice (Zhao *et al.*, 2018).

Tian *et al.* (2019) reported on BBB passaging and glioma targeting *in vitro* and *in vivo*. They constructed dual-targeted curcumin-loaded micelles, functionalized with Tween 80. These micelles could pass the BBB and *target* and *treat* gliomas *via* CD44-mediated endocytosis and glutathione-mediated intracellular curcumin release (Tian *et al.*, 2019). Taken together, localized delivery of curcumin to the tumor site only, aiming to reach therapeutic concentration *via* the use of functionalized nanoparticles, is a highly challenging issue. Because radiotherapy is one of the pillars of the current standard treatment of GBM patients, the most promising additional treatment approach might be the use of functionalized nanoparticles loaded with a combination of curcumin and/or an immune-modulating or targeted radiosensitizing anticancer agent (Narayan *et al.*, 2018; Bikhezar *et al.*, 2020).

Section III

Nanotechnological Strategies in Pancreatic Cancer

Pancreatic ductal adenocarcinoma (PDAC) is the most prevalent tumor type among pancreatic cancers. This tumor has a very poor prognosis, with an overall 5-year survival rate below 10%. Most patients are diagnosed at an advanced stage (Siegel *et al.*, 2020). Patients with locally advanced or metastasized disease are currently treated with combination treatments of deoxycytidine analog gemcitabine with albumin-bound nab-paclitaxel (Abraxane®) or with the cocktail regime (modified) FOLFIRINOX – composed of 5-fluorouracil (5-FU), leucovorin (LV), irinotecan, and oxaliplatin El (Hassouni *et al.*, 2019). Unsurprisingly, the gain in overall survival is only limited to a few months, thus urging better (novel) treatment strategies.

(Pre)clinical research showed that Abraxane® and liposomal irinotecan (Onivyde®) have better safety profiles and pharmacokinetics compared to their non-encapsulated counterparts (Bobo *et al.*, 2016). For instance, the success of liposomal irinotecan lies behind the improved pharmacokinetics, tolerable safety profile, and improvement in overall survival, albeit by 2 months in co-administration with 5-FU/LV, compared to administration of 5-FU/LV only (Frampton, 2020). Nevertheless, PDAC remains very difficult to treat due to inherent resistance against existing therapeutic strategies, including radiotherapy. For this reason, there has been increasing interest in gold nanoparticles (AuNPs) as a possible radiosensitizing agent due to good biocompatibility and interaction with radiation (Tomic *et al.*, 2014; Haume *et al.*, 2016; Penninckx *et al.*, 2020). Briefly, when ionizing radiation (IR) passes through material such as gold, an increased release of Auger electrons could be produced from the interaction, potentially resulting in more DNA damage. It is desirable when AuNPs are selectively taken up in tumor cells, as the released secondary electrons only have a short reach in the distance (McMahon *et al.*, 2011). Several preclinical studies have already demonstrated a potential radiosensitizing effect of this approach in various cancer cell lines (Kumar *et al.*, 2013; Yang *et al.*, 2018).

Interestingly, Bromma and collaborators recently (2020) showed increased uptake of 29 nm AuNPs in cancer-associated fibroblasts (CAFs) instead of normal fibroblasts. Subsequently, elevated DNA damage foci were observed in CAFs, due to the increased accumulation. Although further studies are warranted for the mechanism behind this increased uptake, these results could indicate a good use of AuNPs to target the cancer cells and the microenvironment supporting tumor progression. Especially in PDAC, where the majority of the tumor volume is composed of stroma, the role of CAFs and their interaction with neoplastic cells would need to be taken into careful consideration when applying different therapeutic strategies. In the following section, we would like to focus on a few applications of nanomedicine using AuNPs.

Applications of Gold Nanoparticles in Pancreatic Cancer

The surface coating of AuNPs is incredibly important, as it not only increases its versatility to be used for various purposes but also enhances its bioavailability (Alalaiwe *et al.*, 2017). For diagnostics, the accumulation of gold could enhance contrast imaging (Cheheltani *et al.*, 2016). However, when combined with a targeting moiety, AuNPs could selectively bind to tumors. Notably, Cassano and collaborators (2015) reported the synthesis of 3 nm AuNPs that were arranged in a polymer of poly-l-lysine and finally encompassed by a hollow silica shell. Interestingly, transmission electron microscopy (TEM) showed that the gold polymer array exclusively resides in the inner core. Exposure of these so-called "passion fruit-like" nanoarchitectures (NAs) in zebrafish showed no significant malformations or alterations in survival rate in developing embryos or larvae (d'Amora *et al.*, 2018).

Further modifications enabled the NAs to be functionalized as 1) a drug delivery system *via* covalent linking of, for example, cisplatin prodrug complexes on the polymer array (NAs-cisPt), or 2) for imaging purposes *via* conjugation of fluorescent probes on the surface of the hollow silica shell or in the inner core (Cassano *et al.*, 2016). *In vitro* studies in MiaPaca-2 cells with these NAs-cisPt demonstrated a decrease in cell viability after 48 hours, a time-point when the authors showed complete biodegradation of the NAs after internalization in the PDAC cells *via* TEM imaging. As an improvement, NAs could also be conjugated with a peptide that binds to the transferrin receptor. Mapanao and collaborators demonstrated increased uptake in 3D spheroids comprised of MiaPaca-2 cells with the transferrin-targeting NAs instead of control (Mapanao *et al.*, 2018). Altogether, these multifunctional modifications on the NAs could further fine-tune the application of AuNPs to selectively target tumor cells while exerting the chemotherapeutic effect *via* drugs loaded into the NAs, and radiosensitization *via* the AuNPs (Fig. **3**). However, while promising, these NAs still await further validation of the radiosensitizing effects in appropriate preclinical models.

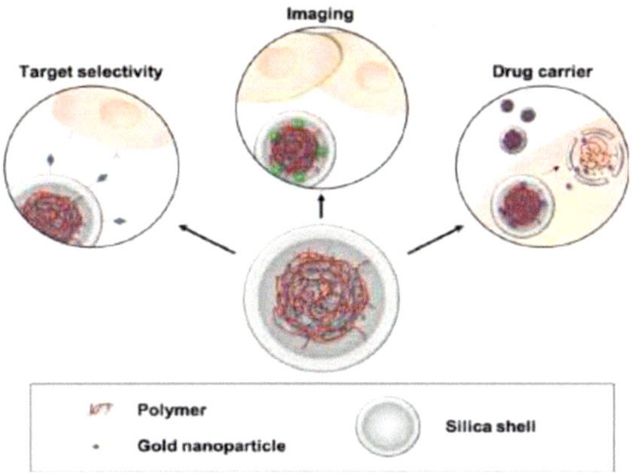

Fig. (3). Overview of possible modifications, where passion fruit-like nanoarchitectures comprised of AuNPs in a polymer array could be functionalized *via* 1) conjugation of targeting moieties to increase selective uptake of NAs in the target cell population, 2) linking of fluorescent probes for cell imaging and tracking or 3) linking of chemotherapeutics. Upon entry into the cellular environment, the NAs are biodegraded and release the AuNPs and drugs. Abbreviations: AuNPs = gold nanoparticles.

Section IV

Perspective for Liver Cancer Therapy

The most common type of primary cancer of the liver is hepatocellular carcinoma (HCC), which is among the leading deadly cancers (Global Burden of Disease Liver Cancer Collaboration, 2017). Over the last years, the role of radiotherapy in the treatment of HCC has progressed substantially (Chen, 2020). While historically, external beam radiotherapy had a limited role in treating liver cancer due to the risk of radiation-induced liver disease, technological advances in radiotherapy have allowed for more precise and dose-escalated treatment regimens (Chen, 2020). With small volume liver treatments, high local tumor control probability with relatively low normal tissue complication probability can be achieved. Therewith, local radiation treatment combined with local or systemic therapy progressively emerges as a promising strategy, including nanotechnology modalities.

Dutta and Mahato (2017) reviewed the various pathways and treatment modalities of HCC, including the developments in nanotechnology. The authors describe experimental findings for passive and receptor-specific active nanoparticle targeting in HCC. Using novel nanocarriers for local delivery of cytotoxic agents at the tumor site, systemic adverse effects might be overcome while tumor response could be enhanced (Dutta and Mahato, 2017).

Hu and colleagues (2019) performed an experimental study on human HCC HepG2 cells and HepG2 tumors in mice using a gadolinium-based nanoparticle

AGuIX. Interestingly, because of the high atomic number of gadolinium, these nanoparticles can be used for enhanced magnetic resonance imaging as well as radiosensitization. Indeed, the nanoparticles provided a better detection of experimental HepG2 tumors for accurate MRI-guided radiotherapy. On cells *in vitro* and in the murine tumors *in vivo*, the nanoparticle itself was found to significantly sensitize for the effect of irradiation (Hu *et al.*, 2019). This study demonstrated that AGuIX could be a promising theranostic nanoparticle for both MRI-guided radiotherapies as well as for radiosensitization. Tang and colleagues (2020) reported on the effectiveness of polyethylene glycol-poly (lactic-c--glycolic acid) (PEG-PLGA) encapsulation and the release of the PI3K/mTOR inhibitor NVP-BEZ235. Notably, they studied the biocompatibility, internalization, and cellular interaction of BEZ235-loaded nanoparticles that were modified with a Glypican-3 (GPC3) antibody (NP-BEZ235-Ab) in hepatoma cells. The nanoparticles could be efficiently loaded with the drug, and they showed high selectivity to GPC3-positive HepG2 liver cancer cells. Synergy was found with irradiation, even better than with the free drug, and therewith these particles were identified as a radiosensitizer (Tang *et al.*, 2020).

Sun and colleagues (2019) reviewed and discussed the opportunities and challenges of nanotechnology in HCC therapy, where individualized treatment with targeted and immune-modulating drugs is gaining ground. Also, emerging preclinical studies offer an encouraging prospect for using nanotechnology to locally deliver radiosensitizing drugs to HCC. Together with local precision radiotherapy, this might finally translate into better clinical outcomes for HCC patients in the future.

CONCLUDING REMARKS

Impressive progress in preclinical research has been made on nanotechnology in the therapy of brain and pancreatic tumors (resp. sections II and III). Clinical studies using nanocarrier-mediated strategies for combination therapy against cancer are emerging. They might finally contribute, *via* widening the therapeutic window, to higher tumor control rates while limiting normal tissue complication rates. The nanotechnology-based treatment approach offers exciting challenges and can lead to breakthroughs in liver cancer therapy. However, a number of technical aspects need further investigation, *e.g.*, regarding nanocarrier drug loading, administration routes to the patient, drug release, the stability of the nanocarriers in tissue fluids, and specific tumor targeting methods. The use of nanoparticles for both imaging and radiosensitization is a promising approach and a great challenge. Important biological issues include nanocarrier/drug dosing, cellular and tissue uptake and biodistribution, scheduling, selectivity, and toxicity. Finally, in view of radiotherapy as the core treatment in oncology, when combining nanocarrier-delivered drugs with radiation, drugs should be selected on their interaction with the Hallmarks of Radiobiology (section I). Exploiting the 6 R's to sensitize for the radiation effect on the molecular, cellular, and tissue level will impact the TCP/NTCP balance positively.

CONSENT FOR PUBLICATION

Not applicable.

CONFLICT OF INTEREST

The authors declare no conflict of interest, financial or otherwise.

ACKNOWLEDGEMENTS

Supported by the Zabawas foundation (grant #CCA 2019-5-55) and Cancer Center Amsterdam (project #2006784)

REFERENCES

Alalaiwe, A, Roberts, G, Carpinone, P, Munson, J & Roberts, S (2017) Influence of PEG coating on the oral bioavailability of gold nanoparticles in rats. *Drug Deliv,* 24, 591-8.
[http://dx.doi.org/10.1080/10717544.2017.1282554] [PMID: 28222611]

Begg, AC, Stewart, FA & Vens, C (2011) Strategies to improve radiotherapy with targeted drugs. *Nat Rev Cancer,* 11, 239-53.
[http://dx.doi.org/10.1038/nrc3007] [PMID: 21430696]

Bikhezar, F, de Kruijff, RM, van der Meer, AJGM, Torrelo Villa, G, van der Pol, SMA, Becerril Aragon, G, Gasol Garcia, A, Narayan, RS, de Vries, HE, Slotman, BJ, Denkova, AG & Sminia, P (2020) Preclinical evaluation of binimetinib (MEK162) delivered *via* polymeric nanocarriers in combination with radiation and temozolomide in glioma. *J Neurooncol,* 146, 239-46.
[http://dx.doi.org/10.1007/s11060-019-03365-y] [PMID: 31875307]

Bobo, D, Robinson, KJ, Islam, J, Thurecht, KJ & Corrie, SR (2016) Nanoparticle-Based Medicines: A Review of FDA-Approved Materials and Clinical Trials to Date. *Pharm Res,* 33, 2373-87.
[http://dx.doi.org/10.1007/s11095-016-1958-5] [PMID: 27299311]

Boustani, J, Grapin, M, Laurent, PA, Apetoh, L & Mirjolet, C (2019) The 6th R of Radiobiology: Reactivation of Anti-Tumor Immune Response. *Cancers (Basel),* 11, 860.
[http://dx.doi.org/10.3390/cancers11060860] [PMID: 31226866]

Bristow, RG, Alexander, B, Baumann, M, Bratman, SV, Brown, JM, Camphausen, K, Choyke, P, Citrin, D, Contessa, JN, Dicker, A, Kirsch, DG, Krause, M, Le, QT, Milosevic, M, Morris, ZS, Sarkaria, JN, Sondel, PM, Tran, PT, Wilson, GD, Willers, H, Wong, RKS & Harari, PM (2018) Combining precision radiotherapy with molecular targeting and immunomodulatory agents: a guideline by the American Society for Radiation Oncology. *Lancet Oncol,* 19, e240-51.
[http://dx.doi.org/10.1016/S1470-2045(18)30096-2] [PMID: 29726389]

Bromma, K, Cicon, L, Beckham, W & Chithrani, DB (2020) Gold nanoparticle mediated radiation response among key cell components of the tumour microenvironment for the advancement of cancer nanotechnology. *Sci Rep,* 10, 12096.
[http://dx.doi.org/10.1038/s41598-020-68994-0] [PMID: 32694592]

Cassano, D, Rota Martir, D, Signore, G, Piazza, V & Voliani, V (2015) Biodegradable hollow silica nanospheres containing gold nanoparticle arrays. *Chem Commun (Camb),* 51, 9939-41. [http://dx.doi.org/10.1039/C5CC02771C] [PMID: 25998799]

Cassano, D, Santi, M, Cappello, V, Luin, S, Signore, G & Voliani, V (2016) Biodegradable Passion Fruit-like NanoArchitectures as Carriers for Cisplatin Prodrug. *Part Part Syst Charact,* 33, 818-24. [http://dx.doi.org/10.1002/ppsc.201600175]

Cheheltani, R, Ezzibdeh, RM, Chhour, P, Pulaparthi, K, Kim, J, Jurcova, M, Hsu, JC, Blundell, C, Litt, HI, Ferrari, VA, Allcock, HR, Sehgal, CM & Cormode, DP (2016) Tunable, biodegradable gold nanoparticles as contrast agents for computed tomography and photoacoustic imaging. *Biomaterials,* 102, 87-97. [http://dx.doi.org/10.1016/j.biomaterials.2016.06.015] [PMID: 27322961]

Chen, CP (2020) Role of External Beam Radiotherapy in Hepatocellular Carcinoma. *Clin Liver Dis,* 24, 701-17. [http://dx.doi.org/10.1016/j.cld.2020.07.006] [PMID: 33012454]

d'Amora, M, Cassano, D, Pocoví-Martínez, S, Giordani, S & Voliani, V (2018) Biodistribution and biocompatibility of passion fruit-like nano-architectures in zebrafish. *Nanotoxicology,* 12, 914-22. [http://dx.doi.org/10.1080/17435390.2018.1498551] [PMID: 30132360]

de Kruijff, RM, van der Meer, AJGM, Windmeijer, CAA, Kouwenberg, JJM, Morgenstern, A, Bruchertseifer, F, Sminia, P & Denkova, AG (2018) The therapeutic potential of polymersomes loaded with ^{225}Ac evaluated in 2D and 3D in vitro glioma models. *Eur J Pharm Biopharm,* 127, 85-91. [http://dx.doi.org/10.1016/j.ejpb.2018.02.008] [PMID: 29428791]

Dutta, R & Mahato, RI (2017) Recent advances in hepatocellular carcinoma therapy. *Pharmacol Ther,* 173, 106-17. [http://dx.doi.org/10.1016/j.pharmthera.2017.02.010] [PMID: 28174094]

Dützmann, S, Schiborr, C, Kocher, A, Pilatus, U, Hattingen, E, Weissenberger, J, Geßler, F, Quick-Weller, J, Franz, K, Seifert, V, Frank, J & Senft, C (2016) Intratumoral concentrations and effects of orally administered micellar Curcuminoids in Glioblastoma patients. *Nutr Cancer,* 68, 943-8. [http://dx.doi.org/10.1080/01635581.2016.1187281] [PMID: 27340742]

El Hassouni, B, Li Petri, G, Liu, DSK, Cascioferro, S, Parrino, B, Hassan, W, Diana, P, Ali, A, Frampton, AE & Giovannetti, E (2019) Pharmacogenetics of treatments for pancreatic cancer. *Expert Opin Drug Metab Toxicol,* 15, 437-47. [http://dx.doi.org/10.1080/17425255.2019.1620731] [PMID: 31100206]

Frampton, JE (2020) Liposomal Irinotecan: A Review in Metastatic Pancreatic Adenocarcinoma. *Drugs,* 80, 1007-18. [http://dx.doi.org/10.1007/s40265-020-01336-6] [PMID: 32557396]

Akinyemiju, T, Abera, S, Ahmed, M, Alam, N, Alemayohu, MA, Allen, C, Al-Raddadi, R, Alvis-Guzman, N, Amoako, Y, Artaman, A, Ayele, TA, Barac, A, Bensenor, I, Berhane, A, Bhutta, Z, Castillo-Rivas, J, Chitheer, A, Choi, JY, Cowie, B, Dandona, L, Dandona, R, Dey, S, Dicker, D, Phuc, H, Ekwueme, DU, Zaki, MS, Fischer, F, Fürst, T, Hancock, J, Hay, SI, Hotez, P, Jee, SH, Kasaeian, A, Khader, Y, Khang, YH, Kumar, A, Kutz, M, Larson, H, Lopez, A, Lunevicius, R, Malekzadeh, R, McAlinden, C, Meier, T, Mendoza, W, Mokdad, A, Moradi-Lakeh, M, Nagel, G, Nguyen, Q, Nguyen, G, Ogbo, F, Patton, G, Pereira, DM, Pourmalek, F, Qorbani, M, Radfar, A, Roshandel, G, Salomon, JA, Sanabria, J, Sartorius, B, Satpathy, M, Sawhney, M, Sepanlou, S, Shackelford, K, Shore, H, Sun, J, Mengistu, DT, Topór-Mądry, R, Tran, B, Ukwaja, KN, Vlassov, V, Vollset, SE, Vos, T, Wakayo, T, Weiderpass, E, Werdecker, A, Yonemoto, N, Younis, M, Yu, C, Zaidi, Z, Zhu, L, Murray, CJL, Naghavi, M & Fitzmaurice, C (2017) The Burden of Primary Liver Cancer and Underlying Etiologies From 1990 to 2015 at the Global, Regional, and National Level: Results From the Global Burden of Disease Study 2015. *JAMA Oncol,* 3, 1683-91. [http://dx.doi.org/10.1001/jamaoncol.2017.3055] [PMID: 28983565]

Good, JS & Harrington, KJ (2013) The hallmarks of cancer and the radiation oncologist: updating the 5Rs of radiobiology. *Clin Oncol (R Coll Radiol),* 25, 569-77. [http://dx.doi.org/10.1016/j.clon.2013.06.009] [PMID: 23850153]

Grover, A, Hirani, A & Sutariya, V (2014) Blood-Brain Barrier Permeation of Glutathione-Coated Nanoparticle. *SOJ Pharm Pharm Sci,* 1, 4.

Harrington, K, Jankowska, P & Hingorani, M (2007) Molecular biology for the radiation oncologist: the 5Rs of radiobiology meet the hallmarks of cancer. *Clin Oncol (R Coll Radiol),* 19, 561-71. [http://dx.doi.org/10.1016/j.clon.2007.04.009] [PMID: 17591437]

Hatcher, H, Planalp, R, Cho, J, Torti, FM & Torti, SV (2008) Curcumin: from ancient medicine to current clinical trials. *Cell Mol Life Sci,* 65, 1631-52. [http://dx.doi.org/10.1007/s00018-008-7452-4] [PMID: 18324353]

Haume, K, Rosa, S, Grellet, S, Śmiałek, MA, Butterworth, KT, Solov'yov, AV, Prise, KM, Golding, J & Mason, NJ (2016) Gold nanoparticles for cancer radiotherapy: a review. *Cancer Nanotechnol,* 7, 8. [http://dx.doi.org/10.1186/s12645-016-0021-x] [PMID: 27867425]

Hu, P, Fu, Z, Liu, G, Tan, H, Xiao, J, Shi, H & Cheng, D (2019) Gadolinium-Based Nanoparticles for Theranostic MRI-Guided Radiosensitization in Hepatocellular Carcinoma. *Front Bioeng Biotechnol,* 7, 368. [http://dx.doi.org/10.3389/fbioe.2019.00368] [PMID: 31828068]

Kanai, M, Imaizumi, A, Otsuka, Y, Sasaki, H, Hashiguchi, M, Tsujiko, K, Matsumoto, S, Ishiguro, H & Chiba, T (2012) Dose-escalation and pharmacokinetic study of nanoparticle curcumin, a potential anticancer agent with improved bioavailability, in healthy human volunteers. *Cancer Chemother Pharmacol,* 69, 65-70. [http://dx.doi.org/10.1007/s00280-011-1673-1] [PMID: 21603867]

Krause, M, Alsner, J, Linge, A, Bütof, R, Löck, S & Bristow, R (2020) Specific requirements for translation of biological research into clinical radiation oncology. *Mol Oncol,* 14, 1569-76. [http://dx.doi.org/10.1002/1878-0261.12671] [PMID: 32175659]

Krishnamoorthy, B, Karanam, V, Chellan, VR, Siram, K, Natarajan, TS & Gregory, M (2014) Polymersomes as an effective drug delivery system for glioma--a review. *J Drug Target,* 22, 469-77. [http://dx.doi.org/10.3109/1061186X.2014.916712] [PMID: 24830300]

Kumar, R, Korideck, H, Ngwa, W, Berbeco, RI, Makrigiorgos, GM & Sridhar, S (2013) Third generation gold nanoplatform optimized for radiation therapy. *Transl Cancer Res,* 2 [PMID: 24392307]

Kunz-Schughart, LA, Dubrovska, A, Peitzsch, C, Ewe, A, Aigner, A, Schellenburg, S, Muders, MH, Hampel, S, Cirillo, G, Iemma, F, Tietze, R, Alexiou, C, Stephan, H, Zarschler, K, Vittorio, O, Kavallaris, M, Parak, WJ, Mädler, L & Pokhrel, S (2017) Nanoparticles for radiooncology: Mission, vision, challenges. *Biomaterials,* 120, 155-84. [http://dx.doi.org/10.1016/j.biomaterials.2016.12.010] [PMID: 28063356]

Louis, DN, Perry, A, Reifenberger, G, von Deimling, A, Figarella-Branger, D, Cavenee, WK, Ohgaki, H, Wiestler, OD, Kleihues, P & Ellison, DW (2016) The 2016 World Health Organization Classification of Tumors of the Central Nervous System: a summary. *Acta Neuropathol,* 131, 803-20. [http://dx.doi.org/10.1007/s00401-016-1545-1] [PMID: 27157931]

Mapanao, AK, Santi, M, Faraci, P, Cappello, V, Cassano, D & Voliani, V (2018) Endogenously Triggerable Ultrasmall-in-Nano Architectures: Targeting Assessment on 3D Pancreatic Carcinoma Spheroids. *ACS Omega,* 3, 11796-801. [http://dx.doi.org/10.1021/acsomega.8b01719] [PMID: 30320273]

Marks, LB, Yorke, ED, Jackson, A, Ten Haken, RK, Constine, LS, Eisbruch, A, Bentzen, SM, Nam, J & Deasy, JO (2010) Use of normal tissue complication probability models in the clinic. *Int J Radiat Oncol Biol Phys,* 76 (Suppl.), S10-9. [http://dx.doi.org/10.1016/j.ijrobp.2009.07.1754] [PMID: 20171502]

McMahon, SJ, Hyland, WB, Muir, MF, Coulter, JA, Jain, S, Butterworth, KT, Schettino, G, Dickson, GR, Hounsell, AR, O'Sullivan, JM, Prise, KM, Hirst, DG & Currell, FJ (2011) Biological consequences of nanoscale energy deposition near irradiated heavy atom nanoparticles. *Sci Rep,* 1, 18. [http://dx.doi.org/10.1038/srep00018] [PMID: 22355537]

Morris, ZS & Harari, PM (2014) Interaction of radiation therapy with molecular targeted agents. *J Clin Oncol,* 32, 2886-93.
[http://dx.doi.org/10.1200/JCO.2014.55.1366] [PMID: 25113770]

Narayan, RS, Fedrigo, CA, Brands, E, Dik, R, Stalpers, LJ, Baumert, BG, Slotman, BJ, Westerman, BA, Peters, GJ & Sminia, P (2017) The allosteric AKT inhibitor MK2206 shows a synergistic interaction with chemotherapy and radiotherapy in glioblastoma spheroid cultures. *BMC Cancer,* 17, 204.
[http://dx.doi.org/10.1186/s12885-017-3193-9] [PMID: 28320338]

Narayan, RS, Gasol, A, Slangen, PLG, Cornelissen, FMG, Lagerweij, T, Veldman, HYYE, Dik, R, van den Berg, J, Slotman, BJ, Würdinger, T, Haas-Kogan, DA, Stalpers, LJA, Baumert, BG, Westerman, BA, Theys, J & Sminia, P (2018) Identification of MEK162 as a Radiosensitizer for the Treatment of Glioblastoma. *Mol Cancer Ther,* 17, 347-54.
[http://dx.doi.org/10.1158/1535-7163.MCT-17-0480] [PMID: 28958992]

Patra, JK, Das, G, Fraceto, LF, Campos, EVR, Rodriguez-Torres, MDP & Acosta-Torres, LS (2018) Nano based drug delivery systems: recent developments and future prospects. *J Nanobiotech ,* 19, 16:71.

Penninckx, S, Heuskin, AC, Michiels, C & Lucas, S (2020) Gold Nanoparticles as a Potent Radiosensitizer: A Transdisciplinary Approach from Physics to Patient. *Cancers (Basel),* 12, E2021.
[http://dx.doi.org/10.3390/cancers12082021] [PMID: 32718058]

Reda, M, Bagley, AF, Zaidan, HY & Yantasee, W (2020) Augmenting the therapeutic window of radiotherapy: A perspective on molecularly targeted therapies and nanomaterials. *Radiother Oncol,* 150, 225-35.
[http://dx.doi.org/10.1016/j.radonc.2020.06.041] [PMID: 32598976]

Schiborr, C, Kocher, A, Behnam, D, Jandasek, J, Toelstede, S & Frank, J (2014) The oral bioavailability of curcumin from micronized powder and liquid micelles is significantly increased in healthy humans and differs between sexes. *Mol Nutr Food Res,* 58, 516-27.
[http://dx.doi.org/10.1002/mnfr.201300724] [PMID: 24402825]

Siegel, RL, Miller, KD & Jemal, A (2020) Cancer statistics, 2020. *CA Cancer J Clin,* 70, 7-30.
[http://dx.doi.org/10.3322/caac.21590] [PMID: 31912902]

Sminia, P, van den Berg, J, van Kootwijk, A, Hageman, E, Slotman, BJ & Verbakel, WFAR (2021) Experimental and clinical studies on radiation and curcumin in human glioma. *J Cancer Res Clin Oncol,* 147, 403-9.
[http://dx.doi.org/10.1007/s00432-020-03432-2] [PMID: 33118056]

Sminia, P & Westerman, BA (2016) Blood-brain barrier crossing and breakthroughs in glioblastoma therapy. *Br J Clin Pharmacol,* 81, 1018-20.
[http://dx.doi.org/10.1111/bcp.12881] [PMID: 26744058]

Steel, GG, McMillan, TJ & Peacock, JH (1989) The 5Rs of radiobiology. *Int J Radiat Biol,* 56, 1045-8.
[http://dx.doi.org/10.1080/09553008914552491] [PMID: 2574214]

Stupp, R, Hegi, ME, Mason, WP, van den Bent, MJ, Taphoorn, MJ, Janzer, RC, Ludwin, SK, Allgeier, A, Fisher, B, Belanger, K, Hau, P, Brandes, AA, Gijtenbeek, J, Marosi, C, Vecht, CJ, Mokhtari, K, Wesseling, P, Villa, S, Eisenhauer, E, Gorlia, T, Weller, M, Lacombe, D, Cairncross, JG & Mirimanoff, RO (2009) Effects of radiotherapy with concomitant and adjuvant temozolomide versus radiotherapy alone on survival in glioblastoma in a randomised phase III study: 5-year analysis of the EORTC-NCIC trial. *Lancet Oncol,* 10, 459-66.
[http://dx.doi.org/10.1016/S1470-2045(09)70025-7] [PMID: 19269895]

Sun, Y, Ma, W, Yang, Y, He, M, Li, A, Bai, L, Yu, B & Yu, Z (2019) Cancer nanotechnology: Enhancing tumor cell response to chemotherapy for hepatocellular carcinoma therapy. *Asian J Pharm Sci,* 14, 581-94.
[http://dx.doi.org/10.1016/j.ajps.2019.04.005] [PMID: 32104485]

Tang, X, Li, A, Xie, C, Zhang, Y, Liu, X, Xie, Y, Wu, B, Zhou, S, Huang, X, Ma, Y, Cao, W, Xu, R, Shen, J, Huo, Z, Cai, S, Liang, Y & Ma, D (2020) The PI3K/mTOR dual inhibitor BEZ235 nanoparticles improve

radiosensitization of hepatoma cells through apoptosis and regulation DNA repair pathway. *Nanoscale Res Lett,* 15, 63.
[http://dx.doi.org/10.1186/s11671-020-3289-z] [PMID: 32219609]

Tian, C, Asghar, S, Hu, Z, Qiu, Y, Zhang, J, Shao, F & Xiao, Y (2019) Understanding the cellular uptake and biodistribution of a dual-targeting carrier based on redox-sensitive hyaluronic acid-ss-curcumin micelles for treating brain glioma. *Int J Biol Macromol,* 136, 143-53.
[http://dx.doi.org/10.1016/j.ijbiomac.2019.06.060] [PMID: 31199976]

Tomić, S, Đokić, J, Vasilijić, S, Ogrinc, N, Rudolf, R, Pelicon, P, Vučević, D, Milosavljević, P, Janković, S, Anžel, I, Rajković, J, Rupnik, MS, Friedrich, B & Colić, M (2014) Size-dependent effects of gold nanoparticles uptake on maturation and antitumor functions of human dendritic cells *in vitro. PLoS One,* 9, e96584.
[http://dx.doi.org/10.1371/journal.pone.0096584] [PMID: 24802102]

United States Government database *Curcumin Bioavailability in Glioblastoma Patients.* NCT01712542. Retrievedfromhttps://clinicaltrials.gov.

van Tellingen, O, Yetkin-Arik, B, de Gooijer, MC, Wesseling, P, Wurdinger, T & de Vries, HE (2015) Overcoming the blood-brain tumor barrier for effective glioblastoma treatment. *Drug Resist Updat,* 19, 1-12.
[http://dx.doi.org/10.1016/j.drup.2015.02.002] [PMID: 25791797]

Wang, G, de Kruijff, RM, Rol, A, Thijssen, L, Mendes, E, Morgenstern, A, Bruchertseifer, F, Stuart, MC, Wolterbeek, HT & Denkova, AG (2014) Retention studies of recoiling daughter nuclides of 225Ac in polymer vesicles. *Appl Radiat Isot,* 85, 45-53.
[http://dx.doi.org/10.1016/j.apradiso.2013.12.008] [PMID: 24374072]

Weiswald, LB, Bellet, D & Dangles-Marie, V (2015) Spherical cancer models in tumor biology. *Neoplasia,* 17, 1-15.
[http://dx.doi.org/10.1016/j.neo.2014.12.004] [PMID: 25622895]

Withers, HR (1975) *The four R's of Radiobiology.* Academic Press, New York, NY.

Yang, C, Bromma, K, Sung, W, Schuemann, J & Chithrani, D (2018) Determining the Radiation Enhancement Effects of Gold Nanoparticles in Cells in a Combined Treatment with Cisplatin and Radiation at Therapeutic Megavoltage Energies. *Cancers (Basel),* 10, E150.
[http://dx.doi.org/10.3390/cancers10050150] [PMID: 29786642]

Zhao, M, Zhao, M, Fu, C, Yu, Y & Fu, A (2018) Targeted therapy of intracranial glioma model mice with curcumin nanoliposomes. *Int J Nanomedicine,* 13, 1601-10.
[http://dx.doi.org/10.2147/IJN.S157019] [PMID: 29588587]

CHAPTER 9

Preclinical Findings for Targeted Nanotherapies to Hepatocellular Carcinoma

Akhil Suresh[1], Chetan H Metha[1], Varalakshmi Velagacherla[1], Srinivas Mutalik[1], Usha Y Nayak[1] and **N. Udupa[1,*]**

[1] *Department of Pharmaceutics, Manipal College of Pharmaceutical Sciences, Manipal Academy of Higher Education, Manipal, Karnataka, India – 576104*

Abstract: Hepatocellular carcinoma (HCC) is considered a major ailment throughout the world, and conventional therapies including chemo and combinational have sub-optimal responses with toxicity and adverse effects. The use of conventional methods becomes challenging, especially when the tumor cells adapt resistance rapidly, which further limits their use. Nanotherapeutics for HCC show their potential with minimal toxicity and enhanced degree of targeted drug delivery, which has attracted researchers across the world to explore the various benefits of nanotherapeutics. This chapter has briefly covered the epidemiology and incidence of HCC, its causes, stages, different ways to diagnose HCC, its pathology, and conventional treatment options. We have explained various targeted nanotherapeutic preclinical approaches such as lipidic nanoparticles, polymeric nanoparticles, and liposomes for HCC. Surface-modified nanoparticles and liposomes can actively target a wide array of overexpressed receptors on the tumor surface. It can be seen from the literature that the nanotherapeutic approach for the management of HCC has a high potential to become the mainstream treatment platform if explored and tweaked appropriately. In almost all the works, promising results were seen. Maximum amount of drug was delivered at the tumor site, drug release at unwanted sites were prevented and selectively caused cell necrosis in the tumors, while not affecting the normal cells. These remarkable outcomes further strengthen the nanotherapeutic platform, showcasing its true potential.

Keywords: Asialoglycoprotein receptor, Cisplatin, Cubosomes, Dendrimers, Diosmin, Doxorubicin, Hepatocellular carcinoma, Irinotecan, Liquid crystalline nanoparticles, Liver cancer, Nanoparticles, Nanostructured lipid carriers, Nanotherapy, Polyester vectors, Selenium nanoparticles, Solid lipid nanoparticles, Sorafenib, Smart nanoparticles, Superparamagnetic iron oxide nanoparticles, Tumor suppressor microRNA.

[*] **Corresponding author N. Udupa:** Department of Pharmaceutics, Manipal College of Pharmaceutical Sciences, Manipal Academy of Higher Education, Manipal, Karnataka, India – 576104; E-mail: n.udupa@manipal

Biswajit Mukherjee (Ed.)

INTRODUCTION

The liver is the largest and essential organ of our body as it plays a prominent role in the metabolism of many substances, including drugs. It helps in eliminating toxic elements from the human body. Liver physiology is unique from other organs as it has super-impossible networks that are one outlet and two inlets (Lorente *et al.* 2020). Apart from metabolism, the liver also aids in the storage of vitamins, and an important fluid in the bile is also secreted by the liver. The liver also aids in thyroid hormone functioning, where it acts as a place for T3 and T4 de-iodination. The prevalence of liver diseases depends on ethnicity, gender, and socioeconomic status. East and North Africa, Latin America, and Caribbean regions are most prone to liver diseases (Aa *et al.*, 2014).

Liver cancer is a type of cancer that affects hepatocytes, and there are three types of liver cancer. Hepatocellular carcinoma (HCC) is the most common type of liver cancer, around 75% of liver cancers belong to this category, and it originates in hepatocytes. Cirrhosis, Hepatitis virus B (HBV), and C (HCV) infections are the main causative reasons for HCC. Cholangiocarcinoma mainly occurs in the tube-like small bile ducts where they carry bile acids to the gallbladder. Around 10 to 20% of hepatocarcinoma arises from Cholangiocarcinoma. Angiosarcoma accounts for about 1% of all types of hepatocarcinoma, and it starts in the blood vessels of the liver and grows fast. Metastatic cancer in the liver develops when primary carcinoma spreads from other part(s) of the body to the liver. Colorectal cancer causes most liver metastases (Types of Liver Cancer: Common, Rare and More Varieties. 2018). HCC is one of the cancers which causes most number of deaths. More than 80% of liver cancers attribute to HCC (El–Serag and Rudolph 2007). Around 85% of cases of HCC are reported in countries like eastern Africa and Asia (Tang *et al.*, 2018). Non-alcoholic steatohepatitis (NASH), HBV and HCV infection, liver cirrhosis, excessive alcohol consumption, and ingestion of Aflatoxin and aristolochic acid are important risk factors for developing HCC (Ma *et al.* 2013). This chapter highlighted the findings of targeted nanotherapeutics to hepatocellular carcinoma from some selective preclinical investigations. Further, in brief description of the causes, staging, diagnostic and therapeutic aspects of HCC has been provided.

CAUSES OF HCC

Viral Hepatitis and Cirrhosis

Around 80% of cases of HCC are due to prolonged infection of HBV and HCV globally (Yang and Roberts 2010; Park *et al.* 2015). In developed countries, most of the HCC cases are developed as a continuation of a prolonged chronic type of hepatitis. Annually, 2 to 5% of HCC cases are reported in cirrhosis patients (Yang *et al.*, 2017a). A Taiwan-based study on 11801 male patients reported an increased chance for the development of HCC. The increased chance was majorly affected by factors like HBV infection, HCV infection, and alcohol consumption at 55.7%, 15.3%, and 2.1%, respectively. This study also reported an association of HBV and HCV infections had enhanced the development of HCC by 1.7%. The combination of HBV infection with alcohol consumption enhances the risk by approximately 4.2% (Liao *et al.*, 2012).

Fatty Liver Disease and Diabetes

Non-alcoholic fatty liver disease (NAFLD) is one of the major causes of liver disease development and increases the risk factor of HCC (Younossi *et al.*, 2016). A range of 10-20% of the HCC cases in the US is accredited to NAFLD. According to a study, NAFLD was associated with a 2.6-fold increased risk to HCC (Younossi *et al.*, 2015). It is also seen that NAFLD-linked HCC frequently occurs even in cases where cirrhosis was absent (Yang *et al.*, 2017b). Obesity and diabetes mellitus also cause an increase in NAFLD (Welzel *et al.*, 2013). A report suggests a 2 to 3-fold increase in the chances of HCC in patients with diabetes mellitus (Huang *et al.*, 2018). Another study reported that diabetes mellitus enhances the chances of HCC in patients with cirrhosis. The resistance of insulin and the production of reactive oxygen species, which triggers the inflammation of the liver, is known to have an important role in hepatocarcinogenesis (Hui *et al.*, 2008).

Alcohol

Cirrhosis caused by alcohol is a common risk factor for HCC. World cancer research fund conducted some studies and reported that consumption of 10 g alcohol a day increases the chances of suffering from HCC by 4%. In contrast, when compared with patients who have chronic viral hepatitis, the patients related to alcoholic cirrhosis have fewer chances of developing the HCC (West *et al.*, 2017). A retrospective cohort study conducted in a single center comprising 450 alcoholic cirrhosis patients revealed independent risk factors (thrombocytopenia and old age) that led to the development of HCC (Mancebo *et al.*, 2013).

Aflatoxin and Aristolochic Acid

Aflatoxins are mycotoxins that have hepatocarcinogenic properties and are adulterated into different kinds of cereal and oilseeds. Ingestion of aflatoxin is one of the risk factors for HCC. Aspergillus sp. produces the aflatoxin B1, which is the main form of the aflatoxins which cause liver carcinogenesis (Wild *et al.* 2015). Mutations at codon 249 in the TP53 tumor suppressor gene caused by Aflatoxin B1 (AGG to AGT) lead to the substitution of arginine for serine

(R249S), which is noticed in HCC (Gouas *et al.* 2009). In hepatic cancers, the interaction of aflatoxin and HBV infection has a major impact (Ross *et al.* 1992). Chronic HBV infection causes increased cytochrome P450 activity, which metabolizes the inactive aflatoxin B1 to the aflatoxin mutagen B1-8,9-epoxide. Chronic regeneration of HBV infection and hepatocyte necrosis also causes the AFB1- induced TP53 mutations (Kew 2003). Aristolochic acid is found in Chinese wild ginger (Aristolochia). It is a highly mutagenic compound. A study of 1400 HCC patients from different regions of the world showed that 78% Taiwan HCC patients, 47% of Chinese HCC patients, 29% of southeast Asian patients, 13% of Korean HCC patients, 4.8% of North American patients, and 1.7% of European HCC patients exhibited the aristolochic acid traces (Ng *et al.* 2017).

Other Causes of Cirrhosis

Metabolic or genetic liver diseases and chronic biliary diseases may lead to cirrhosis and provoke the formation of HCC. However, the percentage of HCC that occurs due to these diseases is low and varies between 5% to 10% (Welzel *et al.*, 2013).

STAGES OF HCC

The staging systems can predict the prognosis of cancer patients for HCC disease. There are various staging systems for the HCC, which include both conventional as well as new systems. However, due to huge limitations in using a conventional staging system, new approaches are proposed that can be used worldwide. Conventional staging systems include Okuda and the tumor node metastases (TNM) staging system. In contrast, in new staging systems, primarily three staging methods have been validated, such as cancer of the Italian Liver Program (CLIP), Barcelona clinic liver cancer (BCLC), and Japan integrated staging (JIS) systems (Pons *et al.* 2005). The different staging used for HCC is shown in Table **1**.

DIAGNOSIS OF HCC

Diagnosis of HCC depends on various aspects such as clinical, radiological, cancer marker proteins like serum α-fetoprotein concentration and biopsy of liver tissue. Among all the parameters, clinical and pathological features are critical which are considered during the diagnosis of HCC. The clinical parameter includes weight loss, upper right quadrant pain, liver function worsening acute abdominal catastrophe due to rupturing of the liver tumor with bleeding from the intra-abdominal region, and rarely extrahepatic manifestations of liver function. These parameters help to decide the presence or absence of the HCC condition.

Radiologic parameters include various techniques that help in the diagnosis of HCC rapidly. It includes radioisotope scans, angiography, ultrasound examination, computed tomography, and magnetic resonance imaging. The presence of intrahepatic masses can be analyzed using radioisotope scanning. But it is not useful for detecting small tumors. Angiography is a highly vascular technique commonly used to diagnose HCC due to the routine evaluation part before resection. But nowadays, its use is limited due to its inability to detect tumors of diameter less than 2 cm. In this case, other imaging techniques help to tackle these problems.

Table 1. HCC Staging System.

Staging System of HCC	Developing Year	No. of Patients Considered	Factors Considered	Advantages	Limitations	Scoring / Stages	References
Okuda	1985	850	Tumor size, liver function (ascites, serum albumin, bilirubin level)	Helpful in identifying stage-III patients (end-stage)	Difficult to differentiate the less advanced patients, not includes a multicentricity or extrahepatic spread of the tumor, vascular invasion, lesser predictive capacity	Three stages, I (not advanced), II (moderately advanced), III (very advanced)	(Shouval 2002)
Barcelona Clinic Liver Cancer (BCLC)	1999	-	Tumor extension (tumors size and their quantity and presence of extrahepatic metastasis or portal vein invasion), liver functional reserve and overall physical status (PS), Child-Pugh grade	First system which recommends evidence-based clinical treatment for every patient at various stages	Developed from the obtained results of RCTs and cohort studies. Unable to predict the HCC patient mortality	Five categories: 0 – very early stage, A – early stage, B – intermediate stage, C – advance stage and D – terminal stage)	(Llovet *et al.* 1999; Pons *et al.* 2005; Forner *et al.* 2012; Subramaniam *et al.* 2013)
Cancer of the Liver Italian Program score (CLIP)	1998	435	Patient Pugh type including tumor characteristics which involves tumor morphology, portal vein extension. Thrombosis and levels of alfa-fetoprotein	Greater predictive power than okude, Easy to calculate, well correlated with survival	Lacks to give information about underlying liver diseases, extrahepatic metastasis, and status of performance.	7 Scores (0, 1, 2, 3, 4, 5 and 6)	(Kudo *et al.* 2003)

(Table 1) cont.....

Staging System of HCC	Developing Year	No. of Patients Considered	Factors Considered	Advantages	Limitations	Scoring / Stages	References
Groupe d'Etude et de Traitement du Carcinoma Hépatocellulaire (GRETCH) system	1999	761	Performance status, Baseline characteristics, Cox regression coefficient	Quite similar to the CLIP	Lacks the information of tumor morphology, Difficult to get the specific therapy, limited prognostic capacity in early HCC.	3 classes A (lower risk to death), B (Intermediate risk to death), and C (High risk to death)	(Cillo *et al.* 2005)
Chinese University Prognostic Index (CUPI)	2002	926	Includes conventional TNM system parameters as well as the function of the liver and tumor load (ascites, serum bilirubin, ALP, AFP serum, and asymptomatic disease)	Better estimation of survival than okuda and CLIP	Not suitable application in western population with predominant HCV infection or alcohol abuse history	3 groups (low-risk, intermediate-risk, and high-risk)	(Zhang *et al.* 2014)
Japan Integrated Staging Score (JIS)	2003	722	Child-Pugh grade with the Japanese TNM (Liver Cancer Study Group of Japan- LCSGJ) which include various parameters vascular invasion, multiple nodules of diameter < *vs.* > 20 mm)	Helps in stratifying the patient's diagnosis at early stages than CLIP system	No liver function evaluation, inaccurate tumor size weighting, and vascular involvement with lack of incorporation of microscopic pathology information	4 Stages (I-IV)	(Kudo *et al.* 2003; Makuuchi *et al.* 2003)
Tokyo	2005	403	tumor nodules size and their quantity in terms of number, serum bilirubin, and albumin values	The equal ability of prediction as CLIP, while better than BCLC classification, Useful for early-stage patients	Not suitable for advanced-stage patients, parameters such as performance status and cancer-related symptoms not included in the study	0-6 scores, o means patients having better prognosis and 6 means five-year survival rates	(Tateishi *et al.* 2005)
Bilirubin-Albumin-AFPL3-AFP-DCP (BALAD)	2006	2600	Indicators such as albumin and bilirubin of liver functional reserve, lens culinaris agglutinin reactive as factors reflecting tumor progression	a simple and objective tool, Comparable with the CLIP and JIS score	-	Six groups	(Makuuchi *et al.* 2003; Toyoda *et al.* 2006)

(Table 1) cont.....

Staging System of HCC	Developing Year	No. of Patients Considered	Factors Considered	Advantages	Limitations	Scoring / Stages	References
Advanced liver cancer prognostic system (ALPCS)	2008	1470	Ascites, abdominal weight loss, pain, child-Pugh grade, ALP, total serum bilirubin, serum AFP, serum urea, tumor size, portal thrombosis, and lung metastasis	A better system than that of the Okuda system and CLIP score	Need to be validated in a western population with predominant HCV infection or alcohol abuse	Three groups (good: score < 8, intermediate: 9-15, and poor: > 16)	(Yau *et al.* 2008)
American Joint Committee on Cancer (AJCC) TNM-7	1977 2002 (Simplified System)	557	Primary tumor extension and lymph node involvement and extrahepatic metastasis, Major and microvascular invasion, severe fibrosis/cirrhosis, multiple tumors with tumor size greater than 5 cm	successfully used by oncologists in several fields	It does not measure the patient's health status and liver function, thus needing to use other scoring systems or other parameters.	10 Stages	(Llovet *et al.* 1998; Marsh *et al.* 2000; Durand *et al.* 2001)
Taipei Integrated Score (TIS)	2010	2030	Burden of a tumor and total tumor volume (TTV), combined with Child-Pugh grade and AFP concentration.	Having superior prognostic value compared with another staging system such as CLIP, BCLC, JIS, and Tokyo, independently of the treatment modality curative or palliative, useful and reliable system	Can not calculate the accurate TTV value as all tumors are not spherical, needs to be externally validated in Western population as includes only HCC patients with HBV infection	Based on TTV – 4 groups, Child-Pugh – 3 groups and Alpha-fetoprotein – 2 groups	(Hsu *et al.* 2010)

(Table 1) cont.....

Staging System of HCC	Developing Year	No. of Patients Considered	Factors Considered	Advantages	Limitations	Scoring / Stages	References
Model to estimate survival in ambulatory HCC patients score (MESSIAH Score)	2012	1381	Scoring for model end-stage liver disease (MELD), age, level of serum albumin, number of tumors and their size, extrahepatic metastasis, and vascular invasion	highly stable, superior predictive accuracy and objectivity and reproducibility of the prognostic factors, independent of the underlying liver disease and treatment modality, better discriminatory ability than BCLC, CLIP, JIS, and Tokyo, one of the most promising staging systems	Limited to the laboratory variables (which are available easily)	-	(Kamath *et al.* 2007; Jd *et al.* 2012; Kim *et al.* 2014)
Hong Kong Liver Cancer (HKLC)	2014	3856	ECOG PS, Child-Pugh grade, liver tumor status, and presence of extrahepatic vascular invasion or metastasis	exhibits better prognostic value than the BCLC classification, better stratify patients	Need to do prospective study in large scale	five main groups and nine subgroups	(Durand *et al.* 2001; Adhoute *et al.* 2015)
ITA.LI.CA integrated staging system (ITALICA)	2016	5000	Tumor diameter and presence of nodules, extra- and intrahepatic macroscopic vascular invasion, extrahepatic metastases, performance status, Child-Pugh score (CPS).	Better discriminant ability	It needs to be validated in prospective studies with more contemporary cohorts	Ten stages by varying the largest tumor diameter, number of tumors, vascular invasion, or metastasis	(Gurda *et al.* 2015; Farinati *et al.* 2016)

Ultrasound imaging can detect very small lesions or tumors in the liver. Currently, magnetic resonance and computed tomography imaging are two techniques preferred worldwide for diagnosing the HCC compared to the other techniques with various modifications such as multiphase contrast enhancement, use of spiral scanners, and many more. In addition to this, measuring the serum (AFP) concentration is also helpful in diagnosing and managing HCC. A concentration above 20 ng/mL is an indication of the presence of HCC. But this method also has limitations due to low specificity to AFP, presence of AFP in different isoforms and its detection, and even higher cut-off values. As discussed earlier, a biopsy of liver tissue is another vital HCC diagnosis technique, including needle biopsy. Still, it has a risk of spreading HCC locally along with needle track.

For diagnosing the nodules with a diameter equal to or more than 1 cm, imaging techniques can be used. If both typical features and clinical criteria are not matching then in this condition, selection of pathological diagnosis is the best option with other parameters such as follow up every three months, imaging repeatedly, and analysis of serum markers (Befeler and Di Bisceglie 2002; Korean Liver Cancer Study Group (KLCSG) and National Cancer Center, Korea (NCC) 2015).

PATHOLOGY OF HCC

Multiple factors are responsible for the pathology of the HCC including hepatotropic viruses, epigenetic factors, genomic alterations, transcriptomic parameters, non-alcoholic fatty liver disease (NAFLD), diabetes and obesity, alcohol and tobacco abuse, an over-dose of iron, environmental toxins, and also autoimmune hepatitis (Streba *et al.* 2014; Streba *et al.* 2018). Fig. (**1**). illustrates the various pathological ways by which HCC onset occurs.

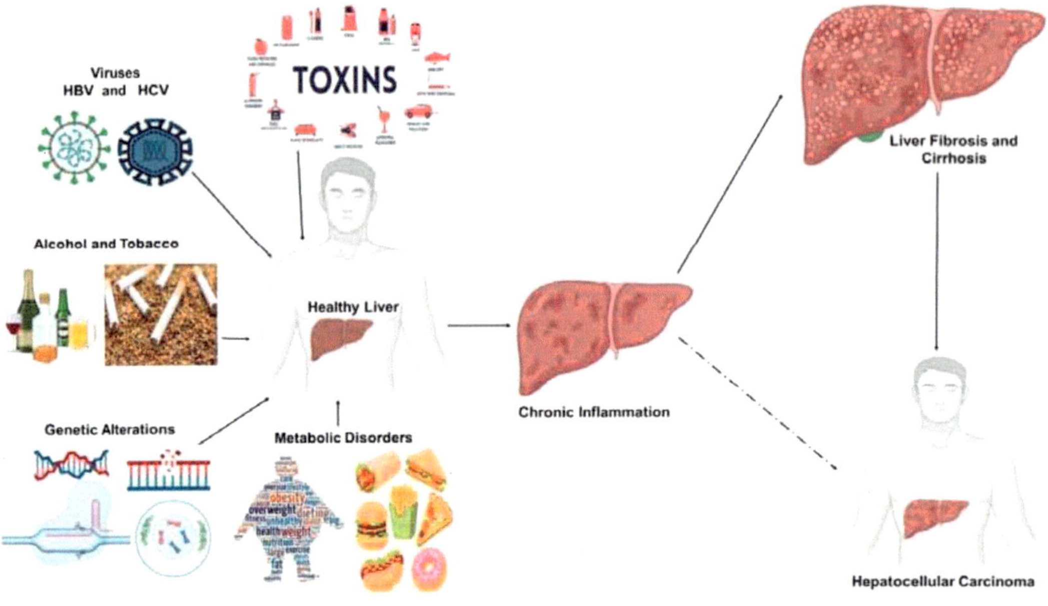

Fig. (1). Risk Factors Involved in Pathogenesis of Hepatocellular Carcinoma.

Hepatotropic Viruses

HBV and HCV are major risk factors for causing HCC that can be characterized by the development of chronic inflammation, viral genome integration into host DNA, and cirrhosis. HBV and HCV are DNA and RNA viruses; respectively, HBV integrates into the host genome and leads to the production of X protein and causes cell proliferation while HCV replicates in the cytoplasm itself. HBV accounts for 50% of the HCC cases. Overall, HBV and HCV lead to the dysfunction of telomere and cellular alteration at micro-and macroenvironment levels, leading to an increase in cellular proliferation, instability of chromosomes, reduction in telomere length, in regenerative liver capacity with hepatocyte regeneration reduction. Finally, it progresses into liver fibrosis followed by cirrhosis that can lead to HCC (Grando-Lemaire *et al.* 1999; Trinchet *et al.* 2004; El–Serag and Rudolph 2007; Tatematsu *et al.* 2009; Geramizadeh *et al.* 2013; Ghouri *et al.* 2017; Zamor *et al.* 2017).

Metabolic Disorders

Diabetes and obesity develop oxidative stress, which damages the DNA, with genomic instability and mutations leading to the development of neoplastic cells, which finally develop into the HCC. Metabolic disorders also lead to the development of non-alcoholic fatty liver disease (NAFLD) or non-alcoholic steatohepatitis (NASH) (Wiklund and Dich 1994; Nair *et al.* 2002; Marrero *et al.* 2005; Toffanin *et al.* 2010).

Alcohol and Tobacco

Chronic alcohol-abusing, tobacco chewing, and smoking are also important factors in causing HCC due to different mechanisms or pathways, including the creation of DNA acetaldehyde, P450 E cytochrome associated ROS species formation with mutation of p53 gene and enhancement in ROS and activation of Kappa-B factors. All these parameters lead to inflammatory and oxidative stress promotion with a reduction in Vitamin A metabolism and, thus, develop into hepatocyte proliferation followed by liver cirrhosis and HCC (Brooks and Theruvathu 2005; Koh *et al.* 2011; Purohit *et al.* 2013).

Environmental Toxins

It includes Aflatoxins and overloading of iron majorly. Aflatoxin is a hepatic carcinogen and a byproduct of fungal contamination of foodstuffs, which acts through mutation of the p53 gene and damaging DNA. There is the generation of free radicals due to overloading of iron, and thus, it leads to oxidative tissue damages to the liver and, finally, the development of HCC (Ludwiczek *et al.*, 2003; Kew 2013; Kew 2014).

Genetic Alterations

As we know, the pathology of HCC includes many factors, and genetic alterations equally contribute to the development of HCC by multiple levels. Genomic somatic mutations and copy number of alterations (CNAs), transcriptomic gene expression level, and changes at the epigenetic level are fundamental in the case of HCC. Various research studies have shown the loss and gains in the chromosome in HCC, which include focal amplifications and focal deletions at oncogenes and tumor suppressors such as MYC, MET, CCND1, TERT and FGF19, and TP53, PTEN, CDKN2B, and CDKN2A, respectively (Thorgeirsson and Grisham 2002; Kumar *et al.* 2011; Kan *et al.* 2013).

There are commonly mutated genes such as TP53 and CTNNB1, associated with HBV infection and are a putative driver for alcoholics. Also, various other mutant genes are responsible for affecting cellular pathways, which include TP53, RB1, and CDKN2A for DNA repair and surveillance, AXIN1 and CTNNB1 for Wnt/β-catenin signaling, RPS6KA3 for signaling of oncogenic mitogen-activated protein kinase (MAPK), KEAP1 and NFE2L2 for oxidative stress, ARID, ARID1A and ARID1B for remodeling of chromatin and MLL, MLL4 and MLL3 for modification of histone (Schulze *et al.* 2015). As discussed earlier, HBV is responsible for 50% of the cases. Also, integrating viral DNA into the human genome leads to disruption of endogenous tumor regulatory and suppressor genes, enhancing proto-oncogenes activity. It leads to an imbalance between the signals responsible for tumor suppression and oncogene, resulting in apoptosis reduction and enhanced proliferation and survival. Finally, it develops into HCC. MLL4, TERT, ROCK1, and CCNE1 are some of the genes which are mostly affected by the integration of HBV (Kremsdorf *et al.* 2006; El-Serag 2011; Ding *et al.* 2012; Jiang *et al.* 2012; Li *et al.* 2013; Lau *et al.* 2014; Ho *et al.* 2015b).

Epigenetic alterations are involved equally in the development of HCC. But it is reversible for modifications and does not include changes in the DNA sequence at the genomic level. Various modulations such as histone modification, DNA methylation, and chromatin remodeling at the gene transcription level help to control the level of gene expression, and different non-coding RNAs such as microRNAs, lncRNAs are also involved in modifications post-transcriptionally (Liu *et al.* 2014a; Ma *et al.* 2014; Saito *et al.* 2014; Younossi *et al.* 2016; De Vincentis *et al.* 2020). Transcriptomic alterations involve the differences in gene expression by upregulation and downregulation of the various genes. FOXM1 and CENPF are two important genes that are found to be upregulated at the transcriptomic level in which FOXM1 is responsible for cell cycle regulation as well as proliferation and repairment of DNA damage, while CENPF is responsible for mitotic segregation and function of the kinetochore. On the other hand, corticotropin-releasing hormone-binding protein (CRHBP), CLEC4G, CLEC4M, and CLEC1B (C-type lecithin family) showed downregulation, which is mainly responsible for adhesion and also acts as receptor signaling for various processes related to the immune system. Overall disturbances at any level, such as genomics, transcriptomic, and epigenetic, alter the various genes expression, and finally, it leads to the HCC development (Huang *et al.* 2011; Lin *et al.* 2014; Ho *et al.* 2015a)

CONVENTIONAL TREATMENT OPTIONS FOR HCC

Depending on the location and size of the HCC tumor, functioning of the liver, and overall health of the patient, treatment options vary from surgical, transplant therapy, destroying the cancer cells with cold or heat treatment, chemo- or radiation therapy, targeted drug therapy, and immunotherapy.

Surgery and transplantation: The tissue surrounding the cancer tissue, along with cancer tissue, can be removed with the help of surgery. But it is limited to people with normal liver function and early-stage liver cancers. If normal surgery is not possible, removing the liver entirely or replacing the liver with the donor's liver may be an option to stop cancer from spreading to other tissues or organs.

Heat or cold therapy for cancer cell termination: People who are unable to go for surgery can try this option of killing the cancer cells within the liver using extreme cold or hot therapy, which includes cryoablation, ablation using alcohol, radiofrequency, and microwaves.

Chemotherapy: Chemotherapy is an important method that is suitable for all patients and easily available. In this therapy, chemotherapeutic drugs such as sunitinib, linifanib, brivanib, tivantinib, and everolimus can be administered to the patients for HCC treatment.

Radiation therapy: X-rays are used as a source of radiation in radiation therapy. Nowadays, a special type of therapy is available called stereotactic body radiotherapy (SBRT) that includes simultaneous targeting of the radiation beams at one of the targeted or specific points in the body. Radioembolization (radiation encapsulated tiny glass sphere) is another option that can be directly provided to the cancer tissues.

Drug Targeted Therapy: Targeted drug delivery mainly works on the principle of direct targeting to the required area or cells or specific delicate protein structures present on the cancer cells. It primarily acts through targeting the particular cells and decreases the disease progression to the final stage. It includes conventional as well as nanoformulations.

Immunotherapy: Antibody against cancer-specific antigen here helps fight the cancer cells, and it helps treat advanced liver cancer (Karaman *et al.* 2014; Hepatocellular carcinoma - Overview - Mayo Clinic).

Among these therapies, chemotherapy is not suitable for advanced hepatoma cases due to poor efficacies of first- and second-line treatments, lack of targeted formulations, and cytotoxic nature of most anticancer drugs (Omata *et al.*, 2017; Vogel *et al.* 2018). In addition to this, clinical trials for targeted molecular therapy are also unable to show satisfactory results. Therefore, recent advances in polymer science and nanoformulation may change the scenario and improve the poor condition associated with conventional therapy. Various modifications such as adsorption, intercalation, encapsulation, polymerization, coupling reactions, and condensation to conjugate or encapsulate the drug on the surface or inside the nanocarriers are being utilized to develop modified nanoformulations against cancer (Ding *et al.* 2013; Chen *et al.* 2020a). These modified nanocarriers have various advantages over conventional formulations or therapies, including admirable compatibility, physically and chemically stable properties, reticuloendothelial system escape (RES), and compatibility for different surface modifications. In addition to this, nanocarriers also possess various unique characteristics such as mechanical, thermal, optical, and magnetic properties, making this formulation for prolonged drug release in a controlled manner with improving their effectiveness. Nanoformulations also have a convertible surface with adaptable size, prolonged blood circulation, and even the accumulation of antineoplastic moieties (Nasir *et al.* 2013; Liu *et al.* 2014b; Liang *et al.* 2015; Sun *et al.* 2015; Chang *et al.* 2016; Chan and Hsiao 2017; Shen *et al.* 2017; Jiang *et al.* 2018; Li *et al.* 2018; Naseema *et al.* 2018; Zhang *et al.* 2018).

TARGETED NANOTHERAPEUTIC SYSTEMS INVESTIGATED AT THE PRECLINICAL STAGE FOR THE TREATMENT OF HCC

Liposomes

Liposomes are spherical, and small vesicles are made up of amphiphilic lipids and enclose an aqueous core, mainly composed of phospholipids such as soya phosphatidylcholine as it forms the bilayer structure, with or without cholesterol. Liposomes have various advantages (including targeted drug delivery, diagnosis suitability, and improved therapeutic index) over other nanoparticles, which make these formulations popular for delivery of various types of pharmaceutically active moieties, which can be hydrophobic, amphiphilic, and hydrophilic drugs (Nounou *et al.* 2008; Güngör *et al.* 2013; Palac *et al.* 2014). Fig. (**2**) illustrates the various nanotherapeutic formulations which are employed in the management of HCC.

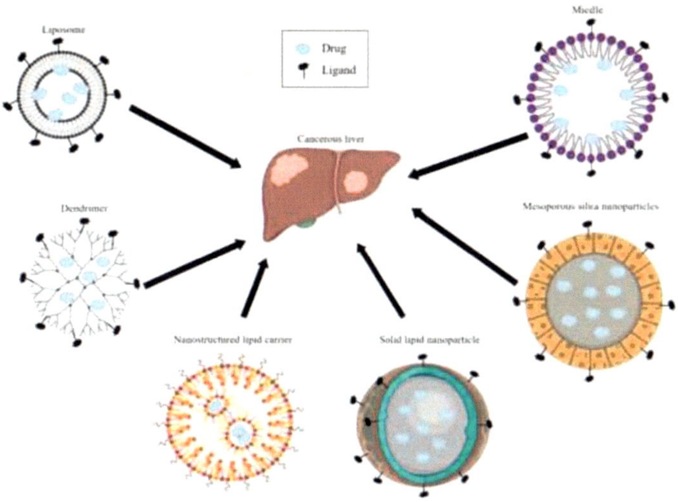

Fig. (2). Various nanocarriers employed for the safe delivery of drugs to the target site.

Zhang *et al.* prepared surface-modified liposomes to improve their permeation and targetability. The penetration of unmodified liposomes to the liver tumor cells is one of the main hurdles in delivering an anticancer drug, Cantharidine. Liposome was surface modified by incorporating peptide BR2 to enhance the cell penetrability, which can effectively and efficiently be targeted to the cells of HCC. In this study, Miha cells (as control) and HepG2 (Malignant hepatocytes) cells were selected for examining the effect of unmodified and surface-modified liposomes on cells using *In vitro* studies. The studies showed a sounder anticancer effect of cantharidine-loaded surface-modified liposomes when compared to the unmodified cantharidine-loaded liposomes. Also, they proved to be stable after incubating with 50% fetal bovine serum for 24 h. *In vitro* cytotoxicity studies showed that BR2-tagged cantharidine showed more toxicity by killing the HepG2 cells compared to untagged cantherdine-loaded liposomes. A cellular uptake study of the modified and normal liposomes was performed, which showed higher uptake of the modified liposomes by HepG2 cells than control cells. Also, cellular uptake and localization studies showed the superior ability of surface-modified liposomes for their entry or penetration and subsequent drug release into the cancerous cells. Substantial accumulation and inhibition of tumor by BR2 modified liposomes were proved after performing *in vivo* efficacy and biodistribution studies. *In vivo* biodistribution studies showed increased fluorescence intensity as time increased, demonstrating the sustained release of drugs and distribution to the various organs. Thus, the surface-modified liposomes effectively helped in the penetration of the liposomes in the tumor cells and its inhibition with cytotoxicity against HepG2 cells compared to unmodified liposomes (Zhang *et al.*, 2017).

Hybrid nanocarriers were developed by AlQahtani *et al.* to avoid the degradation of the liposomes loaded with an anticancer drug such as 5-fluorouracil (5-FU) all through the systemic circulation. Thus, nanoerythrocyte membrane (NEM) coating on liposomes loaded with 5-FU was made, which led to the formation of NEM-5FU-LPs. Various studies were performed for prepared modified liposomes, and results showed that all the liposomes such as NEM-5-FU, NEM-5FUs-LPs, and 5-FU-LPs had the required particle size, polydispersibility index (PDI), and zeta potential. The encapsulation efficiency was analyzed, and it was observed that encapsulation of the drug increased as drug concentration increased while transmission electron microscopy showed the formation of spherical-shaped liposomes. The stability studies showed no or negligible changes in liposome size, PDI, and zeta potential after storage for a longer time, suggesting stability of the formulation. SDS-PAGE studies also proved that accumulation of NEM-5FU-LPs in membrane proteins of erythrocyte and release of the drug was in a sustained manner compared to unmodified liposomes and normal drug solution. In addition to *In vitro* studies, *In vitro* cytotoxicity cell line studies showed late cytotoxic outcomes. Thus, it proved that surface modification helped target cancer cells efficiently and improved stability by minimizing degradation-associated problems (AlQahtani *et al.*, 2019).

Tagaram *et al.* evaluated the *in vivo* efficacy of the antineoplastic agent-loaded C6-ceramide nanoliposomes using *in vivo* human model. The effect of C6-ceramide nanoliposomes in SK-HEP-1 cells was investigated for assessing the activity of caspase 3/7, cell viability, gene expression, AKT phosphorylation, DNA fragmentation, and cell cycle distribution. SK-HEP-1 cells were also injected subcutaneously in the nude mice (athymic), and animals were treated with a C6-ceramide nano-liposomal formulation. The mice were evaluated or examined for tumor size (before removing) and proliferation and vascularization of the tumor, and cellular signaling and apoptosis. Results showed that the modified C6-ceramide liposomal formulation led to apoptotic SK-HEP-1 cell death, reduction in AKT phosphorylation, and improvement in cell accumulation in the G2 phase of the cell cycle. The modified ceramide liposomes were found to have limited toxicity. *In vivo* efficacy studies were performed to check the effect of modified nanoliposomes, and it was seen that the blocking of tumor growth was achieved by reducing the proliferation and vascularization of the tumor, AKT phosphorylation reduction with the induction of tumor cell apoptosis. Thus, it was concluded that C6-ceramide nano-liposomal dispersion was an efficacious anticancerous agent in hepatocellular carcinoma (Tagaram *et al.*, 2011).

Jagwani *et al.* prepared cationic liposomes and evaluated them to improve the site-specific delivery of resveratrol (RSV) in the HCC. The formulation had optimum particle size (145 ± 9.9 nm), zeta potential (38 ± 9.12 mV), PDI (0.359 ±

0.03), and encapsulation efficiency (78 ± 8.04%), and the formulation was found to be stable during the storage conditions. *In vitro* drug release study showed burst release initially, after which the drug release happened in a controlled manner, while drug release kinetics showed the drug release to be following the Hixon-Crowell model, which indicates surface dissolution. *In vitro* cellular uptake and *in vivo* pharmacokinetic and pharmacodynamic studies were performed to analyze the cytotoxicity and efficacy of the formulation. Liposomes loaded RSV showed excellent anticancer activity and better cellular uptake in HepG2 cells compared to the free RSV. *In vivo*, pharmacokinetic and pharmacodynamic studies were performed in N-nitrosodiethylamine induced animal HCC model, which showed accumulation of the highest amount of RSV loaded cationic liposomes in liver tissue as compared to the free RSV drug and in addition to this, reduction in the marker enzymes present in the liver was noticed when compared with the pure drug. The cationic liposomes have a positive charge with the highest affinity towards the cancer cell, having a negative charge bearing phosphophatidylserine. Therefore, it showed the highest accumulation of liposomes in the liver tissue. The prepared cationic liposomes had therapeutic and chemo-preventive action in the diseased model (Jagwani *et al.* 2020).

The anti-miR-221 loaded into liposomes bearing negative charge were prepared by Zhang *et al.* to target the transferrin (Tf) receptor overexpressed in HepG2 cells. Tf was coupled to liposomes in the presence of a linker and catalyst. The optimized formulation with a particle size of 122.5 nm showed a 15-fold enhancement in the efficiency of the drug delivery compared to the non-targeted normal liposomes in HepG2 cells. In addition, it successfully transported anti-miR-221 to the HepG2 cells with upregulation of some proteins such as TIMP3, PTEN, $P27^{KIP1}$, which exhibited higher silencing efficiency as compared to the non-targeted liposome. Cell binding efficiency of these prepared liposomes was determined by adding liposomes to six-well plates having HEPG2 cells and determining active agent concentration after 24 hours. Concentration was determined by fluorescence microscope, and the concentration was more in Tf-loaded liposomes, which was nearly 100 µg/mL of Tf-free liposomes treated cells. The animal model was developed by injecting HepG2 cells intravenously in mice, and mice were treated with the prepared liposomes, which were negatively charged and labeled with anti-miR-221. The study showed successful targeting of the formulation of cancer cells by the formulation with the enhancement of $P27^{kip1}$, PTEN, and TIMP3 expression. MTT assay was conducted by using the 96-well plate method. *In vivo* biodistribution studies were carried out on Kunming mice with the HepG2 xenograft model. It was seen that the drug concentration was more in the tumor of the liver. Thus, it can be concluded from the obtained results that the prepared modified negatively charged liposomes were suitable for gene delivery and can be considered as the probable therapeutic modality in the treatment of HCC (Xiang *et al.*, 2015).

The linoleic acid and propofol (2,6-diisopropyl phenol) conjugate were encapsulated into the nanoliposomes tagged with tuftsin. The conjugate was evaluated for its *in vitro* efficacy in the HepG2 cell lines, which confirmed the effectiveness of conjugate as an antineoplastic agent to induce apoptosis and suppress the migration with HepG2 adhesion. The prepared conjugate was enclosed into the nanoliposome tagged with tuftsin. Liposomes had a particle size of 100-130 nm with a zeta potential of -43.23 mV. TEM images showed that liposomes were spherical, and the surface of the liposomes was smooth. Liposomes have shown sustained drug release up to 144 hours compared to pure drugs (73% of the drug was released from conjugated liposomes at a uniform rate for an extended period). The prepared nanoformulation was tested in the animal model, which reduced COX-2 (highly expressed molecules in HCC) and BCL-2 expressions while upregulating the Bax gene. Also, histopathological results showed significant recovery in the liver architecture and enhanced the cancerous cell apoptosis, specifically at the tumor site. From these results, it can be concluded that the prepared nanoformulation can improve the survival of the mice and hence, can be considered safe, effective, and efficacious in the treatment of liver cancer. The prepared formulation was used for checking apoptotic activity on different proteins. Survival studies were carried by taking certain sets of cancer-induced mice, and it has shown a 60% of survival rate (Khan *et al.* 2016).

Lactoferrin-modified PEGylated doxorubicin liposomes were developed for targeted drug delivery to treat HCC. Lactoferrin has more specificity and more binding capacity towards the asialoglycoprotein receptor. Doxorubicin belongs to the anthracycline class; it acts as one of the important chemotherapeutic agents for treating HCC. As doxorubicin has minimal therapeutic response values, they are formulated into lactoferrin PEGylated liposomes using polyethylene glycol (PEG). PEG has different advantages that will help treat HCC. It can help in the localization of drugs into tissues, increase circulation time, and avoid rapid clearance of the drug from the body, enhancing permeability and retention effect in cancerous cells. Lipids such as soybean phosphatidylcholine,1,2-Distearoyl--n-glycero-3-phosphoethanolamine Poly(ethylene glycol) (DSPE-PEG 2000) were used for the preparation of liposomes by the thin-film hydration method. These nanoliposomes have more significant potential for targeting HCC. Prepared doxorubicin conjugated lactoferrin liposomes have shown a uniform particle size of 200 nm. The zeta potential was 10 mV with high encapsulation efficiency and sustained drug release. The prepared formulation has shown increased anti-proliferative activity, determined by cytotoxicity study (Wei *et al.*, 2015).

Ochi *et al.* prepared nanoliposomes of two drugs, silibinin, and glycyrrhizic acid, with modified PEG. Nanoliposomes were prepared by using lipids such as dipalmitoylphosphatidylcholine (DPPC), cholesterol, and phosphatidylethanolamine. Prepared formulations were evaluated by performing an MTT assay, and its efficacy was determined using fibroblasts cells. Glycyrrhizic acid acted as an hepato-protectant and helped in treating HCC. Prepared formulations had a particle size of 46.3 nm, a zeta potential of -23.25mV, and encapsulation efficiency of 24.37 and 68.78% for silibinin glycyrrhizic acid, respectively, as determined by HPLC analysis. Drug (88%) was released from liposomes within 48 hours. Stability studies were conducted for these liposomes and checked for particle size, zeta potential, and drug release after three months. These mixed liposomes formed were multi-lamellar vesicles. These liposomes have shown better results on cancer cell lines when compared to fibroblasts cell lines. The inhibitory concentration of silibinin was 48.68 μg/ml, and that of glycyrrhizic acid was 485.45 μg/ml (Ochi *et al.*, 2016).

Galactosylated liposomes of doxorubicin/ vimentin were studied along with combining siRNA for treating HCC. A new kind of liposome was formulated by combining chemical drug moiety and therapeutic nucleic acid, siRNA that acts by binding to asialoglycoprotein receptors. Nucleic acid incorporation to liposomes showed synergistic activity against tumors and enhanced transfection efficacy towards cancerous cells. The specificity of galactosylated liposomes towards HCC cells was reported. The fluorescent rhodamine dye conjugated galactosylated liposomes showed target specificity. The antitumor efficacy of the formulations was studied in Huh7 cells and A549 cells. The siRNA formulation had a particle size of 127.54 nm and a zeta potential of 6.4 mV with an encapsulation efficiency of 56%. Cytotoxicity studies were carried out by MTT assay. Cytotoxicity and minimal inhibitory concentration of siRNA labeled drug-loaded liposomes were more. siRNAs transfection efficiency was determined by using a confocal laser scanning microscope, and cytotoxicity of galactosylated lipoplexes was also reported. Antitumor activity and biodistribution studies were performed on tumor-bearing mice. The galactosylated vimentin siRNA liposomes have shown better suppression of HCC tumors. For cellular uptake studies, they used fluorescein-labeled siRNA liposomes, and the intensity was observed for siRNA and liposomes without siRNA. The intensity was more in liposomes conjugated with siRNA (Oh *et al.*, 2016).

Arabinogalactan cholesterol liposomes were developed for targeting HCC through the asialoglycoprotein receptor. The phospholipon 90G and phospholipon 90H were used as lipids. A new ligand was synthesized by binding cholesterol to arabinogalactan by using a spacer compound called alanine. A carbamate bond was formed between cholesterol and arabinogalactan. Molecular dynamic simulations of lipid layers were carried out for 200 nanoseconds and finalized with the above-mentioned lipids. Lipids were selected based on the relativity of lipids to phosphate groups. By molecular dynamic simulation studies, they have figured the effect of cholesterol on membranes. Prepared liposomes had a size of 212 nm, and the PDI was 0.23 while entrapment efficiency was greater than 95%. The liposomes were oval in shape and showed 74% drug release in 48 hours in 7.4 pH. The specificity towards HepG2 cells was more when compared to pure drugs. In biodistribution studies, 95% of the drug was reported in the liver (Pathak *et al.*, 2016).

Hyphenated liposomes in combination with ceramide showed synergistic activity against treating HCC. Sorafenib, an FDA-approved multiple tyrosine kinase inhibitors, alone has not shown satisfactory results against HCC. Therefore, ceramide, which has the property of suppressing tumors, was used in the formulation. The ratio of ceramide and sorafenib was determined after optimizing the formulation through a combination index. Spherical-shaped liposomes were prepared by thin-film hydration method using lipids such as phosphoethanol-amine-N-methoxy PEG 2000 and DSPE-MPEG 2000. Optimized liposomes had a 174 nm particle size, and the zeta potential was -14 mV. After the formulation of liposomes, they are tested on HepG2 cell lines, and the combination of ceramide and sorafenib ratio was also determined on HepG2 cell lines. *In vitro*, cellular uptake studies were carried out by seeding cells into 12-well plates. *In vitro* cytotoxicity studies of the formulation were carried out on HepG2 cells showed improved efficacy (Yin *et al.* 2018).

Nanoliposomes of cisplatin and curcumin were also formulated to test their effectiveness on HCC. Cisplatin is a first-line conventional inorganic chemo-therapeutic agent that acts on DNA but alone, it has not shown idea anti-cancer activity. Hence, cisplatin was combined with curcumin, a polyphenol that possesses anti-cancer, anti-oxidant, and anti-inflammatory properties. To enhance the properties of the drug and to minimize side effects, they were formulated into nanoliposomes. By performing *in vivo* studies, the ratio for a combination of cisplatin and curcumin was determined. Liposomes were prepared by using lipids such as DSPE-PEG 2000, DMPC, and cholesterol. *In vitro* cytotoxicity and cell apoptosis studies were carried out, and the anti-cancer efficacy of cisplatin and curcumin nanoliposomes was checked in HepG2 cell lines. *In vitro* intracellular studies were performed to determine reactive oxidative species. Western blot assay, pharmacokinetic studies, and biodistribution studies were also performed. The combination index was more than 1, and thus, synergistic activity was high. Encapsulation efficiency was 93.4 and 99.5% for curcumin and cisplatin, respectively, while the particle size was 294.6 nm, with a PDI of 0.119, and zeta potential was 10.8 mV. TEM images have shown the prepared formulation had a spherical shape. These nanoliposomes have shown 74.1 and 68.2% of in-vitro drug release of curcumin and cisplatin, respectively, and increased apoptotic activity (Cheng *et al.*, 2018).

Nanoparticles

Nanoparticles are ultrafine particles that lie in the size range of 10 to 1000 nm. They have a wide array of applications in medicine, physics, optics, and electronics. In medical treatment, they are prominently used for drug delivery as spatial and temporal control on the loaded drug can be achieved, which enables the achievement of the desired outcome. Different types of organic and inorganic nanoparticles are studied for treating HCC. Oral doxorubicin (Doxo) protein nanoparticles for target-specific delivery were formulated to overcome the poor bioavailability and toxicity issues of the drug. The proteins employed belong to the transferrin family, and this class of protein receptors is abundantly found on the surface of cancer cells. Apotransferrin and lactoferrin are used to specifically target the Doxo loaded nanoparticles to the cancer cells to increase the effectiveness of the drug. Apotransferrin Doxo nanoparticles (apodoxonano) and lactoferrin Doxo nanoparticles (lactodoxonano) were prepared by the sol-oil chemistry method. The receptor-mediated entry of protein nanoparticles was checked. Apodoxonano and lactodoxonano were tagged with rhodamine, which emitted green fluorescence, while Doxo emitted red fluorescence. Upon analyzing flow cytometry, it was seen that an increased number of fluorescent cells was found when treated with nanoformulations, and it got reduced when preincubation was carried out with receptor antibodies. The same result was confirmed with confocal microscopy. *In vivo,* animal studies were carried out in *Wistar* rats. HCC was induced with the aid of diethylnitrosamine (DENA). The group that received pure Doxo showed a reduction in liver nodule formation with marginal evidence of cancerous growth in the liver. In contrast, in the group which received apodoxonano and lactodoxonano, a significant reduction in the liver nodules was noticed. The histopathological evaluation further confirmed the advantage of using protein nanoparticles as apodoxonano and lactodoxonano formulations treated group that exhibited normal cellular morphology. When Doxo was administered, a significant increase in the creatinine level and poor blood urea elimination were seen, indicating kidney damage. When nanoformulations were administered, a significant reduction in the extent of damage was seen. To understand the extent of damage in the liver, SGOT and SGPT levels were estimated. The group that received Doxo showed elevated SGOT and SGPT, while the group that received nanoformulations showed substantially reduced SGOT and SGPT. Heart toxicity, which is a major concern with Doxo, was evaluated with the measurement of LDH levels. Significantly elevated levels of LDH were seen in the Doxo treatment group, while the level remained minimal in the animals which received nanoformulation. It was evident that apodoxonano and lactodoxonano enhanced the anti-cancer effect of Doxo in HCC *Wistar* rats, which can be carefully implemented in humans (Golla *et al.*, 2013).

Liu *et al.* (2016) developed a dual drug-loaded nanomedicine system with a significant drug synergy and pH-triggered drug release for combating doxorubicin (DOX) resistant HCC cells. The nanomedicine system constituted of arsenite (ATO) prodrug which was obtained by ATO deposition on transitional metal ions in reverse micelles, after which *in-situ* coating of amine-functionalized silica nanoshell was done. DOX molecules were placed on the silica functionalized nanoparticles by imine bonds, a pH-sensitive crosslinking agent. TEM analysis revealed the presence of ATO nanocomplexes clearly inside the silica, and X-ray spectroscopy mapping indicated the presence of iron and silica atoms in the silica shell. It confirmed the fabrication of core-shell nanostructure. The particle size of this nanoparticle was found to be 12.0 ± 1.3 nm and positive zeta potential of +43.2 mV, which could be due to the DOX molecules and amine groups on the silica surface. ATO/ DOX release from the nanoparticles at various pH environments (5.4 and 7.4) was evaluated using inductively coupled plasma spectroscopy (ICP-MS) and fluorescence spectrophotometry, respectively. It was seen that 74.4% and 17.1% of ATO were released within 24 h of incubation at pH 5.4 and 7.5, respectively. In contrast, DOX exhibited faster release in pH 5.4 with 79.0% release at 9 h and achieving 81.9% release after 24 h. However, at pH 7.4, only up to 2.05% release was seen for DOX. It is indicative of the ability of nanoparticles to remain stable in neutral pH while being sensitive to acidic pH, which is beneficial in tumor therapy. To identify the synergistic and anti-drug resistant nature of the formulation, cytotoxicity tests of free DOX and ATO were carried out in wild type Huh-7 and DOX resistant Huh-7/ADM cells for a duration of 24 h. It was noticed that Huh-7/ADM cells showed high resistance towards DOX with an IC_{50} value of 172.90 ± 12.06 μM, which was 100 times that noticed in parent Huh-7 cells. Isobologram equation of Chou-Talalay was used to determine the presence and extent of synergistic effect if any. Cytotoxicity studies were carried out in different groups: the administration of ATO and DOX loaded nanoparticle formulation, free DOX, free ATO, DOX loaded nanoparticle, ATO loaded nanoparticle, and combination of free DOX and ATO. Among all the treatment groups, ATO and DOX-loaded nanoparticle formulation exhibited the best results with an IC_{50} value of 2.2 ± 0.05 μM, 80 folds higher than that of the individual drug. It was concluded that the synthesized dual drug-loaded nanoparticle formulation successfully overcame drug resistance in HCC and would be used in further testing to help in humans. Asialoglycoprotein receptor (ASGPR) was used to target and deliver DOX nanoparticles for the effective treatment of HCC.

Polyethylene sebacate (PES)-Gantrez AN 119 DOX nanoparticles were prepared by a modified nanoparticle precipitation method. To enable a higher level of targeting to ASPGR, the ligands such as pullan (Pul), arabinogalactan (AGn), and a combination of Pul-AGn were attached to the surface of the nanoparticles. Initially, the formulation had an average particle size of 220 nm with PDI <0.62 with a zeta potential of -27 mV. After introducing the selected ligands into the mix, an increase of 22 – 28 nm was noticed in the particle size while the zeta potential was increased by 7 mV. This change confirmed the attachment of ligands onto the surface of the nanoparticles. The entrapment efficiency of >70% was seen along with a biphasic drug release pattern with an initial burst release followed by a sustained release. *In vivo* biodistribution studies were carried out in female *Sprague Dawley* rats which were divided into groups receiving DOX solution, nanoparticle formulation, Pul-nanoparticles, AGn-nanoparticles, and Pul-AGn-nanoparticles. Results indicated significantly lower levels of DOX in the heart tissue of the animals in the groups that received ligand attached nanoparticles when compared with the DOX-free solution group. It is a significant benefit as it has reduced the cardiotoxicity of DOX. When compared with DOX solution, nanoparticles resulted in significantly higher liver uptake. A 38 times increase in liver uptake was seen in the group administered with Pul-AG--nanoparticles at all time points while Pul-nanoparticle and AGn-nanoparticles separately showed only a 20 times increase in their liver uptake. From histopathological evaluation, it was seen that the group which received DOX solution exhibited glycogen infiltration in the liver, severely hemorrhagic spleen, reduced glomerular filtration space, and cloudy swelling of cortical tubules in kidneys. In contrast, the nanoparticles group revealed no abnormal findings and close resemblance to the normal control group. It establishes the safety profile of the formulation. *In vivo* anticancer activity was evaluated in the liver xenograft mouse model, and PLC/PRF/5 cells were subcutaneously injected into the back of the mice to generate tumor-bearing mice. After 45 days of injection, the tumors were extracted, and cancerous tissue was isolated and cut into small pieces of 2mm × 2mm size and transplanted into Nod/Scid mice. The animals were divided into groups after the tumor diameter reached ≥5 mm. All treatment groups showed suppression in tumor growth for up to 12 days. The treatment groups showed regression at varying degrees. Slow regression was exhibited by DOX solution and Pul-nanoparticles for up to 29 days, but beyond day 29, DOX solution showed rapid regression with a comparable tumor volume to that of the Pul-AG--nanoparticle group—the T/C ratio when ≤0.42 was accepted as efficacious. The study showed that Pul-nanoparticles had a T/C value of <0.42 (Pranatharthiharan *et al.*, 2017).

The restoration of tumor suppressor-microRNAs (miRNAs) is an approach that is promising for cancer therapy. But due to its poor efficiency in delivering the miRNA, its use remains unexplored. Yang *et al.* synthesized PEGylated biodegradable charged polyester-based vectors (PEG-BCPVs) as the carrier for providing miR26a and miR122 to treat HCC (Yang *et al.* 2019). Through the electrostatic interactions between positively charged PEG-BCPVs and negatively charged miRNA, the miRNA gets encapsulated in the self-assembled PEG-BCPVs nanocomplexes. TEM analysis revealed the nanocomplexes to possess a spherical morphology with a diameter of 110 nm, further supported by the DLS study, which showed a mean hydrodynamic diameter of around 120 nm. The zeta potential value was at +39 ± 5.3 mV. The nanocomplex should also possess the ability to protect the fragile miRNA molecule from getting degraded. To determine this, naked miRNA and PEG-BCPVs/miRNA were incubated respectively in an RNase-containing solution for a predetermined time, after which the loaded miRNA was completely separated from the nanocomplexes *via* sodium dodecyl sulfate (SDS). Gel electrophoresis assay was used to determine the presence of non-degraded miRNA based on the detached miRNA band brightness. The fluorescence exhibited by the naked miRNA was seen, which was significantly reduced after incubating for one h. At the same time, there was no evident degradation of miRNA encapsulated in the nanocomplex. From HepG2 cancer cell line studies, the nanocomplexes were internalized into the cells, in which miR26a and miR122 were released, resulting in a reduction in cancer cell growth migration and invasion into healthy cells while increasing cancer cell apoptosis and sensitivity towards drugs. These results indicate that PEG-BCPV/miR26a/miR122 can be an effective formulation that can aid in the inhibition of HCC.

Co-encapsulation of cisplatin (CP) and farnesol (FAR) into PLGA nanoparticles (PLGANP) to enhance the anti-cancer activity against HCC was attempted by Mondal and Khuda-Bukhsh (Mondal and Khuda-Bukhsh 2020). CP is among one of the widely accepted chemotherapeutic agents. But due to the cost of the oral administration not yielding the desired result and adverse side effects, its use is restricted. Most cancerous cells increase the efflux of CP, thereby not allowing it to reach DNA and damaging it. FAR belongs to the class isoprenoids. Isoprenoids are a class of phytochemicals that can arrest the cell cycle and cause apoptosis followed by ROS accumulation and mitochondrial degradation. Initially, studies were carried out to determine the effect of CP and FAR on the cancer cells (HepG2) and normal liver cells (WRL68). The cells were treated with varying concentrations of CP and FAR. The LD50 values obtained for CP on HepG2 and WRL68 were 20.12 μM, and 22.16 μM, respectively while for FAR, the LD50 values on HepG2 and WRL68 were 4.4 μg/mL and 11.18 μg/mL respectively. When CP and FAR were combined, the viability of HepG2 cells was reduced to 38.48% by a combination of 4 μM CP and 2.64 μg/mL FAR, which is much below the LD50%, while all other combination doses resulted in the viability above LD50%. The cytotoxicity of the drug combination was also tried on WRL68, and it was seen that 4 μM / 8 μM CP with 2.64 μg/mL FAR had negligible cytotoxicity. Based on the studies, the molar ratio of CP and FAR fixed for the formulation was 2:3. The solvent displacement method was used to prepare PLGANPs. Each drug was individually loaded into the PLGANPs, and both were combined and loaded as well, resulting in CPNPs having a particle size of 145 ± 1.5 nm while FARNPs had a particle size of 123 ± 3.1 nm, but CPFARNPs had the smallest size of 115 ± 2.5 nm. CPNP. FARNP and CPFARNP had a PDI of 0.15, 0.11, and 0.15, respectively, while maintaining a zeta potential value of -15.9 ± 2.3, -13.3 ± 4.1, and -17 ± 1.5 mV, respectively. The PLGANPs exhibited an entrapment efficiency of 78 ± 2.5% for CPNPs, 74 ± 1.4% for FARNPs and 82.7 ± 3.2% for CPFARNPs. Drug release study showed a typical biphasic release pattern. The cumulative drug release under phosphate buffer at pH 6.5 to 7.6 showed a steady increase and reached the plateau phase after 48 h with a drug release of 80% to 96.45%. The anticancer activity of the prepared formulations was tested with flow cytometric studies, and it was seen that CPFARNPs showed the greatest amount of apoptotic cell death when compared with individual drug-loaded NPs while not causing cell death in WRL68 cells, indicating that the formulation is safe to use and is effective. It is concluded that the encapsulated formulation is effective in the case of HCC treatment however needs further testing with cancer in animal models to establish its full potential thoroughly.

Cao *et al.* developed self-assembled sorafenib and curcumin nanoparticles (SCN) to manage HCC (Cao *et al.*, 2015). Sorafenib is an oral multiple kinase inhibitor that is being used in the management of patients with HCC at advanced stages as it is the only approved for molecular targeting medicine for advanced-stage HCC. But due to the low tumor response rate during the clinical application, it is only beneficial for about 30% of patients. PEG derivative of vitamin E succinate (PEG-VES) with alkyl chains and lipophilic phenyl groups is used in the self-assembly and simultaneous delivery of sorafenib and curcumin. SCN self-assembly was aided by the intermolecular hydrophobic interactions existing among lipophilic groups of the drugs and complementary groups in the hydrophobic regions of the amphiphilic PEG-VES. TEM study revealed the morphology of the SCN being uniformly spherical, and from DLS, a particle size of 84.97 ± 6.03 nm with a PDI of 0.176 ± 0.034 was seen. SCN had an encapsulation efficiency of 98.16 ± 0.23% and 91.66 ± 0.53% for sorafenib and curcumin, respectively, while the drug loading efficiency was 6.54 ± 0.01% and 13.58 ± 0.07% respectively for sorafenib and curcumin. Cell apoptosis and *in vitro* antiproliferation study have revealed that the prepared formulation exhibited a dual inhibitory action on the proliferation of cells and tumor angiogenesis, SCN showed an IC_{50} value of 2.34 μM and 8.14 μM for sorafenib and curcumin respectively on BEL-7402 cells, which was 17.8% and 16.2% than that of free sorafenib and curcumin respectively. Whereas in HepG2 cells, SCN showed an IC_{50} value of 3.3 μM and 11.67 μM for sorafenib and curcumin, respectively, which was 38.7% and 52.8% than that from the free sorafenib and curcumin. *In vivo* tissue distribution studies were performed in Balb'c nude mice, and it was seen that the sorafenib concentration from SCN in organs like liver, kidney, and lungs was significantly decreased by 3.48, 3.86, and 3.88 times when compared with the free drug suspension. Particularly in tumor tissues, a significant increase in sorafenib and curcumin concentration was seen, which was 4.23 and 5.85 times greater than that of free drug suspension. Inhibition of tumor growth studies was carried out in BEL-7402 induced tumor graft xenograft models. The SCN treatment group had a 78.8% reduction in tumor growth, 6.0 and 1.5 folds greater than curcumin and sorafenib free-drug solutions. Therefore, it is concluded that the codelivery platform designed can act as a promising platform for anti-cancer agents.

Galactose-modified selenium nanoparticles (GA-SeNPs) loaded with doxorubicin (DOX) for HCC was attempted by Xia *et al.* (Xia *et al.*, 2019). The poor water solubility of DOX and its off-target side effects have limited the use of DOX, which otherwise is an excellent candidate for the management of HCC. Selenium involves in multiple physiological functions and plays an important role in the prevention of cancer. So using it, to design a drug carrier will give an added advantage. Galactose is used to aid the drug carrier in actively targeting HCC. HCC cells have on their surface an overly expressed ASGPR, and these receptors can recognize galactose terminated glycoproteins and glycoconjugates. The prepared SeNPs and GA-DOX-SeNPs had a particle size of 91.3 nm and 95 nm, respectively. From TEM, it was seen that SeNPs had a uniform spherical shape with a diameter in the range of 90 nm and exhibited a tendency to aggregate, but when anchored with GA and loaded with DOX, the drug carrier then showed monodispersed spherical particles in size range of 50 – 150 nm. In order to determine the cellular uptake of the prepared formulation, HepG2 cells were incubated with free DOX, Se-DOX, and GA-DOX-SeNPs for 6 h and then analyzed *via* flow cytometry. Cells, when incubated with GA-DOX-SeNPs, showed greater fluorescence intensity when compared with free DOX and Se-DOX, indicating that better cellular uptake of GA-SeNPs was seen. *In vitro* drug release was carried out in two different pH conditions (pH 5.4 and 7.4) to mimic the cancer cell environment and typical physiological environment. DOX release from the drug carrier in both pH values showed an initial burst release for up to 4 h. GA-DOX-SeNPs released DOX faster in the acidic environment by releasing up to 80.7% for 30 h.

In contrast, the drug release rate in a normal environment was only 49.1%. The acidic environment caused faster drug release, which can be due to the reduction in negative charge on the surface of the drug carrier, which weakened the electrostatic interaction between DOX and the polymer and helped release it from GA-SeNPs. This type of drug release can ensure that the drug carrier will not release the drug in the normal environment but releases the required amount of drug in an acidic or cancerous environment. The cytotoxic ability of the DOX formulation was checked by performing an MTT assay on HepG2 cells. It was seen that at a dose of 8 μg/mL free DOX, DOX-SeNPs and GA-DOX-SeNPs suppressed the proliferation of HepG2 cells with cell viability rates being at 71.4%, 61.3%, and 40.8%, respectively, which indicates that GA-SeNPs might have improved the cellular uptake leading to greater cell toxicity when compared with free DOX and DOX-SeNPs. *In vivo* anti-tumor efficacy studies were carried out in Balb/c nude mice, and a xenograft mouse model was developed by injecting HepG2 cells in saline into the abdomen of mice subcutaneously. After induction of tumors, the mice were divided into groups and treated with GA-DOX-SeNPs, DOX-SeNPs, free DOX, and normal saline. It was seen that when compared with the saline treatment group, free DOX treated group, DOX-SeNPs treatment group, and GA-DOX-SeNPs treatment group, the GA-DOX-SeNPs treated group exhibited significant tumor suppression.

Galactosylated nanostructured lipid carriers (NLCs) were prepared for the delivery of 5-fluorouracil (5-FU) by Varshosaz *et al.* (Varshosaz *et al.* 2012). 5-FU is an anticancer agent that is used in the management of various types of cancer. But due to the issues such as short plasma half-life, improper GI absorption, and resistance development by tumor cells, its use is limited. The NLCs are prepared using a galactosylated lipid and stearyl amine to act as an attachment point for the galactose. This galactose is used to target the ASGPR on HCC. NLCs were prepared by emulsification -solvent diffusion method and had a particle size ranging between 135.7 nm and 187.7 nm with zeta potential between -26.4 mV and -4 mV. Drug loading efficiency ranged between 8.4 and 44.6%. It was clear that the NLCs exhibited a typical initial burst release followed by a more prolonged release phase. SEM analysis revealed a spherical morphology for the NLCs. The MTT assay showed that the prepared formulation increased the mortality of HepG2 cells, and flow cytometry data showed that drug-loaded NLCs showed significant cell uptake.

Pandey *et al.* explored the nano-antioxidant therapy for the treatment of HCC using PLGA nanoparticles loaded with rutin (RT) (Pandey *et al.*, 2018). RT is a natural flavonoid distributed widely in medicinal plants and herbs and possesses anticancer properties and antioxidant and anti-inflammatory properties. RT-loaded PLGA NPs (RT-PLGA-NPs) were prepared by the double emulsion-evaporation method. The optimized RT-PLGA-NPs had a particle size of 211 nm with a PDI of 0.24 and a zeta potential ranging between – 21.3 and – 22.8 mV. SEM and TEM analysis revealed that the prepared RT-PLGA-NPs had spherical morphology. Optimized RT-PLGA-NPs showed a 6.39 ± 0.16% drug loading capacity and an entrapment efficiency of 77.83 ± 1.77%. From *In vitro* drug release studies, it was seen that until a time of 4 h, the drug carrier exhibited a burst release, after which sustained release was attained. A total of 71% of the drug was released in 48 h. *In vivo* animal studies were carried out in male *Wistar* rats. The disease was induced with the injection of DEN. The animals were divided into 6 groups: group 1 was normal control, group 2 was administered with pure RT, group 3 was disease control, group 4 was treated with pure RT at 5 mg/kg body weight, group 5 was treated with pure RT at 100mg/kg body weight, and group 6 was treated with RT-PLGA-NPs at 5mg/kg body weight. The animals which received no DEN possessed a normal liver, while the animals in the disease control group had to have a liver with white nodules on the different lobes of the liver, which is indicative of the development of liver cancer. Group 4 and 5 showed a marked reduction in nodules on the liver and resisted decolorization of the liver. Meanwhile, group 6 showed a complete absence of nodules on the liver. The total number of nodules in the disease control group was 169, and group 4 had 115 nodules, while group 5 had 78 nodules and group 6 had 39 nodules. Histopathological analysis revealed that the disease control group had prominent carcinogenic indications like nuclei enlargement associated with bile duct hyperplasia and widespread hepatic stellate cells in the portal and necrotic, inflammatory cells, and proliferative cells. RT-PLGA-NPs showed less deviation from normal control histopathological findings with less to no necrotic and inflammatory cells. The studies show that the prepared formulation managed HCC, and with further studies and exploration into detailed mechanisms, a better understanding can be attained.

Most currently available anti-cancer agents are poorly water-soluble while requiring oral administration, which will lead to low bioavailability and cause side effects. Wang *et al.* attempted to engineer an injectable polymeric nanoparticle (PN) drug carrier loaded with a multitargeted kinase inhibitor, vandetanib (Van). Biodegradable block copolymer poly (ethylene glycol)-block-poly(D, L lactic acid) (PEG-PLA) was used to nanoprecipitate Van-loaded PN into water-soluble moieties (Wang *et al.* 2016). The drug-loaded nanocarrier (Van-NPs) were prepared by the nanoprecipitation method, and iRGD anchored copolymer was added into the nanocarrier solution to form iRGD anchored nanoparticles (iVan-NPs). Van-NPs had a size of 39.6 ± 1.2 nm, and the size of iVan-NPs was 39.8 ± 0.5 nm. TEM analysis revealed that the prepared formulation was monodispersed with spherical morphology. Drug encapsulation and drug loading were determined for Van-NPs and iVan-NPs, with drug encapsulation values being

83.4 ± 1.1% and 91.0 ± 0.8%, respectively, while percentage drug loading being 3.9 and 4.3 for Van-NPs and iVan-NPs respectively. *In vitro* drug release studies were carried out in two pH conditions at 7.4 and 4.6. The prepared NPs released close to 80% of Van within 8 h in both pH conditions. A cell viability study was carried out using cell counting kit-8 (CCK-8), and the extent of apoptosis was measured by flow cytometry. The cell lines used were BEL-7402, HuH-7, HCC-LM3, and SK-Hep-1. A significant decrease in cell viability was seen when treated with Van-NPs and iVan-NPs for 48 h, and this is possible when there is an efficient release of the drug from the drug carrier, which causes cell apoptosis and inhibits cell proliferation. Labelling NPs with Cy3 fluorescent dye enabled visualization of the internalization of NPs. It was evident from confocal laser scanning microscopy that a significant amount of NPs had been internalized into cells. *In vivo* antitumor efficacy was evaluated on Balb/c nude mice in which subcutaneous injection of BEL-7402 cells into right flanks induced tumors. It was seen that NPs delivering a dose of 20 mg/kg body weight Van was more efficient in reducing tumor growth than those delivering a dose of 30 mg/kg body weight orally administered. The functionalization with iRGD aided in enhanced antitumor action by inhibiting tumor growth by 60%. It can be concluded that the formulated injectable nanomedicine had promising potential to be used in the management of HCC. However, safety and efficacy studies are required to perform in a larger number of animals.

Etoposide (ETO), a potent cytotoxic drug that inhibits topoisomerase II during the cell cycle, is widely used in the case of lung and testicular cancer, off late it is being tested against HCC but is showing poor therapeutic action at around 4-15%, this poor performance can be attributed to the resistance mechanisms exhibited by the cancer cells. Tsend-Ayush *et al.* developed a targeted drug delivery system to explore the untapped potential of ETO with D-α-Tocopheryl polyethylene glycol 1000 succinate (TPGS) conjugated with lactobionic acid (TPGS-LA) nanoparticle to actively seek ASGPR, which is overexpressed on the HCC and by the enhanced permeation and retention effect (EPR) gains access into the cells and released ETO to show its action (Tsend-Ayush *et al.* 2017). ETO-loaded TPGS-LA NPs were prepared by the nanoprecipitation method. DLS determined the particle size and size distribution of NPs. Blank NPs showed a particle size of 198.66 ± 7.86 nm while ETO-TGPS-LA NPs showed a particle size of 141.43 ± 6.67 nm with PDI measuring around 0.287 ± 0.064 and 0.142 ± 0.017 for blank NP and ETO-TPGS-LA NPs, respectively. The possible reason for reduced size while drug loading can be attributed to the hydrophobic interactions between ETO and hydrophobic regions on TPGS-LA. The zeta potential of blank NPs and ETO-TPGS-LA NPs was found to be 14.5 ± 4.75 and 16.01 ± 5.02 mV, respectively. It is beneficial to have a positive zeta potential because these regions of the NP can actively interact with the anionic regions of ASGPR, and negatively charged particles are easily recognized by the Kupffer cells of the liver, which rapidly remove these molecules from blood circulation. TEM analysis revealed the NPs to be monodispersed and spherical in morphology. Drug encapsulation efficiency and drug loading content were determined to be 90.99 ± 0.12% and 13.06 ± 1.3%, respectively. The nanoprecipitation method adopted for the fabrication of the NPs is known to yield smaller particles with greater encapsulation efficiency. *In vitro* drug release studies were performed in two pH conditions to simulate a blood neutral environment at pH 7.4 and an acidic cancerous environment at pH 5.8. By the end of 24 h, ETO-TPGS-LA NPs showed an initial burst release at pH 7.4 (20% drug release), while at pH 5.8, 32% drug release was seen. It can be identified that the drug release from the NPs in an acidic environment is greater than the drug release in a neutral environment. It can be due to the hydrolyzation of the ester bond of TPGS in acidic conditions selectively. After the initial 24 h, the NPs showed a sustained drug release pattern. *In vitro* cytotoxicity study was carried out using HepG2 cells, which were incubated for 24 h with free-ETO, ETO-TPGS-LA NPs, and ETO-TPGS NPs. The results indicated dose-dependent cytotoxicity of ETO. It was noticed that ETO and ETO-TPGS NPs showed no significant difference in the viability of cells. This can be due to the lack of active targeting, which impacts the cell internalization of the drug. The lowest cell viability was observed in ETO-TPGS-LA NPs, which can be attributed to targeting the overexpressed ASPGR on the cell surface, which facilitates the cellular uptake where in ETO released, which showed its action. To determine the extent of cellular uptake, the formulation was encapsulated with C6, a fluorescent molecule, and the labeled formulation was incubated with HepG2 cells and observed under a fluorescence microscope. Deep green fluorescence from the cytoplasm of the HepG2 cells indicated that the C6 encapsulated NPs localized into the cells. The fluorescence intensity increased with an increase in incubation time, which indicates that the cellular uptake of the NPs is directly dependent on the incubation time. While at equal incubation time, the fluorescence intensity from TPGS-LA NPs was more than TPGS NPs, which can be attributed to the receptor-mediated endocytosis through the galactose moiety and ASGPR on HepG2 cells. *In vivo* tumor targeting studies were carried out in Balb/c xenograft-bearing mice. Free-DiR, DiR loaded TPGS-LA NPs, and DiR loaded TPGS NPs were IV administered *via* the tail vein. The animals were monitored using non-invasive near IR optical imaging at various time intervals post-injection. Fluorescence was not observed at the subcutaneous tumor region in the free DiR group, while the NPs groups revealed greater aggregation. When compared between DiR-TPGS-LA NPs and DiR-TPGS NPs, the former showed stronger fluorescence intensity at all time points, with 24 h being the highest intensity. This can be attributed to its ability to target and the EPR nature of the TPGS-LA NPs. Tissue biodistribution was also evaluated, which showed a strong fluorescence intensity in the liver with weaker intensity in the brain, heart, kidney, spleen, and lung upon DiR-TPGS-LA NPs treatments. *In vivo* antitumor efficacy studies showed a significant reduction in tumor volume in all treatment groups when compared with the disease control group. Between free ETO and TPGS loaded ETO NPs, no significant difference in the tumor volume was seen, while ETO-TPGS-LA NPs showed a prominent reduction in tumor volume. The tumor inhibition rates of different treatment groups were checked, and it was seen that the ETO-TPGS-LA NPs treatment group showed the highest inhibition rate at 72.89%, followed by ETO-TPGS NPs at 28.3%, and the least inhibition was seen-in free ETO treatment group at 18.68%. It can be concluded that the prepared formulation is effective in the management of HCC and can be further explored in the treatment of HCC.

Multilayer coated liquid crystalline nanoparticles (LCN) loaded with sorafenib (SOR) for the treatment of HCC was developed by Thapa *et al.* (Thapa *et al.*, 2015). In order to overcome the LCNs drawback of binding to the non-target site due to the bioadhesive property and to overcome rapid elimination from blood circulation, the LNCs were polymer coated with layers of poly-*l*-lysine (PLL) and polyethylene glycol-*b*-polyaspartic acid (PEG-*b*-PAsp). PEGylated drug carriers are known to have benefits like targeted delivery and remain stealthy not to trigger an immune response. The layers of polymer coating will aid in controlling the delivery of the drug. SOR-LCN was prepared by the melting evaporation and sonication method. This was then used to do a layer-by-layer (LbL) polymer coating to form LbL-SOR-LCN. The particle size of the prepared drug-loaded LCN was checked using DLS, while AFM and TEM were employed to better understand the morphology. SOR-LCN showed a particle size of 150.5 ± 0.9 nm with a height of 12.9 ± 3.8 nm in AFM. The change in particle size and height was checked when polymeric layer coating was started. At 2 layers, the size of LbL-SOR-LCN was 154.4 ± 1.0 nm with a height of 16.1 ± 0.2 nm, at 4 layers, the size was 155.1 ± 1.2 nm, and height was 20.1 ± 3.3 nm, and at 6 layers, the size was 160.2 ± 1.1 nm, and height was 24.3 ± 2.2 nm. At low magnification, TEM images revealed cubosomes-like structure. After polymer layers addition, less staining around the LCN was observed, suggesting the polymeric layers' deposition around the LCN. A slight increase in particle diameter was seen, which was reflected in the DLS also. At the optimized conditions, encapsulation efficiency and drug loading were found to be 100% and 2.5%, respectively. *In vitro* drug release studies were carried out in two different pH levels, at pH 7.4 and pH 5.5 for SOR-LCN and LbL-SOR-LCN. In the first 2 h, a burst release was seen with both the formulations. It was followed by a sustained drug release pattern for 48 h. LbL-SOR-LCN showed lesser drug release when compared with SOR-LCN at pH 7.4. This reduced drug release may be due to layers around the LCN that retarded the drug release. The exact opposite observation was noted at acidic pH, where more drugs were released from LbL-SOR-LCN than from SOR-LCN. This may be due to the disassembly of the polymer layers at pH 5.5 due to reduced ionization potential and charge density. Release of SOR from SOR-LCN and LbL-SOR-LCN was greater at pH 5.5 when compared with release at pH 7.4. This can be due to SOR having better solubility in acidic conditions and the occurrence of phase inversion of LCN. *In vitro* cytotoxicity studies were carried out in HepG2 cells for free-SOR, LbL-LCN, LbL-SOR-LCN. Dose-dependent cytotoxicity was seen for free-SOR and LbL-SOR-LCN, while LbL-LCN exhibited minimal cytotoxicity. The IC_{50} values for free-SOR at 24 h, 48 h, and 72 h incubation were found to be >100 μM, 48.30 μM, and 24.58 μM respectively while the same for LbL-SOR-LCN were 27.82 μM, 13.80 μM, and 7.87 μM respectively. To identify intracellular uptake, LCN and LbL-LCN were loaded with coumarin-6. It was seen from confocal microscopy that a time-dependent uptake of LbL-LCN by the HepG2 cells and more intense fluorescence was identified for LbL-LCN compared with LCN. It was concluded that the prepared drug carrier was effective in delivering the drug to HCC. Further investigation is, however, necessary to identify its potential in animals.

In order to improve bioavailability, Chen *et al.* formulated polymeric nanoformulations of sorafenib (SOR) in the management of HCC (Chen *et al.* 2020b). Clinically safe poly(ethylene glycol)-*b*-poly(lactic acid) (PEG-*b*-PLA) was used in the fabrication of the nanoparticle (NP). SOR-loaded NP was prepared by the single emulsion method. The size of blank NP and SOR-NP was analyzed using DLS. It was seen that the size of SOR-NP was smaller than that of blank NP, at 94.7 ± 0.3 nm and 134.5 ± 4.6 nm, respectively. TEM analysis revealed that the prepared NP had spherical morphology and a mean diameter of around 70 nm. The zeta potential of blank NP was around -3 mV, while drug loading into NP made the zeta potential value -1 mV. The drug loading and encapsulation efficiency of SOR-NP were 8.4 ± 1.1% and 82.6 ± 2.6%, respectively. *In vitro* drug release studies were carried out at 3 different pH conditions: pH 7.4, pH 6.8, and pH 5.5. It was seen that the drug release was prolonged for a time duration of 72 h across all three pH values, and a lower pH value facilitated the release of a slightly more amount of drug. This is beneficial as the tumor environment is mostly acidic while the rest of the physiological pH is centered around neutral value. To determine the cellular uptake of the prepared NPs a hydrophobic fluorescent dye was encapsulated into the NP (NP-DiD) by the nanoprecipitation method. Cell uptake studies were carried out on three different cell lines, which were Hepal-6 and H22 (mouse cell lines) and HepG2. Confocal microscopy and flow cytometry were used to understand the cellular uptake mechanism of NP-DiD. Granular red fluorescence was observed around tumor nuclei, which represented NP-DiD uptake by all three cell types. There was a linear relationship between the duration of incubation and the degree of cellular uptake. The mean fluorescence intensity of NP-DiD at 6 h was 100 and 176.6 times greater than what was observed at 0.5 h for HepG2 and Hepal-6, respectively. Similarly, *In vitro* cytotoxicity study and apoptotic effect of SOR-NP on cell lines were determined by MTT assay after incubation for a duration of 24 or 48 h. It was seen that free-SOR and SOR-NP could inhibit the growth of Hepal-6, H22, and HepG2 cells in a drug-concentration-dependent manner. The IC_{50} value for SOR-NP on HepG2 was 10.26 μM, while for Hepal-6, it was 9.99 μM, and the value was 32.96 μM for H22. *The in vivo* antitumor study was carried out in Balb/c and C57BL/6 mice, H22 tumor model was developed in Balb/c mice by subcutaneous injection of H22 cells into the right-back of the animal, while Hepal-6 tumor model was developed in C57BL/6 mice by injecting Hepal-6 cells subcutaneously into the right-back of the animals. The animals were divided into groups; one group was administered with 10 mg/kg body weight while the other was received 30 mg/kg body weight of free-SOR. SOR-NP was administered to a group at a dose of 10 mg/kg body weight. For the H22 tumor model, it was seen that 10 mg/kg free-SOR slightly inhibited the growth of the tumor with statistically significant inhibition in rate of growth between 10 mg/kg free-SOR and SOR-NP, But no statistical significance was seen between 30 mg/kg body weight of free SOR and SOR-NP. The average weight of tumors in SOR-NP was about 54.9% of free-SOR at 10 mg/kg body weight dose. In the case of the Hepal-6 tumor model, when compared with free-SOR, there was a significant inhibition to tumor growth in the SOR-NP treatment group. It can be summarised that the formulated NPs may be useful in the management of HCC. However, further studies are required.

Superparamagnetic iron oxide nanoparticles (SPIONs) were prepared, which were loaded with sorafenib (SOR) for targeted drug delivery to HCC by Tom *et al.* (Tom *et al.*, 2018). SPIONs loaded with SOR were prepared by co-precipitation method to attain iron oxide nanoparticles which are then coated with PVA. Upon analyzing the particle size, it was seen to lie between 5 nm to 15 nm, and TEM analysis revealed that the iron oxide nanoparticles, after getting coated with PVA, had a roughly spherical shape. SOR-SPIONs had a drug encapsulation efficiency of around 76.37%. *In vitro* drug release studies were carried out in pH 7.4. Up to 8 h, SOR was released rapidly (nearly 30%), and then the release was gradually sustained for up to 80 h, wherein almost 66.7% of the drug was released. A cellular uptake study was performed with HepG2 cells, which were incubated with SOR-SPIONs for various time intervals. The cells were then stained with Prussian blue, which is the histology-specific stain for iron. The internalization of SOR was evident by blue dots in the cytoplasm of the incubated cells compared with control cells with no incubation with SOR-SPIONs. *In vitro* cytotoxicity study was carried out by performing an MTT assay. A significant increase in cytotoxicity, which was proportional to the time of incubation and concentration of SOR, was seen when the cells were incubated with free-SOR and SOR-SPIONs. Cells that were incubated with blank SPION were viable along with the cells treated with control and DMSO. The formulation showed an IC_{50} value of 8 μM. By analyzing the intracellular autophagic markers, an estimation of the ability of SOR-SPIONs to cause autophagy of HCC can be understood. Immunofluorescence was used to determine the presence of protein LC3 II. Control cells showed minimal green fluorescence, while LC3 II was indicated in cells treated with SOR-SPIONs. The study concludes that the use of SPION to deliver anti-cancer agents can be a potentially fruitful area for targeted cancer therapy. The location of the magnetic nanoparticles loaded with the drug can be controlled *via* an external magnetic source.

In another study by Depalo *et al.*, a similar attempt was made where SOR - SPIONs were further encapsulated in PEG-modified phospholipid micelles (Depalo *et al.*, 2017). SOR-SPIONs were co-dissolved in chloroform along with PEG. The rapid evaporation of the solvent in a rotatory flask evaporator with 2 mL of phosphate buffer solution at pH 7.4 was introduced, and this mixture was rapidly heated and cooled. It led to the formation of micelles, which are encapsulated SOR-SPION. Depending on the weight of SPION used in the formulation of micelles, a total of 4 types of samples were prepared, with sample 1 being 16%, 2 being 20%, while 3 being 24%, and sample 4 with 28%. Morphological and structural examinations were carried out using DLS and TEM. DLS analysis showed that Sample 1, 2, and 3 existed in a monomodal size distribution where all the dispersed particles were within the same size range and had an average particle size of 48 nm, 50 nm, and 63 nm, respectively, while sample 4 exhibited a bimodal size distribution with the coexistence of smaller and larger particles with size averaging at 51 nm and 212 nm. The drug-loaded SPION micelles had a particle size of 125 nm with monomodal size distribution and possessed a zeta potential -25 ± 2 mV upon drug loading. *In vitro* cytotoxicity assay was performed on HepG2 HCC cells, and MTT assay helped determine cell viability. An IC_{50} value of 58.8 ± 0.2 μg/mL was seen for blank SPION micelles, which indicates that innately these drug carriers did not have any cytotoxicity. While incubating with drug-loaded SPION micelles, it was seen that as the concentration of the drug increased, the cytotoxicity ability of the system also increased. At SOR concentration 22.38 μg/mL, the observed IC_{50} value was 3.20 ± 0.6 μg/mL. The cellular uptake study in the presence of a magnetic field was performed to understand the extent of the effect of the magnetic field. Two separate magnets of different shapes, with one magnet being ring-shaped and the other being square with the same magnetic induction value, were selected to identify which shape would be optimal. HepG2 cells were incubated for a duration of 4 h and 24 h, and cellular uptake happening with and without magnetic field was also checked. Results indicated that exposure to magnetic field strongly increased SIPON micelle uptake, as checked on optical microscopy with the samples stained with Prussian blue. The ring-shaped magnet showed better uptake when compared with the square magnet. The study concluded that the prepared magnetic drug carrier showed good potential for being used in delivering the anti-cancer agent to the cancer site with the aid of an external magnetic field. Further exploration with animal studies can greatly substantiate the findings of this study.

Lipid nanoparticles (LNPs) loaded with doxorubicin (DOX) and sorafenib (SOR) were designed for synergistic targeted therapy for the management of HCC as explored by Duan and Liu (Duan and Liu 2018). In order to overcome the challenges associated with DOX, a prodrug form of the drug was synthesized. N-acetylgalactosamine modified pH selective DOX (NAcGal-DOX) prodrug due to galactose moiety can actively target the HCC, and the selectivity to pH helps in rapid drug release at sites with acidic pH. NAcGal-DOX and SOR-loaded LNPs (NAc-Gal-DOX/SOR LNPs) were synthesized by the single-step nanoprecipitation method. NAc-Gal-DOX/SOR LNPs had a particle size of 121.2 ± 3.5 nm with a zeta potential of -37.4 ± 3.6 mV, and the size and zeta potential of DOX/SOR LNPs were 102.3 ± 2.9 nm and -24.1 ± 2.9 mV. While the size and zeta potential of NAc-Gal-DOX/SOR LNPs and NAc-Gal-DOX LNPs were almost the same, with the latter having a size and zeta potential of 120.8 ± 3.2 nm and -35.9 ± 3.2 mV, respectively. The LNPs with the least particle size was (SOR LNPs), and particle size of blank LNPs was 100.9 ± 2.7 nm and 101.3 ± 2.5 nm, respectively, with a zeta potential of -23.6 ± 3.1 mV and -22.1 ± 2.5 mV, respectively. Drug content, as well as drug loading efficiency, was evaluated for the prepared LNPs, NAc-Gal-DOX/SOR LNPs and DOX/SOR LNPs had drug (DOX) content of 80.7 ± 2.9% and 82.2 ± 3.1% respectively while having SOR of 83.2 ± 3.3% and 82.2 ± 3.1 respectively. For drug loading efficiency, NAc-Ga--DOX/SOR LNPs and DOX/SOR LNPs showed 5.6 ± 0.5% and 7.8 ± 0.8 respectively for DOX and 4.1 ± 0.4% and 6.3 ± 0.6% for SOR respectively. The *In vitro* drug release studies were carried out in two different pH conditions. It was seen that the release of SOR was not influenced by the pH whereas, from NAc-Gal-DOX/SOR LNPs, the amount of DOX released at 36 h was over 80% at pH 5.5, but in neutral pH condition, it took 48 h to release 80% DOX. In HepG2 cellular uptake studies, cells were incubated for a duration of 1h, 3h, 6h, and 9h, and at each time point, the NAc-Gal-DOX/SOR LNPs and NAc-Gal-DOX LNPs gained greater access into the cells, and after 9 h, over 70% of cell uptake was recorded by NAc-Gal-DOX/SOR LNPs. Similar results were seen from the flow cytometry studies as well. Cytotoxicity studies were carried out in HepG2 and HuH7 cells. Significant inhibitory action was seen for NAcGal modified LNPs among all the formulations. DOX-and SOR-loaded LNPs showed better cytotoxic action than the individual drug-loaded LNPs. To identify the ideal ratio of DOX:

SOR concentrations for the optimal synergistic action, synergistic *In vitro* studies were carried out. Based on IC_{50} values, the CI_{50} values were calculated. When the ratio of DOX: SOR was maintained between 10:1 and 1:1, it exhibited a synergistic effect. Ratio 2:1 for DOX: SOR showed the highest synergistic action. *In vivo* tissue distribution studies were carried out in HCC bearing mice model, and 48 h post-administration of LNPs NAc-Gal-DOX/SOR LNPs showed greater DOX and SOR distributions in tumor tissue when compared with DOX/SOR LNPs. Post 2 h of administration, free-DOX and SOR were found to be highly accumulated in the heart and kidney than what was observed for LNP formulations. The antitumor effect of LNPs was checked in HCC bearing Balb/c mice of all groups. Best tumor growth inhibition of 86.9 ± 3.8% was exhibited by the group which received NAc-Gal-DOX/SOR LNPs, which was most potent, while the free drug exhibited a tumor inhibition ratio of 17.1 ± 0.9% for SOR. DOX free-drug had a tumor inhibition of 30.6 ± 1.8%. NAc-Gal-DOX/SOR LNPs and DOX/SOR LNPs had 72.5 ± 3.9% and 63.7 ± 3.2% of tumor inhibition, respectively. It can be summarised that the NAcGal modified pH selective LNPs effectively delivered the drug at the desired region (tumor) while showing promising tumor inhibition. Further studies can lead to this platform being a promising strategy for the delivery of anticancer agents.

Dendrimers

Dendrimers are extensively branched polymeric nanostructured macromolecules known for their well-defined structure and versatile drug delivery properties. They have three standard components, the central core, an internal dendritic structure which is also known as the branches, and an external surface that various groups can functionalize. The name dendrimers come from a Greek word that means tree. Dendrimers directed to ASGPR loaded with curcumin derivative to combat HCC was formulated by Yousef *et al.* Among a few selective ligands which are employed in the targeting of ASGPR, which is overexpressed in HCC is galactosamine (Gal) (Yousef *et al.* 2018). Potent anti-cancer curcumin derivative (CDR) was loaded into polyamidoamine (PAMAM) dendrimers. In order to facilitate targeting specifically to the cancerous cells, the PAMAM dendrimers were anchored with GAL. GAL molecules were attached to the PAMAM *via* a succinic acid linker moiety, after which GAL was introduced, which bound to the free end of succinic acid. CDR was loaded into the dendrimer *via* the equilibrium dialysis method. The amount of drug-loaded into PAMAM-GAL was higher than that loaded into PAMAM, and the drug release was 17.7 ± 5.43% and 13.5 ± 3.70%, respectively. A similar increase was noticed in encapsulation efficiency. PAMAM-GAL showed an encapsulation efficiency of 85 ± 9.8%, while PAMAM showed a value of 75.5 ± 12%. From particle size and zeta potential analysis, it was seen that PAMAM-GAL had a diameter of 48.7 ± 7.03 nm with a zeta potential of -8.3 ± 1.24 mV, while PAMAM had a smaller diameter of 9.97 ± 3.76 nm with a positive zeta potential of 13 ± 3.23 mV. The positive zeta potential can be attributed to the presence of a terminal protonated amine group. Simultaneously, GAL anchored PAMAM had a negative zeta potential because of anionic uncoupled succinic carboxylic groups. TEM analysis was carried out in the dry state. The drug carriers exhibited a spherical morphology, with PAMAM having a size of around 4 nm, while PAMAM-GAL showed a size around 21 nm. MTT assay was carried out to determine the *In vitro* cytotoxicity of CDR along with doxorubicin (DOX), sorafenib (SOR), and cisplatin (CIS) on HCC cell line HepG2. The order of cytotoxicity potential after 48 h was determined, which was CDR> SOR> DOX> CIS with an IC_{50} value of 4 μM, 8 μM, 12 μM, and 22 μM, respectively. The ability of CDR-loaded PAMAM and PAPAM-GAL to showcase their anticancer potential was also tested on ASGPR overexpressed cells *via* MTT assay. CDR-PAMAM-GAL showed an IC_{50} value of 1 ± 0.3 μM, while CDR-PAMAM and CDR showed an IC_{50} value of 2 ± 0.01 μM and 4 ± 0.2 μM, respectively. Rhodamine-B-loaded formulations were prepared to determine cellular uptake, and treated cells were observed under a fluorescence microscope. Higher uptake was seen for PAMAM-GAL-Rhodamine-B, owing to their ASGPR targetability. *In vivo* imaging and biodistribution studies were carried out in 6 – 8 week old female nu/nu mice. Clinically used high contrast structurally symmetrical dye S0456 was conjugated to PAMAM-GAL to form PAMAM-GAL-S0456. Subcutaneous injection of HepG2 human HCC cells led to the formation of a tumor, after which PAMAM-GAL-S0456 was injected, and whole-body imaging was done. It was clear that GAL conjugated PAMAM was distributed predominantly over ASGPR overexpressed HepG2 tumor while PAMAM without GAL showed low tumor uptake. The excretion of the imaging agent was facilitated *via* kidneys, which reduced toxicity. Hence, CDR-PAMA--GAL can act as potential anticancer nanoparticles and aid in imaging. Further investigations are required to translate into humans.

Solid Lipid Nanoparticles

Solid lipid nanoparticles, also known as lipid nanoparticles, are novel pharmaceutical drug delivery systems composed of a phospholipid layer and a solid lipid core. This core is suitable for accommodating lipophilic substances. They are generally spherical and have a diameter in the range of 10 to 1000 nm. Rahman *et al*. formulated diosmin-loaded solid lipid nanoparticles (SLN) to enhance the therapeutic effect on HCC (Rahman *et al.* 2020). Diosmin (Dio) is a flavonoid with various biological properties such as antioxidant, antiviral and anticancer. Despite being a good candidate for managing HCC, Dio is poorly explored due to its biopharmaceutical challenges. Dio-SLNs were prepared by hot homogenization process, Quality by design (QbD) was implemented to yield the best possible formulation. The optimized and prepared Dio-SLNs showed a particle size of 37.48 nm with an entrapment efficiency and drug loading at a range of 61 to 82% and 8.5 to 10%, respectively. The drug carrier exhibited a biphasic drug release mechanism. An initial burst release was seen, which lasted for 6 h, and 100% drug release by 8 h whereas, the Dio drug solution showed only 80% drug release by the end of 25 h. *In vitro* cytotoxicity studies were carried on HepG2 cells. Treatment was carried out with Dio drug solution, Dio-SLN, and plain SLN. The observed IC_{50} values were 38.21 μg/mL for Dio solution at the end of 24 h, while Dio-SLN showed an IC_{50} value of 31.01 μg/mL at the end of 24 h. These values were changed to 33.11 μg/mL and 22.01 μg/mL, respectively, by the end of 48 h. *In vivo* animal studies were carried out in male *Wistar* rats. Cancer was induced by administering an intraperitoneal injection of diethylnitrosamine (Den). The administration of Dio-SLNs facilitated a significant reduction of hepatic nodules compared with the Dio solution and disease control group. Also, the size of the nodules was decreased significantly in the group which received Dio-SLN. It was concluded that Dio-SLNs hold a good potential for managing HCC induced *via* Den. But further studies and testing are essential to confirm the findings of this study.

Tunki *et al.* developed sugar grafted solid lipid nanoparticles (SLNs) loaded with sorafenib (SOR) for the treatment of HCC (Tunki *et al.*, 2019). SOR has poor aqueous solubility, which causes low oral bioavailability, hence low therapeutic efficiency. A ligand having affinity to C-type lectin receptor was used to enable targeting of the SLNs. ASGPR is overexpressed in HCC, and it is a C-type lectin receptor. Emulsification and solvent evaporation method was followed for the fabrication of SLNs. PEGylated galactose is used as the ligand, which enables targeting. The particle size of blank SLN (BSLN) was found to be 59.31 ± 2.99 nm, while SOR-loaded SLN (SSLN) had a particle size of 68.36 ± 3.14 nm and PEGylated galactose attached SOR loaded SLN (PGAL-SSLN) showed the largest particle size of 111.0 ± 6.99 nm. The surface attachment of PEGylated galactose increased the particle size of the SLN by almost 50 nm. The prepared formulations showed zeta potential values of -20.9 ± 1.41 mV, -20.13 ± 1.35 mV, and -19.8 ±1.11 mV for BSLN, SSLN, and PGAL-SSLN, respectively. Encapsulation efficiency did not differ much between SSLN and PGAL-SSLN and was found to be 97.0 ± 1,5% and 95.0 ± 1.8%, respectively. *In vitro* drug release studies were performed in different media such as 0.1N HCl (pH 1.2), phosphate buffer (PB) pH 6.8, sodium acetate buffer (SAB) pH 5.0, and phosphate buffer saline (PBS) at pH 7.4, representing the pH environment which the SLNs will experience post oral administration viz., stomach, the small intestine, tumor environment, and circulation fluid, respectively. Pure drug suspension showed complete release of the drug (over 95%) across all media by the end of 8th h. In comparison, SLN released SOR only up to 25 – 40% by the end of 8th h in various media, indicating that the lipid matrix aided in achieving a sustained release pattern. *In vitro* cell anti-proliferation studies were carried out in HepG2 cells to understand the cytotoxic effect of SOR, BSLN, SSLN, and PGAL-SSLN. The IC_{50} values exhibited by SSLN and PGAL-SSLN were 9.77 ± 1.47 μg/mL and 6.57 ± 0.58 μg/mL respectively, while SOR had an IC_{50} value of 9.48 ± 0.45 μg/mL. A dual staining assay was carried out using annexin V-FITC/propidium iodide to examine the extent of externalization of phosphatidylserine as a measure of the degree of cell apoptosis. HepG2 cells were incubated with SOR, SSLN, PGAL-SSLN for 48 h, and it was noticed that at 5 μg dose, the percentage of apoptosis was at 26.19, 24.48, and 33.03%, respectively, while at a dose of 10 μg, the values were 58.21, 48.56 and 63.29% respectively. In order to figure out cellular uptake, SLN and PGAL-SLN were tagged with C6. After an incubation time of 1, 2, and 4 h with HepG2 cells, the fluorescence intensity of PGAL-SLN was significantly higher than that of SLN at all-time points. This can be attributed to the targeted entry into the HepG2 cells with their overexpressed ASGPR on the cell surface. *In vivo* pharmacokinetic studies were carried out in Balb/c mice for SOR, SSLN, and PGAL-SSLN. The C_{max} obtained for SOR, SSLN and PGAL-SSLN were 6.75 ± 1.07 μg/mL, 25.22 ± 0/50 μg/mL and 28.90 ± 0.13 μg/mL respectively. SOR suspension was not quantifiable in the plasma by the end of 8th h, while the drug release from SSLN and PGAL-SSLN was quantifiable even at the end of 24 h time point. This could be due to the poor water solubility and quicker elimination of the drug from the body while the drug in SLN was protected and entered payer patches in the small intestine and remained more in blood. AUC for SSLN was 272.05 ± 30.60 μg/mL-h while PGAL-SSLN had the value 363.09 ± 32.74 μg/mL.h, which was a significant improvement when compared with SOR suspension. SOR clearance is reduced when released from SSLN and PGAL-SSLN at 7.8 folds and 18.3 folds when compared with SOR suspension. Real-time biodistribution of SLNs was observed post oral administration with the aid of an imaging system that was non-invasive employed near-infrared active die (DiR) loaded SLNs. It was seen that DiR-SLNs had a tendency to reach the lungs and lodged there while DiR-PGAL-SLNs were visualized in hepatocytes even at the end of the 24th h time point. It can be concluded that the SLNs developed with PEGylated galactose can act as an efficient carrier for SOR and show good treatment potential for HCC.

Mesoporous Silica Nanoparticles

Mesoporous silica nanoparticles (MSNs) are silicon dioxide nanoparticles that are spherical in shape with numerous pores of diameter 2 to 50 nm on the surface. Owing to the large surface area of the pores, drugs can easily be incorporated into them and used as drug delivery agents. Plain MSNs have limited permeability across the cell membrane, and many researchers have attempted to modify the surface of these carriers to gain a significant advantage. Li *et al*. designed smart nanoparticles (GPDC-MSNs) that can aggregate in a stepwise fashion within the tumor tissue; due to their ability to selectively enter cancer cells, these nanoparticles are excellent candidates for drug delivery. They can selectively gain access into the cancerous cells due to the tumor microenvironment, which is acidic in nature, and then deliver the encapsulated drug to that region (Li *et al*. 2020). GPDC-MSN comprises of galactosyl-conjugated PEO-PPO-PEO (Gal-P123) for targeting HCC, while having (2E)-4-(dioleostearin)-amino-4-car-onyl-2-butenonic (DC) for selective pH-dependent cellular entry and loaded with irinotecan (CPT-11), finally becoming an anti-tumor drug-loaded mesoporous silica nanoparticle (MSN) for intracellular drug release. The smart nanoparticle was designed to undergo multi-step delivery, with step 1 being the ability to extend circulation due to the anionic charge while targeting into HCC was facilitated by the surface galactosyls units. Once the nanoparticle reaches HCC due to the presence of DC, step 2 occurs, which is the alteration in the surface charge. While in the tumor microenvironment, a change in surface charge from negative was seen to neutral. This change facilitates cellular uptake. Once inside the cell, the acidic endolysosomes cause dissociation of the lipid layer leading to drug release. MSNs were fabricated by a base-catalyzed condensation reaction of TEOS, where templated CTAB was used. CPT-11 was loaded into the MSNs by dispersing the MSNs into a solution of CPT-11 at a 1:1 weight ratio. The solution was centrifuged to remove free CPT-11 to obtain CPT-11-loaded MSNs. CPT-loaded GPDC-MSNs were then formulated by hydration of a lipid film layer consisting of DC, PC-98t, and Gal-P123 phospholipid along with CPT-11-loaded MSNs. TEM analysis indicated that the prepared MSNs had large-sized pores with good dispersity and uniform morphology. At the same time, the SAXRD peaks and N_2 adsorption-desorption isotherms identified that the prepared MSNs have 2-dimensional hexagon-shaped mesostructures with pore size being 8 nm in diameter and 721 m^2/g as surface area. When MSN was added to GPDC, the resultant GPDC-MSNs had a particle size in the range of 70 to 90 nm with a zeta potential value of -28.2 ± 5.6 to -12.2 ± 3.5 mV. *In vitro* cellular uptake studies were carried out in Huh-7 cells which had ASGPR overexpressed and were incubated with Propidium iodide (PI) labeled GPDCMSNs, PDC-MSNs, or GP-MSNs in two different conditions to see the difference with one being simulated physiological condition where the pH will be close to neutral while the other condition being acidic tumor microenvironment. It was seen that the cellular uptake seen for GPDC-MSNs at the acidic microenvironment (pH 6.5) was significantly greater than that observed at physiological conditions (pH 7.4). In contrast, the environmental conditions impacted the internalization of GP-MSNs. Approximately 1.8 folds enhanced uptake was exhibited by GPDC-MSNs at pH 6.5 when compared with PDC-MSNs. *In vitro* drug release demonstrated that

CPT-11 was not released from GPDC-MSNs in buffer at 7.4 pH, while MSNs without the lipid layer released more than half of the drug by the end of 72 h. While in pH 5.0, GPDC-MSNs released 85% drug by the end of 24 h. MTT assay determined the cytotoxicity and cell apoptosis potentials of the prepared formulations. Different formulations were incubated in Huh-7 cells for different periods, and the IC_{50} value was calculated. Drug-loaded nanoparticles had a better IC_{50} value than that of free-drug, and incubating with GPDC-MSNs showed significant enhancement in the cytotoxicity by 19.5 times at pH 6.5. *In vivo* pharmacokinetics and tumor targeting studies were carried out in *Sprague Dawley* (SD) rats. The animals were administered with PDC-MSNs, free-CPT-11, CPT-11 loaded GPDC-MSNs, and GP-MSNs, and longer circulation was exhibited by the group which received GPDC-MSNs, PDC-MSNs, and GP-MSNs when compared with free CPT-11. CPT-11-GPDC-MSNs showed 13 h of elimination half-life while the half-life of free-CPT-11 was close to 1.5 h. The AUC for CPT-1--GPDC-MSNs was 5.5 times greater than the free drug. Tumor targeting efficacy was checked by non-invasive NIRF imaging. The formulations were labeled with DiR dye. DiR labeled GPDC-MSNs aggregated gradually in the liver more than PDC-MSNs and GP-MSNs. It can be concluded that the prepared, smart nanoparticle was successful in gaining access into the tumor cells and releasing the drug at the site. This platform can be further exploited for other drugs to treat cancers.

CONCLUSION

Research to ease the lives of patients suffering from HCC is rapidly being undertaken by scientists worldwide, as it is essential to overcome the common drawbacks faced by the conventional treatment regimen. The ability to design and formulate drug delivery systems for cancer therapy is challenging. It is essential to control various aspects of the delivery system such as the anticancer drug content, the drug release pattern, gaining control over the site at which drug release occurs, drug retention, and drug release duration. Researchers across the world have designed various nanotherapeutic formulations which can address these specific challenges by attaching specific ligands on nanoparticles because of which they can reach the liver and settle at the specific receptors that are overexpressed on the cancerous tissue to aid the release of drugs at the site in a controlled manner. Another approach selected by researchers is to employ pH-sensitive drug release. Since the pH at the cancerous tissue is typically acidic, designing a formulation that triggers the drug release in the acidic pH can prevent unwanted drug release elsewhere. Employing an external magnetic potential to localize the presence of drug-releasing magnetic nanoparticles is also an attractive approach for cancer drug delivery. An emerging number of researchers are delving into the delivery of genetic material at the tumor site. Nanoparticles are being designed with a rugged exterior to safeguard the fragile genetic material that they are carrying on the inside. The future of nanotherapeutic drug delivery for the treatment of HCC will primarily focus on developing formulations that can be marketed in the real world to take full advantage of this nanotechnology for drug delivery to the HCC cells.

CONSENT FOR PUBLICATION

Not applicable.

CONFLICT OF INTEREST

The authors declare no conflict of interest, financial or otherwise.

ACKNOWLEDGEMENT

Declared none.

REFERENCES

Aa, M (2014) https://pubmed.ncbi.nlm.nih.gov/25242656/

Adhoute, X, Penaranda, G, Bronowicki, JP & Raoul, JL (2015) Usefulness of the HKLC *vs.* the BCLC staging system in a European HCC cohort. *J Hepatol,* 62, 492-3.https://linkinghub.elsevier.com/retrieve/pii/S0168827814006229 [http://dx.doi.org/10.1016/j.jhep.2014.08.035] [PMID: 25194894]

AlQahtani, SA, Harisa, GI, Badran, MM, AlGhamdi, KM, Kumar, A, Salem-Bekhit, MM, Ahmad, SF & Alanazi, FK (2019) Nano-erythrocyte membrane-chaperoned 5-fluorouracil liposomes as biomimetic delivery platforms to target hepatocellular carcinoma cell lines. *Artif Cells Nanomed Biotechnol,* 47, 989-96. [http://dx.doi.org/10.1080/21691401.2019.1577887] [PMID: 30873877]

Befeler, AS & Di Bisceglie, AM (2002) Hepatocellular carcinoma: diagnosis and treatment. *Gastroenterology,* 122, 1609-19. [http://dx.doi.org/10.1053/gast.2002.33411] [PMID: 12016426]

Brooks, PJ & Theruvathu, JA (2005) DNA adducts from acetaldehyde: implications for alcohol-related carcinogenesis. *Alcohol,* 35, 187-93. [http://dx.doi.org/10.1016/j.alcohol.2005.03.009] [PMID: 16054980]

Cao, H, Wang, Y, He, X, Zhang, Z, Yin, Q, Chen, Y, Yu, H, Huang, Y, Chen, L, Xu, M, Gu, W & Li, Y (2015) Codelivery of sorafenib and curcumin by directed self-assembled nanoparticles enhances therapeutic effect on hepatocellular carcinoma. *Mol Pharm,* 12, 922-31. [http://dx.doi.org/10.1021/mp500755j] [PMID: 25622075]

Chan, Y-C & Hsiao, M (2017) Protease-activated nanomaterials for targeted cancer theranostics. *Nanomedicine (Lond),* 12, 2153-9. [http://dx.doi.org/10.2217/nnm-2017-0068] [PMID: 28814163]

Chang, H, Yhee, JY, Jang, GH, You, DG, Ryu, JH, Choi, Y, Na, JH, Park, JH, Lee, KH, Choi, K, Kim, K & Kwon, IC (2016) Predicting the *in vivo* accumulation of nanoparticles in tumor based on *in vitro* macrophage uptake and circulation in zebrafish. *J Control Release,* 244, 205-13.http://www.sciencedirect.com/science/article/pii/S016836591630459X [http://dx.doi.org/10.1016/j.jconrel.2016.07.025] [PMID: 27435681]

Chen, F (2020) Recent advances of sorafenib nanoformulations for cancer therapy: Smart nanosystem and combination therapy. *Asian Journal of Pharmaceutical Sciences*

.http://www.sciencedirect.com/science/article/pii/S1818087620303494 a

Chen, Y (2020) Polymeric nanoformulation improves the bioavailability and efficacy of sorafenib for hepatocellular carcinoma therapy. *Biomaterials Science* .https://pubs.rsc.org/en/content/articlelanding/2021/bm/d0bm01881c

Cheng, Y, Zhao, P, Wu, S, Yang, T, Chen, Y, Zhang, X, He, C, Zheng, C, Li, K, Ma, X & Xiang, G (2018) Cisplatin and curcumin co-loaded nano-liposomes for the treatment of hepatocellular carcinoma. *Int J Pharm,* 545, 261-73.
[http://dx.doi.org/10.1016/j.ijpharm.2018.05.007] [PMID: 29730175]

Cillo, U, Vitale, A, Navaglia, F, Basso, D, Montin, U, Bassanello, M, D'Amico, F, Ciarleglio, FA, Brolese, A, Zanus, G, De Pascale, V, Plebani, M & D'Amico, DF (2005) Role of blood AFP mRNA and tumor grade in the preoperative prognostic evaluation of patients with hepatocellular carcinoma. *World J Gastroenterol,* 11, 6920-5.https://www.ncbi.nlm.nih.gov/pmc/articles/PMC4717031/
[http://dx.doi.org/10.3748/wjg.v11.i44.6920] [PMID: 16437593]

De Vincentis, A, Rahmani, Z, Muley, M, Vespasiani-Gentilucci, U, Ruggiero, S, Zamani, P, Jamialahmadi, T & Sahebkar, A (2020) Long noncoding RNAs in nonalcoholic fatty liver disease and liver fibrosis: state-o--the-art and perspectives in diagnosis and treatment. *Drug Discov Today,* 25, 1277-86.http://www.sciencedirect.com/science/article/pii/S1359644620302002
[http://dx.doi.org/10.1016/j.drudis.2020.05.009] [PMID: 32439605]

Depalo, N (2017) Sorafenib delivery nanoplatform based on superparamagnetic iron oxide nanoparticles magnetically targets hepatocellular carcinoma. *Nano Res,* 10, 2431-48.
[http://dx.doi.org/10.1007/s12274-017-1444-3]

Ding, D, Lou, X, Hua, D, Yu, W, Li, L, Wang, J, Gao, F, Zhao, N, Ren, G, Li, L & Lin, B (2012) Recurrent targeted genes of hepatitis B virus in the liver cancer genomes identified by a next-generation sequencing-based approach. *PLoS Genet,* 8, e1003065.https://dx.plos.org/10.1371/journal.pgen.1003065
[http://dx.doi.org/10.1371/journal.pgen.1003065] [PMID: 23236287]

Ding, J, Shi, F, Li, D, Chen, L, Zhuang, X & Chen, X (2013) Enhanced endocytosis of acid-sensitive doxorubicin derivatives with intelligent nanogel for improved security and efficacy. *Biomater Sci,* 1, 633-46.https://pubs.rsc.org/en/content/articlelanding/2013/bm/c3bm60024f
[http://dx.doi.org/10.1039/C3BM60024F] [PMID: 32481836]

Duan, W & Liu, Y (2018) Targeted and synergistic therapy for hepatocellular carcinoma: monosaccharide modified lipid nanoparticles for the co-delivery of doxorubicin and sorafenib. *Drug Des Devel Ther,* 12, 2149-61.
[http://dx.doi.org/10.2147/DDDT.S166402] [PMID: 30034219]

Durand, F, Regimbeau, JM, Belghiti, J, Sauvanet, A, Vilgrain, V, Terris, B, Moutardier, V, Farges, O & Valla, D (2001) Assessment of the benefits and risks of percutaneous biopsy before surgical resection of hepatocellular carcinoma. *J Hepatol,* 35, 254-8.
[http://dx.doi.org/10.1016/S0168-8278(01)00108-8] [PMID: 11580148]

El-Serag, HB (2011) Hepatocellular carcinoma. *N Engl J Med,* 365, 1118-27.
[http://dx.doi.org/10.1056/NEJMra1001683] [PMID: 21992124]

El-Serag, HB & Rudolph, KL (2007) Hepatocellular carcinoma: epidemiology and molecular carcinogenesis. *Gastroenterology,* 132, 2557-76.http://www.sciencedirect.com/science/article/pii/S0016508507007998
[http://dx.doi.org/10.1053/j.gastro.2007.04.061] [PMID: 17570226]

Farinati, F, Vitale, A, Spolverato, G, Pawlik, TM, Huo, TL, Lee, YH, Frigo, AC, Giacomin, A, Giannini, EG, Ciccarese, F, Piscaglia, F, Rapaccini, GL, Di Marco, M, Caturelli, E, Zoli, M, Borzio, F, Cabibbo, G, Felder, M, Sacco, R, Morisco, F, Biasini, E, Foschi, FG, Gasbarrini, A, Svegliati Baroni, G, Virdone, R, Masotto, A, Trevisani, F & Cillo, U (2016) Development and Validation of a New Prognostic System for Patients with Hepatocellular Carcinoma. *PLoS Med,* 13, e1002006.
[http://dx.doi.org/10.1371/journal.pmed.1002006] [PMID: 27116206]

Forner, A, Llovet, JM & Bruix, J (2012) Hepatocellular carcinoma. *Lancet,* 379,

1245-55.https://linkinghub.elsevier.com/retrieve/pii/S0140673611613470 [http://dx.doi.org/10.1016/S0140-6736(11)61347-0] [PMID: 22353262]

Geramizadeh, B, Nikeghbalian, S, Shamsaifar, A, Kazemi, K & Malekhosseini, SA (2013) Hepatocellular carcinoma in two patients with autoimmune hepatitis, a single center experience and review of the literature. *Hepat Mon,* 13, e7957.https://www.ncbi.nlm.nih.gov/pmc/articles/PMC3693535/ [http://dx.doi.org/10.5812/hepatmon.7957] [PMID: 23805159]

Ghouri, YA, Mian, I & Rowe, JH (2017) Review of hepatocellular carcinoma: Epidemiology, etiology, and carcinogenesis. *J Carcinog,* 16, 1. [http://dx.doi.org/10.4103/jcar.JCar_9_16] [PMID: 28694740]

Golla, K, Bhaskar, C, Ahmed, F & Kondapi, AK (2013) A target-specific oral formulation of Doxorubicin-protein nanoparticles: efficacy and safety in hepatocellular cancer. *J Cancer,* 4, 644-52. [http://dx.doi.org/10.7150/jca.7093] [PMID: 24155776]

Gouas, D, Shi, H & Hainaut, P (2009) The aflatoxin-induced TP53 mutation at codon 249 (R249S): biomarker of exposure, early detection and target for therapy. *Cancer Lett,* 286, 29-37. [http://dx.doi.org/10.1016/j.canlet.2009.02.057] [PMID: 19376640]

Grando-Lemaire, V, Guettier, C, Chevret, S, Beaugrand, M & Trinchet, JC (1999) Hepatocellular carcinoma without cirrhosis in the West: epidemiological factors and histopathology of the non-tumorous liver. Groupe d'Etude et de Traitement du Carcinome Hépatocellulaire. *J Hepatol,* 31, 508-13. [http://dx.doi.org/10.1016/S0168-8278(99)80044-0] [PMID: 10488711]

Güngör, S (2013) New Formulation Strategies in Topical Antifungal Therapy. *Journal of Cosmetics. Dermatological Sciences and Applications,* 03, 56-65. [http://dx.doi.org/10.4236/jcdsa.2013.31A009]

Gurda, GT, Zhang, L, Wang, Y, Chen, L, Geddes, S, Cho, WC, Askin, F, Gabrielson, E & Li, QK (2015) Utility of five commonly used immunohistochemical markers TTF-1, Napsin A, CK7, CK5/6 and P63 in primary and metastatic adenocarcinoma and squamous cell carcinoma of the lung: a retrospective study of 246 fine needle aspiration cases. *Clin Transl Med,* 4, 16.https://www.ncbi.nlm.nih.gov/pmc/articles/PMC4417108/ [http://dx.doi.org/10.1186/s40169-015-0057-2] [PMID: 25977750]

Hepatocellular carcinoma - Overview - Mayo Clinic. [no date]. https://www.mayoclinic.org/diseases-conditions/hepatocellular-carcinoma/cdc-20354552

Ho, DW-H, Kai, AK & Ng, IO (2015) TCGA whole-transcriptome sequencing data reveals significantly dysregulated genes and signaling pathways in hepatocellular carcinoma. *Front Med,* 9, 322-30. a [http://dx.doi.org/10.1007/s11684-015-0408-9] [PMID: 26276037]

Ho, DWH, Sze, KM & Ng, IO (2015) Virus-Clip: a fast and memory-efficient viral integration site detection tool at single-base resolution with annotation capability. *Oncotarget,* 6, 20959-63. b [http://dx.doi.org/10.18632/oncotarget.4187] [PMID: 26087185]

Hsu, C-Y, Huang, YH, Hsia, CY, Su, CW, Lin, HC, Loong, CC, Chiou, YY, Chiang, JH, Lee, PC, Huo, TI & Lee, SD (2010) A new prognostic model for hepatocellular carcinoma based on total tumor volume: the Taipei Integrated Scoring System. *J Hepatol,* 53, 108-17.https://linkinghub.elsevier.com/retrieve/pii/S0168827810001923 [http://dx.doi.org/10.1016/j.jhep.2010.01.038] [PMID: 20451283]

Huang, Q, Lin, B, Liu, H, Ma, X, Mo, F, Yu, W, Li, L, Li, H, Tian, T, Wu, D, Shen, F, Xing, J & Chen, ZN (2011) RNA-Seq analyses generate comprehensive transcriptomic landscape and reveal complex transcript patterns in hepatocellular carcinoma. *PLoS One,* 6, e26168. [http://dx.doi.org/10.1371/journal.pone.0026168] [PMID: 22043308]

Huang, SF, Chang, IC, Hong, CC, Yen, TC, Chen, CL, Wu, CC, Tsai, CC, Ho, MC, Lee, WC, Yu, HC, Shen, YY, Eng, HL, Wang, J, Tseng, HH, Jeng, YM, Yeh, CT, Chen, CL, Chen, PJ & Liaw, YF (2018) Metabolic risk factors are associated with non-hepatitis B non-hepatitis C hepatocellular carcinoma in Taiwan, an endemic area of chronic hepatitis B. *Hepatol Commun,* 2,

747-59.https://www.ncbi.nlm.nih.gov/pmc/articles/PMC5983169/
[http://dx.doi.org/10.1002/hep4.1182] [PMID: 29881825]

Hui, L, Zatloukal, K, Scheuch, H, Stepniak, E & Wagner, EF (2008) Proliferation of human HCC cells and chemically induced mouse liver cancers requires JNK1-dependent p21 downregulation. *J Clin Invest,* 118, 3943-53.https://www.ncbi.nlm.nih.gov/pmc/articles/PMC2579707/
[http://dx.doi.org/10.1172/JCI37156] [PMID: 19033664]

Jagwani, S, Jalalpure, S, Dhamecha, D, Jadhav, K & Bohara, R (2020) Pharmacokinetic and Pharmacodynamic Evaluation of Resveratrol Loaded Cationic Liposomes for Targeting Hepatocellular Carcinoma. *ACS Biomater Sci Eng,* 6, 4969-84.https://pubs.acs.org/doi/10.1021/acsbiomaterials.0c00429
[http://dx.doi.org/10.1021/acsbiomaterials.0c00429] [PMID: 33455290]

Yang, JD, Kim, WR, Park, KW, Chaiteerakij, R, Kim, B, Sanderson, SO, Larson, JJ, Pedersen, RA, Therneau, TM, Gores, GJ, Roberts, LR & Park, JW (2012) Model to estimate survival in ambulatory patients with hepatocellular carcinoma. *Hepatology,* 56, 614-21.https://europepmc.org/article/pmc/pmc3564594
[http://dx.doi.org/10.1002/hep.25680] [PMID: 22370914]

Jiang, Y, Fay, JM, Poon, CD, Vinod, N, Zhao, Y, Bullock, K, Qin, S, Manickam, DS, Yi, X, Banks, WA & Kabanov, AV (2018) Nanoformulation of Brain-Derived Neurotrophic Factor with Target Receptor-Triggered-Release in the Central Nervous System. *Adv Funct Mater,* 28, 1703982.
[http://dx.doi.org/10.1002/adfm.201703982] [PMID: 29785179]

Jiang, Z, Jhunjhunwala, S, Liu, J, Haverty, PM, Kennemer, MI, Guan, Y, Lee, W, Carnevali, P, Stinson, J, Johnson, S, Diao, J, Yeung, S, Jubb, A, Ye, W, Wu, TD, Kapadia, SB, de Sauvage, FJ, Gentleman, RC, Stern, HM, Seshagiri, S, Pant, KP, Modrusan, Z, Ballinger, DG & Zhang, Z (2012) The effects of hepatitis B virus integration into the genomes of hepatocellular carcinoma patients. *Genome Res,* 22, 593-601.
[http://dx.doi.org/10.1101/gr.133926.111] [PMID: 22267523]

Kamath, PS & Kim, WR (2007) The model for end-stage liver disease (MELD). *Hepatology,* 45, 797-805.
[http://dx.doi.org/10.1002/hep.21563] [PMID: 17326206]

Kan, Z, Zheng, H, Liu, X, Li, S, Barber, TD, Gong, Z, Gao, H, Hao, K, Willard, MD, Xu, J, Hauptschein, R, Rejto, PA, Fernandez, J, Wang, G, Zhang, Q, Wang, B, Chen, R, Wang, J, Lee, NP, Zhou, W, Lin, Z, Peng, Z, Yi, K, Chen, S, Li, L, Fan, X, Yang, J, Ye, R, Ju, J, Wang, K, Estrella, H, Deng, S, Wei, P, Qiu, M, Wulur, IH, Liu, J, Ehsani, ME, Zhang, C, Loboda, A, Sung, WK, Aggarwal, A, Poon, RT, Fan, ST, Wang, J, Hardwick, J, Reinhard, C, Dai, H, Li, Y, Luk, JM & Mao, M (2013) Whole-genome sequencing identifies recurrent mutations in hepatocellular carcinoma. *Genome Res,* 23, 1422-33.
[http://dx.doi.org/10.1101/gr.154492.113] [PMID: 23788652]

Karaman, B, Battal, B, Sari, S & Verim, S (2014) Hepatocellular carcinoma review: current treatment, and evidence-based medicine. *World J Gastroenterol,* 20, 18059-60.
[http://dx.doi.org/10.3748/wjg.v20.i47.18059] [PMID: 25548509]

Kew, MC (2003) Synergistic interaction between aflatoxin B1 and hepatitis B virus in hepatocarcinogenesis. *Liver Int,* 23, 405-9.http://doi.wiley.com/10.1111/j.1478-3231.2003.00869.x
[http://dx.doi.org/10.1111/j.1478-3231.2003.00869.x] [PMID: 14986813]

Kew, MC (2013) Aflatoxins as a cause of hepatocellular carcinoma. *J Gastrointestin Liver Dis,* 22, 305-10.
[PMID: 24078988]

Kew, MC (2014) Hepatic iron overload and hepatocellular carcinoma. *Liver Cancer,* 3, 31-40.https://www.karger.com/Article/FullText/343856
[http://dx.doi.org/10.1159/000343856] [PMID: 24804175]

Khan, AA, Alanazi, AM, Jabeen, M, Hassan, I & Bhat, MA (2016) Targeted nano-delivery of novel omega-3 conjugate against hepatocellular carcinoma: Regulating COX-2/bcl-2 expression in an animal model. *Biomed Pharmacother,* 81, 394-401.https://linkinghub.elsevier.com/retrieve/pii/S0753332215305151
[http://dx.doi.org/10.1016/j.biopha.2016.04.033] [PMID: 27261618]

Kim, BH, Park, JW, Nam, BH, Kwak, HW & Kim, WR (2014) Validation of a model to estimate survival in ambulatory patients with hepatocellular carcinoma: a single-centre cohort study. *Liver Int,* 34, e317-23.

[http://dx.doi.org/10.1111/liv.12519] [PMID: 24606128]

Koh, W-P, Robien, K, Wang, R, Govindarajan, S, Yuan, JM & Yu, MC (2011) Smoking as an independent risk factor for hepatocellular carcinoma: the Singapore Chinese Health Study. *Br J Cancer,* 105, 1430-5. [http://dx.doi.org/10.1038/bjc.2011.360] [PMID: 21915129]

(2015) 2014 KLCSG-NCC Korea Practice Guideline for the Management of Hepatocellular Carcinoma. *Gut Liver,* 9, 267-317.
[http://dx.doi.org/10.5009/gnl14460] [PMID: 25918260]

Kremsdorf, D, Soussan, P, Paterlini-Brechot, P & Brechot, C (2006) Hepatitis B virus-related hepatocellular carcinoma: paradigms for viral-related human carcinogenesis. *Oncogene,* 25, 3823-33.
[http://dx.doi.org/10.1038/sj.onc.1209559] [PMID: 16799624]

Kudo, M, Chung, H & Osaki, Y (2003) Prognostic staging system for hepatocellular carcinoma (CLIP score): its value and limitations, and a proposal for a new staging system, the Japan Integrated Staging Score (JIS score). *J Gastroenterol,* 38, 207-15.
[http://dx.doi.org/10.1007/s005350300038] [PMID: 12673442]

Kumar, M, Zhao, X & Wang, XW (2011) Molecular carcinogenesis of hepatocellular carcinoma and intrahepatic cholangiocarcinoma: one step closer to personalized medicine? *Cell Biosci,* 1, 5.
[http://dx.doi.org/10.1186/2045-3701-1-5] [PMID: 21711594]

Lau, C-C, Sun, T, Ching, AK, He, M, Li, JW, Wong, AM, Co, NN, Chan, AW, Li, PS, Lung, RW, Tong, JH, Lai, PB, Chan, HL, To, KF, Chan, TF & Wong, N (2014) Viral-human chimeric transcript predisposes risk to liver cancer development and progression. *Cancer Cell,* 25, 335-49.
[http://dx.doi.org/10.1016/j.ccr.2014.01.030] [PMID: 24582836]

Li, S, Zhang, T, Xu, W, Ding, J, Yin, F, Xu, J, Sun, W, Wang, H, Sun, M, Cai, Z & Hua, Y (2018) Sarcoma-Targeting Peptide-Decorated Polypeptide Nanogel Intracellularly Delivers Shikonin for Upregulated Osteosarcoma Necroptosis and Diminished Pulmonary Metastasis. *Theranostics,* 8, 1361-75.
[http://dx.doi.org/10.7150/thno.18299] [PMID: 29507626]

Li, W, Zeng, X, Lee, NP, Liu, X, Chen, S, Guo, B, Yi, S, Zhuang, X, Chen, F, Wang, G, Poon, RT, Fan, ST, Mao, M, Li, Y, Li, S, Wang, J, Jianwang, , Xu, X, Jiang, H & Zhang, X (2013) HIVID: an efficient method to detect HBV integration using low coverage sequencing. *Genomics,* 102, 338-44.
[http://dx.doi.org/10.1016/j.ygeno.2013.07.002] [PMID: 23867110]

Li, Y, Miao, Y, Chen, M, Chen, X, Li, F, Zhang, X & Gan, Y (2020) Stepwise targeting and responsive lipid-coated nanoparticles for enhanced tumor cell sensitivity and hepatocellular carcinoma therapy. *Theranostics,* 10, 3722-36.
[http://dx.doi.org/10.7150/thno.42008] [PMID: 32206118]

Liang, S (2015) Optimizing the Size of Micellar Nanoparticles for Efficient siRNA Delivery. *Adv Funct Mater,* 25, 4778-87.http://doi.wiley.com/10.1002/adfm.201501548
[http://dx.doi.org/10.1002/adfm.201501548]

Liao, S-F, Yang, HI, Lee, MH, Chen, CJ & Lee, WC (2012) Fifteen-year population attributable fractions and causal pies of risk factors for newly developed hepatocellular carcinomas in 11,801 men in Taiwan. *PLoS One,* 7, e34779.https://dx.plos.org/10.1371/journal.pone.0034779
[http://dx.doi.org/10.1371/journal.pone.0034779] [PMID: 22506050]

Lin, K-T, Shann, YJ, Chau, GY, Hsu, CN & Huang, CY (2014) Identification of latent biomarkers in hepatocellular carcinoma by ultra-deep whole-transcriptome sequencing. *Oncogene,* 33, 4786-94.
[http://dx.doi.org/10.1038/onc.2013.424] [PMID: 24141781]

Liu, H, Zhang, Z, Chi, X, Zhao, Z, Huang, D, Jin, J & Gao, J (2016) Arsenite-loaded nanoparticles inhibit PARP-1 to overcome multidrug resistance in hepatocellular carcinoma cells. *Sci Rep,* 6, 31009.
[http://dx.doi.org/10.1038/srep31009] [PMID: 27484730]

Liu, M, Jiang, L & Guan, XY (2014) The genetic and epigenetic alterations in human hepatocellular carcinoma: a recent update. *Protein Cell,* 5, 673-91. a

[http://dx.doi.org/10.1007/s13238-014-0065-9] [PMID: 24916440]

Liu, Y, Feng, L, Liu, T, Zhang, L, Yao, Y, Yu, D, Wang, L & Zhang, N (2014) Multifunctional pH-sensitive polymeric nanoparticles for theranostics evaluated experimentally in cancer. *Nanoscale,* 6, 3231-42. b [http://dx.doi.org/10.1039/c3nr05647c] [PMID: 24500240]

Llovet, JM, Brú, C & Bruix, J (1999) Prognosis of hepatocellular carcinoma: the BCLC staging classification. *Semin Liver Dis,* 19, 329-38.http://www.thieme-connect.de/DOI/DOI?10.1055/s-2007-1007122 [http://dx.doi.org/10.1055/s-2007-1007122] [PMID: 10518312]

Llovet, JM, Bruix, J, Fuster, J, Castells, A, Garcia-Valdecasas, JC, Grande, L, Franca, A, Brú, C, Navasa, M, Ayuso, MC, Solé, M, Real, MI, Vilana, R, Rimola, A, Visa, J & Rodés, J (1998) Liver transplantation for small hepatocellular carcinoma: the tumor-node-metastasis classification does not have prognostic power. *Hepatology,* 27, 1572-7.
[http://dx.doi.org/10.1002/hep.510270616] [PMID: 9620329]

Lorente, S, Hautefeuille, M & Sanchez-Cedillo, A (2020) The liver, a functionalized vascular structure. *Sci Rep,* 10, 16194.https://www.nature.com/articles/s41598-020-73208-8
[http://dx.doi.org/10.1038/s41598-020-73208-8] [PMID: 33004881]

Ludwiczek, S, Aigner, E, Theurl, I & Weiss, G (2003) Cytokine-mediated regulation of iron transport in human monocytic cells. *Blood,* 101, 4148-54.
[http://dx.doi.org/10.1182/blood-2002-08-2459] [PMID: 12522003]

Ma, G (1992) 2013. Hepatocellular carcinoma: epidemiology, biology, diagnosis, and therapies. *Rev Assoc Med Bras,* 59, 514-24.https://europepmc.org/article/med/24041910

Ma, L, Chua, MS, Andrisani, O & So, S (2014) Epigenetics in hepatocellular carcinoma: an update and future therapy perspectives. *World J Gastroenterol,* 20, 333-45.
[http://dx.doi.org/10.3748/wjg.v20.i2.333] [PMID: 24574704]

Makuuchi, M, Belghiti, J, Belli, G, Fan, ST, Lau, JW, Ringe, B, Strasberg, SM, Vauthey, JN, Yamaoka, Y & Yamasaki, S (2003) IHPBA concordant classification of primary liver cancer: working group report. *J Hepatobiliary Pancreat Surg,* 10, 26-30.
[http://dx.doi.org/10.1007/s10534-002-0808-6] [PMID: 12918454]

Mancebo, A, González-Diéguez, ML, Cadahía, V, Varela, M, Pérez, R, Navascués, CA, Sotorríos, NG, Martínez, M, Rodrigo, L & Rodríguez, M (2013) Annual incidence of hepatocellular carcinoma among patients with alcoholic cirrhosis and identification of risk groups. *Clin Gastroenterol Hepatol,* 11, 95-101.
[http://dx.doi.org/10.1016/j.cgh.2012.09.007] [PMID: 22982095]

Marrero, JA, Fontana, RJ, Fu, S, Conjeevaram, HS, Su, GL & Lok, AS (2005) Alcohol, tobacco and obesity are synergistic risk factors for hepatocellular carcinoma. *J Hepatol,* 42, 218-24.
[http://dx.doi.org/10.1016/j.jhep.2004.10.005] [PMID: 15664247]

Marsh, JW, Dvorchik, I, Bonham, CA & Iwatsuki, S (2000) Is the pathologic TNM staging system for patients with hepatoma predictive of outcome? *Cancer,* 88, 538-43.
[http://dx.doi.org/10.1002/(SICI)1097-0142(20000201)88:3<538::AID-CNCR7>3.0.CO;2-H] [PMID: 10649244]

Mondal, J & Khuda-Bukhsh, AR (2020) Cisplatin and farnesol co-encapsulated PLGA nano-particles demonstrate enhanced anti-cancer potential against hepatocellular carcinoma cells *in vitro. Mol Biol Rep,* 47, 3615-28.
[http://dx.doi.org/10.1007/s11033-020-05455-x] [PMID: 32314187]

Nair, S, Mason, A, Eason, J, Loss, G & Perrillo, RP (2002) Is obesity an independent risk factor for hepatocellular carcinoma in cirrhosis? *Hepatology,* 36, 150-5.
[http://dx.doi.org/10.1053/jhep.2002.33713] [PMID: 12085359]

Naseema, (2018) Heat Enhancement Of Heat Exchanger Using Aluminium Oxide(Al2o3), Copper Oxide(Cuo)Nano Fluids With Different Concentrations. *Mater Today Proc,* 5, 6481-8.http://www.sciencedirect.com/science/article/pii/S2214785317332492

[http://dx.doi.org/10.1016/j.matpr.2017.12.261]

Nasir, F (2013) Heat Transfer of Aluminium-Oxide Nanofluids in a Compact Heat Exchanger. *Appl Mech Mater,* 465, 622.
[http://dx.doi.org/10.4028/www.scientific.net/AMM.465-466.622]

Ng, AWT, Poon, SL, Huang, MN, Lim, JQ, Boot, A, Yu, W, Suzuki, Y, Thangaraju, S, Ng, CCY, Tan, P, Pang, ST, Huang, HY, Yu, MC, Lee, PH, Hsieh, SY, Chang, AY, Teh, BT & Rozen, SG (2017) Aristolochic acids and their derivatives are widely implicated in liver cancers in Taiwan and throughout Asia. *Sci Transl Med,* 9, eaan6446.
[http://dx.doi.org/10.1126/scitranslmed.aan6446] [PMID: 29046434]

Nounou, MI, El-Khordagui, LK, Khalafallah, NA & Khalil, SA (2008) Liposomal formulation for dermal and transdermal drug delivery: past, present and future. *Recent Pat Drug Deliv Formul,* 2, 9-18.
http://www.eurekaselect.com/openurl/content.php?genre=article&issn=1872-2113&volume=2&issue=1&spage=9
[http://dx.doi.org/10.2174/187221108783331375] [PMID: 19075893]

Ochi, MM, Amoabediny, G, Rezayat, SM, Akbarzadeh, A & Ebrahimi, B (2016) *In Vitro* Co-Delivery Evaluation of Novel Pegylated Nano-Liposomal Herbal Drugs of Silibinin and Glycyrrhizic Acid (Nano-Phytosome) to Hepatocellular Carcinoma Cells. *Cell J,* 18, 135-48.
[http://dx.doi.org/10.22074/cellj.2016.4308] [PMID: 27540518]

Oh, HR, Jo, HY, Park, JS, Kim, DE, Cho, JY, Kim, PH & Kim, KS (2016) Galactosylated Liposomes for Targeted Co-Delivery of Doxorubicin/Vimentin siRNA to Hepatocellular Carcinoma. *Nanomaterials (Basel),* 6, E141.
[http://dx.doi.org/10.3390/nano6080141] [PMID: 28335269]

Omata, M, Cheng, AL, Kokudo, N, Kudo, M, Lee, JM, Jia, J, Tateishi, R, Han, KH, Chawla, YK, Shiina, S, Jafri, W, Payawal, DA, Ohki, T, Ogasawara, S, Chen, PJ, Lesmana, CRA, Lesmana, LA, Gani, RA, Obi, S, Dokmeci, AK & Sarin, SK (2017) Asia-Pacific clinical practice guidelines on the management of hepatocellular carcinoma: a 2017 update. *Hepatol Int,* 11, 317-70.
[http://dx.doi.org/10.1007/s12072-017-9799-9] [PMID: 28620797]

Palac, Z, Engesland, A, Flaten, GE, Škalko-Basnet, N, Filipović-Grčić, J & Vanić, Ž (2014) Liposomes for (trans)dermal drug delivery: the skin-PVPA as a novel *in vitro* stratum corneum model in formulation development. *J Liposome Res,* 24, 313-22.
[http://dx.doi.org/10.3109/08982104.2014.899368] [PMID: 24646434]

Pandey, P, Rahman, M, Bhatt, PC, Beg, S, Paul, B, Hafeez, A, Al-Abbasi, FA, Nadeem, MS, Baothman, O, Anwar, F & Kumar, V (2018) Implication of nano-antioxidant therapy for treatment of hepatocellular carcinoma using PLGA nanoparticles of rutin. *Nanomedicine (Lond),* 13, 849-70.
[http://dx.doi.org/10.2217/nnm-2017-0306] [PMID: 29565220]

Park, J-W, Chen, M, Colombo, M, Roberts, LR, Schwartz, M, Chen, PJ, Kudo, M, Johnson, P, Wagner, S, Orsini, LS & Sherman, M (2015) Global patterns of hepatocellular carcinoma management from diagnosis to death: the BRIDGE Study. *Liver Int,* 35, 2155-66.
[http://dx.doi.org/10.1111/liv.12818] [PMID: 25752327]

Pathak, P, Dhawan, V, Magarkar, A, Danne, R, Govindarajan, S, Ghosh, S, Steiniger, F, Chaudhari, P, Gopal, V, Bunker, A, Róg, T, Fahr, A & Nagarsenker, M (2016) Design of cholesterol arabinogalactan anchored liposomes for asialoglycoprotein receptor mediated targeting to hepatocellular carcinoma: *In silico* modeling, *in vitro* and *in vivo* evaluation. *Int J Pharm,* 509, 149-58.
[http://dx.doi.org/10.1016/j.ijpharm.2016.05.041] [PMID: 27231122]

Pons, F, Varela, M & Llovet, JM (2005) Staging systems in hepatocellular carcinoma. *HPB (Oxford),* 7, 35-41.https://www.ncbi.nlm.nih.gov/pmc/articles/PMC2023920/
[http://dx.doi.org/10.1080/13651820410024058] [PMID: 18333159]

Pranatharthiharan, S, Patel, MD, Malshe, VC, Pujari, V, Gorakshakar, A, Madkaikar, M, Ghosh, K &

Devarajan, PV (2017) Asialoglycoprotein receptor targeted delivery of doxorubicin nanoparticles for hepatocellular carcinoma. *Drug Deliv,* 24, 20-9.
[http://dx.doi.org/10.1080/10717544.2016.1225856] [PMID: 28155331]

Purohit, V, Rapaka, R, Kwon, OS & Song, BJ (2013) Roles of alcohol and tobacco exposure in the development of hepatocellular carcinoma. *Life Sci,* 92, 3-9.https://linkinghub.elsevier.com/retrieve/pii/S0024320512006121
[http://dx.doi.org/10.1016/j.lfs.2012.10.009] [PMID: 23123447]

Rahman, M (2020) Diosmin-loaded solid nanoparticles as nano-antioxidant therapy for management of hepatocellular carcinoma: QbD-based optimization, *In vitro* and *in vivo* evaluation
[http://dx.doi.org/10.1016/j.jddst.2020.102213]

Ross, RK, Yuan, JM, Yu, MC, Wogan, GN, Qian, GS, Tu, JT, Groopman, JD, Gao, YT & Henderson, BE (1992) Urinary aflatoxin biomarkers and risk of hepatocellular carcinoma. *Lancet,* 339, 943-6.
[http://dx.doi.org/10.1016/0140-6736(92)91528-G] [PMID: 1348796]

Saito, Y, Hibino, S & Saito, H (2014) Alterations of epigenetics and microRNA in hepatocellular carcinoma. *Hepatol Res,* 44, 31-42.
[http://dx.doi.org/10.1111/hepr.12147] [PMID: 23617364]

Schulze, K, Imbeaud, S, Letouzé, E, Alexandrov, LB, Calderaro, J, Rebouissou, S, Couchy, G, Meiller, C, Shinde, J, Soysouvanh, F, Calatayud, AL, Pinyol, R, Pelletier, L, Balabaud, C, Laurent, A, Blanc, JF, Mazzaferro, V, Calvo, F, Villanueva, A, Nault, JC, Bioulac-Sage, P, Stratton, MR, Llovet, JM & Zucman-Rossi, J (2015) Exome sequencing of hepatocellular carcinomas identifies new mutational signatures and potential therapeutic targets. *Nat Genet,* 47, 505-11.
[http://dx.doi.org/10.1038/ng.3252] [PMID: 25822088]

Shen, K, Li, D, Guan, J, Ding, J, Wang, Z, Gu, J, Liu, T & Chen, X (2017) Targeted sustained delivery of antineoplastic agent with multicomponent polylactide stereocomplex micelle. *Nanomedicine,* 13, 1279-88.http://www.sciencedirect.com/science/article/pii/S1549963416302398
[http://dx.doi.org/10.1016/j.nano.2016.12.022] [PMID: 28064009]

Shouval, D (2002) HCC: what's the score. *Gut,* 50, 749-50.https://gut.bmj.com/lookup/doi/10.1136/gut.50.6.749
[http://dx.doi.org/10.1136/gut.50.6.749] [PMID: 12010872]

Streba, C (2018) Introductory Chapter: Etiology and Pathogenesis of Hepatocellular Carcinoma.
[http://dx.doi.org/10.5772/intechopen.78328]

Streba, LAM (2014) Dendritic cells and hepatocellular carcinoma. *Romanian Journal of Morphology and Embryology =. Rev Roum Morphol Embryol,* 55, 1287-93.

Subramaniam, S, Kelley, RK & Venook, AP (2013) A review of hepatocellular carcinoma (HCC) staging systems. *Chin Clin Oncol,* 2, 33.https://cco.amegroups.com/article/view/2528
[PMID: 25841912]

Sun, D, Ding, J, Xiao, C, Chen, J, Zhuang, X & Chen, X (2015) pH-Responsive Reversible PEGylation Improves Performance of Antineoplastic Agent. *Adv Healthc Mater,* 4, 844-55.
[http://dx.doi.org/10.1002/adhm.201400736] [PMID: 25645303]

Tagaram, HRS, Divittore, NA, Barth, BM, Kaiser, JM, Avella, D, Kimchi, ET, Jiang, Y, Isom, HC, Kester, M & Staveley-O'Carroll, KF (2011) Nanoliposomal ceramide prevents *in vivo* growth of hepatocellular carcinoma. *Gut,* 60, 695-701.https://gut.bmj.com/lookup/doi/10.1136/gut.2010.216671
[http://dx.doi.org/10.1136/gut.2010.216671] [PMID: 21193455]

Tang, A, Hallouch, O, Chernyak, V, Kamaya, A & Sirlin, CB (2018) Epidemiology of hepatocellular carcinoma: target population for surveillance and diagnosis. *Abdom Radiol (NY),* 43, 13-25.
[http://dx.doi.org/10.1007/s00261-017-1209-1] [PMID: 28647765]

Tateishi, R, Yoshida, H, Shiina, S, Imamura, H, Hasegawa, K, Teratani, T, Obi, S, Sato, S, Koike, Y, Fujishima, T, Makuuchi, M & Omata, M (2005) Proposal of a new prognostic model for hepatocellular

carcinoma: an analysis of 403 patients. *Gut,* 54, 419-25.
[http://dx.doi.org/10.1136/gut.2003.035055] [PMID: 15710994]

Tatematsu, K, Tanaka, Y, Kurbanov, F, Sugauchi, F, Mano, S, Maeshiro, T, Nakayoshi, T, Wakuta, M, Miyakawa, Y & Mizokami, M (2009) A genetic variant of hepatitis B virus divergent from known human and ape genotypes isolated from a Japanese patient and provisionally assigned to new genotype J. *J Virol,* 83, 10538-47.
[http://dx.doi.org/10.1128/JVI.00462-09] [PMID: 19640977]

Thapa, RK, Choi, JY, Poudel, BK, Hiep, TT, Pathak, S, Gupta, B, Choi, HG, Yong, CS & Kim, JO (2015) Multilayer-Coated Liquid Crystalline Nanoparticles for Effective Sorafenib Delivery to Hepatocellular Carcinoma. *ACS Appl Mater Interfaces,* 7, 20360-8.
[http://dx.doi.org/10.1021/acsami.5b06203] [PMID: 26315487]

Thorgeirsson, SS & Grisham, JW (2002) Molecular pathogenesis of human hepatocellular carcinoma. *Nat Genet,* 31, 339-46.
[http://dx.doi.org/10.1038/ng0802-339] [PMID: 12149612]

Toffanin, S, Friedman, SL & Llovet, JM (2010) Obesity, inflammatory signaling, and hepatocellular carcinoma-an enlarging link. *Cancer Cell,* 17, 115-7.http://www.sciencedirect.com/science/article/pii/S1535610810000346
[http://dx.doi.org/10.1016/j.ccr.2010.01.018] [PMID: 20159605]

Tom, G, Philip, S, Isaac, R, Praseetha, PK, Jiji, SG & Asha, VV (2018) Preparation of an efficient and safe polymeric-magnetic nanoparticle delivery system for sorafenib in hepatocellular carcinoma. *Life Sci,* 206, 10-21.
[http://dx.doi.org/10.1016/j.lfs.2018.04.046] [PMID: 29709652]

Toyoda, H, Kumada, T, Osaki, Y, Oka, H, Urano, F, Kudo, M & Matsunaga, T (2006) Staging hepatocellular carcinoma by a novel scoring system (BALAD score) based on serum markers. *Clin Gastroenterol Hepatol,* 4, 1528-36.
[http://dx.doi.org/10.1016/j.cgh.2006.09.021] [PMID: 17162244]

Trinchet, J (2004) Groupe d'Etude et de Traitement du Carcinome HepatocellulaireRandomized trial of leuprorelin and flutamide in male patients with hepatocellular carcinoma treated with tamoxifen. Hepatology 40: 1361-1369. *Hepatology,* 40, 1361-9.
[http://dx.doi.org/10.1002/hep.20474]

Tsend-Ayush, A, Zhu, X, Ding, Y, Yao, J, Yin, L, Zhou, J & Yao, J (2017) Lactobionic acid-conjugated TPGS nanoparticles for enhancing therapeutic efficacy of etoposide against hepatocellular carcinoma. *Nanotechnology,* 28, 195602.
[http://dx.doi.org/10.1088/1361-6528/aa66ba] [PMID: 28291743]

Tunki, L, Kulhari, H, Vadithe, LN, Kuncha, M, Bhargava, S, Pooja, D & Sistla, R (2019) Modulating the site-specific oral delivery of sorafenib using sugar-grafted nanoparticles for hepatocellular carcinoma treatment. *Eur J Pharm Sci,* 137, 104978.
[http://dx.doi.org/10.1016/j.ejps.2019.104978] [PMID: 31254645]

Types of Liver Cancer: Common, Rare and More Varieties. https://www.cancercenter.com/cancer-types/liver-cancer/types

Varshosaz, J, Hassanzadeh, F, Sadeghi, H & Khadem, M (2012) Galactosylated nanostructured lipid carriers for delivery of 5-FU to hepatocellular carcinoma. *J Liposome Res,* 22, 224-36.
[http://dx.doi.org/10.3109/08982104.2012.662653] [PMID: 22385296]

Vogel, A, Cervantes, A, Chau, I, Daniele, B, Llovet, JM, Meyer, T, Nault, JC, Neumann, U, Ricke, J, Sangro, B, Schirmacher, P, Verslype, C, Zech, CJ, Arnold, D & Martinelli, E (2018) Hepatocellular carcinoma: ESMO Clinical Practice Guidelines for diagnosis, treatment and follow-up. *Ann Oncol,* 29 (Suppl. 4), iv238-55.
[http://dx.doi.org/10.1093/annonc/mdy308] [PMID: 30285213]

Wang, J, Wang, H, Li, J, Liu, Z, Xie, H, Wei, X, Lu, D, Zhuang, R, Xu, X & Zheng, S (2016) iRGD-

Decorated Polymeric Nanoparticles for the Efficient Delivery of Vandetanib to Hepatocellular Carcinoma: Preparation and *in Vitro* and *in Vivo* Evaluation. *ACS Appl Mater Interfaces,* 8, 19228-37.
[http://dx.doi.org/10.1021/acsami.6b03166] [PMID: 27381493]

Wei, M, Guo, X, Tu, L, Zou, Q, Li, Q, Tang, C, Chen, B, Xu, Y & Wu, C (2015) Lactoferrin-modified PEGylated liposomes loaded with doxorubicin for targeting delivery to hepatocellular carcinoma. *Int J Nanomedicine,* 10, 5123-37.https://www.ncbi.nlm.nih.gov/pmc/articles/PMC4540123/
[PMID: 26316745]

Welzel, TM, Graubard, BI, Quraishi, S, Zeuzem, S, Davila, JA, El-Serag, HB & McGlynn, KA (2013) Population-attributable fractions of risk factors for hepatocellular carcinoma in the United States. *Am J Gastroenterol,* 108, 1314-21.
[http://dx.doi.org/10.1038/ajg.2013.160] [PMID: 23752878]

West, J, Card, TR, Aithal, GP & Fleming, KM (2017) Risk of hepatocellular carcinoma among individuals with different aetiologies of cirrhosis: a population-based cohort study. *Aliment Pharmacol Ther,* 45, 983-90.http://doi.wiley.com/10.1111/apt.13961
[http://dx.doi.org/10.1111/apt.13961] [PMID: 28144999]

Wiklund, K & Dich, J (1994) Cancer risks among female farmers in Sweden. *Cancer Causes Control,* 5, 449-57.
[http://dx.doi.org/10.1007/BF01694759] [PMID: 7999967]

Wild, CP (2015). *MYCOTOXIN CONTROL IN LOW- AND MIDDLE-INCOME COUNTRIES.*International Agency for Research on Cancer, Lyon, FR.http://www.ncbi.nlm.nih.gov/books/NBK350558/

Xia, Y, Zhong, J, Zhao, M, Tang, Y, Han, N, Hua, L, Xu, T, Wang, C & Zhu, B (2019) Galactose-modified selenium nanoparticles for targeted delivery of doxorubicin to hepatocellular carcinoma. *Drug Deliv,* 26, 1-11.
[http://dx.doi.org/10.1080/10717544.2018.1556359] [PMID: 31928356]

Zhang, W, Peng, F, Zhou, T, Huang, Y, Zhang, L, Ye, P, Lu, M, Yang, G, Gai, Y, Yang, T, Ma, X & Xiang, G (2015) Targeted delivery of chemically modified anti-miR-221 to hepatocellular carcinoma with negatively charged liposomes. *Int J Nanomedicine,* 10, 4825-36. http://www.dovepress.com/targeted-delivery-of-chemically-modified-anti-mir-221-to-hepatocellula-peer-reviewed-article-IJN
[PMID: 26251599]

Yang, C, Yin, M, Xu, G, Lin, WJ, Chen, J, Zhang, Y, Feng, T, Huang, P, Chen, CK & Yong, KT (2019) Biodegradable Polymers as a Noncoding miRNA Nanocarrier for Multiple Targeting Therapy of Human Hepatocellular Carcinoma. *Adv Healthc Mater,* 8, e1801318.
[http://dx.doi.org/10.1002/adhm.201801318] [PMID: 30829008]

Yang, JD, Mohamed, EA, Aziz, AO, Shousha, HI, Hashem, MB, Nabeel, MM, Abdelmaksoud, AH, Elbaz, TM, Afihene, MY, Duduyemi, BM, Ayawin, JP, Gyedu, A, Lohouès-Kouacou, MJ, Ndam, AW, Moustafa, EF, Hassany, SM, Moussa, AM, Ugiagbe, RA, Omuemu, CE, Anthony, R, Palmer, D, Nyanga, AF, Malu, AO, Obekpa, S, Abdo, AE, Siddig, AI, Mudawi, HM, Okonkwo, U, Kooffreh-Ada, M, Awuku, YA, Nartey, YA, Abbew, ET, Awuku, NA, Otegbayo, JA, Akande, KO, Desalegn, HM, Omonisi, AE, Ajayi, AO, Okeke, EN, Duguru, MJ, Davwar, PM, Okorie, MC, Mustapha, S, Debes, JD, Ocama, P, Lesi, OA, Odeghe, E, Bello, R, Onyekwere, C, Ekere, F, Igetei, R, Mah'moud, MA, Addissie, B, Ali, HM, Gores, GJ, Topazian, MD & Roberts, LR (2017) Characteristics, management, and outcomes of patients with hepatocellular carcinoma in Africa: a multicountry observational study from the Africa Liver Cancer Consortium. *Lancet Gastroenterol Hepatol,* 2, 103-11. a
[http://dx.doi.org/10.1016/S2468-1253(16)30161-3] [PMID: 28403980]

Yang, JD, Ahmed Mohammed, H, Harmsen, WS, Enders, F, Gores, GJ & Roberts, LR (2017) Recent Trends in the Epidemiology of Hepatocellular Carcinoma in Olmsted County, Minnesota: A US Population-based Study. *J Clin Gastroenterol,* 51, 742-8. b
[http://dx.doi.org/10.1097/MCG.0000000000000810] [PMID: 28445235]

Yang, JD & Roberts, LR (2010) Hepatocellular carcinoma: A global view. *Nat Rev Gastroenterol Hepatol,* 7, 448-58.

[http://dx.doi.org/10.1038/nrgastro.2010.100] [PMID: 20628345]

Yau, T, Yao, TJ, Chan, P, Ng, K, Fan, ST & Poon, RT (2008) A new prognostic score system in patients with advanced hepatocellular carcinoma not amendable to locoregional therapy: implication for patient selection in systemic therapy trials. *Cancer,* 113, 2742-51.
[http://dx.doi.org/10.1002/cncr.23878] [PMID: 18853421]

Yin, X, Xiao, Y, Han, L, Zhang, B, Wang, T, Su, Z & Zhang, N (2018) Ceramide-Fabricated Co-Loaded Liposomes for the Synergistic Treatment of Hepatocellular Carcinoma. *AAPS PharmSciTech,* 19, 2133-43.
[http://dx.doi.org/10.1208/s12249-018-1005-4] [PMID: 29714002]

Younossi, ZM, Otgonsuren, M, Henry, L, Venkatesan, C, Mishra, A, Erario, M & Hunt, S (2015) Association of nonalcoholic fatty liver disease (NAFLD) with hepatocellular carcinoma (HCC) in the United States from 2004 to 2009. *Hepatology,* 62, 1723-30.
[http://dx.doi.org/10.1002/hep.28123] [PMID: 26274335]

Younossi, ZM, Koenig, AB, Abdelatif, D, Fazel, Y, Henry, L & Wymer, M (2016) Global epidemiology of nonalcoholic fatty liver disease-Meta-analytic assessment of prevalence, incidence, and outcomes. *Hepatology,* 64, 73-84.
[http://dx.doi.org/10.1002/hep.28431] [PMID: 26707365]

Yousef, S, Alsaab, HO, Sau, S & Iyer, AK (2018) Development of asialoglycoprotein receptor directed nanoparticles for selective delivery of curcumin derivative to hepatocellular carcinoma. *Heliyon,* 4, e01071.
[http://dx.doi.org/10.1016/j.heliyon.2018.e01071] [PMID: 30603704]

Zamor, PJ, deLemos, AS & Russo, MW (2017) Viral hepatitis and hepatocellular carcinoma: etiology and management. *J Gastrointest Oncol,* 8, 229-42.https://www.ncbi.nlm.nih.gov/pmc/articles/PMC5401856/
[http://dx.doi.org/10.21037/jgo.2017.03.14] [PMID: 28480063]

Zhang, JF, Shu, ZJ, Xie, CY, Li, Q, Jin, XH, Gu, W, Jiang, FJ & Ling, CQ (2014) Prognosis of unresectable hepatocellular carcinoma: comparison of seven staging systems (TNM, Okuda, BCLC, CLIP, CUPI, JIS, CIS) in a Chinese cohort. *PLoS One,* 9, e88182.https://dx.plos.org/10.1371/journal.pone.0088182
[http://dx.doi.org/10.1371/journal.pone.0088182] [PMID: 24609114]

Zhang, X, Lin, C, Lu, A, Lin, G, Chen, H, Liu, Q, Yang, Z & Zhang, H (2017) Liposomes equipped with cell penetrating peptide BR2 enhances chemotherapeutic effects of cantharidin against hepatocellular carcinoma. *Drug Deliv,* 24, 986-98.
[http://dx.doi.org/10.1080/10717544.2017.1340361] [PMID: 28644728]

Zhang, Y (2018) Tumor microenvironment-responsive hyaluronate-calcium carbonate hybrid nanoparticle enables effective chemotherapy for primary and advanced osteosarcomas. *Nano Res,* 11, 4806-22.
[http://dx.doi.org/10.1007/s12274-018-2066-0]

CHAPTER 10

Potential Nanoformulation Approaches for Delivery of HCC Therapeutic Agents

Maria Lucia A.D Lestari[1] and **Biswadip Sinha**[2,*]

[1] *Faculty of Pharmacy, Department of Pharmaceutical Science, Universitas Airlangga Surabaya, Surabaya, Indonesia*

[2] *Institute of Pharmacy, Department of Pharmaceutics, Biopharmaceutics & Nutricosmetics, Freie University of Berlin, Berlin, Germany*

Abstract: Hepatocellular carcinoma (HCC) is a major cancer type worldwide. The major challenge with HCC is that it is usually detected at an advanced stage. After the launch of the first drug Sorafenib against HCC in 2007, several other small molecules and monoclonal antibody-based drugs have been launched to fight against HCC. However, the survival rate in HCC is still very poor. This indicates that there is still a necessity for more effective therapy or to increase the efficacy of the existing therapy. Nanoformulation approach refers to such formulation approaches where the particle size of individual particles or vesicles in a formulation range between 1-1000 nm. The individual particle or vesicle could be either single drug particles or nanosphere/nanocapsules having drug entrapped in polymer/lipid matrix or drug connected with metal or metal oxide core. The idea of using nanoformulations for drug targeting first came around the 1950s. Since then, countless research groups across the world have advanced the field to the extent that several products based on the nanoformulation approach have been launched on the market. Besides targeting, nanoparticles can also help circumvent biopharmaceutical challenges of drugs, such as dissolution, limited oral bioavailability issue, or formulating "hard to solubilize" types of molecules for parenteral formulation. This chapter will review different nanoformulation approaches that can be potentially applied for HCC therapy, their manufacturing process, and therapeutic benefits. We will review the application of different nanoformulation approaches for HCC specific therapeutic agents.

Keywords: Liposome, Liquid crystalline nanoparticles (LCN), Micelle, Nano lipid carrier (NLC), Nanocrystal, Nanosuspension, Polymeric nanoparticles, Solid lipid nanoparticle (SLN), Targeted therapy.

* **Corresponding author Biswadip Sinha:** Institute of Pharmacy, Department of Pharmaceutics, Biopharmaceutics & Nutricosmetics, Freie University of Berlin, Berlin, Germany; E-mail: biswadipsinha@gmail.com

Biswajit Mukherjee (Ed.)

INTRODUCTION

Hepatocellular carcinoma (HCC) is the dominant type of liver cancer and, based on recent statistics, is the fourth leading cause of cancer-related death worldwide (El-Serag, 2020). Ten years ago, HCC was the ninth leading cause of cancer death (O'Connor *et al.*, 2010, Balogh *et al.*, 2016). This indicates that despite the progress of science and medicine in the last decade on various fronts, not much progress has been made against the fight with HCC.

In the past decades, scientific research has brought several therapeutic agents against HCC. These are broadly classified under small molecules, monoclonal antibodies (MCA), RNA-based therapeutics (miRNA or siRNA), and peptides. Among them, small molecules and monoclonal antibodies have been approved for HCC by the United States Food and Drug Administration (USFDA or FDA) (Table **1**) and other regulatory agencies. Sorafenib, a protein kinase inhibitor, was the first drug approved for HCC in 2007. Chemically, Sorafenib is a small molecule. After the approval of Sorafenib, it took almost a decade for the second small molecule Regorafenib to be approved for liver cancer.

Besides small molecules, the other classes of drugs that have been approved for HCC are monoclonal antibodies (MCA). Considering the increased number of MCA approved for HCC related to small molecules, it is clearly understood that this class of drugs is in focus for HCC. The major challenge behind HCC therapy is that in the majority of cases, HCC is detected in an advanced stage, when surgical treatments such as resection and transplantation or locoregional treatment such as chemoembolization do not provide much benefit in terms of the overall survival rate of patients (Forner *et al.*, 2018). On the other hand, in such advanced stages, the traditional chemotherapies such as 5-fluorouracil, cisplatin, doxorubicin, or gemcitabine also do not show promising outcomes (Chen *et al.*, 2019). Moreover, since the liver is already in a compromised state in an advanced stage of HCC, any systemic therapy with a chemotherapeutic agent puts additional stress on the liver since those drugs need to be metabolized by the liver to eliminate them from the body. Because of the toxicity related issues, MCA are favored over standard chemotherapeutic agents since MCA can help the immune system to differentiate cancerous cells from healthy cells and destroy them. Because none of the drugs mentioned in Table **1** provides a complete cure, instead only an increase of the survival rate by a few months to years depending on the stage at detection, a significant need exists to explore new therapies. The development of targeted therapy is one such focus area for HCC, especially for advanced HCC (Chen *et al.*, 2019).

In the pharmaceutical area, "Nano" scale particles are defined as particles within the size of 1 – 1000 nm and cover different types of particles depending on their constituent parts and their physical state, which will be covered in more detail in the next sections. Nanoformulations that are formulations comprising "Nano" sized particles are the major types of novel drug delivery systems that can be used for control release, targeted delivery, and increasing therapeutic efficiency. In one of his articles, Professor Kreuter described the historical background of the concept of nanoparticle and drug targeting (Kreuter, 2007). He mentioned that the idea first came to one of the pioneering scientist Paul Ehrlich when he visited Karl Maria von Weber's Opera "Der Freuschütz" in the 1950s. In that opera, the so-called "Freikugeln," made by calling the spirit of the devil, played a central role. This "Freikugeln" particular property always hit the target even if the rifleman did not aim correctly or if the target was out of reach. Paul Ehrlich thought that this idea of targeting could be applied to improve drug delivery significantly. He named the delivery system "Zauberkugeln" or, in English, "Magic Bullet."With the idea of "Zauberkugeln," Paul Ehrlich started the concept of nanoparticle and drug targeting, which was then carried forwarded by several well-known scientists, such as Prof. Peter Paul Speiser from ETH (Swiss Federal Institute of Technology) Zurich, Prof. Patrick Couvreur from Paris, Prof. Robert Gurny from Geneva, Prof. Jörg Kreuter from Frankfurt and many other great scientists across the world (Kreuter, 2007). Since the start in the 1950s, the nanoparticle area has been revolutionized. Around the mid to late 1970s, various research labs across the world started the concept of polymer-drug conjugates or "nano-therapeutics." The three key technologies in the nano-therapeutics area which became successful from the late 1980s till now are PEGylation (polyethylene glycol conjugated drugs or drug carrier), active targeting (by conjugating cell membrane receptor antibodies, peptides, or small molecule cell ligands to the polymer carrier) and the discovery of EPR effect by Hiroshi Maeda in Kumamoto, Japan. EPR effect, or "Enhanced permeation and retention effect," is referred to as the property of nano-scale carrier to get entrapped inside solid tumors because of the leaky vasculature of the fast-growing tumors, which lead to passive targeting of nano-particles to tumors (Hoffman, 2008).

There is also another type of nanoparticles, where the nanosize particles are pure drug particles or nanocrystals. Often such particles are stabilized in suspension or so-called nanosuspension. Nanocrystals or nanosuspensions are used to solve another big challenge of drug discovery: the poor water solubility of compounds. Most of the chemical entities that come out from combinatorial chemistry as a potential therapeutic agent are poorly water-soluble. Therefore, without using advanced formulation techniques, the oral bioavailability of such molecules remains very poor. Because of poor water solubility, formulating those molecules in a parenteral formulation is not always straightforward. One such HCC specific molecule with poor water solubility leading to poor oral bioavailability (59.9%) is Sorafenib or Nexavar®. Nanosuspension can be used to improve their oral bioavailability issues or formulate them in a parenteral suspension formulation.

Although we do not yet see nanotechnology-based drug products in the commercial space for HCC, several research groups are improving drug delivery systems for delivering molecules. In particular, a lot of work is being carried out concerning the targeted delivery of therapeutic molecules.

This chapter will cover different nanoformulation approaches that can be used for improving dissolution limited oral bioavailability challenges or for targeted delivery. The focus will be put on how they are manufactured, the challenges in the manufacturing process, and what therapeutic advantages they bring.

Table 1. Drugs approved for liver cancers(information collected from different sources: cancer.gov, accessdata.fda.gov & epar product information of EMA).

Drug Name	**Type**	**Trade Name**	**Developer**	**Approval Year (USFDA) for Liver Cancer**	**Formulation**
Sorafenib Tosylate	Small molecule	Nexavar?®	Bayer AG & Onyx Pharmaceuticals	2007	Film-coated tablet containing microcrystalline cellulose, croscarmellose, hypromellose, sodium lauryl sulfate, and magnesium stearate
Ramucirumab	Monoclonal antibody	Cyramza®	Eli Lilly	2014	An aqueous parenteral solution containing Histidine, Histidine monohydrochloride, Sodium chloride, Glycine (E640), Polysorbate 80 (E433)
Nivolumab	Monoclonal antibody	Opdivo®	Bristol-Myers Squibb Co.	2017	Aqueous parenteral solution containing Sodium citrate dihydrate, Sodium chloride, Mannitol (E421), Pentetic acid (diethylenetriaminepentaacetic acid), Polysorbate 80 (E433), Sodium hydroxide, Hydrochloric acid
Regorafenib	Small molecule	Stivarga®	Bayer AG	2017	Film-coated tablet, tablet core contains microcrystalline cellulose, Croscarmellose sodium, Magnesium stearate, Povidone (K-25), and colloidal anhydrous silica

(Table 1) cont.....

Drug Name	Type	Trade Name	Developer	Approval Year (USFDA) for Liver Cancer	Formulation
Pembrolizumab	Monoclonal Antibody	Keytruda®	Merck & Co., Inc	2018	An aqueous parenteral solution containing L-histidine, polysorbate 80, and sucrose
LenvatinibMesylate	Small molecule	Lenvima®	Eisai Inc.	2018	Hard gelatin capsule containing Calcium carbonate, Mannitol, Microcrystalline cellulose, Hydroxypropylcellulose, Low-substituted hydroxypropylcellulose, Talc
Cabozantinib-S-Malate	Small molecule	Cabometyx®	Exelixis Inc.	2019	Film-coated tablet with lactose as tablet core excipient
Atezolizumab	Monoclonal Antibody	Tecentriq®	Genentech Inc.	2020	An aqueous parenteral solution containing L-histidine, glacial acetic acid, sucrose, polysorbate 20
Bevacizumab	Monoclonal Antibody	Avastin®	Genentech Inc.	2020	An aqueous parenteral solution containing sodium phosphate, α,α-trehalosedihydrate and polysorbate 20
Ipilimumab with Nivolumab	Monoclonal Antibody	Yervoy® with Opdivo®	Bristol-Myers Squibb Co.	2020	Yervoy® is formulated as an aqueous parenteral solution containing Tris hydrochloride, Sodium chloride, Mannitol (E421) Pentetic acid, Polysorbate 80, Sodium hydroxide, and Hydrochloric acid
Pemigatinib	Small molecule	Pemazyre®	Incyte	2020	Immediate release uncoated tablet containing microcrystalline cellulose, sodium starch glycolate, and magnesium stearate

NANOFORMULATION APPROACHES

The definition of nanodimension differs across different industries. Whereas in the electronics area, size ranges between 1 nm to 100 nm are considered nanodimension, for the pharmaceutical area, the nano-size range is between 1 nm to 1000. Therefore, formulations whose individual molecular aggregates (either of solid particle structure or vesicle structure) fall within 1 nm to 1000 nm can be considered nanoformulation. Several formulation approaches can reach such dimensions. Inside nanoformulation, the drug could be in a solidified form by itself (such as nanocrystals), solidified with polymer or lipids (such as polymeric nanoparticles, different types of lipid nanoparticles), and individual drug molecules attached with a nanometer size core material (metal or metal oxide nanoparticles). Otherwise, the drug could be in a dissolved/dispersed state inside vesicles (such as nanoemulsions, micelles, liposomes, *etc.*). This section will focus on nanoformulations that have been used or could be used for delivering HCC specific drug molecules and how they are manufactured. We will also review the literature to understand different formulation compositions, which have been reported, and the advantage of such nanoformulations. However, this is necessary to highlight that the examples mentioned below are primarily used in a research laboratory. As mentioned earlier, the commercial application of these nanoformulation approaches for HCC therapy has not been established yet.

In this section, we will primarily divide nanoformulations into two primary categories, nanoparticle, and vesicular systems. Nanoparticles have been further divided into inorganic and organic nanoparticles, based on the type of constituent base material which builds the building block of the nanoparticles. When the base material of the nanoparticle contains carbon, such as various polymers, lipids, or only organic drug substances (such nanocrystal), those nanoparticles fall under organic nanoparticles. Otherwise, if the nanoparticles are composed of metal or metal oxide, without any carbon, they fall under inorganic nanoparticles. Vesicular systems are different from the nanoparticle in the way that the primary particles are not solid. However, some of the vesicular structures, such as liposomes, can be solidified by further processing steps. Solutions and formulations approach similar to the solution such as cyclodextrin (cavity size of different type of cyclodextrins are between 4.7 to 8.3 angstrom)complexation, will not be considered, since in those cases the individual element remains in angstrom size range, therefore below the lower than the minimum size of 1 nm that is considered to be the starting range for nanoformulations.

Inorganic Nanoparticles

Inorganic nanoparticles are those which are fabricated from materials without carbon. Such material could be either metal or metal oxides. Metals that have been used to fabricate nanoparticles (NP) are gold (Au), silver (Ag), platinum (Pt), cadmium (Cd), cobalt (Co), iron (Fe), copper (Cu), and zinc (Zn). Among metal oxides, iron oxide (Fe_2O_3), Aluminum oxide (Al_2O_3), zinc oxide (ZnO), silicon dioxide (SiO_2), titanium oxide (TiO_2), cerium oxide (CeO_2), *etc.* have been used for the preparation of NPs.

This section will primarily focus on gold nanoparticles since a vast number of studies can be found on gold nanoparticles for HCC therapy. Among different metallic nanoparticles, gold nanoparticles (AuNPs) are of particular interest since they are biocompatible, the surface can be easily functionalized, and suitable for carrying both small molecule and macromolecules.

Gold nanoparticles theoretically can be produced in two different ways, top-down and bottom-up. As the name suggests, "Top-down" means reducing particle size from bulk gold by applying energy which is not a viable method. The other process, "Bottom-up," is quite a straightforward process for preparing colloidal gold nanoparticles. The particle sizes can be easily controlled by changing the process parameters. Reduction of gold chloride to colloidal gold was reported almost 70 years before by Turkevich and coworkers (Turkevich *et al.*, 1951)(Turkevich *et al.*, 1953). Later on, Frens (Frens 1973) demonstrated how by controlling the process parameters, the particle size of monodisperse gold nanoparticles could be controlled between 16 nm to 150 nm. The process of manufacturing gold nanoparticles involved the reduction of gold chloride solution ($HAuCl_4$) by a reducing agent such as $AgNO_3$, $NaBH_4$, Na_3-citrate, *etc*. Nowadays, glycerol (Nalawade *et al.*, 2013) or thermophilic filamentous fungi (Molnár *et al.*, 2018) have been used for the green synthesis of gold nanoparticles. Usually, the reaction takes place at an elevated temperature and is completed within a minute after the addition of one reactant to others.

Instead of gold, other metals such as selenium, palladium nanoparticles could also be manufactured in quite similar ways. A few examples of such metallic nanoparticles and other metal oxide nanoparticles are provided in Table **2** below.

Various methods can perform surface modification of gold nanoparticles (AuNP). It could be done either by modifying the surface of AuNP by binding of the linker molecule using thiol-based coupling reaction or by sulfur ligands or by modification using phosphine or amine or by using polymer (Mahato *et al.*, 2019). Polymer modification of AuNP offers more excellent stability. A wide variety of polymers can be used. The polymer modification on the surface of AuNPcan is done at various stages of AuNP synthesis and in different ways. The polymer chain can grow from the scaffold attached to the surface of the AuNP ("grafting from" method). In the second method, the Au-NPs are synthesized in polymer aggregates ("grafting to" method). The surface modification can also be done after synthesis ("post-synthetic modification"), where AuNPs are first generated in a conventional way followed by physical adsorption of polymer on the surface (Mahato *et al.*, 2019).

Xue *et al.* (Xue *et al.*, 2016) reported delivery of miR-375 using AuNP to replace miRNA in HCC. miR-375 was covalently linked to AuNPs to form AuNP-mi--375. In a mice model, these nanoparticles demonstrated higher cellular uptake and successfully preserved miR-375's activity. Therefore, and AuNP-miR-375 NP was found to be an effective miR-375 replacement therapy without apparent toxicity.

In a recent study, negatively charged 5-FU was conjugated with AuNP and coated with chitosan. The modified AuNPs were internalized by cancerous cells more easily, and thereby, less drug concentration of AuNPs was required to achieve the same efficacy compared to free 5-FU. The combination of laser irradiation with 5-FU-AuNP significantly increased the effectiveness of killing cancerous cells (Salem *et al.*, 2018).

Besides small molecules, proteins and peptides have also been delivered using gold nanoparticles. AuNP core of 2 nm was conjugated with a peptide having a thiol group (Jha *et al.*, 2017). The peptide conjugated AuNPs were found to be well internalized by HepG2 cells. It could indicate the possible use of these nanoparticles for delivering a suitable therapeutic agent in HCC. The gold cores were synthesized in toluene. A thiol group subsequently displaced the amine on the gold to provide a protective layer around the gold nanoparticles. The thiol group was transferred from the cysteine side chain of the CysPreS1 (21–47) peptide.

The metal of metal oxide nanoparticles has the advantage of being more stable and easier to prepare than liposomes and lipid nanoparticles. However, metal and metal oxide nanoparticles have certain toxicological risks. Because of the size below 100 nm, these particles will be internalized by all cells by endocytosis (Müller *et al.*, 2011). Therefore, these smaller size particles can be considered high-risk particles. Since the metal and metal oxide particles are not biodegradable, they could remain inside the cells. Studies in animal models indicate that gold nanoparticles are slowly excreted through urine without systemic toxicity (Takeuchi *et al.*, 2017, Naz *et al.*, 2016). However, after intracellular uptake of metallic nanoparticles, depending on the type of nanoparticles, the acidic conditions of the cellular compartment could trigger the release of ions from the nanoparticles. These ions are responsible for cascading events, leading to intracellular toxicity (Sabella *et al.*, 2014). However, there is no toxicological data available from clinical studies.

Table 2. Metal or metal oxide nanoparticles for application in HCC.

Therapeutic Agent	Metal or Metal oxide core	Surface Modifier	Method	Mean Size (nm)	Advantage	References
miR-375	Gold	None	Reduction of gold chloride	36-53	High cellular uptake, increased therapeutic efficacy, and no apparent toxicity	(Xue *et al.*, 2016)
5-FU (5-Fluorouracil)	Gold	Chitosan	Reduction of gold chloride with chitosan solution	5-43	Higher cytotoxic effect of 5-F--Chitosan-AuNP compared to free 5-FU	(Salem *et al.*, 2018)
Doxorubicin	Selenium	Galactose	reduction of sodium selenite with Ascorbic acid	50-150	Improved cellular uptake, better proliferation suppression, and increased apoptosis of HepG2 cells	(Xia *et al.*, 2019)
MiR-375+Doxorubicin	Calcium carbonate	Lipid (DOPA or DOTAP & DSPE-PEG)	Reverse microemulsion	91-103	Efficient cellular uptake increased intracellular Dox accumulation and combined anti-tumor activity.	(Zhao *et al.*, 2017)
Sorafenib	iron oxide	PVA	Co-precipitation	5-15	Better anticancer efficiency than free sorafenib	(Tom *et al.*, 2018)

Organic Nanoparticles

Polymer Nanoparticles

A polymeric nanoparticle is composed of organic polymers and ideally has a matrix structure in which the drug is encapsulated. The polymers could be of a natural or synthetic source. Some of the natural polymers which are used in nanoparticles are as follows:

• Polysaccharides o Chitosan o Alginate o Dextran o Agarose o Pullulan	• Proteins o Albumin o Gelatin o Lecithin o Vicillin o Legumin

Among the polymers mentioned above, however, only a few, such as chitosan and albumin, have been used in nanoparticle fabrication. Many of the polymers mentioned above, such as alginate, are quite common in the preparation of microparticles but are not very commonly used in nanoparticle preparation. Chitosan, gelatin, and albumin are some of the natural polymers which are more commonly used in nanoparticle preparation.

Chitosan, a modified natural carbohydrate polymer, is prepared by partial N-deacetylation of crustacean-derived natural biopolymer chitin. Four different methods are commonly used to prepare chitosan nanoparticles: ionotropic gelation, microemulsion, emulsification solvent diffusion, and polyelectrolyte complex (PEC) (Tiyaboonchai, 2013). In the ionotropic gelation method, chitosan is dissolved in acetic acid with or without a stabilizing agent. Polyanion such as tripolyphosphate is added with mechanical stirring to enable the reaction of the amine group of chitosan with the negatively charged group of polyanion, leading to nanoprecipitation of chitosan nanoparticles. In the microemulsion method, chitosan is solubilized in acetic acid and glutaraldehyde and added to a surfactant-containing organic solvent like n-hexane under continuous stirring. Polyelectrolyte complex or PEC is formed when DNA solution is added to an acetic acid solution of chitosan in constant stirring, leading to charge neutralization and forming a self-assembled complex of positively charged polymer and plasmid DNA (Kumari *et al.*, 2010).

Gelatin is chemically a polyampholyte since it has both cationic and anionic groups as well as the hydrophilic group. Gelatin nanoparticles can be manufactured by either desolvation/coacervation or emulsion methods. In the desolvation/coacervation process, natural salt or alcohol is added to a gelatin solution under continuous stirring. It leads to liquid-liquid phase separation, leading to the separation of a transparent solution on the top of a polymer-rich dense phase at the bottom (Kumari *et al.*, 2010).

Similar to gelatin-nanoparticles, albumin-nanoparticles can also be manufactured by desolvation/coacervation or emulsification (Lee *et al.*, 2017). The desolvation/coacervation process is sometimes preferred over the emulsion method since the emulsion method needs organic solvent application (Langer *et al.*, 2003).

Natural polymers, however, suffer from stability issues, could create an immunogenic reaction, and have a batch-to-batch variability. The drawbacks of natural polymers mentioned above can be greatly avoided by using synthetic polymers. The advantage of synthetic polymers is that they are also biodegradable, biocompatible, and non-toxic like natural polymers, but at the same time, they are non-immunogenic and can be obtained with a very high purity grade. However, the biggest advantage of synthetic polymer is that by the flexibility of the synthetic process, the properties of the polymer can be tuned very easily.

Synthetic polymers that can be used in drug delivery are divided into two primary categories: Poly-ester (PE) and poly-alkyl-cyanoacrylates (PAC). Among them, the PE group of polymers is primarily used in drug delivery. PAC polymers are biocompatible as well as biodegradable since they are degraded by esterase in biological fluids. However, their biodegradation produces some toxic products that could stimulate or damage the central nervous system. Therefore the PAC polymer is not authorized for human use (Davis, 2000). We will, therefore, primarily focus on the manufacturing of PE nanoparticles. However, the manufacturing techniques of PAC nanoparticles are quite similar to PE nanoparticles.

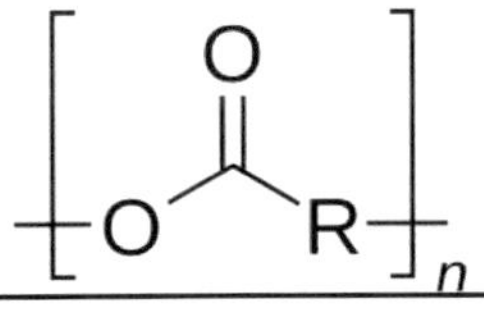	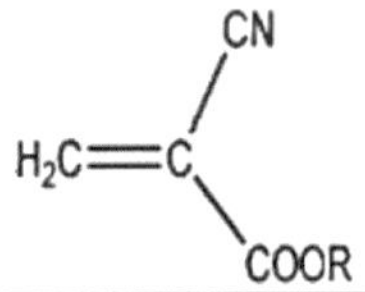
• Polyester o PLA: poly (lactic acid) o PLGA: poly (lactide-co-glycolide) o Polystyrene o Poly (ε -caprolactone)	• Poly (alkyl cyanoacrylates) o Poly(isobutyl cyanoacrylates) o poly (butylcyanoacrylates) o poly methyl (methcyanoacrylates)

In the last few decades, countless work has been carried out in the field of nanoparticle production using biodegradable, biocompatible, and non-toxic polymers. The production methods can be classified under two primary categories depending on whether a polymerization reaction is required or whether a preformed polymer is used to manufacture the nanoparticles (Reis *et al.*, 2006).

The polymerization method could be of two different types, as mentioned in Fig. (**1**). The emulsion polymerization method is a high-speed and easily scalable method. The continuous phase of emulsion could be organic or aqueous, whereas monomers are dispersed into an emulsion or into a material in which the monomer is not soluble. The polymerization process is initiated when a monomer molecule dissolved in the continuous phase collides with an initiator molecule. Polymerization methods have been used for preparing PMMA (polymethyl methacrylate) and PACA (polyalkylcyanoacrylate) nanoparticles (Reis *et al.*, 2006). However, the use of these polymers is restricted for human use.

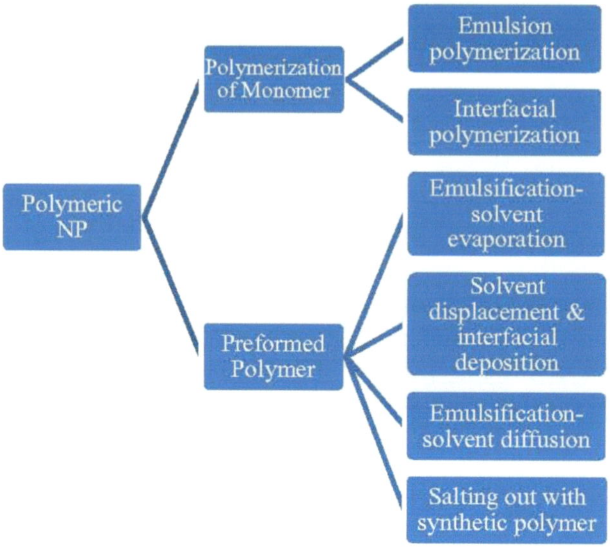

Fig. (1). Different processes for manufacturing polymeric nanoparticles.

Perhaps the most commonly used nanoparticles for drug delivery in humans are made up of preformed polymers. There are several techniques by which nanoparticles from preformed polymers can be manufactured. Primarily they are classified under four different categories: emulsification-solvent evaporation, emulsification-solvent diffusion, solvent displacement, and interfacial deposition, and salting out with synthetic polymers (Reis *et al.*, 2006). In the emulsification-solvent evaporation method, polymer solution in an organic solvent is emulsified into an aqueous phase followed by evaporation of the organic solvent leading to the formation of nanoparticles. Emulsification/solvent diffusion is quite similar to the previous method. The only difference is that the organic phase needs to be miscible with the aqueous phase so that it can diffuse out to the continuous aqueous phase, leading to salting-out or precipitation of the polymeric nanoparticles. The diffusion process can be accelerated by adding an additional aqueous phase. Solvent displacement and interfacial deposition are again similar to emulsification/solvent deposition. In this process, the solvent that solubilizes the polymer phase is mixed with the aqueous phase and diffuses out as soon as the emulsion is formed. However, there is an additional element, which is usually an oil phase, which is dissolved with the organic polymer phase, and that oil phase is not miscible with the aqueous phase. That essentially means that the polymer deposition and solidification happen between the interface of the internal oil phase and the external aqueous phase (Reis *et al.*, 2006). The salting-out process is a modified emulsification/solvent diffusion method, whereas the aqueous phase is an aqueous gel containing salting-out agents such as electrolytes (magnesium chloride, calcium chloride, *etc.*). The oil/water emulsion is diluted with a sufficient amount of water or aqueous phase to enhance the diffusion of the organic phase into the aqueous phase, leading to formation of nano-spheres. Different phases of the emulsions, as mentioned above, can have stabilizer depending on necessity.

We have reviewed below the different polymeric nanoparticles used for delivering therapeutic agents for HCC in Table **3**.

Table 3. Different examples of polymeric nanoparticles for application in HCC.

Therapeutic/Diagnostic Molecule	Polymer	Stabilizer	Surfactant Modifier	NP Method	Mean Size (nm)	DL, EE	Advantage	References
Curcumin+Sorafenib	Copolymers of N-isopropylacrylamide (NIPAAM), with N-vinyl-2-pyrrolidone (VP) and poly(ethyleneglycol)monoacrylate (PEG-A)	None	None	Solvent-antisolvent precipitation	Not available	DL: n/a EE: n/a	Significant decrease of HCC cell	(Hu *et al.*, 2015)
Sorafenib	TPGS-b-poly(caprolactone) &and Pluronic P123	None	anti-GPC3 antibody	Nanoprecipitation	85-99	DL: n/a EE: n/a	higher cellular uptake, greater cytotoxicity	(Gan *et al.*, 2018)
HCC -specific DNA	poly(beta-amino ester)	None	None	Nanoprecipitation	85-157	DL: n/a EE: n/a	high and preferential DNA delivery to HCC cells	(Zamboni *et al.*, 2017)
Vandetanib	copolymer poly(ethylene glycol)-block-poly(D, L-lactic acid)	None	iRGD, a tumor-penetrating peptide	Nanoprecipitation	40	DL: 3.9-4.3% EE: 83-91%	Improved potency compared to oral therapy	(Wang *et al.*, 2016)
Umbelliferone β--galactopyranoside	poly(d,l-lactide-*co*-glycolide)	polyvinyl alcohol / stearic acid / Tween 80	None	Double emulsion solvent technique	190-524	DL: not available EE: 58-90%	Higher hepatic accumulation of the active	(Kumar *et al.*, 2017)
Andrographolide	poly (ethylene glycol)-poly(lacti--co-glycolic acid)	D-α-tocopherol polyethylene glycol 1000 succinate	None	Emulsion solvent evaporation	120	DL: 9.1% EE: 89.6%	Efficient uptake by Hep3B liver cells and long retention in-vivo	(Zhang *et al.*, 2015a)
Apigenin	poly(d,l-lactide-*co*-glycolide)	None	None	multiple emulsion solvent evaporation	270-325	DL: 2-19% EE: n/a	Sustained drug release & successful liver targeting	(Bhattacharya *et al.*, 2018)
Quercetin&superparamagnetic iron oxide nanoparticles (SPION)	methoxy-poly(ethylene glycol)--oligo(ε-caprolacto-ne), mPEG750-b-OCL-Bz	None	None	film hydration method	22-55	Quercetin: DL: 3.5% EE: 70% SPION: DL: 0.8% EE: 15%	HCC Cell Uptake and higher cytotoxici-ty	(Srisa-Nga *et al.*, 2019)
Gemcitabine (GEM)and Antisense-microRNA	poly(d,l-lactide-*co*-glycolide)	None	Poly ethylene glycol	Double emulsion	148-232	DL: ~2% EE: ~40%	The decrease in HCC cell proliferation	(Devulapally *et al.*, 2016)

DL: Drug loading; EE: Encapsulation Efficiency; n/a: not available.

Solid Lipid Nanoparticles/ Nanostructured Lipid Carrier (Sln / Nlc) / Liquid Crystalline Nanoparticles (Lcn)

Lipid-based delivery systems have been widely used for drug targeting, including for the treatment of HCC. Solid Lipid Nanoparticles (SLN) can be considered as an alternative to the colloidal carrier systems such as emulsions, liposomes, and polymeric micro-and nanoparticles. The concept of SLN was firstly introduced in 1991. By definition, SLN is a spherical nanoparticle consisting of a solid lipid core stabilized with surfactants or co-surfactants or emulsifying agents with particle size in average 40 nm to 1000 nm (Mehnert and Mader, 2001, Muchow *et al.*, 2008, Naseri N, 2015). The term solid for the solid lipid refers to the lipid components of SLNs that are solid in the body and at ambient temperature. The solid lipids generally used are triglycerides, partial glycerides, fatty acids, steroids such as cholesterol, and waxes. Those lipids are obtained from physiological lipids; hence the lipid matrix is considered non-toxic (Mehnert and Mader, 2001). Surfactant concentrations used are 0.5 to 5%, and the choice of surfactants or co-surfactants has to be based on the route of administration to be safe for dispensing. In addition, SLNs are prepared in an aqueous environment; therefore, this makes SLNs more advantageous and safer than polymeric carriers, which have to be prepared using organic constituents (Naseri N, 2015). Due to their lipid component, SLNs are ideal for lipophilic drugs with poor aqueous solubility since they can dissolve in the lipid.

Nevertheless, one should also consider drug-lipid melt solubility, the physicochemical structure of solid lipid matrix, and the possibility of the lipid material (Shirodkar *et al.*, 2019). There are some advantages offered by SLNs such as low cost and simple preparation, feasibility for high-scale production, availability of biocompatible as well as biodegradable lipids, and cheaper compared to the polymeric carrier. Despite those advantages, SLNs also hold disadvantages, such as being prone to lipid particle growth, the occurrence of polymeric transitions, and the low drug loading due to the crystalline structure (Naseri N, 2015). In addition, one should carefully consider the occurrence of drug expulsion when using lipids that form particles that are highly crystalline with perfect lattice (Shirodkar *et al.*, 2019). In the later advancement, the concept of nanostructured lipid carrier (NLC) was then introduced to overcome the lack of SLNs, mainly due to drug expulsion.

In contrast to SLNs, NLC combines solid lipids with spatially incompatible liquid lipids, thereby resulting in special nanostructures (Müller *et al.*, 2002). Such nanostructures are the formation of unstructured or imperfect crystal structures; therefore, drug expulsion risk can be avoided during manufacturing and storage. Besides, crystals imperfection provides more space for the drug to dissolve and is also loaded in the liquid lipid part. Consequently, higher loading capacity can be obtained compared to SLNs. Controllable release profiles are also shown by NLCs (Ghasemiyeh and Mohammadi-Samani, 2018). Fig. (**2**) illustrates the lipid structure of SLNs in comparison to NLCs.

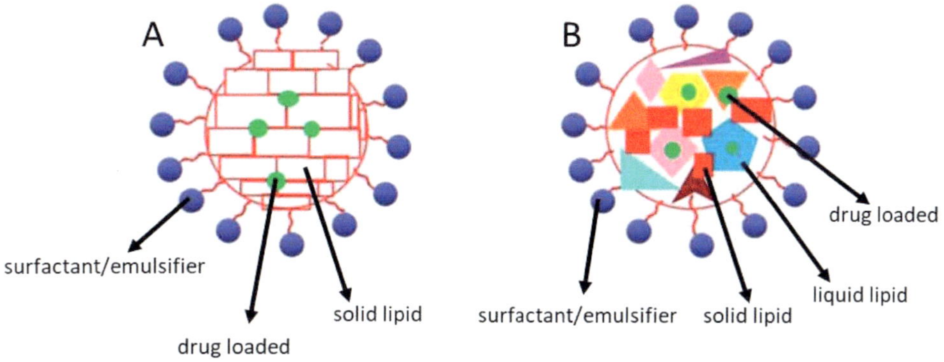

Fig. (2). Theoretical concept of (A) SLN with regular lipid brick-layers; (B) NLC with unstructured crystals.

Lipids in SLNs and NLCs are beneficial for delivering poorly water-soluble drugs and drug targeting to the cells due to the cellular uptake and intracellular trafficking processes of the lipids (Yu B, 2014). Additionally, some ligands targeted for HCC cells and protein materials such as siRNA and miRNA can also be incorporated into lipids with certain modifications. Tables **4** and **5** describe the progress of drug delivery of HCC therapeutic agents based on the SLNs and NLCs platform, respectively.

Table 4. Researches on SLNs for HCC therapeutic agents from the year 2010 to 2020.

Drug and Substance	**Composition**	**Preparation Method**	**DL, EE (%)**	**Zeta Potential and Particle Size**	**References**
Cucurbitacin B N-hexadecyllactobionamide (N-HLBA),	Lipid: Compritol® 888 Emulsifier: soybean lecithin/ Pluronic F 68/Tween 80	HPH	DL: n/a EE: 90.7	123-135 nm; z.p = (-)34.3 mV, (-) 31.6mV	(Wang *et al.*, 2012b)
Plasmid pCMS-EGFP, dextran, protamine	Dotap, Precirol® ATO 5 Surfactant: Tween 80	Solvent emulsification-evaporation method	DL: n/a EE: n/a	284.23 ± 11.87 ; z.p: (+) 30.6 ±6.47	(Delgado *et al.*, 2012)

(Table 4) cont.....

Drug and Substance	Composition	Preparation Method	DL, EE (%)	Zeta Potential and Particle Size	References
Quercetin	Cholesterol/lecithin/cetyl alcohol Surfactant: Tween 80	Lipids phase (in organic solvent) added to tween 20 (aqueous phase)then rotary evaporated.	DL: n/a EE: 99.9	78.0 ± 7.0 nm, the z.p of 22.7 ± 1.3 mV	(Varshosaz *et al.*, 2014)
n/a	Imwitor 900K/Compritol 888 ATO Surfactant: cetyltrimethylammonium bromide (CTAB), poloxamer 188, Miranol® C-32 Ultra	High shear homogenization	DL: n/a EE: n/a	159 to 180 nm ; (+) 60.3 to 64.2	(Doktorovova *et al.*, 2014a, Doktorovová *et al.*, 2014b)
shRNA74 plasmid, protamine, dextran, hyaluronic acid	Dotap, Precirol® ATO 5 Surfactant: Tween 80	solvent emulsification-evaporation method	DL: n/a EE: n/a	208 to 242 nm; z.p: (+/-) 29 to 38.87 mV	(Torrecilla *et al.*, 2014)
Sorafenib, superparamagnetic iron oxide nanoparticles (SPIONs)	Cetylpalmitate Surfactant: Tween 80	Hot homogenization technique	DL: n/a EE: 90	248 ± 113 nm; z.p: −23.0 ± 5.3 mV	(Grillone *et al.*, 2015)
Sorafenib	Glycerylbehenate/soybean lecithin Surfactant: poloxamer 188	high-speed shearing and ultrasonic treatment.	DL: 5.4 EE: 89.9	77.16 nm; z.p: 18.1 mV	(Wang *et al.*, 2018)
shNUPR1 plasmid	Precirol ATO 5 Surfactants: DDAB and Brij 76,	Ethanolic precipitation in combination with high-pressure homogenization	DL: n/a EE: n/a	185 nm ; z.p: 43.3 mV	Botto *et al* 2018, Doktorovova *et al.*, 2014a, Doktorovova *et al.*, 2014b
Ganoderic Acid	CapmulMCMC10 Emulsifier: soy lecithin	hot-homogenization and solvent diffusion method	DL: 11.5 EE: 66	73 nm,	Rahman *et al.*, 2021
Resveratrol	Capmul MCM C10 Surfactants: Cetyltrimethyl ammonium bromide (CTAB),Tween 80	Hot high-pressure homogenization	DL = 24.3 EE = 83.8	139 nm ; z.p: 50.25 mV	Rahman *et al.*, 2020

DL: Drug Loading; EE: Entrapment Efficiency; n/a: not available.

Table 5. Researches on NLCs for HCC therapeutic agents from the year 2010 to 2020.

Drug and Substance	NLC Composition	Preparation Method	DL, EE (%)	Zeta Potential and Particle Size	References
5-fluorouracil (5-FU); N-stearyllactobionamide (N-SALB).	glycerylmonostearate/oleic acid /lecithin glycerylmonostearate/mixture of capric and caprylic acid triglyceride (Labrafac)/lecithin Surfactant: Tween 80 or Solutol® HS15 (polyethylene glycol (PEG) hydroxyl Stearate)	Emulsification solvent diffusion method.	DL: 1.7- 7.2 EE:8.4- 38.7	135.7 nm to 181.0 nm; z.p: (-)26.4 mV to (-)4.0 mV ;	(Varshosaz *et al.*, 2012)
Curcumin, Glycyrrhetinic acid (GA)	Glycerol monostearate / Miglyol 812N Surfactant: Polyoxyethylene 40 Strearate PEGylated with DSPE-PEG_{2000}	Film ultrasound method	DL: 2.2- 2.3 EE: 90.1- 97.1	123.1 nm to 132. 7 nm; z.p: (-)17.1 to (-)14.8 mV	(Chu *et al.*, 2014)
Tyrphostin AG-1478	NLC A: solid un-PEGylated lipid (a mixture of mono-, di- and tri-glycerides of behenic acid; Compritol 888 ATO) NLC B: solid PEGylated lipid (behenoylpolyoxyl-8 glycerides; Compritol HD5ATO) NLC C: a mixture of Tripalmitin with un-PEGylated (glyceryl tri caprylate/caprate medium-chain triglycerides; Captex 355EP/NF) liquid lipid NLC D: a mixture of Tripalmitin with PEGlyated liquid lipid (polyoxyethylenecaprylic/capric glycerides; Acconon CC-)	precipitation method	NLC A: DL: 2.8 EE: 28 NLC B: DL: 1.7 EE: 17 NLC C: DL: 24 EE: 70 NLC D: DL:24 EE: 70	NLC A 176.2 nm; z.p: (-)30.3 ±7.7 NLC B: 80.1nm z.p: (-) 28.5 ± 10.3 NLC C: 209.7 nm; z.p: (-)46.9 ± 8.4 ; NLC D: 189.3 nm; z.p: (-)38.4 ± 6.5	(Bondì *et al.*, 2014)

(Table 5) cont.....

Drug and Substance	NLC Composition	Preparation Method	DL, EE (%)	Zeta Potential and Particle Size	References
Sorafenib	NLC A: Tripalmitin/ Caprylic/ Capric Triglyceride (Captex 355 EP/NF) NLC B: Tripalmitin/Triglycerides, Medium-Chain (Miglyol 812) Emulsifier: Epikuron 200 (lecithin), sodium taurocholate	Precipitation method	NLC-A: DL: 18.5 EE: 100 NLC B: DL: 10.3 EE: 58.5	NLC-A: 221.3 nm ; z.p: (-)40.3 ± 8.74 NLC B: 186 nm ; z.p: (-) 33.5 ± 4.97	(Bondi *et al.*, 2015)
Doxorubicin, Curcumin	Precirol ATO/Labrafac Lipophile WL 1349/ Lipoid S75 Emulsifier: Cremophor RH 40	high pressure microfluidics technique	EE:97.1–99.8	88.8 ±5.6 nm ; z.p: (-)14.3 ±2.4 mV	Zhao 2015

DL: Drug-load; EE:Encapsulation Efficiency ; n/a: not available.

Lipids and Surfactants in SLNs and NLCs

The selection of type and composition of lipids and surfactants/emulsifiers can also be tricky when designing SLNs or NLCs. A higher concentration of surfactant leads to a smaller particle size obtained. Although most of the lipids used are biocompatible and biodegradable, the nature of the lipid and surfactant concentration affects cell viability (Pizzol CD, 2014). About the selection of lipids, better drug solubility was found in medium-chain triglycerides (MCT) compared to long-chain triglycerides (LCD). Stearic acid and its derivatives are commonly used due to its origin as a natural biocompatible fat and safe to use. The ability of stearic acid to penetrate cancer cells and also accumulate in the cytoplasm makes this fat a favorable lipid for the delivery of anti-cancer drugs. For liquid lipids, oleic acid is the most common to be used. The colorless and odorless characteristic of oleic acid enables this lipid to be utilized in drug delivery (Subramaniam, 2020).

About the type of surfactants, an investigation by Silva *et al.*(Silva AH, 2012)reported the high toxicity of SLNs prepared with sodium dodecyl sulfate, an anionic surfactant. In general, non-ionic surfactants are considered to have lower toxicity compared to anionic surfactants. Nevertheless, certain non-ionic surfactants such as Beheneth-25 were found to have stronger irritation potency than SDS(Subramaniam, 2020). Besides, the use of cationic surfactants gives advantages for the delivery of genes. The surface of the gene possesses a negative charge; therefore, interaction with positively charged SLNs would be beneficial for encapsulating the gene into SLNs. There are some problems with the i.v delivery of the naked DNA and they include nuclease digestion, hepatic uptake clearance that causes early elimination of DNA from circulation, and toxicity induction due to aggregation hemagglutination in the transfection process. Delivering the gene using the SLN platform with cationic surfactant can overcome those problems (Delgado *et al.*, 2012). Another advantage of cationic surfactants in comparison to anionic surfactants is their higher serum proteins affinity and cell membranes. It could also facilitate the uptake and interaction of drugs delivered with a cellular receptor (Doktorovová *et al.*, 2014). In another study, Doktorovova *et al.* (Doktorovova *et al*, 2014b) have proven that the use of cationic surfactant CTAB, non-ionic block copolymer poloxamer 188, and an amphoteric surfactant Miranol® C-32 Ultra (Sodium Cocoamphoacetate) showed no genotoxicity and could preserve cells viability. Either SLNs or NLCs can be added with the components that can improve *in vitro* and *in vivo* efficacy by increasing transfection and cellular uptake. Protamine, dextran, oligochitosans and hyaluronic acid are examples of such components (Torrecilla *et al.*, 2014).

Manufacturing of SLNs and NLCs

In general, there are five methods to produce SLNs and NLCs: (1) high-pressure homogenization(HPH); (2) solvent emulsification/evaporation; (3)melt emulsification and ultrasonication; (4) microemulsion; (5) solvent injection (Mehnert and Mader, 2001, Subramaniam, 2020). HPH is the most preferred method and has already been applied for commercial scale. This process can be done in two ways: the hot process and the cold process. The hot process initially started from pre-emulsion preparation by melting drugs and lipids together and mixing with an aqueous emulsifier/surfactants at the same temperature using a high-shear mixer. The pre-emulsion is then passed through the high-pressure homogenizer to obtain SLNs or NLCs, which are then cooled at room temperature or below. Drug solubilized in melted lipid should have high stability against high temperature during melting and the high-pressure homogenization process. For the cold method, lipid and drug are melted together but rapidly cooled using liquid nitrogen or dry ice. Cooled drug-loaded lipid is milled to obtain 50-100 μm in size and suspended in chilled emulsifier solution. The pre-suspension is then nanosized using HPH. Compared to the hot process, the cold process results in bigger and wider particle sizes, but such a method could minimize thermal exposure to the drugs. Besides HPH, nanosizing can also be done using a microfluidizer (Mehnert and Mader, 2001).

The second common approach is solvent emulsification/evaporation. In this method, lipid and drug are dissolved in a miscible organic solvent, evaporated, then dispersed in an aqueous emulsifier or surfactant, and mixed in a high-shear mixer such as ultra-turrax or HPH(Mehnert and Mader, 2001). Nevertheless, this method might not be feasible for a large scale due to the massive organic solvent removal process.

The third approach is based on melt emulsification and ultrasonication. Lipid and drug are melted then dispersed in a hot aqueous surfactant/emulsifier. The temperature of the aqueous surfactant/emulsifier is the same as the temperature of the melted lipid drug. Mixing was conducted with the aid of a stirrer, then continued with a probe sonicator. The dispersion is then rapidly cooled. This method is considered simple with the avoidance of organic solvent, yet the availability of sonicator probes for large scale is the main obstacle for scaling up SLNs or NLCs. In addition, metal contamination of the probe hinders the utilization of this method for a large manufacturing scale [Subramanian 2019]. In the microemulsion method, lipid and drug are melted together and blended into a hot aqueous surfactant/emulsifier solution and then agitated to form a microemulsion then dispersed in cold water to rapidly recrystallize the oil droplets and ultrafiltrated or lyophilized to remove the excess of water. The difficulties in scaling up this method lie in the ultrafiltration process, while lyophilization could modify the physical characteristics of the SLNs and NLCs. In addition, such an approach is time-consuming. The last method is a solvent injection based on precipitation.

The solvent injection method is done by dissolving lipid and drug in a miscible organic solvent, injecting it rapidly into an aqueous surfactant/emulsifier solution using an injection needle. This process will precipitate lipid-drug particles, and precipitants are then filtered. This method can avoid high heat, shear stress, and special equipment, but organic solvent is used (Subramaniam, 2020).

Liquid Crystalline Nanoparticles (LCN) are self-assembled structures formed when polar lipids (*e.g*, monoolein) are exposed to polar environments in the presence of suitable surfactants. The assembled structures are usually of non-lamellar and have both lipophilic and hydrophilic regions, which can carry the drug molecules of different types such as hydrophobic drugs, hydrophilic drugs, and amphiphilic drugs in different layers(Madheswaran *et al.*, 2019). Multiple such single structures can further be assembled together to generate a bigger structure, which has both rigidity and fluidity, which ensures stability, higher drug loading, and sustained drug release. Suppose amphiphilic lipids are self-assembled to produce LCNs. In that case, these can have the advantages of both liposomes and NPs, since they, on the one hand, provide protection of the entrapped compound and, on the other hand, provide sustained release of the compound solubilized in the LCN matrix. Although the LCN could be a very effective targeted drug delivery vehicle, few challenges limit their intravenous administration, namely, bioadhesive leading to adhesion in non-targeted tissues, rapid removal from circulation by MPS (mononuclear phagocytic system), and toxicity leading to excessive hemolysis (Barauskas *et al.*, 2010). However, these challenges could be solved by coating the LCNs, and such surface coating modifies to avoid the adhesion to the non-targeted tissue and thereby reduce the toxicity. Such surface modification can also provide a stealth effect to prevent removal by MPS. Such surface modification can also be done as a single layer or multilayered structure. Liquid crystalline nanoparticles (LCN) have been used to deliver Sorafenib (SF) (Thapa *et al.*, 2015), the first drug approved by the FDA for the treatment of advanced hepatocellular carcinoma. However, the clinical application of Sorafenib is restricted by its poor water solubility and various side effects such as nausea, diarrhea, fatigue, skin rash, hand-foot syndrome, high blood pressure, *etc.* (Xie *et al.*, 2012). Nanoparticles that can control and target the release of SF to the specific tumor site can be used to reduce or overcome the side effects mentioned above (Wang *et al.*, 2011, Zhang *et al.*, 2011a).

The manufacturing of such LCN involves melting the hydrophobic phase besides the drug in the molten hydrophobic phase. In that phase, an aqueous surfactant or stabilizer is added with continuous mixing (Thapa *et al.*, 2015). However, the production process often requires high energy dispersion to enable lipid particles of 1-1000 nm size. High energy dispersion techniques such as ultrasonication, high shear homogenizer (such as Ultra-Turrax™), and high-pressure homogenizer (such as AvestinEmulsiflex™) are used. Especially with a high-pressure homogenizer, a relatively uniform particle size dispersion with particle size below 200 nm is possible to produce within a couple of minutes (Boyd *et al.*, 2009). Particle size can be varied by varying the pneumatic pressure and the time of homogenization. High-pressure homogenization technology also provides the flexibility of scaling up from lab scale (AvestinEmulsiFlex C-5, capacity ca. 1-5L/hr, minimum sample: 7 ml) to pilot scale (AvestinEmulsiFlex C-50, capacity ca. 10-50L/hr, minimum sample 25 ml) to commercial scale (AvestinEmulsiFlex C-500 & C-1000, capacity ca. 500+L/hr, minimum sample 5L) with adjustable pressure control up to 2000 bar (Fig. **3**).

Surface modification is usually achieved by adding polymer solution (PLL, PEG, *etc.*) or derivatized polymer solution to the LCN formulation. Step-by-step addition of different polymer solutions is developed to build the multilayer protection of the surface.

AvestinEmulsiFlex C-5 (source Avestin.com)	AvestinEmulsiFlex C-50 (source Avestin.com)	AvestinEmulsiFlex C-500 (source Avestin.com, the picture is distorted by Avestin to protect intellectual property
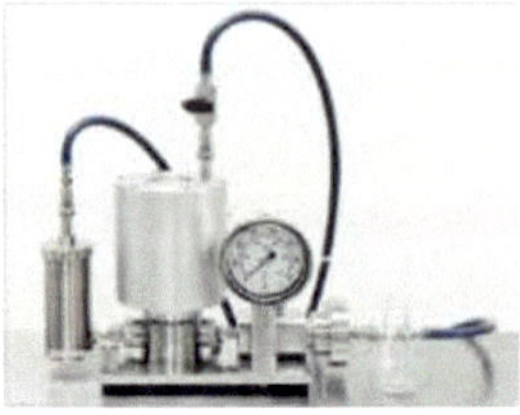	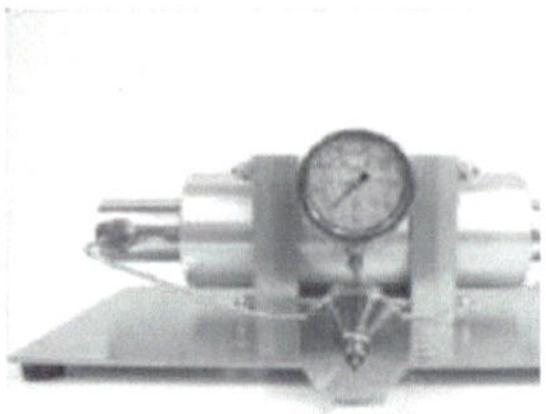	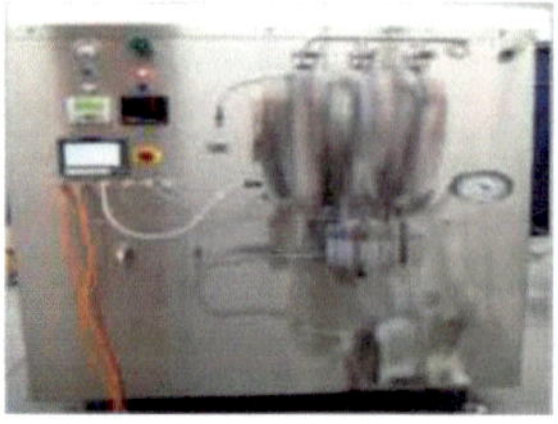

Fig. (3). Different types of equipment for manufacturing lipid nanoparticles.

The primary requirement of the formation of the liquid crystalline phase is the self-assembly of amphiphilic molecules. Monoolein (MO), having the chemical name 1-Monoolein [1-(cis-9-Octadecenoyl)-rac-glycerol] and Phytantriol(PHY) having the chemical name 3,7,11,15-Tetramethylhexadecane-1,2,3-triol, are two such lipids. In contrast, the first one has been widely used in pharmaceuticals, food and the second one in cosmetic and food products (Madheswaran *et al.*, 2019). PHY has no ester linkage and instead contains phytanyl, functional groups. Due to that cause, PHY is less susceptible than MO to be degraded by lipase, and hence PHY can retain a liquid crystalline structure under physiological conditions (Akbar *et al.*, 2017, Tran *et al.*, 2018, Madheswaran *et al.*, 2019).

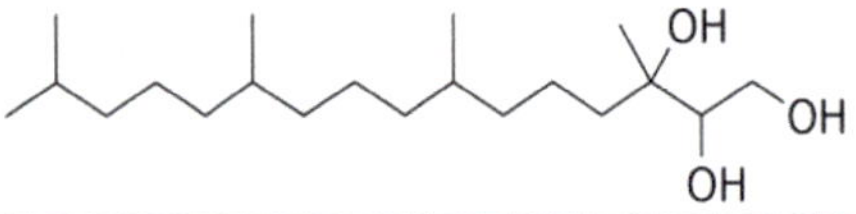	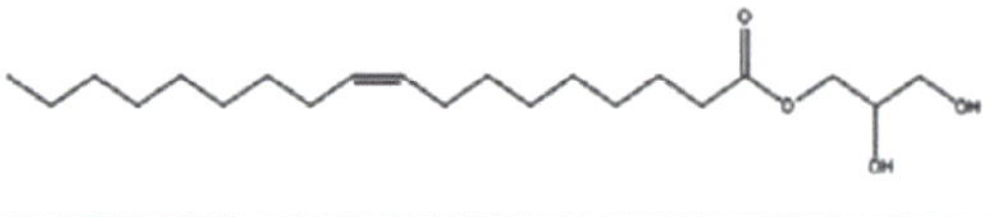
Phytantriol (PHY)	1-Monoolein

Such amphiphilic self-assembled structure forms various mesophases or intermediate phases between liquid and solid. Such mesophases could be of different shapes, such as cubic, micellar, and hexagonal. Among them, hexagonal and cubic phases have been widely studied in drug delivery. The hexagonal phases are composed of 2D hexagonal lattices arranged in micellar cylinder form by lipid self-assembly. Hexagonal phases are classified as either normal (H1) or inverse (H2), depending on whether the hydrocarbon chains are orientated towards the inner core (H1) or whether the chains have a polar head (H2). The H2 phase forms a channel of water inside the micellar cylinder, and there is no contact with water between the inside and outside of the aqueous domain (Madheswaran *et al.*, 2019) (Fig. **4** & Table **6**).

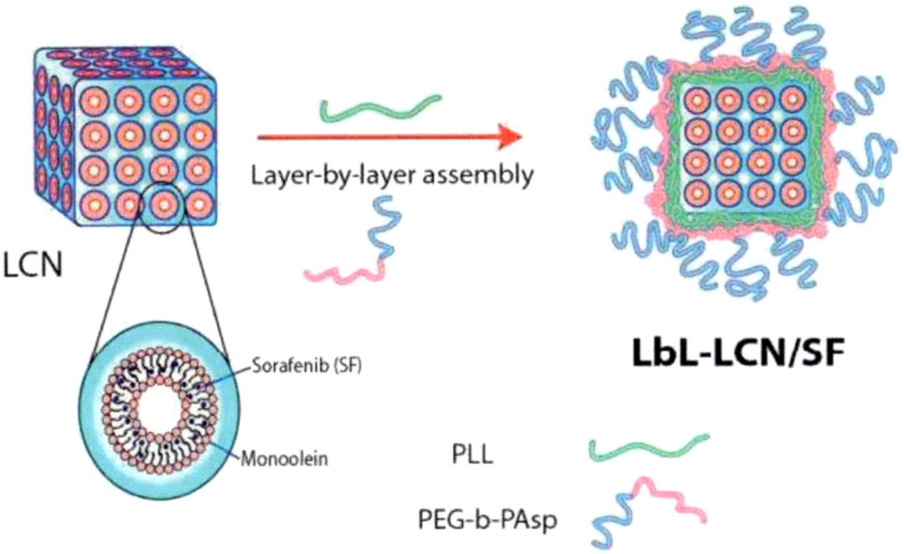

Fig. (4). Schematic representation of fabrication of layer-by-layer polymer-assembled sorafenib-loaded liquid crystalline nanoparticles (LbL-LCN/SF). Reprinted with permission from (Thapa *et al.*, 2015). Copyright (2015) American Chemical Society.

Table 6. Researches on LCNs for HCC Therapeutic Agents from the year 2010 to 2020.

Therapeutic Agent	Lipid Phase	Stabilizer / Surfactant	Surface Modifier	Manufacturing	Mean Size (nm)	Drug Loading (DL) and Encapsulation Efficiency (EE) (%)	Advantage	Refs.
Sorafenib	Monoolein	P407	PEG-b-PAsp	Sonication	140-160	DL:1.9-2.4 EE:80-100	High cellular uptake and greater apoptotic effects in HepG2 cells	(Thapa *et al.*, 2015)
Imatinib Mesylate	Glycerylmonooleate	P407	Lactoferrin + PEG	Sonication	120	DL: 13.6-15.1 EE: 85-96	Superior pharmacokinetic performance and targeted delivery to HCC	(Nisha *et al.*, 2020)
siRNA	(DOA-CA) Dioleostearin-3-amino-1, 2-propanediol (DOA) with citraconic anhydride through ring-opening reaction	Oleic oil	None	Sonication	170 – 286	DL: 50 EE: 100	high siRNA delivery efficiency with low toxicity	(He *et al.*, 2018)
Curcumin	Monoolein	P407	None	Sonication	233 - 271	DL: 2.5 EE: 100	Higher stability and cellular uptake of curcumin	(Baskaran *et al.*, 2014)

(Table 6) cont.....

Therapeutic Agent	Lipid Phase	Stabilizer / Surfactant	Surface Modifier	Manufacturing	Mean Size (nm)	Drug Loading (DL)and Encapsulation Efficiency (EE) (%)	Advantage	Refs.
Curcumin	Monoolein	P407 + SLS	None	Sonication	210-246	DL: 50-70 EE: not available	Hydrotrope formation due to SLS increased NP stability and modified curcumin release profile. No *in vivo* result reported	(de Souza *et al.*, 2020)
Sorafenib+Curcumin	polyethylene glycol (PEG) derivative of vitamin E succinate (PEG-VES)	None	None	Thin-film hydration	85	Sorafenib: DL: 6.5 EE:98.2 Curcumin: DL:13.6 EE:91.7	Improved tissue targeting, *in vitro* cytotoxicity, cell apoptosis in HCC cells, and *in vitro* antiangiogenesis capability	(Cao *et al.*, 2015)
Rapamycin	monoolein	P407	Layer by layer coating with chitosan & hyaluronic acid	Stirring	141	DL: Not available EE: 96.1	Increased bioavailability, higher inhibition of tumor growth, enhanced animal survival, reduced nephrotoxicity	(Freag *et al.*, 2016)

Nanocrystal / Nanosuspension

Drug nanosuspensions are aqueous dispersion of drug crystals in nanometer size, stabilized with stabilizing agents known as surface modifiers. The size of particles in nanosuspensions, in general, is below 1000 nm and is often referred to as colloidal sub-micron. The stabilizing agent can be surfactants (anionic, cationic, nonionic), polymers, or a combination of both (Rabinow, 2004). According to the Noyes-Whitney equation, smaller particle size would increase the surface area; hence, dissolution rate would also increase as explained in the following equation:

$$\frac{dC_x}{d_t} = \frac{D \times A}{h}(C_s - C_x)$$

Dissolution rate (dCx/dt) is equal to the diffusion coefficient (D), surface area (A) and concentration of the dissolved substance at a given time t (Cx), and solubility concentration of the substance (Cs). The h is the thickness of the diffusion layer. In addition to the increasing dissolution rate, solubility significantly increases when the particle size is under 200 nm (Kipp, 2004). As proposed (Butler and Dressman, 2010), there are four biopharmaceutics classification systems of drugs:

BCS class I, BCS class II, BCS class III, and BCS class IV. The BCS class II can be divided into IIa for the drugs with a limited dissolution rate and BCS IIb for the drugs with limited solubility. Based on the Noyes-Whitney equation, nanosuspension is more suitable to overcome BCS class IIa drugs (Möschwitzer, 2013). Nevertheless, this does not limit the possibility that nanosuspension can also overcome drugs with solubility problems.

As the drug particle size decreases, a larger surface area is formed, thus increasing Gibbs free energy (ΔG) as described in the following equation:

$$\Delta G = \Delta A \times \gamma s/l$$

ΔA is the total surface area of the dispersed particles, and $\gamma_{s/l}$ is the interfacial tension of solid/liquid. Accordingly, surface area and interfacial tension should be reduced to maintain free energy at its lowest state. Consequently, reduction of surface area will occur *via* particle agglomerations, and this is unfavorable for nanosuspensions. Therefore, the stabilizing agent is required to prevent agglomerations and to improve the wettability of the hydrophobic drug dispersed and consequently reduce the interfacial tension. The protection mechanism of the stabilizing agent against agglomeration depends on the type of stabilizing agent used in nanosuspensions, as detailed in Fig. (**5**).

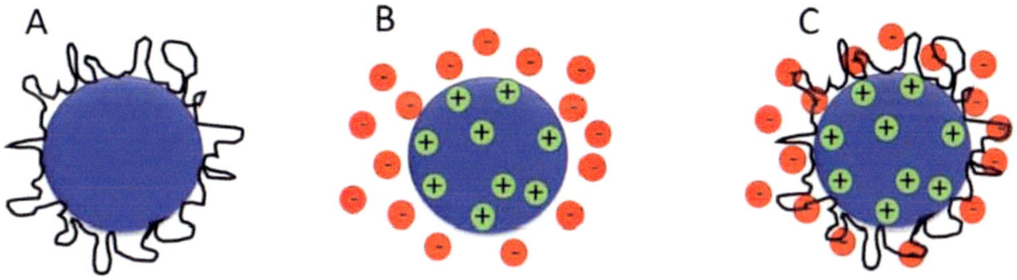

Fig. (5). Stabilization of a dispersed particle by: (A) Steric stabilization; (B) Electrostatic stabilization; (C) Electrosteric stabilization.

Steric stabilization is provided by polymer or nonionic surfactants by the adsorption of stabilizers on the surface of the dispersed particles. The ionic surfactants provide stabilization *via* electrostatic repulsion from the charge of the ions, which are adsorbed on the surrounding of the dispersed particles. Combining polymer or nonionic surfactant with ionic surfactant will form an electrostatic stabilization mechanism (Wu *et al.*, 2011).

Considering that nanosuspensions consist only of pure drug crystals and stabilizing agents, proper selection of the stabilizing agent is critical. For drug delivery, the main criteria of the stabilizing agent are accepted as Generally

Recognized as Safe (GRAS) as listed by the FDA. Based on the GRAS list, there are some ionic surfactants that can be used as stabilizing agents for nanosuspensions. One of those is sodium dodecyl sulfate (SDS). Based on the study conducted to screen potential nanosuspensions stabilizing agents, SDS showed the highest ability to stabilize nanosuspension (Lestari *et al.*, 2015). Nevertheless, SDS use is limited for non-parenteral use, as stated by European Medicines Agency (EMA) due to its irritation effect(EMA, 2017). Nonionic surfactants and polymers are more promising as stabilizing agents for nanosuspensions; thus, they are acceptable as an excipient for both parenteral and nonparenteral routes. Compared to other drug delivery systems based on drug encapsulation, nanosuspensions are considered a non-encapsulation process; hence, 100% drug load efficiency can be achieved, and drug-load can be up to 40% (Liu *et al.*, 2011). Additionally, nanosuspension can be prepared in aqueous media and hence eliminates the need for organic solvent removal (Möschwitzer, 2013).

Nanosuspensions Containing HCC Therapeutic Agents

Research published from the year 2010 to 2020 for nanosuspensions of HCC therapeutic agents is summarized in Table 7. In general, poloxamer as a non-ionic triblock copolymer is frequently utilized as a stabilizing agent for nanosuspensions containing HCC therapeutic agents either for oral or i.v route. Poloxamer 188, a triblock copolymer, has specialty due to its anchor blocks that are partially soluble but strongly adsorbed to the surface of the dispersed particle, and its hydrophilic portions adhere onto the hydrophobic portions. In a study for the macrophageal uptake, after 1h incubation with macrophages and identification using Prussian blue staining, it was observed that nanoparticles coated with poloxamer 188 were not identified by the macrophageal cell, suggesting the ability of poloxamer 188 to avoid the macrophages (Jain *et al.*, 2013). Therefore, poloxamer 188 as stabilizing agent provides an additional benefit for the targeted delivery of nanosuspensions containing therapeutic agents of HCC. In addition to the original concept of nanosuspension, there is lipid-based nanosuspension (Yang *et al.*, 2016, Pang *et al.*, 2019, Zhang *et al.*, 2014a). In this concept, soya lecithin, a water-dispersible phospholipid, is used as a stabilizing agent. The use of phospholipid is more beneficial than nonionic surfactants and polymers due to its higher capability to solubilize poorly soluble and poorly permeable drugs, modification of uptake and release of the drug, and protection from degradation in the GIT tract (Singh *et al.*, 2017). About the size, nanosuspensions with a size less than 100 nm can escape MPS but are susceptible to non-phagocytotic cells, while particle size >100 nm will be eliminated quickly from the bloodstream and taken up by macrophages. Outside the nanometer range (>1000 nm), particles will accumulate in the lungs and cause thrombosis inducing adverse effects post i.v injection (Wang *et al.*, 2012c). An additional feature of drug nanosuspensions is its adhesivity on biological surfaces; hence this could extend absorption time as observed for the absorption of silybin in beagle dogs (Wang *et al.*, 2012c). Lipid-based nanosuspensions also enable PEGylation to give a stealth effect for double protection of the dispersed drug particles *in vivo* and the possibility of ligand attachment for targeted delivery (Pang *et al.*, 2019).

Table 7. Researches on nanosuspension of HCC therapeutic agents from 2010 to 2020.

Drug and Substance	Stabilizing Agent	Method	Size (nm)	References
Glycyrrhizic acid	n/a	SAS and HPH	80. 4	(Zhang *et al.*, 2011b)
Silybin	Poloxamer 188/lecithin/HPMC	HPH	132 to 637	(Wang *et al.*, 2012c)
N3-o-toluyl-fluorouracil	Soya-lecithin	HPH	43.85	(Li *et al.*, 2013)
Berberine	D-α-tocopheryl polyethylene glycol 1000 succinate/ hydroxypropylmethylcellulose	HPH	72.4	(Wang *et al.*, 2014a)
N_3 -O-toluyl-fluorouracil	Soyalecithin	HPH	180.03	(Zhang *et al.*, 2014a)
Curcumin	Poloxamer 188/Hypromellose	HPH	231.2	(Wang *et al.*, 2014b)
Puerarin	Poloxamer 188	HPH	218.5	(Lu *et al.*, 2015)
Sorafenib	Soyphosphatidylcholine	precipitation	164.5	(Yang *et al.*, 2016)
Docetaxel and peptide GCNGRCGC-SH	Lecithin/glycerol	Thin film hydration	100	(Pang *et al.*, 2019)
Betulinic acid	Polyvinylpyrrolidone (PVP) K29-32/sodium dodecyl sulphate	Anti-solvent precipitation method	129.7	(Li *et al.*, 2020a)

n/a: not applicable; SAS: Supercritical anti-solvent; HPH: High-Pressure Homogenization.

Manufacturing of Nanosuspensions

In principle, there are three methods for producing nanosuspensions: (1) bottom-up, (2) top-down, (3) a combination of bottom-up and top-down. The bottom-up method is a basic technique developed to produce nanosuspensions where the drug is first dissolved and then processed for precipitation. Sinha *et al.*(Sinha and Möschwitzer, 2013) classified the bottom-up method as follows: liquid solvent-antisolvent addition precipitation, supercritical fluid precipitation, and solvent removal precipitation with the aid of high energy process. The other method can also be categorized as a combination method (bottom-up and top-down). The liquid solvent-antisolvent precipitation technique is considered the most feasible and economical. According to the process, the drug is dissolved in an appropriate water-miscible solvent and then mixed with a miscible antisolvent, mainly water. The second approach is based on the supercritical fluid in which the drug is dissolved in supercritical solvents such as carbon dioxide, ammonia, fluroroform, ethane, and ethylene. Supercritical antisolvent (SAS) is one of the supercritical fluid methods which is commonly applied. This method overcomes the problem with the drugs which are insoluble in the supercritical fluid by dissolving them in a supercritical antisolvent-miscible organic solvent. The precipitation process was conducted by mixing the drug solution with a compressed fluid as antisolvent either *via* spraying the antisolvent into solution or in reverse. The solvent removal method is the same as the liquid solvent-antisolvent method, but with the addition of cryoprotectant in the antisolvent. The mixing process is then followed by solvent removal treatment, for example, by freeze-drying.

The top-down method is principally particle size reduction using a mechanical process. The top-down approach has two standard techniques: high-pressure homogenization (HPH) and wet beads milling (WBM) using beads size 0.2 to 1.0 mm as milling media. The drug is dispersed in the aqueous surfactant solution and mixed to form a coarse suspension by using ultra-turrax. Following this, the coarse suspension can be processed either using HPH or WBM. There are two types of high-pressure homogenization: micro fluidization and piston-gap homogenizer. The microfluidization requires a high number of passes through microfluidizer, which can be up to 75 cycles.

Additionally, large fractions of microparticles still sometimes remained. The piston-gap homogenizer is more efficient than the microfluidizer by initially applying low to mid pressure (500 bar to 1000 bar) for the suspension to pass the 25 μm gap width followed by higher pressure, in an average 1500 bar. In total, nanosuspension produced with piston-gap requires 20 to 30 cycles only(Keck and Müller, 2006). Furthermore, piston-gap homogenizers have been used widely for the large-scale production of nanosuspensions.

In addition to the top-down method, WBM enables the production of smaller particle sizes of nanosuspensions compared to HPH, and it can be below 400 nm. Principally, nanonizing is obtained from the impaction and attrition of suspension milled with the milling beads. The smaller size of beads with a higher ratio of beads to suspension would produce a smaller particle size. The main consideration of this method is the duration of milling that can last for days to reach a certain particle size, particularly below 200 nm, and the possibility of contamination from beads material (Möschwitzer, 2013). Nevertheless, this can be overcome with the use of abrasive resistance-well beads material such as yttrium-stabilized zirconium beads (Juhnke *et al.*, 2012). In general, characteristics of the nanosized material and stabilizing agent are chosen to determine the success of nanosuspension production (Lestari *et al.*, 2015, Colombo *et al.*, 2017). Fig. (**6**) details the design of wet beads milling utilized for nanosuspensions production.

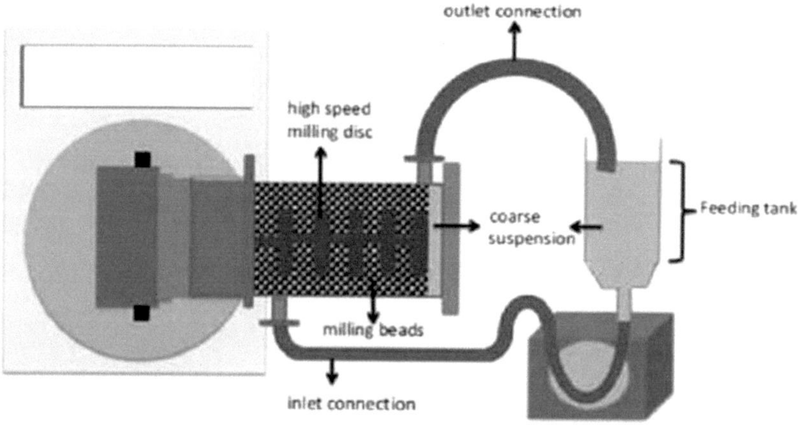

Fig. (6). Schematic representation of a wet beads milling. **Reprinted (adapted) with permission from ref. (Lestari *et al.*, 2019). Copyright (2019) EUREKA SCIENCE (FZC).**

As mentioned above, precipitation in the presence of a high-energy process is also considered a combination method. First, nanosuspension produced *via* precipitation is dried either by using the freeze-drying or spray-drying method. The freeze-drier and the spray dryer should be equipped with solvent entrapment due to the use of organic solvent for precipitation. Following this, the dried nanosuspension is then redispersed in an aqueous solution of stabilizing agent and nanonized using either HPH or wet beads milling (Sinha and Möschwitzer, 2013). The particle size of nanosuspensions obtained with such a method generally could reach below 100 nm.

Nevertheless, the combination method is considered a time-consuming yet expensive process. Overall, the final product obtained from all methods is in liquid form as nanosuspension. Hence, a further drying step is necessary to preserve the stability of nanosuspensions and feasibility if the final dosage form of nanosuspensions is intended as a solid dosage form.

Vesicular Systems

Liposome

Liposomes are composed of natural or synthetic lipids but can also be formed from polymers. Lipid molecules that form liposomes have a self-assembling ability, with each of them containing a hydrophilic head group and hydrophobic tails. Lipid molecules then associate with each other and create leaflets where hydrophobic hydrocarbon tails face each other but still contact with water, while the hydrophilic head groups facing toward the aqueous solution. Leaflets form bilayer membranes where the hydrophobic parts are still in contact with water, causing entropically unfavorable interactions between hydrophobic acyl-chains and aqueous medium. Such condition needs to be minimized by curvature formation of bilayer membrane with a closed aqueous vesicle. This form is known as liposome (Balazs DA, 2011, Laouini *et al.*, 2012). Lipid bilayers also have a core or space between the lipid bilayers that could encapsulate hydrophobic drugs or substances. Therefore, the liposome can entrap both hydrophilic and hydrophobic drugs in each type of its compartments. Liposomes are formed in various sizes from 50 nm to 200 nm, enabling this system to undergo enhanced permeability retention (EPR) effect, which is beneficial for cancer treatment (Kim, 2016). Fig. (**7**) describes the formation and general structure of liposomes.

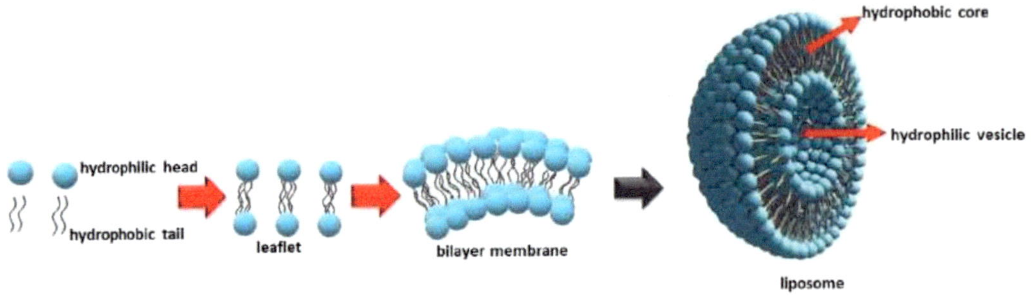

Fig. (7). The stages of liposome assembling and its general structure.

Composition of Liposomes

Hydrophilic Head

The hydrophilic head of lipid can be classified into cationic, anionic, and neutral heads. The cationic head contains a positive charge; hence, it helps attract liposomes to the negatively charged cell membrane and enhances their incorporation rate to the cell. The primary and secondary amines group on the cationic head shows the "proton sponge effect." The protonation will increase osmotic pressure leading to swelling of the endosome, followed by its rupture with releasing its content (Vermeulen *et al.*, 2018). Such an effect helps liposomes to escape lysosomes and prevents degradation of therapeutic active loaded. Cationic lipid also absorbs biological macromolecules having a negative charge and enables double loading. Another advantage is the strong gene transferability of cationic lipids. However, its cytotoxicity should be carefully considered. Reduction of toxicity can be achieved by constructing lipid molecules with endogenous amino acids (Li *et al.*, 2019). Cationic lipid holds disadvantages such as inactivation in the presence of serum and storage instability (Neves *et al.*, 2016). Some common hydrophilic cationic lipids are DOTAP (2,3dioleoyl-propyl)-trimethylamine), DDAB (dimethyl dioctadecyl ammonium bromide), and CTAB (trimethylhexadecyl ammonium bromide (Li *et al.*, 2019). One of the applications of cationic lipids for the delivery of genes was reported by Deng *et al.* (Deng *et al.*, 2011). Their study used DOTAP as a cationic lipid in conjunction with cholesterol to form liposomes loaded with short hair RNA (shRNA) for HCC treatment. Results showed efficient delivery of the shRNA by cationic liposome without the occurrence of *in vivo* toxicity. An earlier study also revealed that the interaction of cationic liposomes with pDNA was dominated by electrostatic attachment between positively charged liposomes with the negatively charged DNA in conjunction with hydrophobic interaction (Zuidam and Barenholz, 1998).

Anionic lipids have better stability in solution with lower aggregation than the neutral charge lipid and increase endocytosis compared to cationic and neutral lipids(Neves *et al.*, 2016). Common anionic lipids used are phospholipids such as phosphatidic acid, phosphatidylglycerol, and phosphatidylserine. The hydrophobic region can contain a broad range of fatty acid chains, which determine the fluidic characteristics of the liposome, such as their behavior and elasticity. Due to its negative charge, anionic lipids are not efficient in gene delivery since the negative charge of the gene will result in electronic repulsion with the anionic lipid. However, this can be overcome by combining anionic lipids with divalent cations, particularly Ca^{2+}, where Ca^{2+} minimizes electrostatic repulsion between DNA and lipids as well as promotes uptake by the cell. The maximum transfection can be achieved by combining anionic lipid with Ca^{2+} with a particle size of 200 nm(Balazs DA, 2011). The combination of neutral lipids with divalent cations also works to increase the interaction ability of neutral lipids with DNA. It is also non-toxic and stable in serum (Angelini *et al.*, 2013). Some neutral lipids which mainly used for assembling liposomes are: phosphatidylethanolamine (PE), neutral phosphatidylcholine (PC) and cholesterol, such as EPC, DPPC (1,2-Dipalmitoyl-sn-Glycero-3-Phosphocoline), DSPE (1,2-distearoyl-sn-glycero-3-phosphoethanolamine), DOPE (1,2-dioleoyl-sn-glycero-3-phosphoethanolamine) (Li *et al.*, 2019).

Hydrophobic Tail

The hydrophobic tail of lipid is composed of hydrocarbon chains, generally two kinds of fatty hydrocarbons and cholesterol. The hydrophobic tail affects the volume of the hydrophobic cavity and the ratio of the hydrophobic part to the hydrophobic region of liposomes (Li *et al.*, 2019). The hydrophilic head and the hydrophobic tail of the liposome are connected *via* a backbone linker. For gene delivery purposes, typically hydrophobic tail comprised of 8 to 18 chains is preferable. A hydrophobic double-tailed portion has less toxicity and better efficiency for gene delivery (Li *et al.*, 2019, Balazs DA, 2011). Some bonds can be ester bonds, ether bonds, and amide bonds between the hydrophobic and hydrophobic ends of lipid molecules.

Furthermore, high transfection efficiency is the primary consideration for delivering nucleic acid, and the ether bonds show this. However, this type of bond is too stable, and the non-degradant parts increase liposome cytotoxicity. Ester and amide bonds are lower in transfection efficiency but biodegradable with lower cytotoxicity (Li *et al.*, 2019).

Formulation of Liposome Loaded with Hepatocellular Carcinoma Therapeutic Agents

There are many pieces of research for the formulation of hepatocellular cancer therapeutic agents using liposomes as the delivery platform. Table **8** extracts research on liposome-based HCC therapeutic agents from the year 2010 to 2020. The aim for formulating HCC therapeutic agents as liposome is mainly for targeting directly to the cancer cells; hence it could increase drug efficacy and decrease toxicity. Nevertheless, there are weaknesses regarding the delivery of conventional liposomes composed of cationic, anionic, or neutral lipid. The main disadvantage is the rapid elimination of such conventional liposomes due to opsonization by the plasma components and uptake by macrophage of the reticuloendothelial system (RES) in the liver and spleen(Sercombe *et al.*, 2015). Thereby modifications of conventional liposomes are required to overcome those problems, viz. sterically stabilized liposomes, ligand-targeted liposomes, or combinations of those two strategies with conventional liposomes. Besides modifications to prolong liposome circulation *in vivo*, another modification can also be done to give additional functions such as attachment of imaging agent of the liposomes. It is known as "theranostic liposome." Fig. (**8**) presents a schematic illustration for conventional liposomes and their modification.

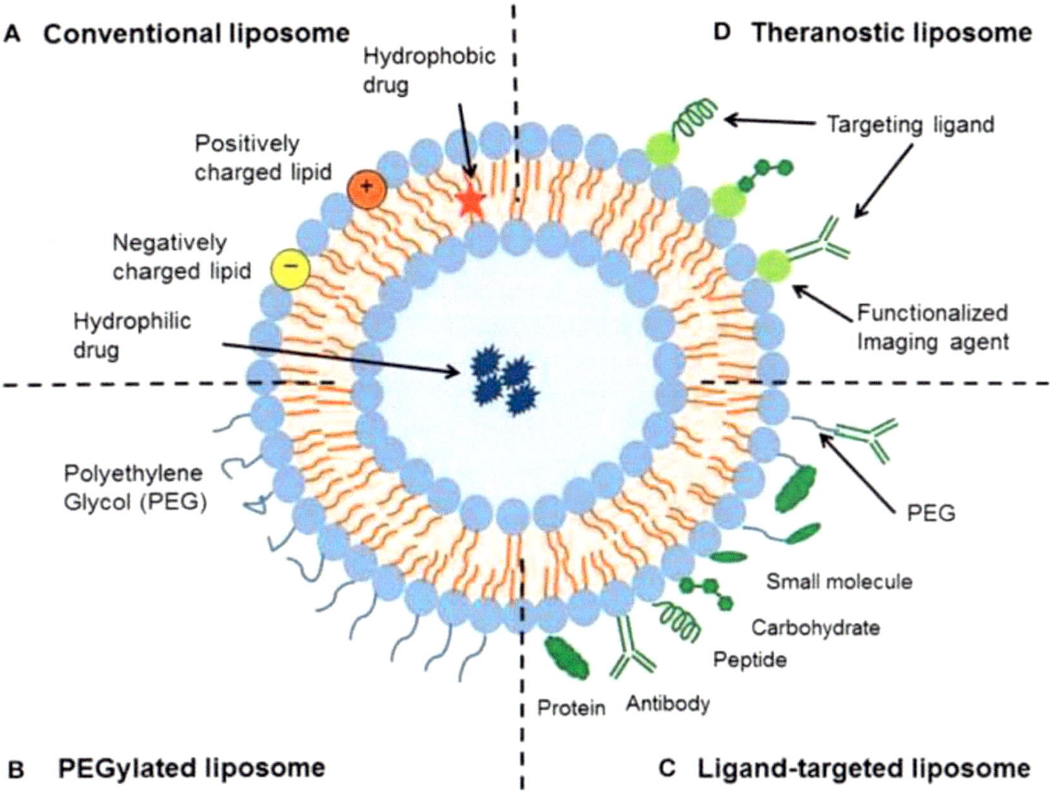

Fig. (8). Schematic representations of conventional liposome and attachment of various substances to modify liposome. **Reprinted (adapted) with permission from ref.** (Sercombe *et al.*, 2015). **Copyright 2015 Sercombe, Veerati, Moheimani, Wu, Sood, and Hua. under the terms of the Creative Commons Attribution License (CC BY).**

Table 8. Representative liposome researches for the delivery of HCC therapeutic agents from 2010 to 2020.

Active Substance	Liposome Composition	Preparation	DL, EE	Size (nm)	References
Green fluorescent protein plasmid DNA (pDNA)	1,2 Dioleoyl 3 trimethylammonium propane (DOTAP)/Chol/MPEG2000 Chol/GA PEG Chol	Thin film formation	n/a	300	(He *et al.*, 2010)
Plasmid (pGL3) encoding luciferase; Homing peptide (HBP) Cys	*Cationic liposome (LP):* DOTAP/Chol/1,2 distearoyl sn glycero 3 phosphoethanolamine N [methoxy(polyethylene glycol) 2000] (DSPE PEG)/1,2 distearoyl sn glycero 3 phosphoethanola ine N [maleimide(polyethylene glycol) 2000] (DSPE PEG maleimide)	Thin film formation	Conjugation efficiency with HBP >95%	103	(Tu and Kim, 2010)
2 methoxyestradiol (2 ME)	Phosphatidylcholine/cholesterol/2 ME	Ether injection method	n/a	167.6 ± 22.0	(Du *et al.*, 2011)
short hairpin RNAs (shRNA)	DOTAP/Chol	Thin film formation	n/a	80 120	(Deng *et al.*, 2011)
9 Nitrocamptothecin (9NC)	Egg yolk lecithin PC 98 (egg yolk phosphatidylcholine)/cholesterol	Film ultrasonic method	Drug:lipid= 1:5 EE − 4.5%	Before lyo. − 162.4±9.4	(Zheng *et al.*, 2011)
siRNA	*Liposome:* Chol T or Chol Q/ Dioleoyl L a phosphatidylethanolamine (DOPE) Cationic lipid added: Cholesteryl b D galactopyranoside (Chol b Gal)	Thin film formation	n/a	30 80	(Dorasamy *et al.*, 2012)
N lactosyl dioleoylphosphatidylethanolamine (Lac DOPE) Calcein (CAL) Doxorubicin (DOX)	*For L DOX or L CAL:* egg phosphatidylcholine/cholesterol/mPEG DSPE *For L Lac DOPE:* egg phosphatidylcholine/cholesterol/ monomethoxy polyethylene glycol 2000 distearoyl phosphatidylethanolamine (mPEG DSPE)/Lac DOPE	Thin film formation	drug:lipid − 1:20 EE − 90%	Lac L DOX − 96 ± 39 L DOX − 124 ± 49	(Zhou *et al.*, 2012)

(Table 8) cont.....

Active Substance	Liposome Composition	Preparation	DL, EE	Size (nm)	References
Doxorubicin (DOX) Palmitoylatedarabinogalactan (PAG) ;	Lipoid S 100 /Lipoid S PC 3 /Cholesterol	Thin film formation; reverse phase evaporation vesicle	EE = 94.22-94.88%	184.3-185.2	(Shah *et al.*, 2014)
miR-221 antisense oligonucleotide (anti-miR-221)	HSPC/CHOL/mPEG-DSPE/DSPE-mPEG2000-NH_2 = 55:40:4:1	Thin film dispersion method	EE = 70%	122.5	Zhang *et al.*, 2015c
Lactoferrin (Lf)	*Liposome:* Soybean phosphatidylcholine / Cholesterol *PEGylation liposome* Lipid: 1,2-distearoyl-sn-glycero-3-phosphoethanolamine-N-[methoxy (polyethylene glycol)-2000] (DSPE-PEG_{2000})/ 1,2-distearoyl-sn-glyce-o-3-phosphoethanolamine-N-[methoxy(polyethylene glycol)-2000](ammonium salt) (DSPE-PEG 2000-COOH)	Thin film hydration	EE = 85.17 86.48%	151-159 nm	(Wei *et al.*, 2015)
Paclitaxel (PTX); Arg-Gly-Asp (RGD) ligand	*LP PTX:* Soybean lecithin phosphatidylcholine (SPC)/ cholesterol *RGD Modified LP:* DSPE-PEG2000-Maleimide (Mal)/Cys-RGD *RGD LP PTX:* 1) 1,2-distearoylphosphatidylethanolamine methylated polyethyleneglycol 2000 (DSPE-mPEG2000)/RGD-modified LP 2) + LP-PTX mixed then prepared for liposome	Thin film hydration	EE LP-PTX = 87.79±2.45% EE RGD-LP=PTX = 88.48±3.61%	LP-PTX 123.6±11.8 RGD-LP-PTX 117.4±12.1	(Chen *et al.*, 2015)
Cisplatin	Phosphatidylcholine (PC)/Cholesterol (CHO)/ 5-cholestene-3-beta-ol-3-hemisuccinate (CHO-HS):methoxypolyeythyleneglycol-stearic acid (MPEG-ST)/acetyl glycyrrhetinic acid-poly(ethylene glycol)-stearic acid (AGA-PEG-ST)	Thin film hydration	DL = 23.2 26.7% EE = 51.5 61.7%	120-180 nm	(Zhang *et al.*, 2016)
Diacid metabolite of norcantharidin (DM-NCTD), Folic Acid	DSPC/cholesterol/DSPE-PEG2000/DSPE-PEG2000-FA	Reverse phase evaporation	EE ≥ 80%	200	(Liu *et al.*, 2016)
Oxaliplatin Ligand: lactobionicacid	HSPC/cholesterol/DSPE	Thin-film formation	EE = 45 ± 3.89%	310 ± 7.24	(Bansal *et al.*, 2014)
Cantharidin; cell-penetrating peptide BR2	SPC/DSPEPEG2000/DSPE-PEG2000-BR2	Hydration	n/a	10	(Zhang *et al.*, 2017)
Coumarin 6 (Cou6)	18α-GA-PEG-DSPE (18α-GA-Cou6-Lip)	thin film lipid formation	DL = 20.40± 0.27 EE = 76.50% ±1.02	169.9± 14.1	(Sun *et al.*, 2018)
Cantharidin, 3-Galactosidase-30-stearyl deoxyglycyrrhetinic acid (11-DGA-3-O-Gal)-	soybeanphospholipids (SPC)/cholesterol	thin film lipid formation	EE = 90.63± 1.66%	107.17± 6.12	(Zhou *et al.*, 2019a)
Doxorubicin	Soy lecithin/cholesterol/DSPE-PEG2000-GA/ DSPE-PEG2000-PNA	Thin film lipid formation	DL = 9.3 ± 0.37% EE = 94.1 ± 3.65%	108 ± 1.28	(Li *et al.*, 2020b)

DL: Drug-load ; EE: Encapsulation Efficiency; n/a: not available.

Sterically Stabilized Liposome

PEG has a flexible chain that anchors *via* cross-linked with the hydrophilic lipid and then occupies space of the hydrophilic surface of the liposome, as seen in Fig. (**8**). Such a chain will sterically protect the liposome by excluding other molecules from the surrounding area, hindering access and binding of blood plasma opsonins/opsonization and avoiding interactions with MPS, reducing the uptake by the reticuloendothelial system (RES). Those mechanisms will prolong *in vivo* circulation of liposomes, thus enabling the passive accumulation of drug-loaded liposomes inside other tissues or organs. In addition, steric stabilization of PEG overcomes Van der Waals attraction force hence minimizing aggregation of liposomes (Immordino *et al.*, 2006). The PEG-coated liposomes or PEGylated liposomes are also known as "stealth liposomes."PEGylation of liposome offers several advantages, for example, prolonged circulation time, avoidance of RES that causes rapid clearance, and functioning of EPR by passive targeting.

Nevertheless, it lacks specific interaction with target cells, so maximum uptake cannot be achieved. Therefore, surface modification is required by using targeting ligands (Wei *et al.*, 2015). In general, three methods are used to attach PEG to the liposome, namely, physical adsorption on the vesicle surface, incorporating PEG with lipid conjugates in the preparation process, or covalent attachment reactive groups onto the surface of preformed liposomes (Immordino *et al.*, 2006).

Ligand-targeted Liposome

Binding liposomes enhance the delivery of drug-loaded liposomes for the tumor with specific ligands such as transferrin, folic acid, peptides, and antibodies. These ligands work by being selectively recognized and then binding to the specific receptors that overexpressed on tumor cells hence increasing delivery of liposomes to the right target, thus reducing toxicity (Chen *et al.*, 2015). In contrast to passive transport of PEGylated liposomes, ligands actively transport drug-loaded liposomes to the target cells.

There are some overexpressed specific receptors for HCC that can be utilized. The most common specific receptor is the asialoglycoprotein receptor (ASGPR) which resides exclusively on the sinusoidal face of the plasma membrane of liver parenchymal cells (Dorasamy *et al.*, 2012). ASGPR is a receptor of membrane glycoprotein that binds to terminal galactose and *N*-acetylgalactosamine residues on serum glycoproteins. ASGPR is expressed in hepatocellular carcinoma and exhibits receptor-mediated endocytosis, and thereby it is a specific receptor for ligand binding and can be effective for the delivery of drugs to HCC for treatment. There are several ligands that can be bound to ASGPR, such as palmitoylatedarabinogalactan (PAG), galactose, lactose, acetylgalactosamine, asialofetuin, and lactoferrin. Those are natural ligands and hepatocyte-specific carriers for drug and gene delivery (Wei *et al.*, 2012, Shah *et al.*, 2014). Besides natural ligands, some synthetic galactose polymer ligands such as poly-(--vinylbenzyl-O-β-Dgalactopyranosyl-[1-4]-D-gluconamide showed higher affinity to ASGPR (Shah *et al.*, 2013, Shah *et al.*, 2014). In addition, the normal cellular membrane of hepatocytes shows the presence of abundant Glycyrrhetinic Acid (GA) receptors, and their numbers are increasing in tumor tissue up to 5-fold than in normal tissue. Moreover, protein kinase C-α is reported to be highly expressed in HCC cells, and this kinase is a target binding protein of GA (Sun *et al.*, 2018). Another specific receptor is integrin, a transmembrane heterodimer and main receptor proteins, that binds to the cells and hence the cell can respond to the extracellular matrix (Alberts *et al.*, 2002). There are few types of integrins, but the type αvβ3 and αvβ5 are particularly overexpressed on the angiogenic endothelium of diseased tissue and various types of malignant tumor, including hepatocellular carcinoma. Targeting this receptor can be done by utilizing one of the peptides known as cyclic argininine-glycin-aspartic acid (cRGDFK/RGD). RGD comprises of extracellular matrix which is functioning as an adherence site of various types of integrin, particularly αvβ3 and αvβ5 (Chen *et al.*, 2015).

In the latest study, modification of liposomes by combining with dual ligand was reported. In their study, Li *et al.* (Li *et al.*, 2020b) applied two types of ligands: glycyrrhetinic acid [GA] and peanut agglutinin (PNA), a plant lectin protein. PNA is known to bind with mucin 1 (MUC1), a high-molecular-weight and highly glycosylated protein that overexpresses in epithelial cancer cells. The dual ligand modification was aimed to target hepatoma cells as well as to circumvent damage of the normal hepatocytes.

Combination Strategy

In addition to PEGylated liposome and ligand-targeted liposome, a combination of conventional liposome with one or both methods mentioned above has also been explored. One of the potential treatments given for HCC is gene therapy which is based on the induction of "suicide" of cancer cells. The delivered gene encodes an enzyme, and consequently, such encoding transforms a non-toxic prodrug into a toxic drug within the transduced cells. Concerning HCC, therapeutic genes will selectively bind to HCC, and to obtain that, the delivery is aided by incorporating the therapeutic genes with HCC-specific ligands. One of the ligands is a homing peptide (HBP) carried by cationic liposomes. In conjunction with a cationic liposome, HBP considerably increases cellular internalization of plasmid DNA, increasing transgene expression in the human hepatocarcinoma cell line (HepG2 cells). HBP is bound to a hepatocarcinoma-cell-specific membrane receptor, as proven by its high result of transfection assay. Free-HBP inhibited luciferase expression while, in contrast, the targeted liposome did not significantly change luciferase expression levels. It suggests an involvement of a receptor-mediated internalization process in targeted liposome uptake (Tu and Kim, 2010).

The combination of ligand-cationic-stealth liposomes was studied by He *et al.*(He *et al.*, 2010). Cationic liposomes are considered as the most representative non-viral gene delivery vectors due to many advantages over the viral-vectors, such as low-immunogenicity, non-oncogenicity, large DNA capacity with non-restriction on DNA molecule size, avoidance of random integration of DNA vector into the host chromosome, and ability to be produced in large scale. Additionally, at physiological pH, cationic liposomes can interact with negatively charged plasmids *via* electrostatic attractions. Such interaction forms positively charged lipid-DNA complexes (lipoplexes). A negatively charged membrane will endocytose these lipoplexes; therefore, their permeability into the cell membrane will enhance.

Nevertheless, interactions between lipoplexes and cells or tissue led to a non-specific cell or tissue uptake as well as a non-specific immune response. This causes problems with the use of lipoplexes due to their low efficiency and short-circulating time in the biological system. Some researchers showed that attaching cationic liposomes with targeting ligands could improve its efficiency with less toxicity for the targeted gene delivery system. Some ligands are already reported for such a purpose, *e.g.*, folate, galactosyl, integrins, sigma ligands, estradiol, transferrin, TAT, and glycyrrhetinic acid (GA). In a more defined manner, the target binding sites of GA are protein kinase C (PKC), which overexpresses in HCC cells. In their study, a combination of the ligand with modified PEGylated cationic liposomes (GA–PEG–CLs) was then loaded with pDNA. This study found that 5% GA–PEG–CLs showed the highest transfection efficiency as gene vectors in serum-free or serum-containing medium. Additionally, it also showed the lowest cytotoxicity on human normal hepatocyte cell line L0.

A combination of anionic-PEGlyated liposomes in conjunction with ligand was reported by Zhang *et al.* (Zhang *et al.*, 2016). In this study, they utilized acetyl glycyrrhetinic acid (AGA), a ligand in the group of glycyrrhetinic acid (GA) which can be bound to the receptors on the hepatocytes. This ligand was combined with PEG anchored with the aid of stearic acid to form a PEGylated anionic liposome (5-cholestene-3-beta-ol-3-hemisuccinate (CHO-HS)). Confocal laser scanning microscopy observation and flow cytometric measurement further confirmed that AGA modified liposomes had a stronger affinity to HepG2 cells than liposomes without AGA. In addition, liposomes with the PEG segment have higher storage stability and long *in vivo* circulation.

Preparation and Scale-Up

There are two standard techniques for preparing liposomes at a bench scale: thin-film hydration and reverse-phase evaporation method. The thin-film hydration is considered more feasible, with shorter steps required. In this method, lipids are dissolved in organic solvent then evaporated to form a film which was then hydrated and extruded using polycarbonate membrane, generally 0.10 – 0.22 μm pore size. For the reverse-phase evaporation method, lipids are dissolved in an organic solvent and then emulsified with an aqueous solvent such as buffer, homogenized using a sonicator, and evaporated using a rotary evaporator to form liposome suspension. Following this, an extrusion is generally conducted by using a polycarbonate membrane in a range of 0.10 μm to 0.22 μm pore size (Liu *et al.*, 2016). Other techniques are the ethanolic injection method and the ultrasonic film method. The ethanolic injection method was done by dissolving lipids in an organic solvent or aqueous organic solvent. The solution was then dropped into an aqueous phase containing surfactant while being stirred rapidly under low-pressure N_2 (Batzri and Korn, 1973). The other method, which is also applied, is the film-ultrasonic method, where the lipids are dispersed in an organic solvent, for example, chloroform. The active substance is dissolved in another organic solvent which is more polar like ethanol. Both are then mixed and evaporated to form a thin film, hydrated, and probe-sonicated to form liposomes. A combination of ethanolic injection technique and probe sonication was also conducted by Du *et al.*, but the solvent chosen was ether (Du *et al.*, 2011).

Two latest articles published in 2019 and 2020 (Shah *et al.*, 2019, Schmidt *et al.*, 2020)reported using a novel laboratory-scale device to mix lipids followed by drug loading. The device, namely NanoAssemblr™ or micromixer, is based on a microfluidizer, but the parts are translated into a cartridge with a smaller capacity starting from 1.5 mL to 4 mL. The method utilized by this device is also known as extrusion. Shah *et al.* (Shah *et al.*, 2019) compared liposome preparation at laboratory bench using NanoAssemblr™ and with a conventional laboratory-scale microfluidizer. Liposome preparation using microfluidizer still required a purification process by filtration using Sephadex. The final liposome size produced using microfluidizer was smaller than using NanoAssemblr™; however, liposomes obtained from both the methods showed identical results for their *in vitro* and *in vivo* performance.

For a larger scale, two options are available based on those laboratory bench methods. The first approach is based on thin-film hydration, followed by mixing in a high shear mixer and high-pressure homogenization by using a microfluidizer to produce liposomes with particle size 0.16 micron at 4000 mL scale (Vemuri *et al.*, 1990). The second approach is based on the ethanol injection method. Pham *et al.* (Pham *et al.*, 2012) reported the production of liposomes at a 750 mL scale. The aqueous phase is pumped into the Shirazu Porous Glass (SPG) tubular membranes at 0.9 μm pore size. Active substances and lipids are dispersed in an organic solvent in the pressurized vessel under the nitrogen stream and circulated into SPG. When the aqueous phase arrives in the membrane, the aqueous phase is pumped. Once both the phases were in contact, the spontaneous nanovesicles were formed. The suspension containing nanovesicles was then stirred to stabilize them. In a newer scale-up, Charcosset *et al.* (Charcosset *et al.*, 2015) reported the ethanol injection method for 600 mL capacity and pilot-scale at 3 L. For the pilot scale, the organic phase is filtered through the SPG membrane and then pumped to the jacketed reactor while the aqueous phase is flown from the other channel. Mixing to form liposomes is done with the aid of a propeller mixer inside the double jacketed reactor and under a vacuum system. Evaporation is conducted by reducing the pressure of vacuum system and if necessary, separated rotary evaporation process was also conducted as the second stage of evaporation. Fig. (**9**) illustrates schematic design for large scale production of liposomes.

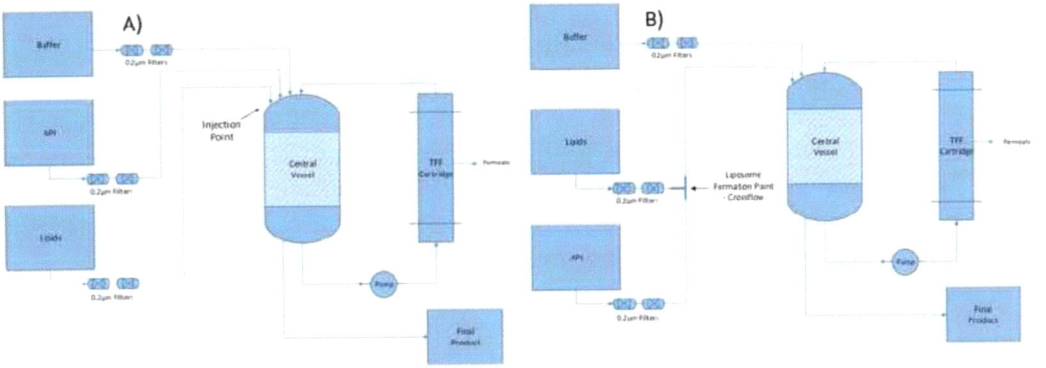

Fig. (9). Schematic batch production for large-scale production of liposomes. (A) Filtration is conducted for each solution component and aqueous phase. ; (B) crossflow method where API and liposome are mixed prior to precipitation by aqueous phase in the central vessel—reprinted (adapted) from ref (Worsham *et al.*, 2019) under Creative Commons Attribution License. Copyright 2018 The Authors. Biotechnology Journal Published by Wiley-VCH Verlag GmbH & Co. KGaA.

In general, the feasibility of producing liposomes into production scale and its reproducibility is an ultimate advantage of this delivery platform despite the relatively expensive cost for lipids as constituents for liposome formation. Several therapeutic products primarily for cancer therapy based on liposomes are already approved by the FDA and available on the market. However, liposomes-based delivery for HCC treatment is not available yet.

Micelles

Micelles are structured amphiphiles with both hydrophilic and lipophilic parts that form aggregates in a particular solvent at a specific concentration higher than its Critical Micelle Concentration/CMC. The lipophilic part of amphiphiles is a long saturated or unsaturated hydrocarbon chain (known as "tail"), whilst the hydrophilic part, or namely the "head", is an ionic (anionic or cationic), zwitterionic, or non-ionic surfactants (Hashidzume and Harada, 2015). In addition to surfactant micelles, polymeric micelles have been long introduced since the 80s as a more promising alternative for drug delivery (Bader *et al.*, 1984). Polymeric micelles are composed of amphiphilic polymers that can be obtained *via* two ways: (1) partial derivatization of water-soluble polymer with hydrophobic side chain units to form copolymers with hydrophilic and hydrophobic sites(Bader *et al.*, 1984); (2) utilization of block copolymers or graft copolymers. A block copolymer contains two or more polymer chains attached at their ends, while a graft copolymer comprises two polymer chains. One acts as a backbone and another one as a 'grafted' part. Both block copolymer and graft copolymer have amphiphilic properties (Kulthe *et al.*, 2012). The amphiphilic di-block (hydrophilic-hydrophobic) or tri-block (hydrophilic-hydrophobic-hydrophilic) polymers and graft (hydrophilic-g-hydrophobic) or also ionic (hydrophilic-ionic) copolymers are commonly used for drug delivery purposes (Owen *et al.*, 2012). Polymeric micelle is formed primarily *via* hydrophobic interactions between the hydrophobic chains. It occurred when the amphiphilic concentration containing hydrophobic and hydrophilic chains exceeded its Critical Aggregation Concentration (CAC) (Zhang *et al.*, 2014b). The core of micelle is formed from the hydrophobic portion of the copolymer or block copolymer, while the shell or corona of the micelles is formed by the hydrophilic portion, as described in Fig. (**10**). There are many hydrophilic blocks to form the shell or corona of polymeric micelles. The most frequently used hydrophilic block is poly(ethylene oxide) (PEO), commonly known as poly(ethylene glycol) (PEG). For the core-forming blocks, there are some hydrophobic blocks that have been reported, such as poly(propylene oxide) (PPO), poly ε-caprolactone (PCL), poly (L-lactide), poly(lactide-co-glycolic acid) (PLGA), poly(L-aspartic acid) (pAsp), poly(L-histidine) (pHis), poly (β-amino ester) (PbAE) (Jhaveri and Torchilin, 2014).

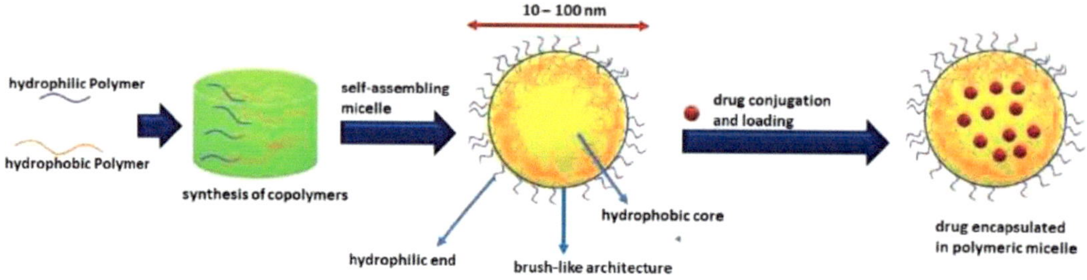

Fig. (10). Schematic representation of polymeric micelle.

Compared to conventional surfactant micelles, polymeric micelles have a covalent linkage within a hydrophobic core composed of individual polymer molecules. Such a link hinders the dynamic exchange of monomers between the free solution and the micellar pseudo-phase. Its condition assures stability and rigidity of the micelles. The hydrophilic part has a brush-like architecture that could prevent the biological invasion of the hydrophobic portion and minimize protein adsorption on the micelle (Ahmad *et al.*, 2014). In general, the size of the polymeric micelles is slightly bigger than surfactant micelles, ranging from 10 nm to 100 nm. The smallest size of polymeric micelles is above 5.5 nm as the threshold for kidney filtration; hence this could avoid fast renal clearance. Such small size also enables avoidance of mononuclear phagocytic system (MPS) in the liver; therefore, it could prolong drug circulation in the blood (Lu and Park, 2013, Ahmad *et al.*, 2014).

Additionally, the uptake mechanism of polymer is based on the endocytosis mechanism; therefore, it provides passive transport of the drug carried in this system (Bader *et al.*, 1984). Another advantage of the polymeric micelles is higher drug solubilization and bigger drug loading, particularly with the bigger size of the hydrophobic core (Kulthe *et al.*, 2012). The ability of micelle, in particular polymeric micelles, to solubilize hydrophobic drugs is beneficial to solubilize chemotherapeutics agents, which are typically hydrophobic. Besides, their very small size (10-100 nm) is ideal for passive targeting to solid tumors and poorly vascularized tumors. Circulation time and systemic toxicity of cancer drugs also require this drug to be delivered directly to the targeted cell (Zhang *et al.*, 2014c), and this can be achieved by encapsulating the anti-cancer drug in polymeric micelles. Table **9** details the kinds of research that have been published for HCC therapeutic agents using the polymeric micelles platform.

Table 9. Researches of HCC therapeutic agents-loaded micelles from the year 2010 to 2020.

Therapeutic Agent	Polymeric Micelle Composition And Preparation	Conjugation Process	Drug Loading (DL), Encapsulation Efficiency (EE) %	Particle Size (nm)	References
Doxorubicin (DOX)	PEG-PLGA	Chemical reaction, dialysis, and lyophilization	DL: 2.4 EE: 91.7	54.97	(Cheng Jin *et al.*, 2010)
Sorafenib (SOR)	a,b-poly(N-2hydroxyethyl)-D,L-aspartamide (PHEA)-ethylenediamine (EDA) - Poly-lacticacid(PLA)-Galactosylated (GAL)	Thin layer film and lyophilization.	DL:3.6 EE: not available	In PBS: 125.7 in NaCl0.9%: 101.8	(Craparo *et al.*, 2014)
Epirubicin (EPI)	PEG-poly(α,β-aspartic acid) (NC 6300)	Precipitation and filtration	DL = 9 per molecule of polymer conjugate	n/a	Takahashi *et al.*, 2013
SOR, folate and Superpara - magnetic iron oxide nanoparticles (SPIONs) Triptolide (TRIP) and folate	Polyethylene glycol-block-poly(ε-caprolactone) (PEG-PCL) Octadecylamine-p(API-Asp)$_{10}$ API: 1-(3- aminopropyl)imidazole Asp: aspartate	Dialysis and filtration Folic acid prepared in Pluronic F127 Thin film formation and dialysis	DL SOR = 6.2 DL SPIONs = 16.3 DL: 9 EE: 94	74 120	(Zhang *et al.*, 2013) (Ling *et al.*, 2014)

(Table 9) cont.....

Therapeutic Agent	Polymeric Micelle Composition And Preparation	Conjugation Process	Drug Loading (DL), Encapsulation Efficiency (EE) %	Particle Size (nm)	References
Paclitaxel (PTX) and galactose	PEG-b-P(TMBPEC-co-AC) diblock copolymer TMBPEC: Mono-2,4,6-trimethoxybenzylide-e-pentaerythritol carbonate AC: acryloylcarbonate	Gal polymer: Dialysis + Irgacure 2959 cross-linker solution irradiated by UV light at an intensity of 100 mW/cm for 10 min. PTX loaded micelles: dialysis and cross-linked as for Gal-polymer.	DL: 6.17 8.36 EE: 65.8 91.2	92.1 136.3	(Wu *et al.*, 2012, Zou *et al.*, 2014)
Doxorubycin (DOX)	Pluronic 123-tocopherylsuccinate (TOS)	Dialysis and lyophilization	DL: 21.2 EE: n/a	100	(Li *et al.*, 2015)
Epirubicin (EPI)	mPEG-b-PGA diblock copolymer	Dialysis and lyophilization	DL: 14.7 EE:72.5	90	(Zhang *et al.*, 2015b)
Andrographolide (AGP)	Glycyrrhetinic acid (GA)-poly(L-Histidine) conjugated with poly(ethylene glycol)-poly(lacti--co-glycolic acid)	AGP was loaded to GA-PPP by dialysis and filtration.	DL: 9.1 EE: 89.6	126	(Zhang *et al.*, 2015a)
Doxorubicin	glycyrrhetinic acid modified gelatin (GA-GEL)	emulsion-solvent evaporation method followed by filtration and lyophilization.	DL:8.3 12.5 EE:63.6 96.2	195-235	(Fan *et al.*, 2018)
Sorafenib (SOR)	PEG-poly (ε-caprolactone) [PEG-PCL]	dialysis	DL: 20.8 EE: > 90	11.73	(Su *et al.*, 2018)
UrsolicAcid (UA)	Methoxy poly (ethylene glycol)-poly(L-lactic acid) (mPEG-PLA),	Thin layer film formation	n/a	29.35	(Zhou *et al.*, 2019b)
Galangin (GAL)	Galactosylated- pluronic F68 (F68-Gal) copolymer.	dialysis.	DL: 4.35 EE: 77.50	242	(Patil *et al.*, 2019)
Niclosamide (NIC)	Pluronic F108	Cloudy suspension of NIC in acetone + deionized water added with pluronic F108, frozen and lyophilized (nanoprecipitation).	DL: 16.4 EE: 39.4	437.2	(Zeyada *et al.*, 2020)

Polymer Composing Micelles

Based on Table **9**, PEG is the hydrophilic polymer that is mainly used to compose polymeric micelles. The FDA has approbated this polymer for use in an oral, topical, and intravenous formulation, and it has a broad range of molecular weights (Zhang *et al.*, 2014b). Typically, PEGs with molecular weight less than 40 kDa are used for surface conjugation and crosslinking. PEG with a large molecular weight (20-50 kDa) can avoid rapid renal clearance, while small molecular weight PEG (2-5 kDa) could extend the blood half-life of nanoparticles (Verhoef and Anchordoquy, 2013). PEG is soluble in water as well as in most organic solvents. This makes easier use of PEG for end-group modification (Knop *et al.*, 2010).

Furthermore, the hydrophilicity of PEG generates a hydrated cloud which sterically protects the nanoparticles formed from the neighboring environment, including preventing interactions with blood components, protein adsorption and interactions including enzymatic degradation or opsonization, and causing slower uptake by the organs of the reticuloendothelial system (RES) such as liver and spleen (Knop *et al.*, 2010, Zhang *et al.*, 2014b). Additionally, the hydrated cloud shields the charge in the carrier systems causing near-neutral zeta potential and decreasing charge-induced interactions within the body. It will avoid opsonization since the immune system cannot recognize it. Such property is known as the "stealth effect." The hydrated cloud is obtained from the highly flexible polymer chains, providing several possible conformations. It is influenced by these factors: molar mass of PEG, surface density, and conformation form of PEG to the surface, such as brush-like or mushroom-like (Knop *et al.*, 2010). Although PEG is biocompatible, the main drawback of PEG is non-biodegradability.

Nevertheless, researches related to this matter are still limited. A recent study was conducted by Ulbricht *et al.* (Ulbricht *et al.*, 2014) for *in vitro* degradation study of PEG by reacting it with the system of $H_2O_2/Cu(II)$ as a source of Reactive Oxygen Species (ROS). They suggested that there is a possibility that the ROS generated in phagocytes enables *in vivo* degradation of polymers. Despite considering its biodegradability, PEG is biocompatible, enhancing the permeability and retention (EPR) effect. Hypervascularization with loosely connected endothelial cells and reduction of lymphatic drainage of the tumor as well as the inflamed tissues will enable the entrance of PEGylated drugs (Joralemon *et al.*, 2010). In order to overcome the biodegradability problem, it is advised to use PEG with a molar mass bigger than 400 Da since oxidative degradation decreases significantly as the molar mass increases. One should also consider the molar mass limit between 20 kDa to 60 kDa with a hydrodynamic radius of approximately 3.5 nm since this corresponds to the albumin excretion limit. In addition, a molar mass below 40-60 kDa prevents accumulation since below that limit PEG is efficiently secreted *via* urine (Knop *et al.*, 2010).

There are several options for the biodegradable and biocompatible hydrophobic polymer conjugates that form copolymers or block copolymers with PEG and other hydrophilic polymers composing micelles. The formation of polymeric self-assemble micelle is primarily influenced by the size of the hydrophobic domain in the amphiphilic molecules. When the size of the hydrophobic domain increases, this will increase hydrophobic interaction and enhance micellization. This is the analog with the surfactant micelles, in which the CMC decreases with an increasing number of carbon atoms, which are notably hydrophobic, irrespective of the polar head group. In this matter, size corresponds to the mass and composition of the copolymer backbone and also the concentration of the polymer chains (Owen *et al.*, 2012). As observed in Table **9**, three hydrophobic polymers are commonly used to form copolymers. Those hydrophobic polymers are biocompatible and biodegradable and have been approved by the FDA. Those are poly ε-caprolactone (PCL), poly (lactic acid), and poly(lactide-co-glycolic acid) (PLGA).

The most frequent hydrophobic polymer used for polymeric micelles is PLGA, a polymer composed of lactic acid (LA) and glycolic acid (GA) with an equal ratio of D- and L-lactic acid. Synthesis of PLGA involves random ring-opening copolymerization of two different monomers in the presence of a catalyst. Ester linkages link together the monomer unit of LA and GA. Hence it could degrade in the body *via* hydrolysis into endogenous monomers and then be further degraded without toxicity into water and carbon dioxide (Pandey and Jain, 2015). The ratio of LA and GA may vary, resulting in a broad range of PLGA from below 10,000 to 200,000 g/mol. PLGA can also be prepared as a wholly amorphous or highly crystalline form. The amorphous form has low mechanical strength. Therefore, it is more suitable for drug delivery. PLGA containing 70% of LA is amorphous (Sun *et al.*, 2017). Copolymerization of crystalline LA with GA tends to reduce the degree of crystallinity of the PLGA obtained. Higher content of GA also results in the increasing rate of hydration and hydrolysis as well as the rates of degradation. In contrast, PLGA containing the higher composition of LA degrades slower due to the presence of hydrophobic methyl side groups of LA. It causes PLGA copolymers to become less hydrophilic, and thus, they absorb less water. PLGA is soluble in a wide range of organic solvents with hydrophobic methyl side groups in LA (Makadia and Siegel, 2011).

In general, degradation and drug release of a PLGA-based polymer are influenced by the following factors: initial molecular weight, the ratio of LA/GA, processing method, type of the incorporated drug, and pH of the release medium. Types of PLGA can be identified based on their monomer ratio; for example, PLGA 75/25 consists of 75 wt% LA and 25 wt% GA (Xu *et al.*, 2017). In addition to PEG and PLGA, poloxamer is used. As detailed in the nanosuspensions/nanocrystals section, poloxamer can avoid macrophages, which is beneficial for the targeted drug delivery.

Furthermore, the ideal polymeric micelles should meet the following criteria for the successful delivery of cancer drugs: (1) small enough (size 10-100 nm) to penetrate tissue; (2) avoid being recognized by the mononuclear phagocyte system (MPS), and therefore accumulate in target tissue; (3) enable elimination from the organism by degradation or dissolution process; (4) could reach the location of target cells and interact with those cells; (5) stable; (6) able to improve pharmacokinetics (PK) of the encapsulated drug; (7) high drug loading capacity; (8) less complicated, inexpensive and reproducible synthesis process (Owen *et al.*, 2012). In addition, polymers composing micelles have to fulfill the main requirement, which has complete biocompatibility and *in vivo* biodegradation into non-toxic products. The biodegradation enables micelles to control drug release as well as prevent the accumulation of polymers in the human tissues and organs, which are prone to long-term toxicity (Deng *et al.*, 2012). With regard to the delivery route, intravenous injection is the chosen route for targeted delivery. This route has a few major challenges that need to be overcome by the correct selection and composition of polymeric composing micelles. Those challenges are (1) extensive dilution in the blood that affects *in vivo* stability of polymeric micelles. Additionally, blood pool interaction could cause dissociation or aggregation of the polymeric micelle, causing the occurrence of the initial bursting release of a drug, and hence the drug cannot reach the targeted tumor; (2) stiff extracellular matrix (ECM) of the tumor, high interstitial fluid pressure (IFP) and affinity of the tumor cell in the peripheral region of a solid tumor mass that hinder the intratumoral penetration; (3) the existence of naturally surface shields of polymers which cause inefficient drug uptake from the micelles by target tumor cells; (4) intracellular drug release will occur slowly and become inadequate to reach the amount required to be taken up by tumor cells (Deng *et al.*, 2012). With regard to the encapsulation ability, one should consider the compatibility of micelle core – bioactive moiety (Deshmukh *et al.*, 2017). In addition, aggregation number also rules the drug loading efficiency where a greater aggregation number of micelles shows higher loading capacity (Ahmad *et al.*, 2014). Another consideration is the hydrophilic-lipophilic balance (HLB) of the block copolymer as well as a polymer-drug ratio (Deshmukh *et al.*, 2017).

Manufacturing of Polymeric Micelle and Loading Drug

Despite the promising results obtained for delivering a drug to hepatocellular carcinoma based on polymeric micelle, there are some obstacles for manufacturing drug-loaded polymeric micelles, particularly for hepatocellular carcinoma treatment. The major hindrance is the high cost of preparation for building copolymers or block copolymer micelles. In addition, the scalability and reproducibility of the process also come with difficulty in the drug-loading process (Kulthe *et al.*, 2012, Bresseleers *et al.*, 2019). In principle, when the polymer is hydrophilic enough, mostly highly hydrophilic, both polymers and drugs can be dissolved directly to yield drug-loaded polymeric micelles. Nevertheless, this method generally results in low drug loading. As seen in Table **9**, almost all of the amphiphilic polymers have to be dissolved in an organic solvent prior to conjugation with the drug. In principle, there are three methods for drug conjugation with polymeric micelles: direct dissolution, evaporation, and dialysis. Direct dissolution can only be applied if both polymeric micelles and drugs are well solubilized in water and form self-assembly micelles. An increase in temperature is often applied to enhance the conjugation process. The second approach is emulsification, also known as the solution-casting technique. Both polymeric micelles and drugs are dissolved in a volatile organic solvent, and the solvent is then evaporated mainly using a rotary evaporator to obtain a thin film. In this method, the composition of solvent used will influence the average diameter of self-assembled micelles obtained as well as improve the efficiency of the drug encapsulation in the hydrophobic part. Another standard method used is the dialysis method, where both polymeric micelles and drugs are dissolved in an organic solvent, then stirred and undergone dialysis with water. The process requires a relatively long duration, more than 24h to ensure efficient loading and water replenishment regularly. One strategy that can be applied is to use a mixture of water and organic solvent to dissolve polymer and drug (Kulthe *et al.*, 2012). Since the solution is less likely stable, the drying process is needed, and this is usually conducted by lyophilization.

The product obtained is then further redispersed with a suitable vehicle before dispensing. Additionally, the dialysis method is ideal for the long core-forming blocks with more hydrophobic characteristics. Such a structure is more beneficial to load large amounts of poorly water-soluble drugs (Kulthe *et al.*, 2012, Varela-Moreira *et al.*, 2017). To this date, only one product, Genexol® PM, based on polymeric micelle, has been approved by the FDA already available on the market. However, this product is not for hepatocellular carcinoma therapy. Until recently, other drug-loaded polymeric micelles are still in the clinical trial phase, either phase II or III (NanoCarrier Co® ., 2021, Varela-Moreira *et al.*, 2017). Nonetheless, the polymeric micelles platform for hepatocellular carcinoma treatment is not yet on the list.

THERAPEUTIC BENEFITS OF NANOFORMULATION APPROACHES IN HCC TREATMENT

As discussed in the earlier sections, significant progress has been made in terms of nanoformulation approaches that can be exploited to improve the delivery of therapeutic agents targeted for HCC. The nanoformulation approaches can primarily provide two distinct types of advantages. The first advantage, which is more applicable to small organic molecules, is to solve the challenge of poor solubility in water or other biocompatible non-aqueous medium and the dissolution limited oral bioavailability of such molecules. The use of polymers and lipids in the nanometer domain also prolongs circulation of the delivered drug in blood by avoiding macrophageal uptake of the RES. The second advantage is applicable for all types of molecules, including small organic molecules, proteins, peptides, RNAs, and genes, to make the delivery more precise to the targeted tissue or organ. When the therapeutic agent has relatively higher toxicity, it is targeted to the cancer cells, where it is required. The third advantage is that it reduces the overall systemic toxicity of the molecule. In this part, we will cover various benefits, which can be obtained from nanoformulation approaches.

Drug-ability of Therapeutic Agent with Poor Water Solubility

A decade ago, similar to other therapeutic areas, small organic molecules were the primary therapeutic agents for HCC. It is evident from the approval of Sorafenib, the first drug approved in 2007 against HCC. However, since then, several drugs have been launched against HCC, which are not small molecules, rather monoclonal antibodies (biologic drugs). Biologic drugs have drawn considerable attention in the last decade because of their higher success rate in drug approval than the small molecule therapies, partly due to high target specificity and the ability to modulate targets in unmet medical needs (Khanna, 2012). In the last 2-3 years, few other organic small molecule drugs have been launched against HCC (Table **1**). It indicates that although there is a high interest in biomolecules (biologic drugs), the small molecule will continue to interest the pharmaceutical industry. It is evident that 77% of the drugs approved by the FDA between 2007 and 2016 were small-molecule drugs, and 23% of them were biologic drugs (Beall *et al*., 2019, Khanna, 2012).

Small molecules are developed by combinatorial chemistry and high throughput screening. To increase their specificity to the biological target, often those molecules contain chemical groups which are extremely hydrophobic. These molecules demonstrate excellent activity in *in vitro* assays but show a significant challenge to a formulator since those molecules, having several hydrophobic groups, become very poorly soluble in water, and therefore, their oral bioavailability becomes significantly low. In many cases, such molecules are even poorly soluble with standard co-solvent approaches, such as using polypropylene glycol, polyethylene glycol. Therefore, it becomes difficult to formulate them for parenteral administration for pre-clinical and clinical studies. Nanoformulation approaches provide options to develop those molecules to be administered through oral and parenteral routes in pre-clinical and clinical studies, thereby offering those molecules to become the successful drug of the future.

Drug nanosuspension technique or drug nanocrystal technology can be used to nanonize drug molecules to reduce their particle size between 1-1000 nm size ranges. By reducing the particle size, the surface area can be significantly improved, thereby increasing the dissolution rate, which leads to increasing oral bioavailability. Nanosuspension technology has been used for several compounds on a commercial scale (Möschwitzer, 2013). Nanosuspension technology, especially the top-down approach (such as wet milling), has matured to an extent where it can be applied from the pre-clinical stage of formulation development up to the commercial scale. Nanosuspension also has the advantage that it can be easily transferred into solid dosage form using conventional drying techniques such as spray drying, fluidized bed granulation, or coating onto inert tablet cores (Möschwitzer, 2013). Nanosuspension technology can also be used for the parenteral route of administration (Jacob *et al.*, 2020). It is beneficial for those molecules with solubility problems even in the presence of co-solvents and other solubilizing excipients.

Lipid-based simple formulations such as nanoemulsion or micelles formulations are the other options that can be beneficial at the earlier stage of drug development for drugs with poor water solubility. These formulations can be easily manufactured by solubilizing the drug in the lipid phase and then converting them to nanoemulsion or micelle formulation by simply mixing or homogenizing them at high speed. These types of formulations are typically used for *in-vitro* studies or pre-clinical animal studies to test the efficacy or safety of new compounds. Although liposomes and lipid complex-based formulations have been available on the market for decades, they often have the drawbacks such as low drug loading, stability, and toxicity-related issues.

Targeted Delivery of Therapeutic Agents

As highlighted in the earlier sections, targeted delivery of therapeutic agents is an area where nanoformulations such as polymeric or lipid-based nanoformulations have a significant impact. The approval of lipid nanoparticle-based mRNA delivery as SARS-CoV-2 vaccine has catapulted the interest in the lipid nanoparticle area (Batty *et al.*, 2021). Targeted delivery systems using polymeric and lipid-based nanoformulations serve two purposes. It can protect the active agent inside the nanostructure, and by targeted delivery, it can increase the concentration of the therapeutic agent to the targeted site, thereby increasing the efficacy of the therapy.

Why the targeted therapy using nanoparticles could be beneficial for HCC treatment can be answered by understanding the physiological and biological properties of HCC. HCC tumors are solid spheres or oval shapes and present as a single tumor of a large mass or multiple small ones in various liver segments. Some of the pathological and physiological features of HCC are similar to other malignant tumors, such as leaky vascular structure, low pH, hypoxic microenvironment, and stiffer extracellular matrix (Khawar *et al.*, 2015). Vascular leakiness is one of the physiological defects of tumor tissue that happens due to the fact of angiogenesis or creation of a new vascular system (neovasculature) which usually sprouts from capillaries, and their structure is disordered, discontinuous, and highly fenestrated (Lu *et al.*, 2018). When nanoparticles circulate to such neovasculature, they are prone to accumulate in the tumor site through extravasation. It is one of the ways how passive targeting with nanoparticles works for cancer treatment. The acidic microenvironment of the tumor can be used as a biomarker to trigger drug release from nanoparticles containing ionizable functional groups, and this could be easily achieved based on pH-induced charge and hydrophilicity transformation (Lu *et al.*, 2018).

The other type of targeting, namely active targeting, is accomplished by attaching some targeting ligand on the nanoparticle surface. The nanoparticles with targeting ligands can be taken up by HCC cells through the overexpressed receptors located on the HCC cell membrane. Different types of receptors are proliferated on the HCC cells. Folate receptor and asialoglycoprotein receptor (ASGPR) are, for example, two small-molecule receptors which are overexpressed on the hepatic cell surface, and sugars such as galactose or lactose and sugar derivatives can be, for example, be used as a ligand to bind to the glycoprotein receptor(Shi *et al.*, 2013, Lu *et al.*, 2018). Protein receptors such as transferrin receptor (also known as CD71), epithelial growth factor receptor (EGF), AF-20 antigen receptor, a cluster of differentiation 44 (CD44) antigen receptor also found to overexpress on HCC cells. Nanoparticles modified with ligand demonstrated to effectively target HCC tumors (Inoue *et al.*, 1993, Gao *et al.*, 2014, Wang *et al.*, 2012a). Several other types of receptors, such as specific peptide receptors or aptamer receptors, are overexpressed on the HCC cells and can be targeted.

The drug can be entrapped inside the core, which could be of a different type, either polymeric (polymeric nanoparticle) or lipidic (lipid nanoparticle) or metal or metal oxide nanoparticle. The protective surface around the core could be a single layer or multilayered. As soon as the nanoparticles reach the bloodstream, plasma protein builds up around the particle surface and forms a protein corona around the particle. Protein corona formation around the particle can be significantly influenced. For example, by PEGylating the surface, protein absorption could be significantly reduced. The type of protein adsorbed on the surface is also dependent on the surface property of the particles. The type of protein adsorbed on the surface also determines the fate of the nanoparticles afterward (Alexis *et al.*, 2010). Adsorption of albumin (a dysopsonin) can prolong blood circulation. In contrast, adsorption of opsonins such as fibrinogen and immunoglobulin G increases the detection by mononuclear phagocyte system (MPS), leading to rapid removal from the body. By modifying the size and surface properties of the particles, the targeting properties of nanoparticles can be significantly altered.

Although the commercially available drug products against HCC have not used such targeted therapy until now, a vast amount of research has been carried out in the last several decades to demonstrate that such targeted therapy is technically possible. Possibly this work will pave the way for nanoformulation-based commercial products to deliver therapeutic agents for HCC (Fig. **11**).

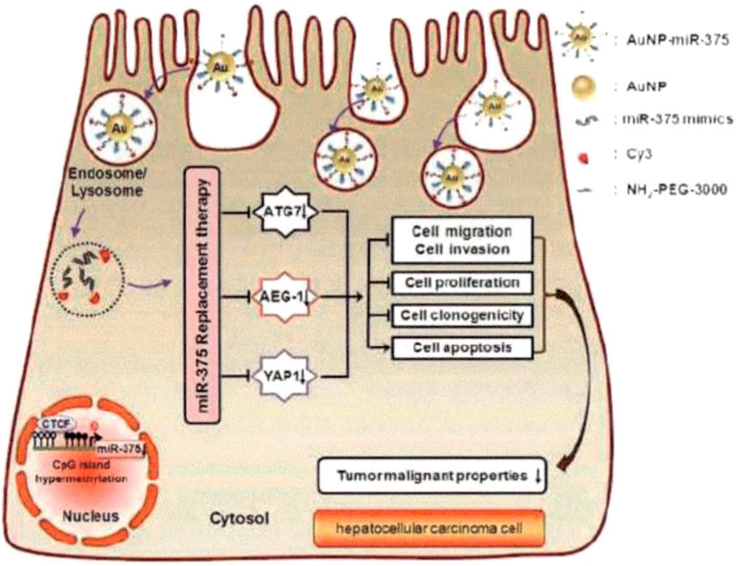

Fig. (11). Schematic illustration of gold nanoparticles delivered miR-375 for replacement therapy in hepatocellular carcinoma (HCC). AuNP-miR-375 nanoparticles escape from the endosome/lysosome, and mature miR-375 is released to the cytoplasm after being taken up by hepatoma cells. Released miR-375 acts on its target genes like AEG-1, YAP1, and ATG7 and suppresses malignant tumor phenotypes of HCC cells. It was reprinted (adapted) from (Xue *et al.*, 2016) under Creative Commons Attribution 3.0 License.

CONCLUSION AND FUTURE OUTLOOK

Hepatocellular carcinoma is on the rise and is currently considered one of the major types of cancer across different geographies. Although several drugs have been approved in the last two decades after the approval of the first drug Sorafenib against HCC in 2007, the improvement of the overall survival rate in HCC has not increased much. This indicates that there is still an unmet need for effective therapy against HCC. Several nanoformulation approaches are currently available, which can support not only better targeting of the HCC therapeutic agent on the commercial scale but can also support the development of such therapeutic agents from the early stage of drug development. Although approaches such as nanoemulsion, nano-lipid carrier formulations, nanosuspension, *etc*., are more investigated in pre-clinical drug development in the pharmaceutical industry than their commercial use, it is essential to acknowledge the contribution of these nano-formulations, in general, for drug development and drug development specific to HCC.

Advanced nanoformulation could be beneficial for targeted drug delivery in HCC. Although the use of nano-formulations in the commercial space for HCC therapy is not yet observed, a vast amount of research is ongoing in various academic and industrial research laboratories to establish proof of higher targeting efficiency than the standard therapy available in the market. The primary reason for using any targeted nanoformulation approach for commercialized drugs is that the drug molecules, either the small organic molecules or the biologics, are designed to identify specific mutations in the targeted cancer cells and attack them. Nanoformulations provide benefits in terms of both passive and active targeting. The availability of different types of nanoformulations, such as polymeric nanoparticles, liposomes, micelle, *etc*., provides various alternatives to formulators to deliver different types of drug molecules individually or as multiple drug combinations. Targeted therapy using nano-formulations is beneficial when a non-specific anticancer molecule, such as Doxorubicin targets cancer cells. By using nanoformulation approaches, such molecules can be targeted to the desired cancer cell target. At the same time, the toxicity to the healthy cells or tissues can be avoided.

Nevertheless, nanosuspension approaches designed to improve dissolution limited oral bioavailability might be necessary for future small molecules for HCC having dissolution rate-limited oral bioavailability. Additionally, if those molecules are also poorly soluble in mediums suitable for the parenteral application, then possibly the nanosuspension approach could be one of the few remaining options to deliver such molecules.

CONSENT FOR PUBLICATION

Not applicable.

CONFLICT OF INTEREST

The authors declare no conflict of interest, financial or otherwise.

ACKNOWLEDGEMENT

Declared none.

REFERENCES

Ahmad, Z, Shah, A, Siddiq, M & Kraatz, H-B (2014) 'Polymeric micelles as drug delivery vehicles'. *RSC Advances,* 4, 17028.
[http://dx.doi.org/10.1039/C3RA47370H]

Akbar, S, Anwar, A, Ayish, A, Elliott, JM & Squires, AM (2017) Phytantriol based smart nano-carriers for drug delivery applications. *Eur J Pharm Sci,* 101, 31-42.
[http://dx.doi.org/10.1016/j.ejps.2017.01.035] [PMID: 28137471]

Alberts, B, Johnson, A, Lewis, J, Raff, M, Roberts, K & Walter, P (2002) *Molecular Biology of the Cell 4th edition New York: Garland Science; 2002 Integrins.* https://www.ncbi.nlm.nih.gov/books/NBK26867/

Alexis, F, Pridgen, EM, Langer, R & Farokhzad, OC (2010) Nanoparticle technologies for cancer therapy'. In: Schäfer-Korting, M (ed.) *Handb Exp Pharmacol.*Heidelberg: Springer, Berlin.
[http://dx.doi.org/10.1007/978-3-642-00477-3_2]

Takahashi, A, Yamamoto, Y, Yasunaga, M, Koga, Y, Kuroda, J, Takigahira, M, Harada, M, Saito, H, Hayashi, T, Kato, Y, Kinoshita, T, Ohkohchi, N, Hyodo, I & Matsumura, Y (2013) NC-6300, an epirubicin-incorporating micelle, extends the antitumor effect and reduces the cardiotoxicity of epirubicin. *Cancer Sci,* 104, 920-5.
[http://dx.doi.org/10.1111/cas.12153] [PMID: 23495762]

Angelini, G, Pisani, M, Mobbili, G, Marini, M & Gasbarri, C (2013) Neutral liposomes containing crown ether-lipids as potential DNA vectors. *Biochimica et Biophysica Acta 1828,* 2506-12.
[http://dx.doi.org/10.1016/j.bbamem.2013.06.003]

Bader, H, Ringsdorf, H & Schmidt, B (1984) 'Watersoluble Polymers in Medicine '. *Die Angewandte Makromolekulare Chemie,* 123/124, 457-85.
[http://dx.doi.org/10.1002/apmc.1984.051230121]

Balazs, DA & Godbey, W (2011) Liposomes for use in gene delivery. *J Drug Deliv,* 2011, 326497.
[http://dx.doi.org/10.1155/2011/326497] [PMID: 21490748]

Balogh, J, Victor, D, III, Asham, EH, Burroughs, SG, Boktour, M, Saharia, A, Li, X, Ghobrial, RM & Monsour, HP, Jr (2016) Hepatocellular carcinoma: a review. *J Hepatocell Carcinoma,* 3, 41-53.
[http://dx.doi.org/10.2147/JHC.S61146] [PMID: 27785449]

Bansal, D, Yadav, K, Pandey, V, Ganeshpurkar, A, Agnihotri, A & Dubey, N (2016) Lactobionic acid coupled liposomes: an innovative strategy for targeting hepatocellular carcinoma. *Drug Deliv,* 23, 140-6.
[http://dx.doi.org/10.3109/10717544.2014.907373] [PMID: 24786484]

Barauskas, J, Cervin, C, Jankunec, M, Špandyreva, M, Ribokaitė, K, Tiberg, F & Johnsson, M (2010) Interactions of lipid-based liquid crystalline nanoparticles with model and cell membranes. *Int J Pharm,* 391, 284-91.
[http://dx.doi.org/10.1016/j.ijpharm.2010.03.016] [PMID: 20214966]

Baskaran, R, Madheswaran, T, Sundaramoorthy, P, Kim, HM & Yoo, BK (2014) Entrapment of curcumin into monoolein-based liquid crystalline nanoparticle dispersion for enhancement of stability and anticancer activity. *Int J Nanomedicine,* 9, 3119-30.
[PMID: 25061290]

Batty, CJ, Heise, MT, Bachelder, EM & Ainslie, KM (2021) Vaccine formulations in clinical development for the prevention of severe acute respiratory syndrome coronavirus 2 infection. *Adv Drug Deliv Rev,* 169, 168-89.
[http://dx.doi.org/10.1016/j.addr.2020.12.006] [PMID: 33316346]

Batzri, S & Korn, ED (1973) Single bilayer liposomes prepared without sonication. *Biochim Biophys Acta,* 298, 1015-9.
[http://dx.doi.org/10.1016/0005-2736(73)90408-2] [PMID: 4738145]

Beall, RF, Hwang, TJ & Kesselheim, AS (2019) Pre-market development times for biologic *versus* small-molecule drugs. *Nat Biotechnol,* 37, 708-11.
[http://dx.doi.org/10.1038/s41587-019-0175-2] [PMID: 31213674]

Bhattacharya, S, Mondal, L, Mukherjee, B, Dutta, L, Ehsan, I, Debnath, MC, Gaonkar, RH, Pal, MM & Majumdar, S (2018) Apigenin loaded nanoparticle delayed development of hepatocellular carcinoma in rats. *Nanomedicine,* 14, 1905-17.
[http://dx.doi.org/10.1016/j.nano.2018.05.011] [PMID: 29802937]

Bondì, ML, Azzolina, A, Craparo, EF, Botto, C, Amore, E, Giammona, G & Cervello, M (2014) 'Entrapment of an EGFR inhibitor into nanostructured lipid carriers (NLC) improves its antitumor activity against human hepatocarcinoma cells'. *J Nanobiotechnology,* 12, 1-9.
[http://dx.doi.org/10.1186/1477-3155-12-21]

Bondì, ML, Botto, C, Amore, E, Emma, MR, Augello, G, Craparo, EF & Cervello, M (2015) Lipid nanocarriers containing sorafenib inhibit colonies formation in human hepatocarcinoma cells. *Int J Pharm,* 493, 75-85.
[http://dx.doi.org/10.1016/j.ijpharm.2015.07.055] [PMID: 26211902]

Botto, C, Augello, G, Amore, E, Emma, MR, Azzolina, A, Cavallaro, G, Cervello, M & Bondì, ML (2018) Cationic Solid Lipid Nanoparticles as Non Viral Vectors for the Inhibition of Hepatocellular Carcinoma Growth by RNA Interference. *J Biomed Nanotechnol,* 14, 1009-16.
[http://dx.doi.org/10.1166/jbn.2018.2557] [PMID: 29883570]

Boyd, BJ, Dong, Y-D & Rades, T (2009) Nonlamellar liquid crystalline nanostructured particles: advances in materials and structure determination. *J Liposome Res,* 19, 12-28.
[http://dx.doi.org/10.1080/08982100802691983] [PMID: 19515004]

Bresseleers, J, Bagheri, M, Storm, G, Metselaar, JM, Hennink, WE, Meeuwissen, SA & van Hest, JCM (2019) Scale-Up of the Manufacturing Process To Produce Docetaxel-Loaded mPEG-*b*-p(HPMA-Bz) Block Copolymer Micelles for Pharmaceutical Applications. *Org Process Res Dev,* 23, 2707-15.
[http://dx.doi.org/10.1021/acs.oprd.9b00387] [PMID: 32952390]

Butler, JM & Dressman, JB (2010) The developability classification system: application of biopharmaceutics concepts to formulation development. *J Pharm Sci,* 99, 4940-54.
[http://dx.doi.org/10.1002/jps.22217] [PMID: 20821390]

Cao, H, Wang, Y, He, X, Zhang, Z, Yin, Q, Chen, Y, Yu, H, Huang, Y, Chen, L, Xu, M, Gu, W & Li, Y (2015) Codelivery of sorafenib and curcumin by directed self-assembled nanoparticles enhances therapeutic effect on hepatocellular carcinoma. *Mol Pharm,* 12, 922-31.
[http://dx.doi.org/10.1021/mp500755j] [PMID: 25622075]

Charcosset, C, Juban, A, Valour, J-P, Urbaniak, S & Fessi, H (2015) 'Preparation of liposomes at large scale using the ethanol injection method: Effect of scale-up and injection devices'. *Chem Eng Res Des,* 9, 508-15.
[http://dx.doi.org/10.1016/j.cherd.2014.09.008]

Chen, L, Liu, Y, Wang, W & Liu, K (2015) Effect of integrin receptor-targeted liposomal paclitaxel for hepatocellular carcinoma targeting and therapy. *Oncol Lett,* 10, 77-84.
[http://dx.doi.org/10.3892/ol.2015.3242] [PMID: 26170980]

Chen, S, Cao, Q, Wen, W & Wang, H (2019) Targeted therapy for hepatocellular carcinoma: Challenges and opportunities. *Cancer Lett,* 460, 1-9.

[http://dx.doi.org/10.1016/j.canlet.2019.114428] [PMID: 31207320]

Jin, C, Qian, N, Zhao, W, Yang, W, Bai, L, Wu, H, Wang, M, Song, W & Dou, K (2010) Improved therapeutic effect of DOX-PLGA-PEG micelles decorated with bivalent fragment HAb18 F(ab')(2) for hepatocellular carcinoma. *Biomacromolecules,* 11, 2422-31.
[http://dx.doi.org/10.1021/bm1005992] [PMID: 20831277]

Chu, Y, Li, D, Luo, Y-F, He, X-J & Jiang, M-Y (2014) Preparation and in vitro evaluation of glycyrrhetinic acid-modified curcumin-loaded nanostructured lipid carriers. *Molecules,* 19, 2445-57.
[http://dx.doi.org/10.3390/molecules19022445] [PMID: 24566313]

Colombo, M, Orthmann, S, Bellini, M, Staufenbiel, S & Bodmeier, R (2017) Influence of Drug Brittleness, Nanomilling Time, and Freeze-Drying on the Crystallinity of Poorly Water-Soluble Drugs and Its Implications for Solubility Enhancement. *AAPS PharmSciTech,* 18, 2437-45.
[http://dx.doi.org/10.1208/s12249-017-0722-4] [PMID: 28168626]

Craparo, EF, Sardo, C, Serio, R, Zizzo, MG, Bondì, ML, Giammona, G & Cavallaro, G (2014) Galactosylated polymeric carriers for liver targeting of sorafenib. *Int J Pharm,* 466, 172-80.
[http://dx.doi.org/10.1016/j.ijpharm.2014.02.047] [PMID: 24607205]

Davis, S (2000) 'Drug delivery systems'. *Interdiscip Sci Rev,* 25, 175-83.
[http://dx.doi.org/10.1179/030801800679206]

de Souza, JF, da Silva Pontes, K, Alves, TFR, de Barros, CT, Amaral, VA, de Moura Crescencio, KM, Rios, AC, Batain, F, Souto, EB & Severino, P (2020) 'Structural comparison, physicochemical properties, and *in vitro* release profile of curcumin-loaded lyotropic liquid crystalline nanoparticle: Influence of hydrotrope as interface stabilizers'. *J Mol Liq,* 306, 112861.
[http://dx.doi.org/10.1016/j.molliq.2020.112861]

Delgado, D, Gascón, AR, Del Pozo-Rodríguez, A, Echevarría, E, Ruiz de Garibay, AP, Rodríguez, JM & Solinís, MÁ (2012) Dextran-protamine-solid lipid nanoparticles as a non-viral vector for gene therapy: *in vitro* characterization and *in vivo* transfection after intravenous administration to mice. *Int J Pharm,* 425, 35-43.
[http://dx.doi.org/10.1016/j.ijpharm.2011.12.052] [PMID: 22226874]

Deng, C, Jiang, Y, Cheng, R, Meng, F & Zhong, Z (2012) 'Biodegradable polymeric micelles for targeted and controlled anticancer drug delivery: Promises, progress and prospects'. *Nano Today,* 7, 467-80.
[http://dx.doi.org/10.1016/j.nantod.2012.08.005]

Deng, H, Jiang, Q, Yang, Y, Zhang, S, Ma, Y, Xie, G, Chen, X, Qian, Z, Wen, Y, Li, J, Yang, J, Chen, L, Zhao, X & Wei, Y (2011) Intravenous liposomal delivery of the short hairpin RNAs against Plk1 controls the growth of established human hepatocellular carcinoma. *Cancer Biol Ther,* 11, 401-9.
[http://dx.doi.org/10.4161/cbt.11.4.14178] [PMID: 21150280]

Deshmukh, AS, Chauhan, PN, Noolvi, MN, Chaturvedi, K, Ganguly, K, Shukla, SS, Nadagouda, MN & Aminabhavi, TM (2017) Polymeric micelles: Basic research to clinical practice. *Int J Pharm,* 532, 249-68.
[http://dx.doi.org/10.1016/j.ijpharm.2017.09.005] [PMID: 28882486]

Devulapally, R, Foygel, K, Sekar, TV, Willmann, JK & Paulmurugan, R (2016) 'Gemcitabine and antisense-microRNA co-encapsulated PLGA PEG polymer nanoparticles for hepatocellular carcinoma therapy'. *ACS Appl Mater Interfaces,* 8, 33412-22.
[http://dx.doi.org/10.1021/acsami.6b08153] [PMID: 27960411]

Doktorovová, S, Santos, DL, Costa, I, Andreani, T, Souto, EB & Silva, AM (2014a) Cationic solid lipid nanoparticles interfere with the activity of antioxidant enzymes in hepatocellular carcinoma cells. *Int J Pharm,* 471, 18-27.
[http://dx.doi.org/10.1016/j.ijpharm.2014.05.011] [PMID: 24836663]

Doktorovova, S, Silva, AM, Gaivão, I, Souto, EB, Teixeira, JP & Martins-Lopes, P (2014b) Comet assay reveals no genotoxicity risk of cationic solid lipid nanoparticles. *J Appl Toxicol,* 34, 395-403.
[http://dx.doi.org/10.1002/jat.2961] [PMID: 24243595]

Dorasamy, S, Narainpersad, N, Singh, M & Ariatti, M (2012) Novel targeted liposomes deliver sirna to hepatocellular carcinoma cells *in vitro*. *Chem Biol Drug Des,* 80, 647-56.
[http://dx.doi.org/10.1111/j.1747-0285.2012.01446.x] [PMID: 22783887]

Du, B, Wang, SY, Shi, XF, Zhang, CF & Zhang, ZZ (2011) The effect of 2-methoxyestradiol liposome on growth inhibition, angiogenesis and expression of VEGF and Ki67 in mice bearing H22 hepatocellular carcinoma. *Tumori,* 97, 660-5.
[http://dx.doi.org/10.1177/030089161109700520] [PMID: 22158500]

Fan, D, Yu, J, Yan, R, Xu, X, Wang, Y, Xie, X, Liu, C, Liu, Y & Huang, H (2018) Preparation and evaluation of doxorubicin-loaded micelles based on glycyrrhetinic acid modified gelatin conjugates for targeting hepatocellular carcinoma. *Journal of Nanomaterials.*
[http://dx.doi.org/10.1155/2018/8467169]

El-Serag, HB (2020) Epidemiology of hepatocellular carcinoma. *The Liver: Biology and Pathobiology,* 758-72.
[http://dx.doi.org/10.1002/9781119436812.ch59]

EMA. 'Nexavar EPAR European Medicines Agency' [Online] Available: https://www.ema.europa.eu/en/documents/scientific-discussion/nexavar-epar-scientific-discussion_en.pdf retrieved: 30 January 2021. [viewed].

EMA. (2017). 'Sodium laurylsulfate used as an excipient. European Medicines Agency' [Online]. European Medicines Agency. Available: https://www.ema.europa.eu/en/documents/report/sodium-laurilsulfate-used-excipient-report-published-support-questions-answers-sodium-laurilsulfate_en.pdf retrieved: 30 January 2021 [viewed]

Forner, A, Reig, M & Bruix, J (2018) Hepatocellular carcinoma. *Lancet,* 391, 1301-14.
[http://dx.doi.org/10.1016/S0140-6736(18)30010-2] [PMID: 29307467]

Freag, MS, Elnaggar, YS, Abdelmonsif, DA & Abdallah, OY (2016) Layer-by-layer-coated lyotropic liquid crystalline nanoparticles for active tumor targeting of rapamycin. *Nanomedicine (Lond),* 11, 2975-96.
[http://dx.doi.org/10.2217/nnm-2016-0236] [PMID: 27785978]

Frens, G (1973) 'Controlled nucleation for the regulation of the particle size in monodisperse gold suspensions'. *Nat Phys Sci (Lond),* 241, 20-2.
[http://dx.doi.org/10.1038/physci241020a0]

Gan, H, Chen, L, Sui, X, Wu, B, Zou, S, Li, A, Zhang, Y, Liu, X, Wang, D, Cai, S, Liu, X, Liang, Y & Tang, X (2018) Enhanced delivery of sorafenib with anti-GPC3 antibody-conjugated TPGS-b-PCL/Pluronic P123 polymeric nanoparticles for targeted therapy of hepatocellular carcinoma. *Mater Sci Eng C,* 91, 395-403.
[http://dx.doi.org/10.1016/j.msec.2018.05.011] [PMID: 30033270]

Gao, J, Xia, Y, Chen, H, Yu, Y, Song, J, Li, W, Qian, W, Wang, H, Dai, J & Guo, Y (2014) Polymer-lipid hybrid nanoparticles conjugated with anti-EGF receptor antibody for targeted drug delivery to hepatocellular carcinoma. *Nanomedicine (Lond),* 9, 279-93.
[http://dx.doi.org/10.2217/nnm.13.20] [PMID: 23721168]

Ghasemiyeh, P & Mohammadi-Samani, S (2018) Solid lipid nanoparticles and nanostructured lipid carriers as novel drug delivery systems: applications, advantages and disadvantages. *Res Pharm Sci,* 13, 288-303.
[http://dx.doi.org/10.4103/1735-5362.235156] [PMID: 30065762]

Grillone, A, Riva, ER, Mondini, A, Forte, C, Calucci, L, Innocenti, C, de Julian Fernandez, C, Cappello, V, Gemmi, M, Moscato, S, Ronca, F, Sacco, R, Mattoli, V & Ciofani, G (2015) 'Active targeting of sorafenib: preparation, characterization, and *in vitro* testing of drug-loaded magnetic solid lipid nanoparticles'. *Adv Healthc Mater,* 4, 1681-90.
[http://dx.doi.org/10.1002/adhm.201500235] [PMID: 26039933]

Hashidzume, A & Harada, A (2015) Micelles and Vesicles. In: Kobayashi, S., Müllen, K., (Eds.), *Encyclopedia of Polymeric Nanomaterials.*Springer, Berlin.
[http://dx.doi.org/10.1007/978-3-642-29648-2_56]

He, S, Fan, W, Wu, N, Zhu, J, Miao, Y, Miao, X, Li, F, Zhang, X & Gan, Y (2018) 'Lipid-based liquid crystalline nanoparticles facilitate cytosolic delivery of siRNA *via* structural transformation'. *Nano Lett,* 18, 2411-9.
[http://dx.doi.org/10.1021/acs.nanolett.7b05430] [PMID: 29561622]

He, ZY, Zheng, X, Wu, XH, Song, XR, He, G, Wu, WF, Yu, S, Mao, SJ & Wei, YQ (2010) Development of glycyrrhetinic acid-modified stealth cationic liposomes for gene delivery. *Int J Pharm,* 397, 147-54.
[http://dx.doi.org/10.1016/j.ijpharm.2010.06.029] [PMID: 20667672]

Hoffman, AS (2008) The origins and evolution of "controlled" drug delivery systems. *J Control Release,* 132, 153-63.
[http://dx.doi.org/10.1016/j.jconrel.2008.08.012] [PMID: 18817820]

Hu, B, Sun, D, Sun, C, Sun, Y-F, Sun, H-X, Zhu, Q-F, Yang, X-R, Gao, Y-B, Tang, W-G, Fan, J, Maitra, A, Anders, RA & Xu, Y (2015) A polymeric nanoparticle formulation of curcumin in combination with sorafenib synergistically inhibits tumor growth and metastasis in an orthotopic model of human hepatocellular carcinoma. *Biochem Biophys Res Commun,* 468, 525-32.
[http://dx.doi.org/10.1016/j.bbrc.2015.10.031] [PMID: 26482853]

Immordino, ML, Dosio, F & Cattel, L (2006) Stealth liposomes: review of the basic science, rationale, and clinical applications, existing and potential. *Int J Nanomedicine,* 1, 297-315.
[PMID: 17717971]

Inoue, T, Cavanaugh, PG, Steck, PA, Brünner, N & Nicolson, GL (1993) Differences in transferrin response and numbers of transferrin receptors in rat and human mammary carcinoma lines of different metastatic potentials. *J Cell Physiol,* 156, 212-7.
[http://dx.doi.org/10.1002/jcp.1041560128] [PMID: 8314858]

Jacob, S, Nair, AB & Shah, J (2020) Emerging role of nanosuspensions in drug delivery systems. *Biomater Res,* 24, 3.
[http://dx.doi.org/10.1186/s40824-020-0184-8] [PMID: 31969986]

Jain, D, Athawale, R, Bajaj, A, Shrikhande, S, Goel, PN & Gude, RP (2013) Studies on stabilization mechanism and stealth effect of poloxamer 188 onto PLGA nanoparticles. *Colloids Surf B Biointerfaces,* 109, 59-67.
[http://dx.doi.org/10.1016/j.colsurfb.2013.03.027] [PMID: 23608470]

Jha, S, Ramadori, F, Quarta, S, Biasiolo, A, Fabris, E, Baldan, P, Guarino, G, Ruvoletto, M, Villano, G, Turato, C, Gatta, A, Mancin, F, Pontisso, P & Scrimin, P (2017) 'Binding and uptake into human hepatocellular carcinoma cells of peptide-functionalized gold nanoparticles'. *Bioconjug Chem,* 28, 222-9.
[http://dx.doi.org/10.1021/acs.bioconjchem.6b00441] [PMID: 27771945]

Jhaveri, AM & Torchilin, VP (2014) Multifunctional polymeric micelles for delivery of drugs and siRNA. *Front Pharmacol,* 5, 77.
[http://dx.doi.org/10.3389/fphar.2014.00077] [PMID: 24795633]

Joralemon, MJ, McRae, S & Emrick, T (2010) PEGylated polymers for medicine: from conjugation to self-assembled systems. *Chem Commun (Camb),* 46, 1377-93.
[http://dx.doi.org/10.1039/b920570p] [PMID: 20162127]

Juhnke, M, Märtin, D & John, E (2012) Generation of wear during the production of drug nanosuspensions by wet media milling. *Eur J Pharm Biopharm,* 81, 214-22.
[http://dx.doi.org/10.1016/j.ejpb.2012.01.005] [PMID: 22269938]

Keck, CM & Müller, RH (2006) Drug nanocrystals of poorly soluble drugs produced by high pressure homogenisation. *Eur J Pharm Biopharm,* 62, 3-16.
[http://dx.doi.org/10.1016/j.ejpb.2005.05.009] [PMID: 16129588]

Khanna, I (2012) Drug discovery in pharmaceutical industry: productivity challenges and trends. *Drug Discov Today,* 17, 1088-102.
[http://dx.doi.org/10.1016/j.drudis.2012.05.007] [PMID: 22627006]

Khawar, IA, Kim, JH & Kuh, H-J (2015) Improving drug delivery to solid tumors: priming the tumor microenvironment. *J Control Release,* 201, 78-89.
[http://dx.doi.org/10.1016/j.jconrel.2014.12.018] [PMID: 25526702]

Kim, J-S (2016) 'Liposomal drug delivery system'. *J Pharm Investig,* 46, 387-92.
[http://dx.doi.org/10.1007/s40005-016-0260-1]

Kipp, JE (2004) The role of solid nanoparticle technology in the parenteral delivery of poorly water-soluble drugs. *Int J Pharm,* 284, 109-22.
[http://dx.doi.org/10.1016/j.ijpharm.2004.07.019] [PMID: 15454302]

Knop, K, Hoogenboom, R, Fischer, D & Schubert, US (2010) Poly(ethylene glycol) in drug delivery: pros and cons as well as potential alternatives. *Angew Chem Int Ed Engl,* 49, 6288-308.
[http://dx.doi.org/10.1002/anie.200902672] [PMID: 20648499]

Kreuter, J (2007) Nanoparticles--a historical perspective. *Int J Pharm,* 331, 1-10.
[http://dx.doi.org/10.1016/j.ijpharm.2006.10.021] [PMID: 17110063]

Kulthe, SS, Choudhari, YM, Inamdar, NN & Mourya, V (2012) 'Polymeric micelles: authoritative aspects for drug delivery'. *Des Monomers Polym,* 15, 465-521.
[http://dx.doi.org/10.1080/1385772X.2012.688328]

Kumar, V, Bhatt, PC, Rahman, M, Kaithwas, G, Choudhry, H, Al-Abbasi, FA, Anwar, F & Verma, A (2017) Fabrication, optimization, and characterization of umbelliferone β-D-galactopyranoside-loaded PLGA nanoparticles in treatment of hepatocellular carcinoma: *in vitro* and *in vivo* studies. *Int J Nanomedicine,* 12, 6747-58.
[http://dx.doi.org/10.2147/IJN.S136629] [PMID: 28932118]

Kumari, A, Yadav, SK & Yadav, SC (2010) Biodegradable polymeric nanoparticles based drug delivery systems. *Colloids Surf B Biointerfaces,* 75, 1-18.
[http://dx.doi.org/10.1016/j.colsurfb.2009.09.001] [PMID: 19782542]

Lestari, LAD (2015) 'Systematic Screening of Different Surface Modifiers for the Production of Physically Stable Nanosuspensions'. *J Pharm Sci,* 104, 1128-40.
[http://dx.doi.org/10.1002/jps.24266]

Langer, K, Balthasar, S, Vogel, V, Dinauer, N, von Briesen, H & Schubert, D (2003) Optimization of the preparation process for human serum albumin (HSA) nanoparticles. *Int J Pharm,* 257, 169-80.
[http://dx.doi.org/10.1016/S0378-5173(03)00134-0] [PMID: 12711172]

Laouini, A, Jaafar-Maalej, C, Limayem-Blouza, I, Sfar, S, Charcosset, C & Fessi, H (2012) 'Preparation, Characterization and Applications of Liposomes: State of the Art'. *Journal of Colloid Science and Biotechnology,* 1, 147-68.
[http://dx.doi.org/10.1166/jcsb.2012.1020]

Lestari, MLAD, Müller, RH & Möschwitzer, JP (2019) The Scalability of Wet Ball Milling for The Production of Nanosuspensions. *Pharm Nanotechnol,* 7, 147-61.
[http://dx.doi.org/10.2174/2211738507666190401142530] [PMID: 30931866]

Li, M, Du, C, Guo, N, Teng, Y, Meng, X, Sun, H, Li, S, Yu, P & Galons, H (2019) Composition design and medical application of liposomes. *Eur J Med Chem,* 164, 640-53.
[http://dx.doi.org/10.1016/j.ejmech.2019.01.007] [PMID: 30640028]

Li, M, Zhang, J, Feng, L, Zhang, L & Zhang, N (2013) The in vitro anti-tumor efficacy and the pharmacokinetics of N3-o-toluyl-fluorouracil loaded nanosuspension (TFu-LNS). *J Biomed Nanotechnol,* 9, 801-10.
[http://dx.doi.org/10.1166/jbn.2013.1586] [PMID: 23802409]

Li, S, Zhang, J, Fang, Y, Yi, J, Lu, Z, Chen, Y & Guo, B (2020) Enhancing Betulinic Acid Dissolution Rate and Improving Antitumor Activity *via* Nanosuspension Constructed by Anti-Solvent Technique. *Drug Des Devel Ther,* 14, 243-56. a [http://dx.doi.org/10.2147/DDDT.S233851] [PMID: 32021108]

Li, X, Diao, W, Xue, H, Wu, F, Wang, W, Jiang, B, Bai, J, Lian, B, Feng, W, Sun, T, Yu, W, Wu, J, Qu, M, Wang, Y & Gao, Z (2020) Improved efficacy of doxorubicin delivery by a novel dual-ligand-modified liposome in hepatocellular carcinoma. *Cancer Lett,* 489, 163-73. b
[http://dx.doi.org/10.1016/j.canlet.2020.06.017] [PMID: 32592729]

Li, YJ, Dong, M, Kong, FM & Zhou, JP (2015) 'Enhanced therapeutic efficacy and cytotoxicity of doxorubicin-loaded vitamin E Pluronic micelles against liver cancer'. *RSC Advances,* 5, 43965-71.
[http://dx.doi.org/10.1039/C5RA04027B]

Ling, D, Xia, H, Park, W, Hackett, MJ, Song, C, Na, K, Hui, KM & Hyeon, T (2014) pH-sensitive nanoformulated triptolide as a targeted therapeutic strategy for hepatocellular carcinoma. *ACS Nano,* 8, 8027-39.
[http://dx.doi.org/10.1021/nn502074x] [PMID: 25093274]

Liu, MC, Liu, L, Wang, XR, Shuai, WP, Hu, Y, Han, M & Gao, JQ (2016) Folate receptor-targeted liposomes loaded with a diacid metabolite of norcantharidinenhance antitumor potency for h22 hepatocellular carcinoma both *in vitro* and *in vivo International Journal of Nanomedicine,* 11, 1395-412.

Liu, P, Rong, X, Laru, J, van Veen, B, Kiesvaara, J, Hirvonen, J, Laaksonen, T & Peltonen, L (2011) Nanosuspensions of poorly soluble drugs: preparation and development by wet milling. *Int J Pharm,* 411, 215-22.
[http://dx.doi.org/10.1016/j.ijpharm.2011.03.050] [PMID: 21458552]

Lu, J, Wang, J & Ling, D (2018) 'Surface engineering of nanoparticles for targeted delivery to hepatocellular carcinoma'. *Small,* 14, 1702037.
[http://dx.doi.org/10.1002/smll.201702037]

Lu, W-l, Shi, H-z, Wang, Y-f, Zhou, Q, Wang, Z-p, Xiong, S & Zhang, Y-j (2015) '*In vitro* Antitumor Efficacy of Puerarin Nanosuspension Against Human HepG2 Cells '. *Adv Mat Res,* 1083, 27-31.
[http://dx.doi.org/10.4028/www.scientific.net/AMR.1083.27]

Lu, Y & Park, K (2013) Polymeric micelles and alternative nanonized delivery vehicles for poorly soluble drugs. *Int J Pharm,* 453, 198-214.
[http://dx.doi.org/10.1016/j.ijpharm.2012.08.042] [PMID: 22944304]

Madheswaran, T, Kandasamy, M, Bose, RJ & Karuppagounder, V (2019) Current potential and challenges in the advances of liquid crystalline nanoparticles as drug delivery systems. *Drug Discov Today,* 24, 1405-12.
[http://dx.doi.org/10.1016/j.drudis.2019.05.004] [PMID: 31102731]

Mahato, K, Nagpal, S, Shah, MA, Srivastava, A, Maurya, PK, Roy, S, Jaiswal, A, Singh, R & Chandra, P (2019) Gold nanoparticle surface engineering strategies and their applications in biomedicine and diagnostics. *3 Biotech,* 9, 57.
[http://dx.doi.org/10.1007/s13205-019-1577-z]

Makadia, HK & Siegel, SJ (2011) Poly Lactic-co-Glycolic Acid (PLGA) as Biodegradable Controlled Drug Delivery Carrier. *Polymers (Basel),* 3, 1377-97.
[http://dx.doi.org/10.3390/polym3031377] [PMID: 22577513]

Mehnert, W & Mäder, K (2001) Solid lipid nanoparticles: production, characterization and applications. *Adv Drug Deliv Rev,* 47, 165-96.
[http://dx.doi.org/10.1016/S0169-409X(01)00105-3] [PMID: 11311991]

Molnár, Z, Bódai, V, Szakacs, G, Erdélyi, B, Fogarassy, Z, Sáfrán, G, Varga, T, Kónya, Z, Tóth-Szeles, E, Szűcs, R & Lagzi, I (2018) Green synthesis of gold nanoparticles by thermophilic filamentous fungi. *Sci Rep,* 8, 3943.
[http://dx.doi.org/10.1038/s41598-018-22112-3] [PMID: 29500365]

Möschwitzer, JP (2013) Drug nanocrystals in the commercial pharmaceutical development process. *Int J Pharm,* 453, 142-56.
[http://dx.doi.org/10.1016/j.ijpharm.2012.09.034] [PMID: 23000841]

Muchow, M, Maincent, P & Müller, RH (2008) Lipid nanoparticles with a solid matrix (SLN, NLC, LDC) for oral drug delivery. *Drug Dev Ind Pharm,* 34, 1394-405.
[http://dx.doi.org/10.1080/03639040802130061] [PMID: 18665980]

Müller, RH, Gohla, S & Keck, CM (2011) State of the art of nanocrystals--special features, production, nanotoxicology aspects and intracellular delivery. *Eur J Pharm Biopharm,* 78, 1-9.
[http://dx.doi.org/10.1016/j.ejpb.2011.01.007] [PMID: 21266197]

Müller, RH, Radtke, M & Wissing, SA (2002) Nanostructured lipid matrices for improved microencapsulation of drugs. *Int J Pharm,* 242, 121-8.
[http://dx.doi.org/10.1016/S0378-5173(02)00180-1] [PMID: 12176234]

Nalawade, P, Mukherjee, T & Kapoor, S (2013) Green Synthesis of Gold Nanoparticles Using Glycerol as a Reducing Agent. *Advances in Nanoparticles,* 2, 78-86.
[http://dx.doi.org/10.4236/anp.2013.22014]

NanoCarrier® (2021) https://www.nanocarrier.co.jp/en/pipeline/ [viewed 30 January 2021]

Naseri, N, Valizadeh, H & Zakeri-Milani, P (2015) Solid Lipid Nanoparticles and Nanostructured Lipid Carriers: Structure, Preparation and Application. *Adv Pharm Bull,* 5, 305-13.
[http://dx.doi.org/10.15171/apb.2015.043] [PMID: 26504751]

Naz, F, Koul, V, Srivastava, A, Gupta, YK & Dinda, AK (2016) Biokinetics of ultrafine gold nanoparticles (AuNPs) relating to redistribution and urinary excretion: a long-term *in vivo* study. *J Drug Target,* 24, 720-9.
[http://dx.doi.org/10.3109/1061186X.2016.1144758] [PMID: 26837799]

Neves, LFF, Duan, J, Voelker, A, Khanal, A, McNally, L, Steinbach-Rankins, J & Ceresa, BP (2016) Preparation and optimisation of anionic liposomes for delivery of small peptides and cDNA to human corneal epithelial cells. *J Microencapsul,* 33, 391-9.
[http://dx.doi.org/10.1080/02652048.2016.1202343] [PMID: 27530524]

Nisha, R, Kumar, P, Kumar, U, Mishra, N, Maurya, P, Singh, S, Singh, P, Guleria, A, Saha, S & Saraf, SA (2021) Fabrication of imatinib mesylate-loaded lactoferrin-modified pegylated liquid crystalline nanoparticles for mitochondrial-dependent apoptosis in hepatocellular carcinoma. *Mol Pharm,* 18, 1102-20.
[PMID: 33356314]

O'Connor, S, Ward, J, Watson, M, Momin, B & Richardson, L (2010) Hepatocellular carcinoma - United States, 2001-2006. *MMWR Morb Mortal Wkly Rep,* 59, 517-20.
[PMID: 20448528]

Owen, SC, Chan, DPY & Shoichet, MS (2012) 'Polymeric micelle stability'. *Nano Today,* 7, 53-65.
[http://dx.doi.org/10.1016/j.nantod.2012.01.002]

Pandey, A & Jain, DS (2015) Poly Lactic-Co-Glycolic Acid (PLGA) Copolymer and Its Pharmaceutical Application. In: Thakur, V.K., Thakur, M.K., (Eds.), *Handbook of Polymers for Pharmaceutical Technologies: Processing and Applications* Wiley-Scrivener, Beverly, MA.
[http://dx.doi.org/10.1002/9781119041412.ch6]

Pang, X, Wang, T, Jiang, D, Mu, W, Zhang, B & Zhang, N (2019) Functionalized docetaxel-loaded lipid-based-nanosuspensions to enhance antitumor efficacy in vivo. *Int J Nanomedicine,* 14, 2543-55.
[http://dx.doi.org/10.2147/IJN.S191341] [PMID: 31114190]

Patil, S, Ujalambkar, V, Rathore, A, Rojatkar, S & Pokharkar, V (2019) Galangin loaded galactosylated pluronic F68 polymeric micelles for liver targeting. *Biomed Pharmacother,* 112, 108691.
[http://dx.doi.org/10.1016/j.biopha.2019.108691] [PMID: 30798131]

Pham, TT, Jaafar-Maalej, C, Charcosset, C & Fessi, H (2012) Liposome and niosome preparation using a membrane contactor for scale-up. *Colloids Surf B Biointerfaces,* 94, 15-21.
[http://dx.doi.org/10.1016/j.colsurfb.2011.12.036] [PMID: 22326648]

Pizzol, CD, Filippin-Monteiro, FB, Restrepo, JA, Pittella, F, Silva, AH, Alves de Souza, P, Machado de Campos, A & Creczynski-Pasa, TB (2014) Influence of surfactant and lipid type on the physicochemical properties and biocompatibility of solid lipid nanoparticles. *Int J Environ Res Public Health,* 11, 8581-96. [http://dx.doi.org/10.3390/ijerph110808581] [PMID: 25141003]

Rabinow, BE (2004) Nanosuspensions in drug delivery. *Nat Rev Drug Discov,* 3, 785-96. [http://dx.doi.org/10.1038/nrd1494] [PMID: 15340388]

Rahman, M, Almalki, WH, Afzal, O, Alfawaz Altamimi, AS, Kazmi, I, Al-Abbasi, FA, Choudhry, H, Alenezi, SK, Barkat, MA, Beg, S, Kumar, V & Alhalmi, A (2020) Cationic Solid Lipid Nanoparticles of Resveratrol for Hepatocellular Carcinoma Treatment: Systematic Optimization, *in vitro* Characterization and Preclinical Investigation. *Int J Nanomedicine,* 15, 9283-99. a [http://dx.doi.org/10.2147/IJN.S277545] [PMID: 33262588]

Rahman, M, Beg, S, Alharbi, KS, Alruwaili, NK, Alotaibi, NH, Alzarea, AI, Almalki, WH, Alenezi, SK, Altowayan, WM & Alshammari, MS (2020) 'Implications of Solid Lipid Nanoparticles of Ganoderic Acid for the Treatment and Management of Hepatocellular Carcinoma'. *J Pharm Innov,* 1-12. b

Reis, CP, Neufeld, RJ, Ribeiro, AJ & Veiga, F (2006) Nanoencapsulation I. Methods for preparation of drug-loaded polymeric nanoparticles. *Nanomedicine,* 2, 8-21. [http://dx.doi.org/10.1016/j.nano.2005.12.003] [PMID: 17292111]

Sabella, S, Carney, RP, Brunetti, V, Malvindi, MA, Al-Juffali, N, Vecchio, G, Janes, SM, Bakr, OM, Cingolani, R, Stellacci, F & Pompa, PP (2014) A general mechanism for intracellular toxicity of metal-containing nanoparticles. *Nanoscale,* 6, 7052-61. [http://dx.doi.org/10.1039/c4nr01234h] [PMID: 24842463]

Salem, DS, Sliem, MA, El-Sesy, M, Shouman, SA & Badr, Y (2018) Improved chemo-photothermal therapy of hepatocellular carcinoma using chitosan-coated gold nanoparticles. *J Photochem Photobiol B,* 182, 92-9. [http://dx.doi.org/10.1016/j.jphotobiol.2018.03.024] [PMID: 29653312]

Schmidt, ST, Christensen, D & Perrie, Y (2020) Applying Microfluidics for the Production of the Cationic Liposome-Based Vaccine Adjuvant CAF09b. *Pharmaceutics,* 12, 1237. [http://dx.doi.org/10.3390/pharmaceutics12121237] [PMID: 33352684]

Sercombe, L, Veerati, T, Moheimani, F, Wu, SY, Sood, AK & Hua, S (2015) Advances and Challenges of Liposome Assisted Drug Delivery. *Front Pharmacol,* 6, 286. [http://dx.doi.org/10.3389/fphar.2015.00286] [PMID: 26648870]

Shah, SM, Goel, PN, Jain, AS, Pathak, PO, Padhye, SG, Govindarajan, S, Ghosh, SS, Chaudhari, PR, Gude, RP, Gopal, V & Nagarsenker, MS (2014) Liposomes for targeting hepatocellular carcinoma: use of conjugated arabinogalactan as targeting ligand. *Int J Pharm,* 477, 128-39. [http://dx.doi.org/10.1016/j.ijpharm.2014.10.014] [PMID: 25311181]

Shah, SM, Pathak, PO, Jain, AS, Barhate, CR & Nagarsenker, MS (2013) Synthesis, characterization, and in vitro evaluation of palmitoylated arabinogalactan with potential for liver targeting. *Carbohydr Res,* 367, 41-7. [http://dx.doi.org/10.1016/j.carres.2012.11.025] [PMID: 23298829]

Shah, VM, Nguyen, DX, Patel, P, Cote, B, Al-Fatease, A, Pham, Y, Huynh, MG, Woo, Y & Alani, AW (2019) Liposomes produced by microfluidics and extrusion: A comparison for scale-up purposes. *Nanomedicine,* 18, 146-56. [http://dx.doi.org/10.1016/j.nano.2019.02.019] [PMID: 30876818]

Shi, B, Abrams, M & Sepp-Lorenzino, L (2013) Expression of asialoglycoprotein receptor 1 in human hepatocellular carcinoma. *J Histochem Cytochem,* 61, 901-9. [http://dx.doi.org/10.1369/0022155413503662] [PMID: 23979840]

Shirodkar, RK, Kumar, L, Mutalik, S & Lewis, S (2019) 'Solid Lipid Nanoparticles and Nanostructured Lipid Carriers: Emerging Lipid Based Drug Delivery Systems'. *Pharm Chem J,* 53, 440-53. [http://dx.doi.org/10.1007/s11094-019-02017-9]

Silva, AH, Filippin-Monteiro, FB, Mattei, B, Zanetti-Ramos, BG & Creczynski-Pasa, TB (2012) *In vitro* biocompatibility of solid lipid nanoparticles. *Sci Total Environ,* 432, 382-8. [http://dx.doi.org/10.1016/j.scitotenv.2012.06.018] [PMID: 22750185]

Singh, RP, Gangadharappa, HV & Mruthunjaya, K (2017) 'Phospholipids: Unique carriers for drug delivery systems'. *Technology (Singap),* 39, 166-79.

Sinha, B, Müller, RH & Möschwitzer, JP (2013) Bottom-up approaches for preparing drug nanocrystals: formulations and factors affecting particle size. *Int J Pharm,* 453, 126-41.
[http://dx.doi.org/10.1016/j.ijpharm.2013.01.019] [PMID: 23333709]

Srisa-Nga, K, Mankhetkorn, S, Okonogi, S & Khonkarn, R (2019) 'Delivery of superparamagnetic polymeric micelles loaded with quercetin to hepatocellular carcinoma cells'. *J Pharm Sci,* 108, 996-1006.
[http://dx.doi.org/10.1016/j.xphs.2018.08.008] [PMID: 30121312]

Su, Y, Wang, K, Li, Y, Song, W, Xin, Y, Zhao, W, Tian, J, Ren, L & Lu, L (2018) Sorafenib-loaded polymeric micelles as passive targeting therapeutic agents for hepatocellular carcinoma therapy. *Nanomedicine (Lond),* 13, 1009-23.
[http://dx.doi.org/10.2217/nnm-2018-0046] [PMID: 29630448]

Subramaniam, B, Siddik, ZH & Nagoor, NH (2020) 'Optimization of nanostructured lipid carriers: understanding the types, designs, and parameters in the process of formulations'. *J Nanopart Res,* 22, 141.
[http://dx.doi.org/10.1007/s11051-020-04848-0]

Sun, X, Xu, C, Wu, G, Ye, Q & Wang, C (2017) 'Poly(Lactic-co-Glycolic Acid): Applications and Future Prospects for Periodontal Tissue Regeneration'. *Polymers (Basel),* 9, 189.
[http://dx.doi.org/10.3390/polym9060189]

Y, sun, C, Dai, M, Yin, Ye, Q, J, Lu, H, Hu & D, Chen (2018) Hepatocellular carcinoma-targeted effect of configurations and groups of glycyrrhetinic acid by evaluation of its derivative-modified liposomes. *International Journal of Nanomedicine,* 13, 1621-32.

Takeuchi, I, Nobata, S, Oiri, N, Tomoda, K & Makino, K (2017) Biodistribution and excretion of colloidal gold nanoparticles after intravenous injection: Effects of particle size. *Biomed Mater Eng,* 28, 315-23.
[http://dx.doi.org/10.3233/BME-171677] [PMID: 28527194]

Thao, LQ, Lee, C, Kim, B, Lee, S, Kim, TH, Kim, JO, Lee, ES, Oh, KT, Choi, HG, Yoo, SD & Youn, YS (2017) Doxorubicin and paclitaxel co-bound lactosylated albumin nanoparticles having targetability to hepatocellular carcinoma. *Colloids Surf B Biointerfaces,* 152, 183-91.
[http://dx.doi.org/10.1016/j.colsurfb.2017.01.017] [PMID: 28110040]

Thapa, RK, Choi, JY, Poudel, BK, Hiep, TT, Pathak, S, Gupta, B, Choi, H-G, Yong, CS & Kim, JO (2015) 'Multilayer-coated liquid crystalline nanoparticles for effective sorafenib delivery to hepatocellular carcinoma'. *ACS Appl Mater Interfaces,* 7, 20360-8.
[http://dx.doi.org/10.1021/acsami.5b06203] [PMID: 26315487]

Tiyaboonchai, W (2013) 'Chitosan nanoparticles: a promising system for drug delivery'. *Naresuan University Journal: Science and Technology,* 11, 51-66. [NUJST].

Tom, G, Philip, S, Isaac, R, Praseetha, PK, Jiji, SG & Asha, VV (2018) Preparation of an efficient and safe polymeric-magnetic nanoparticle delivery system for sorafenib in hepatocellular carcinoma. *Life Sci,* 206, 10-21.
[http://dx.doi.org/10.1016/j.lfs.2018.04.046] [PMID: 29709652]

Torrecilla, J, del Pozo-Rodríguez, A, Apaolaza, PS, Solinís, MÁ & Rodríguez-Gascón, A (2015) Solid lipid nanoparticles as non-viral vector for the treatment of chronic hepatitis C by RNA interference. *Int J Pharm,* 479, 181-8.
[http://dx.doi.org/10.1016/j.ijpharm.2014.12.047] [PMID: 25542984]

Tran, N, Mulet, X, Hawley, AM, Fong, C, Zhai, J, Le, TC, Ratcliffe, J & Drummond, CJ (2018) 'Manipulating the ordered nanostructure of self-assembled monoolein and phytantriol nanoparticles with unsaturated fatty acids'. *Langmuir,* 34, 2764-73.
[http://dx.doi.org/10.1021/acs.langmuir.7b03541] [PMID: 29381863]

Tu, Y & Kim, JS (2010) Selective gene transfer to hepatocellular carcinoma using homing peptide-grafted cationic liposomes. *J Microbiol Biotechnol,* 20, 821-7.

[PMID: 20467260]

Turkevich, J, Stevenson, PC & Hillier, J (1951) 'A study of the nucleation and growth processes in the synthesis of colloidal gold'. *Discuss Faraday Soc,* 11, 55-75.
[http://dx.doi.org/10.1039/df9511100055]

Turkevich, J, Stevenson, PC & Hillier, J (1953) 'The formation of colloidal gold'. *J Phys Chem,* 57, 670-3.
[http://dx.doi.org/10.1021/j150508a015]

Ulbricht, J, Jordan, R & Luxenhofer, R (2014) On the biodegradability of polyethylene glycol, polypeptoids and poly(2-oxazoline)s. *Biomaterials,* 35, 4848-61.
[http://dx.doi.org/10.1016/j.biomaterials.2014.02.029] [PMID: 24651032]

Varela-Moreira, A, Shi, Y, Fens, MHAM, Lammers, T, Hennink, WE & Schiffelers, RM (2017) 'Clinical application of polymeric micelles for the treatment of cancer'. *Mater Chem Front,* 1, 1485-501.
[http://dx.doi.org/10.1039/C6QM00289G]

Varshosaz, J, Hassanzadeh, F, Sadeghi, H & Khadem, M (2012) Galactosylated nanostructured lipid carriers for delivery of 5-FU to hepatocellular carcinoma. *J Liposome Res,* 22, 224-36.
[http://dx.doi.org/10.3109/08982104.2012.662653] [PMID: 22385296]

Varshosaz, J, Jafarian, A, Salehi, G & Zolfaghari, B (2014) Comparing different sterol containing solid lipid nanoparticles for targeted delivery of quercetin in hepatocellular carcinoma. *J Liposome Res,* 24, 191-203.
[http://dx.doi.org/10.3109/08982104.2013.868476] [PMID: 24354715]

Vemuri, S, Yu, C-D, Wangsatorntanakun, V & Roosdorp, N (1990) 'Large-Scale Production of Liposomes by a Microfluidizer'. *Drug Dev Ind Pharm,* 16, 2243-56.
[http://dx.doi.org/10.3109/03639049009043797]

Verhoef, JJF & Anchordoquy, TJ (2013) Questioning the Use of PEGylation for Drug Delivery. *Drug Deliv Transl Res,* 3, 499-503.
[http://dx.doi.org/10.1007/s13346-013-0176-5] [PMID: 24932437]

Vermeulen, LMP, De Smedt, SC, Remaut, K & Braeckmans, K (2018) The proton sponge hypothesis: Fable or fact? *Eur J Pharm Biopharm,* 129, 184-90.
[http://dx.doi.org/10.1016/j.ejpb.2018.05.034] [PMID: 29859281]

Wang, H, Wang, H, Yang, W, Yu, M, Sun, S & Xie, B (2018) 'Improved oral bioavailability and liver targeting of sorafenib solid lipid nanoparticles in rats'. *AAPS PharmSciTech,* 19, 761-8.
[http://dx.doi.org/10.1208/s12249-017-0901-3] [PMID: 28983849]

Wang, J, Wang, H, Li, J, Liu, Z, Xie, H, Wei, X, Lu, D, Zhuang, R, Xu, X & Zheng, S (2016) 'iRGD-decorated polymeric nanoparticles for the efficient delivery of vandetanib to hepatocellular carcinoma: preparation and *in vitro* and *in vivo* evaluation'. *ACS Appl Mater Interfaces,* 8, 19228-37.
[http://dx.doi.org/10.1021/acsami.6b03166] [PMID: 27381493]

Wang, L, Su, W, Liu, Z, Zhou, M, Chen, S, Chen, Y, Lu, D, Liu, Y, Fan, Y, Zheng, Y, Han, Z, Kong, D, Wu, JC, Xiang, R & Li, Z (2012) CD44 antibody-targeted liposomal nanoparticles for molecular imaging and therapy of hepatocellular carcinoma. *Biomaterials,* 33, 5107-14. a
[http://dx.doi.org/10.1016/j.biomaterials.2012.03.067] [PMID: 22494888]

Wang, W, Zhao, X, Hu, H, Chen, D, Gu, J, Deng, Y & Sun, J (2010) Galactosylated solid lipid nanoparticles with cucurbitacin B improves the liver targetability. *Drug Deliv,* 17, 114-22. b
[http://dx.doi.org/10.3109/10717540903580176] [PMID: 20148709]

Wang, XQ, Fan, JM, Liu, YO, Zhao, B, Jia, ZR & Zhang, Q (2011) Bioavailability and pharmacokinetics of sorafenib suspension, nanoparticles and nanomatrix for oral administration to rat. *Int J Pharm,* 419, 339-46.
[http://dx.doi.org/10.1016/j.ijpharm.2011.08.003] [PMID: 21843612]

Wang, Y, Wang, L, Liu, Z, Zhang, D & Zhang, Q (2012) *In vivo* evaluation of silybin nanosuspensions targeting liver. *J Biomed Nanotechnol,* 8, 760-9. c
[http://dx.doi.org/10.1166/jbn.2012.1444] [PMID: 22888746]

Wang, Z-p, Wu, J-b, Zhou, Q, Wang, Y-f & Chen, T-s (2014) 'Anti-hepatocarcinoma effects of berberine nanosuspension against human HepG2 and Huh7 cells as well as H22 tumor bearing mice'. *Proc SPIE,* 9230 a
[http://dx.doi.org/10.1117/12.2067978]

Wang, Z, Wu, J, Chen, T, Zhou, Q, Fan, H & Wang, Y (2014) '*In vitro* and *in vivo* Antitumor Efficacy of Curcumol Nanosuspension Against H22 Tumor '. *Adv Mat Res,* 998-999, 151-5. b
[http://dx.doi.org/10.4028/www.scientific.net/AMR.998-999.151]

Wei, M, Guo, X, Tu, L, Zou, Q, Li, Q, Tang, C, Chen, B, Xu, Y & Wu, C (2015) Lactoferrin-modified PEGylated liposomes loaded with doxorubicin for targeting delivery to hepatocellular carcinoma. *Int J Nanomedicine,* 10, 5123-37.
[PMID: 26316745]

Wei, M, Xu, Y, Zou, Q, Tu, L, Tang, C, Xu, T, Deng, L & Wu, C (2012) Hepatocellular carcinoma targeting effect of PEGylated liposomes modified with lactoferrin. *Eur J Pharm Sci,* 46, 131-41.
[http://dx.doi.org/10.1016/j.ejps.2012.02.007] [PMID: 22369856]

Worsham, RD, Thomas, V & Farid, SS (2019) Potential of Continuous Manufacturing for Liposomal Drug Products. *Biotechnol J,* 14, e1700740.
[http://dx.doi.org/10.1002/biot.201700740] [PMID: 29781114]

Wu, L, Zhang, J & Watanabe, W (2011) Physical and chemical stability of drug nanoparticles. *Adv Drug Deliv Rev,* 63, 456-69.
[http://dx.doi.org/10.1016/j.addr.2011.02.001] [PMID: 21315781]

Wu, Y, Chen, W, Meng, F, Wang, Z, Cheng, R, Deng, C, Liu, H & Zhong, Z (2012) Core-crosslinked pH-sensitive degradable micelles: A promising approach to resolve the extracellular stability *versus* intracellular drug release dilemma. *J Control Release,* 164, 338-45.
[http://dx.doi.org/10.1016/j.jconrel.2012.07.011] [PMID: 22800578]

Xia, Y, Zhong, J, Zhao, M, Tang, Y, Han, N, Hua, L, Xu, T, Wang, C & Zhu, B (2019) Galactose-modified selenium nanoparticles for targeted delivery of doxorubicin to hepatocellular carcinoma. *Drug Deliv,* 26, 1-11.
[http://dx.doi.org/10.1080/10717544.2018.1556359] [PMID: 31928356]

Xie, B, Wang, DH & Spechler, SJ (2012) Sorafenib for treatment of hepatocellular carcinoma: a systematic review. *Dig Dis Sci,* 57, 1122-9.
[http://dx.doi.org/10.1007/s10620-012-2136-1] [PMID: 22451120]

Xu, Y, Kim, C-S, Saylor, DM & Koo, D (2017) Polymer degradation and drug delivery in PLGA-based drug-polymer applications: A review of experiments and theories. *J Biomed Mater Res B Appl Biomater,* 105, 1692-716.
[http://dx.doi.org/10.1002/jbm.b.33648] [PMID: 27098357]

Xue, H-Y, Liu, Y, Liao, J-Z, Lin, J-S, Li, B, Yuan, W-G, Lee, RJ, Li, L, Xu, C-R & He, X-X (2016) Gold nanoparticles delivered miR-375 for treatment of hepatocellular carcinoma. *Oncotarget,* 7, 86675-86.
[http://dx.doi.org/10.18632/oncotarget.13431] [PMID: 27880727]

Yang, S, Zhang, B, Gong, X, Wang, T, Liu, Y & Zhang, N (2016) *In vivo* biodistribution, biocompatibility, and efficacy of sorafenib-loaded lipid-based nanosuspensions evaluated experimentally in cancer. *Int J Nanomedicine,* 11, 2329-43.
[PMID: 27307733]

Yu, B, Wang, X, Zhou, C, Teng, L, Ren, W, Yang, Z, Shih, CH, Wang, T, Lee, RJ, Tang, S & Lee, LJ (2014) Insight into mechanisms of cellular uptake of lipid nanoparticles and intracellular release of small RNAs. *Pharm Res,* 31, 2685-95.
[http://dx.doi.org/10.1007/s11095-014-1366-7] [PMID: 24740244]

Zamboni, CG, Kozielski, KL, Vaughan, HJ, Nakata, MM, Kim, J, Higgins, LJ, Pomper, MG & Green, JJ (2017) Polymeric nanoparticles as cancer-specific DNA delivery vectors to human hepatocellular carcinoma.

J Control Release, 263, 18-28.
[http://dx.doi.org/10.1016/j.jconrel.2017.03.384] [PMID: 28351668]

Zeyada, MS, Abdel-Rahman, N, El-Karef, A, Yahia, S, El-Sherbiny, IM & Eissa, LA (2020) Niclosamide-loaded polymeric micelles ameliorate hepatocellular carcinoma *in vivo* through targeting Wnt and Notch pathways. *Life Sci,* 261, 118458.
[http://dx.doi.org/10.1016/j.lfs.2020.118458] [PMID: 32961231]

Zhang, J-Y, He, B, Qu, W, Cui, Z, Wang, YB, Zhang, H, Wang, J-C & Zhang, Q (2011) Preparation of the albumin nanoparticle system loaded with both paclitaxel and sorafenib and its evaluation *in vitro* and *in vivo*. *J Microencapsul,* 28, 528-36. a
[http://dx.doi.org/10.3109/02652048.2011.590614] [PMID: 21702701]

Zhang, J, Li, M, Liu, Z, Wang, L, Liu, Y & Zhang, N (2014) Preclinical studies of N_3-O-toluyl-fluorouraril-loaded lipid-based nanosuspensions in H_{22}-bearing mice. *Int J Nanomedicine,* 9, 2741-51. a
[http://dx.doi.org/10.2147/IJN.S59338] [PMID: 24920908]

Zhang, J, Zhang, M, Ji, J, Fang, X, Pan, X, Wang, Y, Wu, C & Chen, M (2015) 'Glycyrrhetinic acid-mediated polymeric drug delivery targeting the acidic microenvironment of hepatocellular carcinoma'. *Pharm Res,* 32, 3376-90. a
[http://dx.doi.org/10.1007/s11095-015-1714-2] [PMID: 26148773]

Zhang, K, Tang, X, Zhang, J, Lu, W, Lin, X, Zhang, Y, Tian, B, Yang, H & He, H (2014) PEG-PLGA copolymers: their structure and structure-influenced drug delivery applications. *J Control Release,* 183, 77-86. b
[http://dx.doi.org/10.1016/j.jconrel.2014.03.026] [PMID: 24675377]

Zhang, L, Gong, F, Zhang, F, Ma, J, Zhang, P & Shen, J (2013) Targeted therapy for human hepatic carcinoma cells using folate-functionalized polymeric micelles loaded with superparamagnetic iron oxide and sorafenib *in vitro*. *International Journal of Nanomedicine,* 8, 1517-24.
[http://dx.doi.org/10.2147/IJN.S43263]

Zhang, L, Kuang, Y, Jia Liu, ZL, Huang, S & Zhuo, R (2016) 'Long circulating anionic liposomes for hepatic targeted delivery of cisplatin†'. *RSC Advances,* 6, 76905-14.
[http://dx.doi.org/10.1039/C6RA08566K]

Zhang, L, Wei, W, Zhao, X, Zu, Y, Yang, L & Zu, B (2011) 'Comparative study on effects of GA nanoparticles suspension and unprocessed GA solution on oral bioavailability, hepatic function and liver antioxidant enzymes activities in carbon tetrachloride induced liver damage rats '. *Mater Sci Forum,* 694, 423-9. b
[http://dx.doi.org/10.4028/www.scientific.net/MSF.694.423]

Zhang, Q, Ding, J, Lv, C, Xu, W, Sun, X & Meng, X (2015) 'Epirubicin-Complexed Polypeptide Micelle Effectively and Safely Treats Hepatocellular Carcinoma'. *Polymers (Basel),* 7, 2410-30. b
[http://dx.doi.org/10.3390/polym7111521]

Zhang, X, Lin, C, Lu, A, Lin, G, Chen, H, Liu, Q, Yang, Z & Zhang, H (2017) Liposomes equipped with cell penetrating peptide BR2 enhances chemotherapeutic effects of cantharidin against hepatocellular carcinoma. *Drug Deliv,* 24, 986-98.
[http://dx.doi.org/10.1080/10717544.2017.1340361] [PMID: 28644728]

Zhang, Y, Huang, Y & Li, S (2014) Polymeric micelles: nanocarriers for cancer-targeted drug delivery. *AAPS PharmSciTech,* 15, 862-71. c
[http://dx.doi.org/10.1208/s12249-014-0113-z] [PMID: 24700296]

Zhao, P, Wu, S, Cheng, Y, You, J, Chen, Y, Li, M, He, C, Zhang, X, Yang, T, Lu, Y, Lee, RJ, He, X & Xiang, G (2017) MiR-375 delivered by lipid-coated doxorubicin-calcium carbonate nanoparticles overcomes chemoresistance in hepatocellular carcinoma. *Nanomedicine,* 13, 2507-16.
[http://dx.doi.org/10.1016/j.nano.2017.05.010] [PMID: 28577837]

Zhao, X, Chen, Q, Li, Y, Tang, H, Liu, W & Yang, X (2015) Doxorubicin and curcumin co-delivery by lipid nanoparticles for enhanced treatment of diethylnitrosamine-induced hepatocellular carcinoma in mice. *Eur J*

Pharm Biopharm, 93, 27-36.
[http://dx.doi.org/10.1016/j.ejpb.2015.03.003] [PMID: 25770771]

Zheng, S, Chang, S, Lu, J, Chen, Z, Xie, L, Nie, Y, He, B, Zou, S & Gu, Z (2011) Characterization of 9-nitrocamptothecin liposomes: anticancer properties and mechanisms on hepatocellular carcinoma *in vitro* and *in vivo*. *PLoS One,* 6, e21064.
[http://dx.doi.org/10.1371/journal.pone.0021064] [PMID: 21695227]

Zhou, L, Zou, M, Zhu, K, Ning, S & Xia, X (2019) 'Development of 11-DGA-3-O-Gal-Modified Cantharidin Liposomes for Treatment of Hepatocellular Carcinoma'. *Molecules,* 24, 3080. a
[http://dx.doi.org/10.3390/molecules24173080]

Zhou, M, Yi, Y, Liu, L, Lin, Y, Li, J, Ruan, J & Zhong, Z (2019) Polymeric micelles loading with ursolic acid enhancing anti-tumor effect on hepatocellular carcinoma. *J Cancer,* 10, 5820-31. b
[http://dx.doi.org/10.7150/jca.30865] [PMID: 31737119]

Zhou, X, Zhang, M, Yung, B, Li, H, Zhou, C, Lee, LJ & Lee, RJ (2012) Lactosylated liposomes for targeted delivery of doxorubicin to hepatocellular carcinoma. *Int J Nanomedicine,* 7, 5465-74.
[PMID: 23093902]

Zou, Y, Song, Y, Yang, W, Meng, F, Liu, H & Zhong, Z (2014) Galactose-installed photo-crosslinked pH-sensitive degradable micelles for active targeting chemotherapy of hepatocellular carcinoma in mice. *J Control Release,* 193, 154-61.
[http://dx.doi.org/10.1016/j.jconrel.2014.05.016] [PMID: 24852094]

Zuidam, NJ & Barenholz, Y (1998) 'Electrostatic and structural properties of complexes involving plasmid DNA and cationic lipids commonly used for gene delivery1A preliminary report of this study was presented at the 3rd annual conference: Artificial Self-Assembling Systems for Gene Delivery'. *Biochimica et Biophysica Acta (BBA) -. Biomembranes,* 1368, 115-28.
[http://dx.doi.org/10.1016/S0005-2736(97)00187-9]

W, Zhang,, F, Peng,, T, Zhou,, Y, Huang,, L, Zhang,, P., Ye,, M, Lu,, G, Yang,, Y, Gai,, T, Yang,, X, Ma, & G, Xiang, (2015) Targeted delivery of chemically modified anti-miR-221 to hepatocellular carcinoma with negatively charged liposomes. *International journal of nanomedicine* 4825-36.
[http://dx.doi.org/https://doi.org/10.2147/IJN.S79598]

CHAPTER 11

Recent Patents and Commercially Available Nanotherapeutics on Hepatocellular Carcinoma

Susanthi Jayasinghe[1], **Imalka Munaweera**[2,3], **Disni Dedunupitiya**[1], **Chamalki Madhusha**[2], **Nilwala Kottegoda**[2,4] and **Veranja Karunaratne**[1,*]

[1] *Department of Chemistry, Faculty of Science, University of Peradeniya, Peradeniya, Sri Lanka*

[2] *Department of Chemistry, Faculty of Applied Sciences, University of Sri Jayewardenepura, Gangodawila, Nugegoda, Sri Lanka*

[3] *Instrument Center, Faculty of Applied Sciences, University of Sri Jayewardenepura, Gangodawila, Nugegoda, Sri Lanka*

[4] *Center for Advanced Materials Research (CAMR), Faculty of Applied Sciences, University of Sri Jayewardenepura, Gangodawila, Nugegoda, Sri Lanka*

Abstract: Hepatocellular carcinoma (HCC) remains a significant reason for cancer-associated deaths. The diagnostic methods for early-stage detection are insufficient, and there are limited treatments available for the late stages. Thus, novel approaches from nanotechnology have gained much attention to overcome the major hurdles in designing nanoscale materials that could be used in both diagnosis and treatments. Recently approved patents showed that progress had been made with nanotechnology in both diagnosis and therapy. The invention of HCC biomarkers, such as alpha-fetoprotein, liver carboxylesterase 1, glypican-3, endoglin, or CD105, has made significant progress in the area of diagnosis. On the other hand, methods for enhancing the sensitivity and specificity of imaging in nuclear magnetic resonance using Ga^{3+} and nanogold Computed Tomography (CT) contrast agents are noteworthy in the accuracy of cancer imaging. Nanodrugs have long-circulating times inside the body while enhancing the bioavailability of these drugs and improving efficacy without higher doses. Polymer-based nanoparticles, liposomal nanoparticles, and magnetic nano-drug vehicles are used in therapeutics to transport drugs like paclitaxel, docetaxel, doxorubicin, and mitomycin. Antisense oligodeoxynucleotides of midkine, phosphoryl N-fatty acyl nucleosides, siRNAs, and polypeptides have all been used. The long period between clinical trials and commercialization of nanotherapeutics and key issues related to clinical development should be addressed by eliminating the regulatory hurdles limiting nanotherapeutics for HCC in the market.

Keywords: Cancer chemotherapy, Cancer nanotechnology, Clinical trial, Commercial nanotherapeutics, Computed tomography, Diagnosis, Doxorubicin,

[*] **Corresponding author Veranja Karunaratne:** Department of Chemistry, Faculty of Science, University of Peradeniya, Peradeniya, Sri Lanka; E-mail: veranjaK@slintec.lk

Drug delivery, EPR effect, FDA, Hepatocellular carcinoma, Liposomes, Liver cancer, Nanoparticles, Nanotherapeutics, Nanomedicine, Nuclear magnetic resonance, Patents, Treatments.

INTRODUCTION

Hepatocellular carcinoma (HCC) is the fifth most common malignant tumor and is the third leading cause of cancer-related deaths globally. It is mainly a significant issue in Asian and African countries. Usually, the lifetime of HCC patients is around five years after being diagnosed with HCC. It is basically due to the lack of symptoms at an early stage, and most of the time, the symptoms appear in the middle and late stages. Therefore, treatment is difficult and results in poor curative effects with a very low five-year survival rate (3%-5%).

Liver transplantation or resection is the curative therapeutic approach for HCC. The transplanting in Barcelona Clinic Liver Cancer (BCLC) stages 0, A, and probably B can be implemented, and the tumor resection is only applicable in stage 0. Hence, most of the late-stage tumors would only be treated with local ablation procedures (Laser-induced thermotherapy (LITT), transarterial chemoembolization (TACE)), or systemic palliative treatment (chemotherapy with sorafenib). The initial finding of cancer is thus essential for effective treatment.

The usual diagnosis techniques such as ultrasonography (US), multiphase computerized tomography (CT), and magnetic resonance imaging (MRI) cannot be used to detect the small HCC nodules ≤2 cm with good sensitivity. (Balogh *et al.*, 2016). Hence, the key to an effective treatment for liver cancer is early detection, early diagnosis, and early treatment. They are often called "three early," the most important in the early diagnosis. Before clinical symptoms are developed or before the cancer is penetrated, it achieves a higher cure rate and decreases the mortality rate. In this context, engineered nanoparticles-based drug delivery systems have recently been developed for cancer therapy and other biomedical applications (Munaweera *et al.*, 2015a, Munaweera *et al.*, 2015b, Munaweera *et al.*, 2014). An ideal controlled drug delivery vehicle should be equipped with factors such as prolonged circulation of drug molecules in the blood, targeting into the tumor sites, response to local stimuli such as pH/temperature, *etc.*, and efficient delivery of drugs into the tumor sites (El-Sawy *et al.*, 2018).

Nanotechnology-based discoveries play a significant role in HCC diagnosis, therapeutics, and drug delivery, mainly due to the significant drawbacks and limitations in conventional pharmaceutical agents, formulations, and drug delivery systems (Kumari *et al.*, 2016, Mulik *et al.*, 2016). One of the critical problems in conventional therapeutics for HCC is the non-specific drug delivery and toxicity of conventional drug formulations. Nanopharmaceuticals have become a promising solution for the issues mentioned earlier, and several drug formulations based on nanotechnology have been developed in the market now. Several properties of these nanotherapeutics make them applicable for delivering active drugs to the target tumor tissue. Small molecule drugs, like most chemotherapies, have very short circulation time inside the body. The incorporation of nanoparticles can overcome this drawback. These nanodrugs can be made to have a long-circulating time inside the body while enhancing the bioavailability of these drugs and thus improving efficacy without the need for higher doses. Further, nanoparticles offer the ability to control the release of the encapsulated payload. In this regard, a high percentage of the trapped drug is released after the nanoparticles have reached their target tissue. This striking controlled release property of nanoparticles can improve the efficacy of the drugs while reducing off-target toxic effects.

Nanoparticles can be preferentially and easily delivered to the HCC tissues and cells by overcoming the shortcomings of conventional treatment and diagnostic approaches (Munaweera *et al.*, 2016). Nanoparticles have the targeting ability to reach the tumor area in tissue, and they invariably control the dose limit of the active drug. Multiple delivery strategies are included in a well-designed nanosystem by paving the way to reach a higher accumulation in a tumor area. Typically, extensive angiogenesis with defective vascular structure can be seen (Kalyane *et al.*, 2019). Further, a damaged lymphatic drainage system can also be seen. Therefore, increased permeability to circulating nanoparticles is provided through vascular networks of HCC. As a result, a higher concentration of nanoparticles resides in HCC tumor interstitial spaces. This phenomenon is called the enhanced permeation and retention (EPR) effect, and it is the basis for achieving passive targeting of most of the nanosystems (Stylianopoulos, 2013) (Fig. **1**).

This book chapter focuses on patents approved for nanoparticles and other nanoformulations developed for the diagnosis and therapy for HCC and those having commercial applications. Tables **1**, **2**, and **3** present a summary of the patents that have been covered in this book chapter.

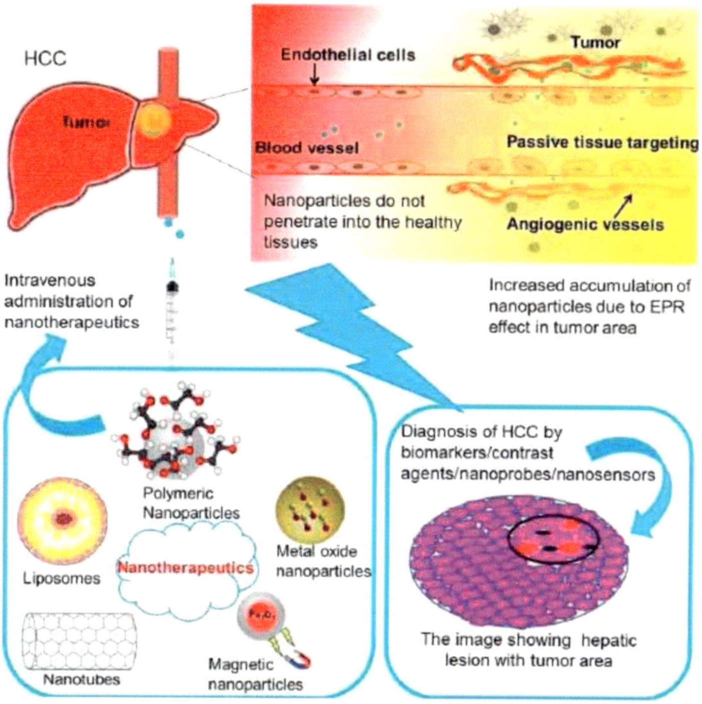

Fig. (1). Schematic illustration of EPR effect of nanotherapeutics in a tumor area and diagnosis of HCC by nanodiagnostic methods.

Table 1. Recent patents regarding diagnosis and nanotherapeutics on hepatocellular carcinoma.

Type of Nanoparticle	Patent Number(s)	Year	Authors	Description	Type
Biomarkers and diagnosis kits	CN101358973A	2007	Guangfu *et al.*	Use of a ZnO nanorod detection kit with anti-APF protein, anti- AFP alpha ferroprotein, anti-sugar protein 19-9, and anti-sugar protein 125 for the early diagnosis of liver cancer.	**Diagnosis**
	US2011097738A1	2010	Na and Paik.	Plasma biomarker tool to determine the presence of liver carboxylesterase 1 in human plasma for the diagnosis of HCC at an early stage.	
	CN104090103A	2014	Liu *et al.*	An antibody modified Zn-Se nanocrystalline kit for detection of the unique HCC marker GPC3.	

(Table 1) cont.....

Type of Nanoparticle	Patent Number(s)	Year	Authors	Description	Type
Aptamer related innovations	CN107029252A	2017	Huang *et al.*	A specific target magnetic endoglin aptamer imaging probe system(mEND-Fe_3O_4@CMCS) can bind to neo-tumor vascular endothelial cells of HCC.	**Diagnosis**
Contrast agents	WO2012113733A1	2012	Knobloch *et al.*	Nanoparticles as MRT contrast media for the diagnosis of HCC	
	CN105797173A	2016	Hu *et al.*	Human serum albumin (HSA) and PGLA loaded with a nano-gold compound as an improved contrasting agent in the MRT of HCC.	
Nano Probes/sensors and chips	CN103721271A	2013	Huang *et al.*	Au-ICG (gold-indocyanine green) lipidsome multifunctional nanoprobe for multimodal images and photothermal therapy of liver cancer.	
	CN105267992A	2015	Chen *et al.*	Superparamagnetic iron oxide nano-MRI probe,which could be used in early detection of liver cancer and lesions. With no cytotoxicity to HCC cell line HepG2.	
	CN105486679A	2016	Du *et al.*	Alpha fetoprotein electrochemiluminescence sensor based on gold hybrid carbon black intercalation with reduced graphene for the detection of hepatoma marker alpha-fetoprotein antigen.	
	CN106841164A	2017	Han *et al.*	Glycoprotein detection chip based on combination of SERS (surface enhanced Raman scattering) with an ability to improve the diagnosis.	

(Table 1) cont.....

Type of Nanoparticle	Patent Number(s)	Year	Authors	Description	Type
Polymer-based	CN101254308A	2008	Chuangnian *et al.*	Nano-formulated glycyrrhetinic acid-polyethylene glycol/chitosan as a liver-specific drug carrier.	**Delivery**
	CN101732721A	2010	Juan *et al.*	Adriamycin and a biocompatible drug carrier polymer nanoparticles which can effectively and selectively enter the abnormal cells of liver cancer tissues.	**Delivery**
	CN102198083A	2011	Cheng *et al.*	Nanomicelles and freeze-dried preparations of diblock polymer-supported taxane medicines which target HCC.	**Treatment**
	CN102920660A	2012	Chen *et al.*	Treatment with a physical and biological double-targeting effect by coupling docetaxel nanoparticles with ultrasonic irradiation.	**Treatment**
	CN103371974A	2012	Ma *et al.*	Carboplatin sustained release polymeric microspheres prepared based on micro-fluidic technology causing apoptosis of liver cancer cells.	**Delivery**
	CN104840947A	2015	Wang *et al.*	PLGA loaded DCN antioncogene plasmid nano-formulation, which targets the liver cancer cells.	**Treatment**
Liposomal	CN101716352A	2009	Hang *et al.*	An antisense oligonucleotide nano-preparation for treatment of primary hepatocellular carcinomaprepared from cation nano-liposome and an antisense oligonucleotide having amplified anti-tumor-suppressing function on HepG2.	**Treatment**
	CN102989007A	2012	Dai and Zhong	Midkine antisense oligodeoxynucleotide nanoliposomes for injection, stable and having enhanced anti-liver effect.	**Treatment**
	CN104211742A	2014	Du *et al.*	Phosphoryl N-fatty acyl nucleoside analog which is prepared by mixing liposomes and niosomes for treating viral hepatitis and liver cancers.	**Treatment**

(Table 1) cont.....

Type of Nanoparticle	Patent Number(s)	Year	Authors	Description	Type
Magnetic	CN1416812A	2001	Chen J.	Mitomycin, adsorbed in a nano-level magnetic fluid to selectively target primary liver cancers.	**Treatment**
Other	CN1243538C	2002	Yi-Yimu	Nanoparticle powder injection of ursolic acid having a high dispersion and good stability as a liver targeting agent.	**Treatment**
	US9370494B2	2011	Wong and Yeo	Nanoparticles of taxane and albumin as the effective agent for the treatment of HCC.	**Treatment**
	CN103976956A	2014	Liu *et al.*	Reduced selenium nanoparticle loaded anisomycin and hyaluronic acid for the treatment of HCC. The polysaccharide framework of hyaluronic acid targets the tumor cells.	**Treatment**
	CN103976950A	2014	Li *et al.*	A nanodispersion of adriamycin in a solid lipid and liquid lipid in a fat soluble emulsifier which selectively targets liver cancer cells.	**Treatment**
	CN104587473A	2015	Cheng *et al.*	Mesoporous apatite nanodrug carrier with reduction responsiveness and the ability to target liver cancer cells.	**Delivery**
	KR20180047442A	2016	Hyun and Lee	A siRNA nanodelivery carrier that targets CD 44 receptors in liver cancer for oral administration.	**Delivery**
	CN107596430A	2017	Gao *et al.*	A microsphere composite comprising of an inorganic nanomaterial, and its application in chemoembolization of liver cancer.	**Treatment**
	CN107778367A	2017	Cai *et al.*	A medicine containing a polypeptide which can construct a nanomaterial by carrying out tandem two-step self-assembly under the action of ALP and GSH.	**Treatment**

Table 2. Commercially available nanotherapeutics on hepatocellular Carcinoma.

Type	Commercial Name	Patent Number(s)	Year	Patent Description	Manufacturer	Type of Nanotherapeutics	Clinical Trial Number	References
Diagnosis	Sonazoid	WO2015150354A1	2015	Ultrasound contrast agent based on microbubbles (MB) containing perfluorobutane (PFB) gas	GE Health care Oslo, Norway	Liposomes; F-butane encapsulated in a lipid shell	NCT04006275	(Henriksen *et al.*, 2017)
Drug delivery	ADI-PEG 20	US9333268B2	2016	Depletes the external supply of arginine, causing arginine-dependent cancer cells to die	Polaris group	Polymeric nanosystem	NCT01287585	(Bomalaski and Wu, 2016)
	Thermodox	US10251901B2	2019	Heat-sensitive liposome to release doxorubicin directly into and around the targeted tumor	Celsion corporation	Lyso-thermosensitive liposomal doxorubicin	NCT02112656	(Reed and Daishui, 2019)
	Doxil	WO1988009168A1	1989	Encapsulated doxorubicin hydrochloride liposome	Ben Venue Laboratories	Liposomal formulation	NCT00079027	(Barenholz and Gabizon, 1990)
	Livatag	WO2017144548A1	2017	Doxorubicin in the form of lyophilised polyisohexylcyanoaerylate (PIHCA) nanoparticles, to be delivered to the liver by intra-arterial infusion.	BioAlliance Pharma SA	nanoparticle formulation of lyophilised polyisohexylcyanoaerylate	NCT01655693	(Dixon and Trochon-joseph, 2020)
	DCR-MYC	US8513207B2	2013	Double-stranded RNA in a stable lipid particle suspension for down regulation of oncogene c-myc	Dicema Pharmace-uticals	lipid nanoparticle	NCT02314052	(Brown, 2013)
	MRX 34	WO2016161196A1	2015	Double-stranded RNA which mimics microRNA-34a (miR-34a) within liposomal NPs causing down regulation of miR-34a targets	Mirna Therapeutics	lipid nanoparticle	NCT01829971	(Bader *et al.*, 2015)
	MTL-CEBPA	US10633659B2	2019	Short activating RNAs (saRNA) within liposomal NPs causing down regulation of CCAAT enhancer binding protein alpha (CEBPA) gene	Mirna Therapeutics	liposome	NCT02716012	(Saetrom, 2019)
Treatment	Hensify®	WO2013087920A1	2013	Crystalline hafnium oxide nanoparticle	NANOBIOTIX	Crystalline hafnium oxide nanoparticle	NCT02379845	(Pottier *et al.*, 2014)
	Zinostatin Stimalaer	CA1327161C	1994	Lipophilic intra-arterial chemotherapeutic agent for HCC	Yamanouchi	Lipophilic nanosystem	UMIN C000000111	(Kobayashi *et al.*, 1991)
	TKM□080301	US9139554B2	2015	Lipid nanoparticle (LNP) formulation of a siRNA directed against human PLK1 mRNA	Arbutus Biopharma	lipid nanoparticle (LNP) formulation	NCT02191878	(Hope *et al.*, 2015)

Nanotherapeutics: The Future of Hepatocellular Carcinoma Treatment

Table 3. Patents applied in 2019/2020 regarding diagnosis and nanotherapeutics on HCC.

Type	Patent Number	Year	Authors	Description
Treatment	CN201710554782A	2017	Chen and Ju	Gene therapy against HCC by targeting interleukin-22, which is widely distributed in normal pancreas, liver, small intestine, colon, and kidney.
Treatment	CN110302153A	2018	Fu *et al.*	Sorafenib nanomicelles, using polyethylene glycol-polycaprolactone block copolymer. The invention increases the drug concentration at the tumor site, significantly increases the therapeutic effect, reduces the toxicity of the drug to normal tissues, and reduces side effects.
Treatment	CN110772496A	2018	Bai *et al.*	Paclitaxel nanoparticle applied to the interventional treatment of liver cancer.
Delivery	CN109276559A	2018	Zhang	T Silver nanoparticles loaded microRNA, a non-chemotherapy drug, with less toxic side effects, multidrug resistance is avoided.
Treatment	CN110522922A	2019	Chen *et al.*	Nano-particles coupled with ginsenosides, and the application of Fe_2O_3 nanoparticles coupled with ginsenosides for preparing anti-liver cancer drug
Diagnosis	CN109701039A	2019	Ai *et al.*	Dual-targeted magnetic nanoparticles for liver cancer. Superparamagnetic iron oxide (SPIO) nanoparticles are currently the ideal magnetic resonance tracer. The researchers used MR tracing SPIO-labeled stem cells to achieve success in animal models of various organ damage and disease.
Delivery	CN110420221A	2019	Qu	A natural nanovesicle application in regulating cell transfer and TGF-β signal pathway inhibitors.
Treatment	CN111568879A	2020	Hu *et al.*	Anti-hepatoma drug nanoparticle-based on pH and redox dual response prepared by grafting urocanic acid and alpha-lipoic acid with a polysaccharide.

Diagnosis of HCC

Nanostructured materials have gained much attention as innovative bioimaging, diagnostic and therapeutic agents in the biomedical sector. They have unique characteristics such as superparamagnetic or fluorescent properties and smaller sizes compared to biomolecules. Several new findings include new detection kits, new contrast agents, nanoprobe/sensors, aptamer imaging devices, and nano-liquid chromatography coupled to tandem mass spectrometry (nanoLCMS), which are based on nanostructured material, especially for detection of HCC at early stages.

Biomarkers and Diagnosis Kits

Alpha-fetoprotein (AFP) serum markers have been used to detect HCC since 1968 (Wong *et al.*, 2014). Only the cancerous hepatocytes synthesize AFP, but not the normal liver cells. Thus, this increased AFP concentration level could be used as an indicator for cancer detection at an early stage. However, it has been identified that AFP could be elevated in acute hepatitis, cirrhosis, colitis, germ cell tumors, and intrahepatic cholangiocarcinoma conditions, resulting in poor sensitivity and specificity. Therefore, detection of AFP alone would not be accurate, and it would be better to detect Carcino Embryonic Antigen (CEA) related to liver cancer tumors.

Guangfu *et al.* in 2007 have patented an invention of a ZnO nanorod array detection kit with anti-AFP protein, anti-sugar protein 19-9 (CA19-9), and anti-sugar protein 125 (CA125) for early diagnosis of liver cancer. The CA19-9 and CA125 markers have also been included to improve the accuracy of detection. The kit consists of an enhanced ZnO nanorod array film-coated by four kinds of proteins described above, a bottom plate, a micro field device (with an electrophoresis tank and a pair of electrodes), a buffer solution. The ZnO nanorod array film has been formed on the glass substrate by gel method, and then the antibody and protein were chemically covalently bonded to the surface of the ZnO nanorod by a polypeptide condensation technique. Further, the detectable signal is a photoluminescence signal of ZnO nanorods. Guangfu *et al.* have reported that the kit could be used to diagnose primary liver cancer tumors, particularly for the detection of early clinical primary liver cancer, and could also be used for the chemotherapeutic monitoring and the prognostic evaluation after the operation on the liver cancer. Besides, they have further claimed that the invention has various features such as high speed, sensitivity, accuracy, reliability, simplicity of the procedure, and suitability for the primary health care units and hospitals of multiple levels (Guangfu *et al.*, 2007).

Even though the biomarkers alpha-fetoprotein (AFP), des-gamm--carboxyprothrombin (DCP), glypican-3 (GPC3), alpha-1-fucosidase, and transforming growth factor-b1 have been utilized, alone or in combination, for the clinical screening of HCC patients, the lack of sensitivity and the specificity of those, indeed urge the recent developments with enhanced sensitivity and specificity for early diagnosis of HCC.

Na and Paik have invented a new plasma biomarker tool to determine the presence of liver carboxylesterase 1 (hCE1) in human plasma to diagnose HCC at an early stage (Na and Paik, 2010). The hCE1 is an N-linked glycosylated protein that is a specific biomarker for HCC. Even though hCE1 is expressed in small amounts in HCC tissues relative to normal liver tissues, there are no reliable conventional methods reported for direct detection of hCE1 in human plasma. In the reported invention, the proteomics techniques, 2-D DIGE, and nano-L--MS/MS system, were applied, and it showed that hCE1 is present in the plasma of both healthy and HCC patients. However, according to this invention, the amount of biomarker protein secreted into plasma is measured. It is considered an indicator of the existence and early diagnosis of HCC, allowing for timely therapeutic intervention and thus increasing the survival rate of patients with HCC.

Liu *et al.* (2014a) reported an invention of an antibody-modified Zn-Se nanocrystalline-based kit to detect HCC marker glypican-3 (GPC-3). GPC-3 is a member of the glypican family, a group of heparan sulfate proteoglycans linked to the cell surface through a glycosyl-phosphatidyl inositol-anchor. It has been found that glypicans interact with growth factors, modify their activities and perform an essential role in cell growth, differentiation, and migration. However, according to the recent findings, it is only expressed in most HCC but weakly expressed or not expressed in normal liver tissues and liver lesions. Moreover, GPC-3 seems to function differently in various cancers, whereas GPC-3 is downregulated in breast cancer, ovarian cancer, and lung adenocarcinoma. It is upregulated in HCC (Filmus and Capurro, 2008, Sung *et al.,* 2003). Besides, inventors have observed that DCP-3 was detected in 33% of HCC patients seronegative for AFP and DCP (Nakatsura *et al.*, 2003). Importantly, GPC-3 expression seems to be independent of the tumor size, as GPC-3 showed a sensitivity of 56% in patients with initial stage cancers that are < 3 cm in size (Tangkijvanich *et al.*,2010). Hence it is believed that GPC-3 has high sensitivity and specificity for the diagnosis of HCC.

Nevertheless, the concentration of GPC-3 in serum samples is generally as low as parts per billion (ppb). Hence, rapid, sensitive, and straightforward PC-3 protein serum analysis and detection technology are not quite ordinary. Authors claimed that the given invention has combined immunoassay technology with novel Zn-Se nanocrystals to develop a rapid, specific, and highly sensitive detection method for liver cancer markers (GPC-3). The kit, which is patented, contains Zn-Se nanocrystals with the surface cross-linking modified GPC-3 antibody, zinc ion fluorescent probe solution, GPC-3 antibody, and GPC-3 protein standard. The Zn-Se nanocrystal and the GPC-3 detection antibody may be directly or indirectly cross-linked, preferably directly, and the Zn-Se nanocrystal has a particle diameter of 1 to 10 nm. Further, the kit utilized a combination of double-antibody sandwich immunoassay method and cation exchange reaction of Zn-Se nanocrystalline, where it recognizes an increase of the GPC-3 detection signal in immunoreaction, and thus has the benefits of stable signal, high sensitivity, low detection limit of the HCCmarker GPC-3 (Liu *et al.*, 2014a).

Aptamer Related Innovations

Molecular targeting therapy with oligonucleotide nanomedicine to detect HCC is another powerful method for the early diagnosis of HCC with high efficiency. This method uses aptamers, single-stranded RNA, or DNA oligonucleotides with low molecular weight (6-30 kDa). Since the aptamers have a flexible configuration, it has a high binding affinity and specificity to small and large target molecules in the intracellular and extracellular environment with agonist or antagonist function. Besides, their stability at room temperature and in non-physiological environments, no immunogenicity and toxicity, suitable for frequent long-term administration, greater capacity for bio-distribution in biological fluids, and high capability to enter and persist in the tumor site as well as the cost-effectiveness in synthesis than antibody production, have focused much attention in developing these nanomedicines as diagnostic and therapeutic tools (Ladju *et al.*, 2017).

Endoglin (also known as CD105) is a cell membrane glycoprotein with a molecular weight of about 68 kD. It is prominently expressed on the endothelial cells of tumor neovasculature but not on normal blood vessels (Minhajat *et al.*, 2006). Endogl in which is a component of the transforming growth factor-beta (TGF-β) receptor complex, accompanied by the propagation of vascular endothelial cells. It also stimulates vascularization *via* triggering the anti-apoptotic pathway in hypoxic endothelial cells. Therefore, CD105 could be used as a possible application in the diagnosis and treatment of HCC.

Huang *et al.* in 2017 identified a method to prepare a target-specific magnetic endoglin aptamer imaging probe system (mEND-Fe_3O_4@CMCS), which can specifically bind to neo-tumor vascular endothelial cells of HCC. In this invention, the magnetic endoglin aptamer imaging probe, mEND-Fe_3O_4@CMCS, is prepared by modifying the surface of Fe_3O_4@CMCS with an endoglin aptamer by the cross-linking action of sulfo-SMCC. Fe_3O_4@CMCS are ready using magnetic Fe_3O_4 nano-particles (equipped with the hydrothermal method) and carboxymethyl chitosan nanoparticle emulsification and cross-linking methods with glutaraldehyde as the cross-linking agent. The magnetic endoglin aptamer imaging probe, mEND-Fe_3O_4@CMCS, has an average particle size of about 87.15 ± 1.66 nm and a surface potential of -31.9 ± 0.5 mV with no apparent accumulation. Authors claimed that the preparation method has the advantages such as easy and simple preparation, large-scale industrial production, small particle size, high saturation magnetic susceptibility, stable suspension and dispersion, low toxicity, high relaxation rate, good biocompatibility, and targeting to the liver and spleen. Further, they have demonstrated that mEND-Fe_3O_4@CMCS can successfully target mouse tumor angiogenesis endothelial cell (mTEC) surface CD105 molecules and has hepatic transplantable tumor mouse MRI imaging capability (Huang *et al.*, 2017).

Contrast Agents

Molecular imaging techniques can be used as an early diagnostic method to detect early biological characteristics of tumors when clinical symptoms have not yet occurred. Current methods commonly used for tumor diagnosis in clinical practices include: magnetic resonance imaging (MRI), computed tomography (CT), ultrasound imaging, near-infrared imaging, *etc*., often use contrast agents for non-invasive imaging. Enhancing the sensitivity and specificity of the above imaging techniques to reach diagnostic imaging at the cellular or molecular level is the core and key to the early diagnosis of liver cancer. Currently, several types of auxiliary contrast enhancers have been commonly used in clinical practice to increase the sensitivity and specificity of the above imaging techniques.; For example, metal complexes based on Gd^{3+} have been effectively used in MRI. However, toxic side effects such as increased tissue osmotic pressure and tissue edema could be observed after injection. Additionally, poor sensitivity can lead to high-dose injections and increase toxic side effects. Hence, the sensitivity of most of the contrast agents presently used in clinical practice needs to be further improved.

HCC frequently progresses at the beginning of cirrhosis of the liver, mainly due to hepatitis B and hepatitis C viral infections, aflatoxins, and alcohol abuse. Hence, patients with liver cirrhosis and suspicious nodules are considered at high risk of becoming HCC patients in the future. In HCC diagnosis with contrast MR or CT, small HCCs are rarely being detected. Thus, the clinically critical differentiation between small HCCs and regenerated and dysplastic nodules in the cirrhotic liver is an urgent need. The challenges presented are on the methods to improve magnetic resonance tomography (MRT) performance in the diagnosis of HCC. Knobloch *et al.* developed nanoparticles, comprising a gadolinium compound and/or incorporated perfluorooctyl bromide, to be used as contrast media with high specificity and sensitivity in MRT to detect liver diseases, predominantly of HCC of a size smaller than 1.5 cm. Nanoparticles made from the polymers such as human serum albumin (HSA) and poly (D, L-lactic-co-glycolic) acid (PLGA) were loaded with a gadolinium compound (Gd-DTPA) and used productively for improved contrasting in the MRT of HCC. The contrast agent given in this invention contains a physiologically compatible aqueous medium and is provided in an injection solution. The MRT examination was carried out using a 3-Tesla tomograph. The advantage of these nanoparticle-based contrast media is reduced toxicity. There is no undesired long-term accumulation of these carrier systems in the body since the body breaks down both the HSA and PLGA nanoparticles.

Further, the authors claimed that the nanoparticles of the present invention have surprisingly advantageous properties, which favor a contrast of the HCC caused by the EPR effect, which is known as the deposition of the macromolecular substances such as nanoparticles in the tumor tissue as tumor vessels have increased permeability. As a result, it empowers prior recognition of even minor HCC and permits the distinction of HCC and cirrhotic regenerated lumps (Knobloch *et al.,* 2012).

One of the methods used in diagnosing liver cancer is the use of Computed Tomography (CT). The imaging contrast agents used in current CT are mainly iodine small molecules, which have several limitations in the early diagnosis of liver cancer, such as poor specificity, low signal intensity, and specific toxicity. Therefore, developing effective, sensitive, and nontoxic contrast agents is crucial for the early diagnosis and precise diagnosis of liver cancer. Hu *et al.*, in 2016, revealed a method for preparing a nanogold CT contrast agent that could be used for the early diagnosis of HCC. Here, they have used pH-sensitive lipoic acid-modified N-diisopropylethanediamine (LA-N(iPr)2), lipoic acid polyethylene glycol-modified glycyrrhetinic acid (LA-PEG3.5k-GA), and lipoic acid linked polyethylene glycol (LA-PEG2k) are modified on the surface of gold nanoparticles (AuNPs) with a mass ratio of the n(LA-N(iPr)2) to the n(LA-PEG3.5k-GA) to the n(LA-PEG2k) is at 1 to 1 to (3-5). Authors claimed that as the nanogold has a high electron density and a two-time higher X-ray absorption coefficient than the iodine, it could accurately diagnose the HCC.

Additionally, smaller particles (18-25 nm) result in effective penetration in tumor tissues and attachment of liver targeted pH-sensitive ligands that could be reversible by the "shield-deshield" process pH changes of the tumor site. Thus, utilizing active and passive targeting gives this method an added advantage over other contrast agents for the early diagnosis of HCC. Authors have applied the present contrast agent to detect mouse H22 HCC (Hu *et al.*, 2016).

NanoProbes/Sensors and Chips

Modern medicine is generally required to create various imaging data for accurate cancer diagnosis. However, clinically used contrast agents have no multi-modal, multi-angle imaging ability; hence, numerous contrast injections may have to be used to obtain the final diagnosis. As a result, the contrast agents' side effects could be increased, leading to the patient's adverse health effects and increased economic burden. Therefore, the development of very sensitive multimodal molecular imaging contrast agents to increase the sensitivity and specificity of diagnosis is highly important. The combinations of different nanostructured materials with various characteristics could provide synergistic multifunctional nanomedical platforms, making it possible to achieve multimodal imaging and simultaneous diagnosis and therapy. Multifunctional nanomaterials have been produced by combining different types of nanomaterials. Furthermore, the conjugation of targeting moieties on these multifunctional nanomaterial surfaces provides them with specifically targeted imaging and therapeutic features. However, many concerns, including the biocompatibility, toxicity in humans, the effectiveness of the *in vivo* targeting, and the long-term stability of the multifunctional nanoparticles, must be addressed.

Huang *et al.* in 2013 reported an Au-ICG (gold-indocyanine green) liposome multifunctional nanoprobe suitable for MRI, CT imaging, near-infrared fluorescence imaging, and targeted photothermal therapy for liver cancer. This Au-ICG liposome multifunctional nanoprobe comprises of a core and a shell; the core is surface coated with a polydopamine (PDA) layer and adsorbed with indocyanine green (ICG) nanogold particles, the outer shell is DSPE-PEG (polyethylene glycol-di-stearoyl phosphatidylethanolamine) liposome coupled with lactobionic acid (LA) and chelated with a Gd^{3+} ion membrane. The Au-PD--ICG nanoparticles can be excited by 808 nm near-infrared light for near-infrared fluorescence imaging. The gold nanoparticles have a significant molecular weight (higher than medical iohexol) and have strong X-ray absorption ability (higher than medical iohexol), slow blood removal (lower than medical iohexol), so it can effectively improve the spatial resolution of CT, reduce the X-ray radiation dose and prolong the CT imaging time. Authors claimed that the Au-ICG liposome multifunctional nanoprobe could be used for various image modes such as MRI (magnetic resonance imaging), CT (computed tomography) imaging, and near-infrared fluorescence imaging of liver cancer. Hence, various diagnosis effects can be acquired. Furthermore, as the sensitivity is improved, the use of contrast agents can be reduced, and thus the toxic side effect could be minimized. Besides, as the ICG molecule can effectively convert light energy into heat energy, producing excessive heat of 60 °C to 70 °C, liver cancer cells can be killed thermally as well. Hence, in the present invention, the multifunctional nanoprobe has the advantage of being able to be used both as a multimodal contrast agent for liver cancer diagnosis and as a photo-thermal therapeutic agent in liver cancer (Huang *et al.*, 2013).

Chen *et al.* in 2015 reported another superparamagnetic iron oxide nano MRI probe that could be used in the early detection of liver cancer and lesions. The present invention comprised of superparamagnetic iron oxide (SPIO), PEG (polyethylene glycol), and CTX (chloride channel toxin), and the MRI probe has been abbreviated as SPIO-PEG-CTX. Authors claimed that the present invention had not shown any cytotoxicity to human HCC cell line HepG2 (Chen *et al.*, 2015).

There are many clinical methods for detecting alpha-fetoprotein (a tumor marker and an important indicator widely used in diagnosing early stages of HCC), such as enzyme-linked immunosorbent assay radioimmunoassay, chemiluminescence immunoassay, *etc*. Radioactive contamination, low sensitivity, long detection, and cumbersome steps are some of the aforementioned methods-related disadvantages. Du *et al.* 2016 reported a new invention that disclosed a method for preparing an alpha-fetoprotein electrochemiluminescence sensor based on gold hybrid carbon black intercalation of reduced graphene. In this report, they have mixed the carbon black and graphene and obtained reduced graphene to minimize agglomeration of the graphene sheet layer and improve the sensing platform conductivity. The reduced graphene of the carbon black intercalation layer was further functionalized with gold sol to enhance the sensor's electrochemiluminescence performance. Trisbipyridine ruthenium is used as the electrochemiluminescence signal source. The carrier content of an antibody is improved by good biocompatibility and a large specific surface area of gold hybrid carbon black intercalation reduced graphene. Nano-porous silver is taken as the second antibody marker and is obtained by the de-alloying method. The hepatoma marker alpha-fetoprotein antigen is identified based on the intensity changes of the electrochemiluminescence signal as the concentration of tested substances changes (Du *et al.*, 2016).

Han *et al.* in 2017 reported another new finding, a glycoprotein detection chip that could read AFP-L3 heterogeneous body resolution. AFP-L3 is specifically expressed in liver cancer cells, and if the total amount of AFP-L3 accounts for more than 10% of AFP, it has been diagnosed as early liver cancer. The present invention utilized the combination of Surface-Enhanced Raman Scattering (SERS) displacement and detecting technique, an ultra-sensitive surface analysis method. The latest quantitative method (displacement of Raman characteristic peaks) and an old quantitative method (internal standard and characteristic peak relative intensity) are combined for the first time quantitatively for detecting the read variant %. Moreover, antibody nanogold and a silver assembly membrane with Raman activity and good biocompatibility have been used as substrates for the first time. Authors claimed that the protein chip could significantly improve the diagnosis accuracy due to the high distinguishing capacity for AFP (alpha-fetoprotein). Hence, it could be the protein chip application with the most potential in early liver cancer diagnosis (Han *et al.*, 2017).

Nanotherapeutics on HCC

Nanoparticle therapies are emerging technologies which is undergoing active research all over the world. In this connection, clinically noteworthy studies involving nanoparticle technologies are currently being reported. Therefore, making sense of these innovations at this stage of the technology is essential in understanding cancer chemotherapy. This truism applies to HCC as well, and perhaps more so, as therapies for HCC are still at an embryonic stage. Therefore, taking stock of the patents and commercially used medicines in the control and cure of HCC provides a different perspective to this emergent area. The size of nanoparticles used in HCC varies from 5-100 nm (Dawar *et al.*, 2013). There are many materials from which nanoparticles can be fabricated. Organic polymers such as Poly-lactide-coglycolide (PLGA) and Poly-caprolactone (PCL) are common. Also, metal nanoparticles from gold, iron, silver, and other components such as silica are used. Thus, the variety of materials used also expands the variety of possible functional groups that can be incorporated onto the surface of nanoparticles. Here, numerous targeting agents can be conjugated to the surface or into the core, depending on the nanoparticle's structural and other features. It is optimal that these nanoparticles can curtail rapid metabolism and clearance, leading to sustained delivery of therapeutics (Brannon-Peppas and Blanchette, 2004). Besides, it is also essential that these nanoparticles improve the therapeutic index of drugs by enhancing the drug's efficacy and increasing the tolerance of therapies involved (Cortes and Saura, 2010). Nanoparticle therapies can significantly improve the bioavailability of hydrophobic drugs, thereby minimizing delivery drawbacks related to hydrophobic drugs (Katsumi *et al.*, 2012). When the functionalized nanoparticles possess targeting abilities, therapeutics delivery to the intended site of action is enhanced, leading to low side-effects accompanied with most therapeutic procedures (McMillan *et al.*, 2011).

Active Targeting of the Therapeutic Agent

Delivery modes of drugs can be of active or passive types. Passive targeting fundamentally based on the tumor microenvironment involves the systemic and lymphatic systems for drug delivery. The increased EPR effect primarily enables the tumor microenvironment. EPR effect occurs due to poorly separated vasculature and inadequate lymphatic drainage, leading to weak, unstable, and leaky vasculature (Maeda, 2001b, 2012). On the other hand, active targeting engages ligand or receptor facilitated drug delivery. Targeting ligands comprise many agents such as antibodies, aptamer, siRNA, peptides, proteins, and small molecules. The targeting ligands can be covalently bonded to a drug or held onto the carrier surface, such as nanoparticles, liposomes, and nanomicelles, through electrostatic forces (Pohl *et al.*, 1974; Bae and Park, 2011). In addition, nanoparticles range from 50-300 nm in diameter with a polydispersity index between 0.1-0.4 and zeta potential of ± 30 mV.

Nanomedicine carriers are one of the essential areas of research in the field of nanomedical research. Many studies have reported that nano-drug carriers can promote the accumulation of drugs in tumor tissues. Because the microenvironment of tumor tissues is considerably different from normal tissues, they are dilated and curved in terms of the layout of blood vessels. The absence of lymphatic reflux makes the pressure inside tumor tissues considerably higher than the surrounding normal tissues. These differences are not favorable to the delivery of small molecule drugs through the blood vessels to the deep part of the tumor tissue, and the drugs do not easily reach the tumor cells and the target of the action. However, because of the discontinuity of tumor neovascular endothelial cells, nanoparticles with a particle size of less than 200 nm can enter the interstitial space *via* the blood vessel wall. Therefore, loading drugs into nanoparticles can enhance their efficacy through penetration and retention. It is estimated that the inclusion of anticancer drugs in nanoparticles can increase the drug's improvement at the tumor site by 5-10 times. If the surface of the nanoparticles is further decorated with tumor cell-specific ligands with targeting ability, the drug can be further enhanced in tumors. Enrichment, to a great extent, reduces the toxic and side effects of the drug and improves the quality of life of patients. The fabrication of highly efficient and low-toxic nano-drug carriers that can address penetration and cell targeting provides valuable strategies in the clinical treatment of tumors. However, serious challenges are still remaining (Shilpi, 2018).

Targeting Agents

Polymer-Based Nanoparticles

Polymer nanoparticle research has developed rapidly as drug transport vehicles in recent years. They possess several advantages, such as the availability of various structures, ease of preparation, rapid quality control, superior biocompatibility, and degradation amenable to structural control. They are known to enhance the drug *in vivo* activity significantly. Recently, more amphiphilic polymer materials have been studied, which can spontaneously aggregate in aqueous solution to form nanoparticles with distinctive structures, such as micelles and vesicles suitable for the delivery of drugs both hydrophilic and hydrophobic. One such example is the block polymers of polyethylene glycol-polyaspartic acid derivatives for delivering the anticancer drug paclitaxel (Kataoka *et al.*, 2012). Polyethylene glycol is used as the hydrophilic portion. Polyaspartic acid derivatives act as the hydrophobic segment, which self-assembles into nanoparticles. A problem that cannot be ignored is that the structure of the self-assembled nanoparticles of amphiphilic polymers strongly depends on the relative amounts of the hydrophilic and hydrophobic components because their stability tends to be less. Such self-assembled nanoparticles are easily dissociated after dilution in body fluids or blood. As such, their breakup often results in a burst release of the drug before the nanoparticles reach the target site. Therefore, added chemical or physical cross-linking is applied to make the structures more stable to enhance drug release and drug delivery performance. Among them, chemical cross-linking is generally used to synthesize amphiphiles with cross-linkable functional groups.

Chuangnian *et al.* in 2008 described nanoformulated glycyrrhetinic acid-polyethylene glycol/chitosan or chitosan derivative as a liver-specific drug carrier. Glycyrrhetinic acid, a triterpenoid saponin much sweeter than sucrose, is the main biologically active ingredient in licorice (Nassiri and Hosseinzadeh, 2008) is known for its anti-inflammatory, hepatoprotective, and antiviral activity (Graebin *et al.*, 2018). Glycyrrhetinic acid and polyethylene glycol in the presence of chitosan and a cross-linking agent spontaneously forms nanoparticles by electrostatic interactions. *In-vitro* experiments revealed potent binding to liver cells and cell kill (Chuangnian *et al.*, 2008).

A biocompatible drug carrier polymer nanoparticles containing an organic phospholipid was described by Juan *et al.* in 2010. It can carry doxorubicin effectively to liver cancer cells. Doxorubicin, along with the nanoparticle, is more effective than doxorubicin itself. The nanoparticle biocompatibility makes it a drug conveying carrier, making the method convenient for further decorating the nanoparticle with other ligands. The nanoparticle is used for transferring drugs in a targeted manner. These nanoparticles can carry doxorubicin to effectively and selectively enter abnormal cells of liver cancer tissues. It makes the nanoparticle treatment method better than doxorubicin itself (Juan *et al.*, 2010).

A nanomicelle preparation of freeze-dried preparations of diblock polymer-supported taxane was reported by Cheng *et al.* in 2011. This formulation, among many cancer types, was able to target liver cancer. The nanomicellar formulation was prepared by taking 1.5 to 99 parts of methoxypolyethylene glycol and polycaprolactone diblock polymer and 1 part of the taxane paclitaxel (Taxol) and docetaxel (Taxotere), which are known to disrupt the microtubule formation. The micelles and freeze-dried formulations of taxanes can be used for treating cancers, Kaposi sarcoma, malignant tumors, tissues, and cell hyperplasia. This preparation mainly targets hepatocellular carcinoma, ovarian cancer, and breast cancer (Cheng *et al.*, 2011).

The ability of paclitaxel to be effective against various malignant tumor cells such as breast cancer, melanoma, and ovarian cancer, its efficacy against HCC has been doubted. For example, a phase II clinical trial of paclitaxel for HCC patients concluded that paclitaxel had no significant anti-cancer effect in HCC patients (Chao *et al.*, 1998). Docetaxel, on the other hand, was reported to be more potent against HCC than paclitaxel. A novel approach to liver cancer treatment with a physical and biological double-targeting effect was reported by Chen *et al.* in 2012. Here, docetaxel nanoparticles with an average particle size of 209 nm were prepared by mixing in hydrophilic mono-methoxypolyoxyethylene glycol, poly (lactic-co-glycolic acid), docetaxel, and galactosidated cholesterol. *In vivo* anti-tumor target experiments show that the treatment gives better efficacy by coupling docetaxel nanoparticle treatment with ultrasonic irradiation, where the anti-tumor activity reached 74.2% (Chen *et al.*, 2012).

Ma *et al.* in 2012 revealed a sustained release drug prepared using polymeric microspheres based on microfluidic technology. Here, polylactic acid-hydroxyacetic acid (PLGA) copolymer microspheres monodispersed into a honeycomb structure containing water-soluble anti-cancer drugs prepared by a micro-fluidic chip. The microspheres prepared possess unique structures with homogeneous nanoscale thin film layers on the surface and inner micron level water-soluble drugs such as carboplatin, which continuously released the latter with the degradation of polymer carrier (Ma *et al.*, 2012). Carboplatin-loaded microspheres induce apoptosis of liver cancer cells. Carboplatin has been used as a chemotherapeutic agent against several cancers such as ovarian cancer, lung cancer, head and neck cancer, brain cancer, and neuroblastoma (Apps *et al.*, 2015).

HCC gene-targeted therapy has become a hot spot in cancer clinical research. However, so far, the functional gene transfection lacks cell targeting ability. The target gene carried by the vector is often destroyed by enzyme digestion in the cell where the action time is short, leading to low utility issues. These problems have led to the poor efficiency of traditional gene therapy, which has become a bottleneck limiting its applications (Yazdani *et al.*, 2018). On the other hand, nanogene carriers are novel gene carrier systems that use nanoparticles to encapsulate the therapeutic gene in the nanoparticle or adsorbed on the surface. The nanoparticle enters the cell and releases the therapeutic gene through intracellular injection. Wang *et al.* in 2015 disclosed that AFP monoclonal antibodies, biodegradable macromolecular biomaterials such as PLGA-loaded Decorin (DCN) antioncogene plasmids act as a nanotherapy against liver cancer. When the liver targeting nanomedicine is combined with liver cells, the therapeutic effect was slowly realized, inhibiting the liver cancer cells. This nanoformulation has the advantage in that the gene transfection efficiency is improved coupled with long-term inhibition of targeted genes in cancer cells is achieved (Wang *et al.*, 2015).

Liposomal Nanoparticles

Liposomes are vesicles made of phospholipid bilayers highly dispersed in an aqueous solution and assist as carriers of a range of drugs. Their high dispersibility allows targeting and sustained release of the drug in the body. They possess lymphatic tropism in oral administration, allowing them to carry drugs across the blood-brain barrier, and they enter cells with ease by fusion and endocytosis. The phospholipid bilayer membrane of the liposome vesicles separates the inner drug encapsulated aqueous phase from the external aqueous phase and remains hydrophobic within the bilayer. Generally, the water-soluble drug is encapsulated in the inner aqueous phase, and the fat-soluble drug is in the film layer. During their preparation, phospholipid molecules self-assemble in water, and the volume ratio of the inner and outer aqueous phases cannot be large. These factors determine the encapsulation rate of water-soluble drugs (<50%), and whether the encapsulated drug leaks into the outer aqueous phase. In the presence of a suitable fat-soluble group (such as a fatty chain), the fat-soluble drug molecule can be incorporated into the phospholipid bilayer, where the binding is relatively firm, and the drug molecule is embedded well, leading to high drug encapsulation rates. If the liposome is used for carrying a fat-soluble nucleoside prodrug, the encapsulation rate can be increased, and the prodrug can be made to penetrate the cell easily.

Midkine (MK or MDK), also known as neurite growth-promoting factor 2 (NEGF2), is a protein that in humans is encoded by the MDK gene. Midkine is an essential heparin-binding growth factor having low molecular weight. It is a retinoic acid-responsive gene product that is important for development and induced during mid-gestation, hence the name midkine. It is restricted to specific tissues in the average adult and is induced strongly during oncogenesis, inflammation, and tissue repair. MK appears to enhance the angiogenic and proliferative activities of cancer cells (Kato *et al.*, 2000), and its expression is elevated in various cancer types, such as neuroblastoma, glioblastoma, colorectal, liver, ovary, bladder, breast, lung, esophageal, stomach, and prostate cancers. Hang *et al.* (2009) disclosed an antisense oligonucleotide nanomedicine with the potential of treating the primary HCC, which resists the MK factor. It is prepared from cation nanoliposome and antisense oligonucleotide (CCCCGGGCCGCCCTTCTTCA). The nano-preparation has an amplified anti-tumor suppressing function to HepG2 liver cancer cells; moreover, an in-vivo pharmacodynamical analysis result shows that it has an obvious suppressing function to the primary liver cancer and has the advantages of less toxicity or side effects, little possibility of generating drug resistance, and good biological compatibility. The nanopreparation can be used for target transportation and is degraded *in vivo* (Hang *et al.*, 2009).

These nanoliposomes in the range of 100-500 nm possess an anti-hepatoma effect. These nanoparticles, which are easy to prepare, can be scaled up easily. The invention relates to preparing midkine antisense oligodeoxynucleotidenano-liposomes for injection, which is stable while it has an enhanced anti-liver cancer effect. The technique is simple in process, easy to realize, amplified, and suitable for industrial production (Dai and Zhong, 2012).

Nucleotides and nucleic acids are carriers of genetic information. The most important genetic material, DNA and RNA, is assembled from nucleotides. Nucleoside analogs are an essential class of compounds whose structural features are similar to those of nucleosides. A variety of nucleoside analogs have been synthesized, and many of them have been reported to have pharmacological activities such as antiviral action, cytotoxicity, immunosuppressive effects (Senanayake *et al.*, 2011). A phosphoryl N-fatty acyl nucleoside analog containing nanomedicine was developed by Du *et al.* in 2014. This system is prepared by mixing liposomes and niosomes, non-ionic surfactant-based vesicles, with nucleoside analogs such as lamivudine, adenine arabinoside, cidofovir, gemcitabine, cytosine arabinoside, azacitidine, and fludarabine attached to the fatty acid chain at N. This nucleoside analog targets liver cancer and viral hepatitis (Du *et al.*, 2014).

Magnetic Nanoparticles (MNPs)

MNPs have achieved enormous attention for theranostic cancer functions due to their unique physicochemical properties, MRI contrast, facile synthesis, easy surface functionalization, low toxicity, and good biodegradability that aid them to function as excellent imaging agents and delivery vehicles in cancer theranostics (Mukherjee *et al.*, 2020). Mitomycin is a broad-spectrum anti-tumor drug and a potent DNA cross-linker with exceptional outcomes on digestive tract tumors (Tomasz, 1995). However, mitomycin does not exclusively target tumor cells, and clinically applied mitomycin injections result in systemic toxic side effects. Therefore, its therapeutic dose does not achieve the expected results. As early as 2001, it was reported that mitomycin, adsorbed in a nanolevel magnetic fluid, was used to selectively target primary liver cancers. The liver-targeted mitomycin magnetic nanoparticle was prepared as an intravenously injected lyophilized powder injection. It has natural liver targeting function and liver tissue distribution after intravenous administration without an external magnetic field at a rate of 54-70%. However, mitomycin distribution in the liver is significantly enhanced under an external magnetic field of intensity greater than 0.35T. Therefore, it can increase the local blood concentration of the liver cancer area, thereby controlling and killing the cancer cells and reducing the blood concentration in other organs, thereby reducing the systemic toxicity of the drug (Chen, 2001).

Other Types of Nanoparticles

Yi-Yimu, in 2002, disclosed nanoparticles of ursolic acid as a liver targeting agent. Ursolic acid is known as an anti-inflammatory, anti-oxidant, anti-apoptotic, and anti-carcinogenic compound which can be used as an unconventional medicine for the management of cancer, obesity/diabetes, cardiovascular disease, brain disease, liver disease, and muscle wasting (sarcopenia) (Seo *et al.*, 2018). At present, the pharmacological effects of ursolic acid have not gained therapeutic potential, and there are no ursolic acid-based medicines on the market. Ursolic acid shows low water solubility, and absorption through oral administration is not viable. This innovation is the first application of nano-ursolic acid. Here, the nanoparticle powder injection used has the advantages of high dispersion and good stability (Yi-Yimu, 2002).

Albumin-based nanoparticle compositions have been developed as a drug delivery system for delivering water-insoluble drugs such as taxanes (Neil *et al.,* 2000). Such nanoparticles can transport and deliver water-insoluble drugs to the disease target because of the natural properties of albumin. Because albumin-based nanoparticle technology improves drug solubility, it avoids the need for toxic chemicals, such as solvents, thus, potentially improving safety by eliminating solvent-based side effects. Wong and Yeo reported another method of nano intervention against HCC using taxane in 2011. Here, nanoparticles of taxane and albumin are used as the effective agent. This treatment can also be applied as a combination therapy. Paclitaxel is known to bind to the β subunit of tubulin, the building blocks of microtubules, leading to hyper-stabilization of the microtubules (Wong and Yeo, 2011). The ensuing paclitaxel/microtubule structure cannot disassemble, leading to mitosis arresting and inhibiting angiogenesis.

Liver cancer stem cell research is a popular and current intervention method in the field of medicine. In addition to the basic features of normal stem cells, namely self-renewal and multi-directional differentiation, liver cancer stem cells also have the properties of tumor cells, and therefore can maintain the proliferation and growth of tumors and escape the mechanism of endogenous and exogenous regulation of their internal environment stability. It takes part in the incidence, development, metastasis, and recurrence of tumors through various signal transduction and regulatory pathways. The newly discovered liver cancer surface marker, CD44, is on the liver cancer stem cell surface. Its expression in liver cancer tissues is significantly higher than in adjacent tissues, normal liver tissues, and other tissues. Besides, the CD44 receptor molecule has a high affinity for the polysaccharide hyaluronic acid (Sackstein, 2011). Reduced selenium nanoparticle-loaded anisomycin and hyaluronic acid were reported for the treatment of HCC as disclosed in 2014 by Liu *et al.* Here, the polysaccharide framework of hyaluronic acid targets the tumor cells, especially liver cancer stem cells. In addition, toxic side effects to the normal cells are reduced compared to cancer cells in an effective pharmaceutical dosage range. Anisomycinis, an antibiotic, inhibits eukaryotic protein synthesis (Grollman, 1967). Mode of action of anisomycin (Liu *et al.*, 2014b).

Li *et al.* in 2014 disclosed a solution to the multidrug resistance problem by using a nanodispersion of doxorubicin, a known chemotherapeutic agent, in a solid lipid and liquid lipid in a fat-soluble emulsifier, in an organic solvent. After the evaporation of the solvent, the mixture is taken up in the water, followed by emulsification in oil and homogenization under high pressure to obtain an agent that will selectively target liver cancer cells. Specifically, his invention provides a doxorubicin nanodrug-loading system. This preparation method will co-deliver a chemotherapy sensitizer such as curcumin and doxorubicin, a chemotherapeutic drug, through a nano-drug-loading system. This makes chemotherapy sensitizers work synergistically with chemotherapeutic drugs to reverse multidrug resistance and enhance tumor cell killing. This innovation has the potential of solving the current anticancer drug issues, especially anti-hepatocarcinoma drugs, which are limited in efficacy and are prone to drug resistance (Li *et al.*, 2014).

Although mesoporous silicon is widely used as a drug carrier in intelligent drug-controlled release systems due to its excellent performance, it degrades slowly as a drug carrier. Therefore, its excessive use of carriers may cause side effects, such as cell mutation, chronic bronchitis, and even lung cancer; thus, new drug carrier construction is still a big challenge (Salonen *et al.*, 2008). In this connection, Cheng *et al.*in 2015 disclosed mesoporous apatite nano-drug carriers with reduced responsiveness and the ability to target liver cancer cells. This invention alleviates drug carrier problems such as high toxicity, side effects, and low biodegradability after normal cellular uptake. Since the drug is released slowly and quantitatively to the cancer cells, the utilization period is enhanced (Cheng *et al.*, 2015).

Small interfering RNAs (siRNAs), used for specific down-regulation of targeted genes, have gained considerable interest as an attractive new class of drugs for broad clinical applications. Hyun and Lee, in 2016, disclosed a siRNA nanodelivery carrier that targets liver cancer for oral administration. Specifically, it targets CD 44 receptors in liver cancer cells. The nanocarrier contains taurocholic acid (TCA)-hyaluronic acid (HA) complex, which allows it to easily pass the gastrointestinal tract upon oral administration. It is absorbed through the distal ileum of the small intestine and therefore has the benefit of moving to the liver *via* enterohepatic circulation. An added advantage is that it has no cellular cytotoxicity because a siRNA-protamine protein complex is made using nontoxic nuclear proteins, such as protamines. In addition, because of facilitated liposomal escape, it has the outstanding therapeutic gene silencing ability of siRNAs (Hyun and Lee, 2016).

Gao *et al.* in 2017 disclosed a method of synthesis of a microsphere composite comprising of an inorganic nanomaterial and its application in chemoembolization of liver cancer. The microsphere synthesis is accomplished by mixing the inorganic nanomaterial, such as silver nanowire, dispersed in water with chitosan in acetic acid. The nanomaterial/chitosan mixture and a span/cyclohexane mixture are respectively sucked into the syringe and then injected into the NaOH/ethanol solution, forming a micro NaOH/ethanol solution. After purification, this mixture is dried by supercritical drying to obtain powdery nanomaterial/chitosan composite microspheres. The microsphere is of uniform size and has good biosafety. It can be used as an embolization agent in the intervention chemoembolization of liver cancer and as a blood vessel CT (computed tomography) contrast agent of a liver cancer area (Gao *et al.*, 2017).

Peptide self-assembled nanostructures are very popular in many biomedical applications. Drug delivery is one of the most promising applications among them. Tremendous advantages for self-assembled peptide nanostructures include good biocompatibility, low cost, tunable bioactivity, high drug loading capacities, chemical diversity, specific targeting, and stimuli-responsive drug delivery at disease sites (Fan *et al.*, 2017). Such a self-assembly method to deliver a polypeptide was disclosed by Cai *et al.* in 2017. The polypeptide with a specific sequence (NBD-GFFpYssERGD) can initiate a tandem self-assembly process by the action of alkaline phosphatase (ALP) and glutathione (GSH) to obtain nanomaterials. Simultaneously, liver cancer cells have extracellular ALP, and the simultaneous high expression of intracellular GSH makes the polypeptide show strong selectivity. It can form nanofibers in hepatoma cells and inhibit the growth of hepatoma cells (Cai *et al.*, 2017).

Commercially Available Nanotherapeutics on Hepatocellular Carcinoma

Over the past few decades, the US FDA has approved about 100 commercial nanotherapeutics products for various applications. Even though the FDA has approved about 100 nanotherapeutics and many different articles and review papers cover nanotechnology applications in HCC, there has not been sufficient information/explanations regarding the commercially available nanotherapeutics in this field (Farjadian *et al.*, 2019). Herein, the commercially available nanotherapeutics in HCC, related patent information, and clinical trials have been addressed concisely.

Diagnosis

Currently, clinical practice guidelines highly recommend semiannual surveillance for patients at a high risk of having HCC to better their health condition (Maruyama *et al.,* 2016). In this regard, ultrasonography contrast agents are used in a standard examination for HCC surveillance. Sonazoid is one of the ultrasonography contrast agents, and it is a second-generation lipid-stabilized suspension of a perfluorobutane gas microbubble contrast agent (Numata *et al.*, 2010). The most significant feature in this contrasting agent is Kupffer phase imaging (Numata, 2015). When it gets into the action of sonazoid inside the liver, it has some unique characteristic features. Kupffer cells are commonly identified as liver-specific macrophages. Those cells phagocytize the perfluorobutane and amplify the ultrasound scattering to generate the amplified sound wave (Maruyama *et al.,* 2016). As a result, the number of Kupffer cells in a hepatic lesion is either significantly decreased or absent and shows a defect on ultrasonography during the Kupffer phase. Sonazoid-enhanced ultrasonography with defect reperfusion imaging is a breakthrough technique in the diagnosis and treatment of HCC.

On the other hand, this Kupffer cell imaging technique, using sonazoid, is only applicable in Japan, Korea, China, and Norway (Salvatore *et al.*, 2016). In this respect, sonazoid should be made more available worldwide for the treatment of HCC. The most prominent feature in this sonazoid diagnosing drug is, it facilitates stable Kupffer phase imaging for a repeated scanning time frame of 10 to 60 minutes after the injection. At the same time, it can create real-time blood flow images at low acoustic power (Li *et al.*, 2017).

Drug Delivery

Arginine depletion is a prominent characteristic in HCC and more often lacks argininosuccinate synthetase, which is the arginine-repleting enzyme (Baboci *et al.*, 2020). Moreover, multiple cancers, including HCC, have been reported to have a high degree of arginine dependency (Garcia-Bermudez *et al.*, 2020). ADI-PEG 20 is a cloned arginine degrading enzyme consisting of arginine deiminase-conjugated with polyethylene glycol. More interestingly, it has been found that arginine dependency of HCC can potentially be treated with ADI-PEG 20 (Harding *et al.*, 2018). Typically, arginine is essential for the protein synthesis and survival of cells in a healthy person. But cancer cells become dependent upon an external supply of arginine to survive and grow in a patient with HCC (Phillips *et al.*, 2013). Therefore, it is designed to deplete the arginine's external supply, causing arginine-dependent cancer cells to die while leaving the patient's normal healthy cells unharmed.

The human trial of ADI-PEG 20 (pegylated arginine deiminase), an arginine degrading enzyme, *versus* placebo in patients with HCC who failed prior systemic treatment (chemotherapy), was conducted. HCC has been found to require arginine, an amino acid, as previously explained (Baboci *et al.*, 2020). Thus this hypothesis that by restricting arginine with ADI-PEG 20, HCC cells would die. In the clinical trials, patients were randomized as 2:1 to study the drug *versus* placebo. More importantly, safety and tolerability were assessed, as well as pharmacodynamics (peripheral blood levels of arginine and citrulline), pharmacokinetics (peripheral blood levels of ADI-PEG 20), and immunogenicity (antibodies to ADI-PEG 20) in these clinical trials (Synakiewicz *et al.*, 2014).

ThermoDox is a commonly used cancer drug for HCC, and it uses LTSL (lysolipid thermally sensitive liposome) technology to encapsulate doxorubicin (Mohamed *et al.*, 2017). The significant features of this drug are that it is delivered by IV infusion, and the drug should be used in combination with heat-based treatments, such as microwave thermal therapy, radiofrequency thermal ablation, or high-intensity focused ultrasound (Svenson, 2012). The ultimate goal of such heat-based treatments is to expand the effective treatment zone to capture micrometastases, which are most commonly responsible for post-treatment disease recurrence.

When heated to 40 °C - 45 °C, the heat-sensitive liposomes rapidly change the outer lay structure by creating openings in the liposome (Nardecchia *et al.*, 2019). As a result, doxorubicin is released directly into and around the targeted tumor (Gasselhuber *et al.*, 2010). Tumors have leaky vasculature, which is permeable to liposomes and enables their accumulation within tumors. When heated, blood vessels in tumors become even more permeable, further increasing the accumulation of liposomes in tumors before releasing the doxorubicin (Pattni *et al.*, 2015).

Doxil® is the first drug delivery system based on PEGylated liposome technology (Park, 2002). It consists of encapsulated doxorubicin hydrochloride, an anticancer drug of the anthracycline family (Gabizon *et al.*, 2003). This liposomal formulation induces caspase-dependent apoptosis in cancer cells through oxidative DNA damage by blocking topoisomerase II. It is an enzyme needed by cancer cells to divide and grow (Jiang *et al.*, 2011). The enzyme also generates free radicals such as reactive oxygen species, leading to lipid peroxidation and membrane impairment. A liposomal formulation was approved by the US Food and Drug Administration (FDA) in 1995, and it was the first nanosized liposomal product to obtain regulatory approval in the US (Barenholz, 2012).

Livatag® (doxorubicin Transdrug™) contains doxorubicin in the form of lyophilized polyisohexylcyanoaerylate (PIHCA) nanoparticles to be delivered to the liver by intra-arterial infusion (Merle *et al.,* 2017). The significant breakthrough in this drug is the treatment of a variety of cancers. The first intervention of this drug formulation is in primary liver cancer. Transdrug technology uses nanoparticles to help fight against chemotherapy resistance, a major mechanism in the failure of some anticancer drugs, facilitating the penetration of the drug into the tumor cell and increasing cellular exposure to the drug (Svenson, 2012). In this novel therapeutic approach, cancer cells can be directly targeted because the anticancer agent's masking prevents them from being expelled from the cell.

Further, this trans-drug technology offers a controlled release of the active ingredient to extend its effect over a prolonged period (Marchal *et al.*, 2015). When we consider the human trials of Livatag®, the main objective is to determine whether it is effective in treating patients suffering from advanced HCC after failure or intolerance to sorafenib. The most striking feature in this trans-drug is overcoming the multidrug resistance (MDR) *in vitro* and *in vivo* models. Further, it has been identified that the doxorubicin trans drug is more effective than doxorubicin on both resistant and sensitive tumor models (Sobot *et al.*, 2016).

DCR-MYC is also another drug delivery mode that is used for HCC. It consists of a novel synthetic double-stranded RNA in a stable lipid nanoparticle suspension directly targeting the oncogene MYC (Nikam and Gore, 2018). This MYC oncogene activation is essential to the growth of many hematologic and solid tumor malignancies. When it gets into the drug-delivering mechanism of DCR-MYC, it delivers siRNA molecules to multiple tumor types, including HCC (Scarabel *et al.*, 2017). In the clinical trials of this drug, the primary purpose was to assess the safety and tolerability of the DCR-MYC. In addition, in recent studies, greater attention has been given to the study of DCR-MYC and its ability to inhibit MYC and thereby inhibit cancer cell growth (Baboci *et al.,* 2020).

MRX34 is a liposomal mimic of microRNA-34a. It is a synthetic version of miR-34a with a double-stranded structure (Zhang *et al.*, 2019). It is encapsulated in a liposomal nanoparticle with a diameter of approximately 110 nm. The liposomal component contains amphoteric lipids by ensuring the stability of liposomal nanoparticles. Cationic species are generated during liposome formation under acidic conditions, but the encapsulation of the negatively charged miR-34a mimic is ensured (Hong *et al.*, 2016).

On the other hand, in anionic conditions, it gets into neutral pH *in-vivo* by minimizing the particle aggregation and electrostatic adherence to the cellular membranes of endothelial cells (Baumann and Winkler, 2014). Consistent with these outstanding biochemical attributes, MRX34 has a prolonged circulation time in blood and delivers high numbers of miR-34a mimics to the liver (Anselmo and Mitragotri, 2019). In clinical trials, the safety, pharmacokinetics, and pharmacodynamics of the micro ribonucleic acid (microRNA) MRX34 in patients with HCCwas investigated. MRX34 was administered daily x 5 with 2 weeks off (total of 21 days) for three cycles, followed by a no-treatment observation period (Hong *et al.*, 2020).

MTL-CEBPA is a lipid-based nanoparticle formulation composed of liposomes encapsulating a small oligonucleotide encoding a small activating RNA (saRNA). It targets the CCAAT enhancer-binding protein alpha (CEBPA; C/EBP-a) gene with potential antineoplastic activity (Wiradharma *et al.*, 2009). This CEBPA gene is downregulated in most cancer cells, including liver cancer cells, and saRNA upregulates its gene expression. After administering this MTL-CEBPA liposome, it binds specially to a DNA regulatory target region for the CEBPA gene. Then, CEBPA gene transcription will be restored, increasing both CEBPA mRNA levels and protein expression. As a result, the expression of tumor suppressor genes is be activated, and the proliferation of tumor cells is reduced. This upregulation of CEBPA in tumor cells will prevent liver failure by reducing liver cancer cell proliferation.

The clinical trials of MTL-CEBPA were held in two parts; dose escalation followed by a dose expansion (Setten *et al.*, 2018). In both parts of the study, it recruited advanced HCC patients with cirrhosis. This first-in-human and first-i--class multicenter phase I dose and dose-escalation study of the RNA oligonucleotide MTL-CEBPA has shown the drug to be well tolerated with no maximum tolerated dose (MTD) reached (Sarker *et al.*, 2018). Based on a combination of safety, pharmacokinetics, and pharmacodynamics, the recommended dose of MTL-CEBPA for further evaluation is 130 mg/m2 QW. The toxicity profile was favorable and comparable with the other drugs used in this patient population, including sorafenib, regorafenib, and nivolumab (Sarker *et al.*, 2020).

Treatment

NBTXR3/Hensify is a crystalline hafnium oxide nanoparticle with a negatively charged phosphate coating (Anselmo and Mitragotri, 2019). Further, this Hensify drug gets into action on hafnium's natural radio enhancing properties by enhancing external radiotherapy *via* a physical mode of action. The interaction between the hafnium oxide nanoparticles and ionization radiation provides a more significant energy deposit. That energy deposit is significantly higher than the ionization radiation without hafnium oxide nanoparticles. This greater interaction provides more electrons, resulting in the enhancement of radiation-mediated cell death (Baboci *et al.*, 2020).

In the clinical trials of Hensify associated radiation therapy, it has been found that the drug kills more cancer cells by increasing the tumor shrinkage. This shrinkage facilitates better local control of the tumor while leading to easier surgeries. In phase II/III trials, patients were randomly allowed to receive either Hensify as an intratumor injection, activated by an external beam of radiation therapy, or an external radiation therapy beam alone. When this radiotherapy treatment was completed, tumor surgeries were performed successfully (Svenson, 2012).

Zinostatinstimalamer (SMANCS) is a lipophilic intra-arterial chemotherapeutic agent for HCC, and it was marketed in Japan in 1993 (Maeda, 2001a). Zinostatinstimalamer is administered *via* embolization (it is injected into the artery supplying the hepatoma), and in clinical trials, a response rate of 35.9% has been achieved (Okusaka *et al.*, 2002). The drug is given in combination with iodized poppy oil fatty acid ethyl ester, increasing its duration in tumor tissues (Ishii *et al.*, 2003).

TKM-080301 consists of a lipid nanoparticle formulation of a siRNA directed against human PLK1 mRNA (Semple *et al.*, 2011). The lipid components of TKM-080301 play a significant role, and it protects the siRNA from degradation by plasma and tissue nucleases. As a result, it enables effective intracellular uptake of the PLK1-targeting siRNA into cancer cells (Wan *et al.*, 2014). PLK1 siRNA formulated in lipid nanoparticle formulation resulted in a potent anti-proliferative activity. Gene-specific silencing in many cancer cell lines is another striking feature of PLK1 siRNA-developed lipid nanoparticle formulations (Semple *et al.*, 2011).

Further, TKM-080301 exhibited intense anti-tumor activity in several human cancers, including tumors implanted intra-hepatically. The rapid inducing of mitotic arrest and apoptosis in proliferating cancer cells has shown *in vitro* data by the inhibition of PLK1. In this regard, cancer cell sensitivity to the cytotoxic effects of chemotherapy is increased (Llovet *et al.*, 2015). Human trials were carried out to determine the safety, pharmacokinetics, and preliminary anti-tumor activity of intravenous TKM-080301 in subjects with HCC (El Dika *et al.*, 2019).

CONCLUDING REMARKS

Applications of nanomaterials in HCC diagnosis and treatment are a new avenue to overcome the many hurdles associated with early diagnosis of HCC and treatments. Nanostructured materials could offer greater potential in the future in the biomedical field, developing new imaging facilities, multimodal imaging, and detecting devices. They inherited unique properties such as superparamagnetic or fluorescent properties and smaller sizes. Current innovations patented are the robust base for future developments, leading to applying those into clinical trials (Table **3**). As a global requirement, these new applications and technologies should be supported to bring them to practical use in the early diagnosis of HCC.

Even though there are many patents on different modes for diagnostics and interventions, such as nano-formulations and nano-delivery systems for HCC, chemotherapy has been issued in the last decade. However, much needs to be done to improve the treatment in tackling adsorption/distribution/metabolism/ excretion (ADME), toxicity, and long-term control of this difficult-to-treat disease. Furthermore, there is a paucity of commercially available nano-treatments for HCC. Therefore, lacking a set of benchmark treatments makes it difficult to assess the efficacy of the claims made in these patients.

In order to move nanotherapeutics on HCC from the laboratories to the market, several experimental challenges need to be addressed. It is mainly regulated within the conventional framework governed by the key regulatory authority of each country (*e.g.*, FDA, TGA, and EMA). On the other hand, the pace for the clinical translation of nanotherapeutics on HCC has been relatively slow as the development phases are very costly, complex, and time-consuming. This should consider the complexity of the nanotherapeutics, route of administration to the liver, pharmacokinetics, pharmacodynamics, and safety profile. Further, the most appropriate clinical trial design and patient selection should be carefully implemented. In this regard, it is apparent that the process requires considerable time to obtain regulatory approval for the nanotherapeutics going from bench to market. By considering the significant and positive impact on HCC by nanotherapeutics, the lag time between clinical trials and commercialization should be decreased to obtain the maximum benefits. On the other hand, pharmaceutical investors should be appropriately informed about the risk-t--benefit conditions of nanotherapeutics on HCC. The emerging and potential commercialization of nanotherapeutics on HCC has a great potential to advance significantly and even potentially revolutionize various aspects of treatment on HCC.

Despite the evident growth of research of nanomaterials to target HCC, preclinical trials are not reaching clinical trials at an acceptable rate. It is the latter that leads to FDA approval and commercialization. The patent applications indicate that while the scientific community is continually attempting to formulate the best possible nanomaterial to be used as anticancer drug carriers, no USFDA-approved therapeutic nanomaterial targeting HCC has been disclosed. For drug-loaded nanoparticles to be commercially accessible, the process typically needs to be chemically and physically characterized before proceeding to thorough *in vitro* and *in vivo* assessments. Those nanoparticles are finally introduced to patients through another lengthy phase of clinical trials.

It is too early to make a prognosis of the successful outcomes of the available patent scenario in HCC. However, the emerging patents suggest that the small molecules and other interventions used in normal cancer therapy are being applied to HCC through nanotechnology.

CONSENT FOR PUBLICATION

Not applicable.

CONFLICT OF INTEREST

The authors declare no conflict of interest, financial or otherwise.

ACKNOWLEDGEMENT

Declared none.

REFERENCES

Ai, J, Chen, X, Ren, Z, Sun, J, Wu, L, Zhang, Y, Zhou, G, Zhou, M, Zhou, T & Zhu, T (2019) Method for preparing double target magnetic nanoparticle of liver cancer. CN109701039A

Anselmo, AC & Mitragotri, S (2019) Nanoparticles in the clinic: An update. *Bioeng Transl Med,* 4, e10143. [http://dx.doi.org/10.1002/btm2.10143] [PMID: 31572799]

Apps, MG, Choi, EHY & Wheate, NJ (2015) 'The state-of-play and future of platinum drugs' *Endocrine-Related Cancer* BioScientifica Ltd. R219-33. [http://dx.doi.org/10.1530/ERC-15-0237]

Baboci, L, Capolla, S, Di Cintio, F, Colombo, F, Mauro, P, Dal Bo, M, Argenziano, M, Cavalli, R, Toffoli, G & Macor, P (2020) The Dual Role of the Liver in Nanomedicine as an Actor in the Elimination of Nanostructures or a Therapeutic Target. *J Oncol,* 2020, 4638192. [http://dx.doi.org/10.1155/2020/4638192] [PMID: 32184825]

Bader, A, Zhao, J & Kelnar, K (2015) Mirna Therapeutics Inc *Combination cancer treatments utilizing micrornas and egfr-tki inhibitors,.* WO2016161196A1.

Bae, Y H & Park, K (2011) Targeted drug delivery to tumors: Myths, reality and possibility *Journal of Controlled Release* Elsevier B.V 198-205. [http://dx.doi.org/10.1016/j.jconrel.2011.06.001]

Bai, L, Jiang, Y & Jin, C (2018) Paclitaxel nanoparticles applied to liver cancer interventional therapy. CN110772496A.

Balogh, J, Victor, D, III, Asham, EH, Burroughs, SG, Boktour, M, Saharia, A, Li, X, Ghobrial, RM & Monsour, HP, Jr (2016) Hepatocellular carcinoma: a review. *J Hepatocell Carcinoma,* 3, 41-53.
[http://dx.doi.org/10.2147/JHC.S61146] [PMID: 27785449]

Barenholz, Y & Gabizon, A (1990) Hadassah Medical Organization and Yissum Research Development Co of Hebrew University.

Barenholz, Y (2012) Doxil®--the first FDA-approved nano-drug: lessons learned. *J Control Release,* 160, 117-34.
[http://dx.doi.org/10.1016/j.jconrel.2012.03.020] [PMID: 22484195]

Baumann, V & Winkler, J (2014) miRNA-based therapies: strategies and delivery platforms for oligonucleotide and non-oligonucleotide agents. *Future Med Chem,* 6, 1967-84.
[http://dx.doi.org/10.4155/fmc.14.116] [PMID: 25495987]

Bomalaski, JS & Wu, BW (2016) Methods of treatment with arginine deiminase *US9333268B2*

Brannon-Peppas, L & Blanchette, JO (2004) 'Nanoparticle and targeted systems for cancer therapy', *Advanced Drug Delivery Reviews* Elsevier 1649-59.
[http://dx.doi.org/10.1016/j.addr.2004.02.014]

Brown, BD (2013) Dicerna Pharmaceuticals Inc. Extended dicer substrate agents and methods for the specific inhibition of gene expression, US8513207B2.

Cai, Y, Yang, Z & Zhan, J (2017) Polypeptide, application thereof and medicine containing polypeptide CN107778367A

Capurro, M, Wanless, IR, Sherman, M, Deboer, G, Shi, W, Miyoshi, E & Filmus, J (2003) Glypican-3: a novel serum and histochemical marker for hepatocellular carcinoma. *Gastroenterology,* 125, 89-97.
[http://dx.doi.org/10.1016/S0016-5085(03)00689-9] [PMID: 12851874]

Capurro, MI, Xiang, YY, Lobe, C & Filmus, J (2005) Glypican-3 promotes the growth of hepatocellular carcinoma by stimulating canonical Wnt signaling. *Cancer Res,* 65, 6245-54.
[http://dx.doi.org/10.1158/0008-5472.CAN-04-4244] [PMID: 16024626]

Chao, Y, Chan, W-K, Birkhofer, MJ, Hu, OY, Wang, S-S, Huang, Y-S, Liu, M, Whang-Peng, J, Chi, KH, Lui, WY & Lee, SD (1998) Phase II and pharmacokinetic study of paclitaxel therapy for unresectable hepatocellular carcinoma patients. *Br J Cancer,* 78, 34-9.
[http://dx.doi.org/10.1038/bjc.1998.438] [PMID: 9662247]

Chen, J (2001) Liver-targeting mitomycin magnetic nano particle and its preparation and application in medicine. CN1416812A.

Chen, W & Ju, D (2017) Nanogene drug targeting interleukin-22 for treating liver injury. CN201710554782A.

Chen, X, Chen, X, Ren, Z, Song, Y & Yue, Z (2019) Application of nanoparticle coupled ginsenoside in preparation of anti-liver cancer drugs. CN110522922A.

Chen, Z, Lin, L & Xue, E (2012) Novel liver cancer treatment preparation with physical and biological double targeting effect. CN102920660A.

Chen, Z, Xiao, E & Zeng, W (2015) Superparamagnetic iron oxide nano MRI (magnetic resonance imaging) probe and preparation method and application thereof. CN105267992A.

Cheng, W, He, J, Huang, Y, Li, D, Li, J & Wei, F (2015) Preparation method of mesoporous apatite nano-drug carrier with reduction responsiveness and cellular targeting property for hepatoma cell. CN104587473A.

Cheng, W, Xia, Z, Yuquan, W & Zhiyong, Q (2011) Micelles and freeze-dried preparations of diblock polymer-supported taxane medicines and preparation and use thereof. CN102198083A.

Chuangnian, Z, Qin, T, Tong, L, Wei, H, Xiaoting, H, Yue, C, Yue, Z & Zhi, Y (2008) Biogastrone acid-polyethyleneglycol /chitosan liver target composite drug administration system and preparation thereof. CN101254308A.

Cortes, J & Saura, C (2010) Nanoparticle albumin-bound (nab™)-paclitaxel: improving efficacy and tolerability by targeted drug delivery in metastatic breast cancer. *Eur J Cancer, Suppl,* 8, 1-10. [http://dx.doi.org/10.1016/S1359-6349(10)70002-1]

Dai, L & Zhong, J (2012) Method for massively preparing midkine antisense oligodeoxynucleotide nano-liposomes for injection. CN102989007A.

Dawar, S, Singh, N, Kanwar, RK, Kennedy, RL, Veedu, RN, Zhou, SF, Krishnakumar, S, Hazra, S, Sasidharan, S, Duan, W & Kanwar, JR (2013) Multifunctional and multitargeted nanoparticles for drug delivery to overcome barriers of drug resistance in human cancers. *Drug Discov Today,* 18, 1292-300. [http://dx.doi.org/10.1016/j.drudis.2013.09.009] [PMID: 24055842]

Dixon, G & Trochon-joseph, V (2020) Combination therapies comprising Immuno-Oncologyagents and belinostat. WO2017144548A1.

Du, B, Fan, D, Hu, L, Ma, H, Pang, X, Sun, X, Wei, Q, Wu, D, Zhang, Y & Zhu, W (2016) Method for preparing alpha fetoprotein electrochemiluminescence sensor based on gold hybrid carbon black intercalation reduced graphene. CN105486679A.

Du, LN, Jin, Y & Wang, S (2014) Phosphoryl N-fatty acyl nucleoside analogue for treating viral hepatitis and liver cancer. CN104211742A.

El Dika, I, Lim, HY, Yong, WP, Lin, CC, Yoon, JH, Modiano, M, Freilich, B, Choi, HJ, Chao, TY, Kelley, RK, Brown, J, Knox, J, Ryoo, BY, Yau, T & Abou-Alfa, GK (2019) An Open-Label, Multicenter, Phase I, Dose Escalation Study with Phase II Expansion Cohort to Determine the Safety, Pharmacokinetics, and Preliminary Antitumor Activity of Intravenous TKM-080301 in Subjects with Advanced Hepatocellular Carcinoma. *Oncologist,* 24, 747-e218. [http://dx.doi.org/10.1634/theoncologist.2018-0838] [PMID: 30598500]

El-Sawy, HS, Al-Abd, AM, Ahmed, TA, El-Say, KM & Torchilin, VP (2018) Stimuli-responsive nano-architecture drug-delivery systems to solid tumor micromilieu: past, present, and future perspectives. *ACS Nano,* 12, 10636-64. [http://dx.doi.org/10.1021/acsnano.8b06104] [PMID: 30335963]

Fan, T, Yu, X, Shen, B & Sun, L (2017) Peptide Self-Assembled Nanostructures for Drug Delivery Applications *Journal of Nanomaterials.* Hindawi Limited [http://dx.doi.org/10.1155/2017/4562474]

Farjadian, F, Ghasemi, A, Gohari, O, Roointan, A, Karimi, M & Hamblin, MR (2019) Nanopharmaceuticals and nanomedicines currently on the market: challenges and opportunities. *Nanomedicine (Lond),* 14, 93-126. [http://dx.doi.org/10.2217/nnm-2018-0120] [PMID: 30451076]

Filmus, J & Capurro, M (2008) The role of glypican-3 in the regulation of body size and cancer. *Cell Cycle,* 7, 2787-90. [http://dx.doi.org/10.4161/cc.7.18.6672] [PMID: 18787398]

Fu, S, Li, J, Li, Y, Lu, L, Su, Y & Zhan, M (2018) Method for preparing sorafenib nano micelle CN110302153A

Gabizon, A, Shmeeda, H & Barenholz, Y (2003) Pharmacokinetics of pegylated liposomal Doxorubicin: review of animal and human studies. *Clin Pharmacokinet,* 42, 419-36. [http://dx.doi.org/10.2165/00003088-200342050-00002] [PMID: 12739982]

Gao, H, Li, F, Lu, Y, Lyu, X, Pan, Z, Pu, T, Shang, X, Song, Y, Su, Y, Wang, X, Yan, X & Yan, Y (2017) Synthesis method of composite microsphere comprising inorganic nanomaterial, and application of composite microsphere in intervention chemoembolization of liver cancer CN107596430A.

Garcia-Bermudez, J, Williams, RT, Guarecuco, R & Birsoy, K (2020) Targeting extracellular nutrient

dependencies of cancer cells. *Mol Metab,* 33, 67-82.
[http://dx.doi.org/10.1016/j.molmet.2019.11.011] [PMID: 31926876]

Gasselhuber, A, Dreher, MR, Negussie, A, Wood, BJ, Rattay, F & Haemmerich, D (2010) Mathematical spatio-temporal model of drug delivery from low temperature sensitive liposomes during radiofrequency tumour ablation. *Int J Hyperthermia,* 26, 499-513.
[http://dx.doi.org/10.3109/02656731003623590] [PMID: 20377363]

Graebin, CS (2018) The Pharmacological Activities of Glycyrrhizinic Acid ("Glycyrrhizin") and Glycyrrhetinic Acid In *Sweeteners* Nature Publishing Group 245-61.
[http://dx.doi.org/10.1007/978-3-319-27027-2_15]

http://www.jbc.org/

Guangfu, Y, Xiaoming, L, Yadong, Y, Yunqing, K & Zongbing, H (2007) Hepatocarcinoma early diagnosis kit based on ZnO nano-bar array CN101358973A

Han, X, Ma, H & Zhao, B (2017) Variant distinguishing glycoprotein detection chip based on combination of SERS (surface enhanced Raman scattering) displacement and intensity CN106841164A

Hang, Y, Jing, Z, Licheng, D & Xiang, W (2009) Antisense oligonucleotide nano preparation resisting middle-period factor, preparation and application thereof CN101716352A.

Harding, JJ, Do, RK, Dika, IE, Hollywood, E, Uhlitskykh, K, Valentino, E, Wan, P, Hamilton, C, Feng, X, Johnston, A, Bomalaski, J, Li, CF, O'Reilly, EM & Abou-Alfa, GK (2018) A phase 1 study of ADI-PEG 20 and modified FOLFOX6 in patients with advanced hepatocellular carcinoma and other gastrointestinal malignancies. *Cancer Chemother Pharmacol,* 82, 429-40.
[http://dx.doi.org/10.1007/s00280-018-3635-3] [PMID: 29971467]

Henriksen, I, Kvale, S, Tokerud, OJ, Per, S & Kiserud, MSN GE Healthcare AS (2017) Ultrasound precursor preparation method, WO2015150354A1

Hong, DS, Kang, Y-K, Borad, M, Sachdev, J, Ejadi, S, Lim, HY, Brenner, AJ, Park, K, Lee, J-L, Kim, T-Y, Shin, S, Becerra, CR, Falchook, G, Stoudemire, J, Martin, D, Kelnar, K, Peltier, H, Bonato, V, Bader, AG, Smith, S, Kim, S, O'Neill, V & Beg, MS (2020) Phase 1 study of MRX34, a liposomal miR-34a mimic, in patients with advanced solid tumours. *Br J Cancer,* 122, 1630-7.
[http://dx.doi.org/10.1038/s41416-020-0802-1] [PMID: 32238921]

Hong, DS, Kang, Y-K, Brenner, AJ, Sachdev, JC, Ejadi, S, Borad, MJ, Kim, T-Y, Lim, HY, Park, K & Becerra, C (2016) MRX34, a liposomal miR-34 mimic, in patients with advanced solid tumors: Final dose-escalation results from a first-in-human phase I trial of microRNA therapy. American Society of Clinical Oncology.

Hope, MJ, Semple, SC, Chen, J, Madden, TD, Cullis, PR, Ciufolini, MA & Mui, BLS (2015) University of British Columbia and Tekmira Pharmaceuticals Corp, *Amino lipids and methods for the delivery of nucleic acids.* US9139554B2.

Hu, J, Wang, X & Xu, Y (2020) Preparation method of anti-hepatoma drug nanoparticles on pH and redox dual response CN111568879A.

Hu, Z, Ma, J, Tian, Z, Wang, W & Yuan, Z (2016) Nano-gold CT contrast agent for early diagnosis of hepatocellular carcinoma and preparation method of contrast agent CN105797173A

Huang, A, Liu, J, Liu, X & Zhang, D (2013) Multifunctional nano probe for multimodal images and photothermal therapy of liver cancer and application of multifunctional nano probe CN103721271A

Huang, Y, Huang, Y, Zhao, Y & Zhou, S (2017) Method for preparing specific magnetic Endoglin aptamer imaging probe system CN107029252A.

Hyun, EJ & Lee, YK (2016) siRNA Liver Cancer Targeted siRNA Nano-transporter System For Oral Administration And Manufacturing Method Thereof, KR20180047442A.

Ishii, H, Furuse, J, Nagase, M, Maru, Y, Yoshino, M & Hayashi, T (2003) A phase I study of hepatic arterial infusion chemotherapy with zinostatin stimalamer alone for hepatocellular carcinoma. *Jpn J Clin Oncol,* 33,

570-3.
[http://dx.doi.org/10.1093/jjco/hyg106] [PMID: 14711981]

Jiang, W, Lionberger, R & Yu, LX (2011) *In vitro* and *in vivo* characterizations of PEGylated liposomal doxorubicin. *Bioanalysis,* 3, 333-44.
[http://dx.doi.org/10.4155/bio.10.204] [PMID: 21320053]

Juan, W, Menghua, X & Wang, J (2010) Biocompatibility nanoparticle and application thereof as drug conveying carrier CN101732721A.

Kalyane, D, Raval, N, Maheshwari, R, Tambe, V, Kalia, K & Tekade, RK (2019) Employment of enhanced permeability and retention effect (EPR): Nanoparticle-based precision tools for targeting of therapeutic and diagnostic agent in cancer. *Mater Sci Eng C,* 98, 1252-76.
[http://dx.doi.org/10.1016/j.msec.2019.01.066] [PMID: 30813007]

Kato, M, Maeta, H, Kato, S, Shinozawa, T & Terada, T (2000) Immunohistochemical and *in situ* hybridization analyses of midkine expression in thyroid papillary carcinoma. *Mod Pathol,* 13, 1060-5.
[http://dx.doi.org/10.1038/modpathol.3880195] [PMID: 11048798]

Kataoka, K, Harada, A & Nagasaki, Y (2012) 'Block copolymer micelles for drug delivery: Design, characterization and biological significance', *Advanced Drug Delivery Reviews* Elsevier 37-48.
[http://dx.doi.org/10.1016/j.addr.2012.09.013]

Katsumi, Y, Otabe, O, Matsui, F, Kidowaki, S, Mibayashi, A, Tsuma, Y & Ito, H (2012) Effect of a single inhalation of laninamivir octanoate in children with influenza. *Pediatrics,* 129, e1431-6.
[http://dx.doi.org/10.1542/peds.2011-2054] [PMID: 22614774]

Knobloch, T, Koeberle, V, Korkusuz, H, Kreuter, J, Langer, K, Piiper, A, Ulbrich, K & Vogel, TJ (2012) Nanoparticles as MRT contrast media for the diagnosis of hepatocellular carcinoma, *WO2012113733A1.*

Kobayashi, M, Ohtani, G, Sekino, J, Konno, T & Maeda, H Yamanouchi Pharmaceutical Co Ltd (1991) Lyophilized pharmaceutical composition of neocarzinostatin derivative CA1327161C

Kumari, P, Ghosh, B & Biswas, S (2016) Nanocarriers for cancer-targeted drug delivery. *J Drug Target,* 24, 179-91.
[http://dx.doi.org/10.3109/1061186X.2015.1051049] [PMID: 26061298]

Ladju, RB, Pascut, D, Massi, MN, Tiribelli, C & Sukowati, CHC (2017) Aptamer: A potential oligonucleotide nanomedicine in the diagnosis and treatment of hepatocellular carcinoma. *Oncotarget,* 9, 2951-61.
[http://dx.doi.org/10.18632/oncotarget.23359] [PMID: 29416827]

Libbrecht, L, Severi, T, Cassiman, D, Vander Borght, S, Pirenne, J, Nevens, F, Verslype, C, van Pelt, J & Roskams, T (2006) Glypican-3 expression distinguishes small hepatocellular carcinomas from cirrhosis, dysplastic nodules, and focal nodular hyperplasia-like nodules. *Am J Surg Pathol,* 30, 1405-11.
[http://dx.doi.org/10.1097/01.pas.0000213323.97294.9a] [PMID: 17063081]

Li, P, Hoppmann, S, Du, P, Li, H, Evans, PM, Moestue, SA, Yu, W, Dong, F, Liu, H & Liu, L (2017) Pharmacokinetics of perfluorobutane after intra-venous bolus injection of Sonazoid in healthy Chinese volunteers. *Ultrasound Med Biol,* 43, 1031-9.
[http://dx.doi.org/10.1016/j.ultrasmedbio.2017.01.003] [PMID: 28283327]

Li, Y, Liu, W, Tang, H, Wan, J, Yang, X & Zhao, X (2014) Adriamycin nano drug delivery system as well as preparation method and application thereof *CN103976950A*

Liu, J, Liu, X, Wei, X, Huang, A, Wang, Q & Zeng, Y (2014) Antibody Modified ZnSe Nanocrystalline Based Kit For Detection of Hepatocellular Carcinoma Marker Gpc3 a CN103976956A

Liu, J, Xia, J, Xiao, J & Xing, F (2014) Targeted anti-hepatoma nanoparticle and preparation method and application thereof b CN103976956A

Llovet, JM, Villanueva, A, Lachenmayer, A & Finn, RS (2015) Advances in targeted therapies for hepatocellular carcinoma in the genomic era. *Nat Rev Clin Oncol,* 12, 408-24.

[http://dx.doi.org/10.1038/nrclinonc.2015.103] [PMID: 26054909]

Ma, J, Qin, J & Zhang, M (2012) Drug sustained release polymeric microspheres prepared based on micro-fluidic technology and application CN103371974A

Maeda, H (2001) SMANCS and polymer-conjugated macromolecular drugs: advantages in cancer chemotherapy. *Adv Drug Deliv Rev,* 46, 169-85. a
[http://dx.doi.org/10.1016/S0169-409X(00)00134-4] [PMID: 11259839]

Maeda, H (2001) The enhanced permeability and retention (EPR) effect in tumor vasculature: the key role of tumor-selective macromolecular drug targeting. *Adv Enzyme Regul,* 41, 189-207. b
[http://dx.doi.org/10.1016/S0065-2571(00)00013-3] [PMID: 11384745]

Maeda, H (2012) Vascular permeability in cancer and infection as related to macromolecular drug delivery, with emphasis on the EPR effect for tumor-selective drug targeting *Proc Jpn Acad Ser B Phys Biol Sci,* 53-71.
[http://dx.doi.org/10.2183/pjab.88.53]

Marchal, S, El Hor, A, Millard, M, Gillon, V & Bezdetnaya, L (2015) Anticancer drug delivery: an update on clinically applied nanotherapeutics. *Drugs,* 75, 1601-11.
[http://dx.doi.org/10.1007/s40265-015-0453-3] [PMID: 26323338]

Maruyama, H, Sekimoto, T & Yokosuka, O (2016) Role of contrast-enhanced ultrasonography with Sonazoid for hepatocellular carcinoma: evidence from a 10-year experience. *J Gastroenterol,* 51, 421-33.
[http://dx.doi.org/10.1007/s00535-015-1151-3] [PMID: 26694825]

McMillan, J, Batrakova, E & Gendelman, HE (2011) Cell delivery of therapeutic nanoparticles.*Progress in Molecular Biology and Translational Science* Elsevier B.V. 563-601.
[http://dx.doi.org/10.1016/B978-0-12-416020-0.00014-0]

Merle, P, Camus, P, Abergel, A, Pageaux, GP, Masliah, C, Bronowicki, JP, Zarski, JP, Pelletier, G, Bouattour, M, Farloux, L, Dorval, E, Verset, G, Si-Ahmed, SN, Doffoel, M, Couzigou, P, Taieb, J, Vasseur, B & Attali, P (2017) Safety and efficacy of intra-arterial hepatic chemotherapy with doxorubicin-loaded nanoparticles in hepatocellular carcinoma. *ESMO Open,* 2, e000238.
[http://dx.doi.org/10.1136/esmoopen-2017-000238] [PMID: 29104762]

Minhajat, R, Mori, D, Yamasaki, F, Sugita, Y, Satoh, T & Tokunaga, O (2006) Organ-specific endoglin (CD105) expression in the angiogenesis of human cancers. *Pathol Int,* 56, 717-23.
[http://dx.doi.org/10.1111/j.1440-1827.2006.02037.x] [PMID: 17096728]

Mohamed, NK, Hamad, MA, Hafez, MZ, Wooley, KL & Elsabahy, M (2017) Nanomedicine in management of hepatocellular carcinoma: Challenges and opportunities. *Int J Cancer,* 140, 1475-84.
[http://dx.doi.org/10.1002/ijc.30517] [PMID: 27861850]

Mukherjee, S, Liang, L & Veiseh, O (2020) 'Recent advancements of magnetic nanomaterials in cancer therapy', *Pharmaceutics* .MDPI AG.
[http://dx.doi.org/10.3390/pharmaceutics12020147]

Mulik, RS, Bing, C, Ladouceur-Wodzak, M, Munaweera, I, Chopra, R & Corbin, IR (2016) Localized delivery of low-density lipoprotein docosahexaenoic acid nanoparticles to the rat brain using focused ultrasound. *Biomaterials,* 83, 257-68.
[http://dx.doi.org/10.1016/j.biomaterials.2016.01.021] [PMID: 26790145]

Munaweera, I, Hong, J, D'Souza, A & Balkus, KJ (2015) Novel wrinkled periodic mesoporous organosilica nanoparticles for hydrophobic anticancer drug delivery. *J Porous Mater,* 22, 1-10. a
[http://dx.doi.org/10.1007/s10934-014-9897-1]

Munaweera, I, Koneru, B, Shi, Y, Di Pasqua, AJ, Balkus, J & Kenneth, J (2014) Chemoradiotherapeutic wrinkled mesoporous silica nanoparticles for use in cancer therapy. *APL Mater,* 2, 113315.
[http://dx.doi.org/10.1063/1.4899118]

Munaweera, I, Shi, Y, Koneru, B, Saez, R, Aliev, A, Di Pasqua, AJ & Balkus, KJ, Jr (2015) Chemoradiotherapeutic magnetic nanoparticles for targeted treatment of nonsmall cell lung cancer. *Mol*

Pharm, 12, 3588-96. b
[http://dx.doi.org/10.1021/acs.molpharmaceut.5b00304] [PMID: 26325115]

Munaweera, I, Trinh, M, Hong, J & Balkus, KJ (2016) Chemically powered nanomotor as a delivery vehicle for biologically relevant payloads. *J Nanosci Nanotechnol,* 16, 9063-71.
[http://dx.doi.org/10.1166/jnn.2016.12904]

Na, K & Paik, Y-K (2010) Plasma biomarker tool for the diagnosis of liver cancer comprising liver carboxylesterase 1 and liver cancer screening method US2011097738A1

Nakatsura, T, Yoshitake, Y, Senju, S, Monji, M, Komori, H, Motomura, Y, Hosaka, S, Beppu, T, Ishiko, T, Kamohara, H, Ashihara, H, Katagiri, T, Furukawa, Y, Fujiyama, S, Ogawa, M, Nakamura, Y & Nishimura, Y (2003) Glypican-3, overexpressed specifically in human hepatocellular carcinoma, is a novel tumor marker. *Biochem Biophys Res Commun,* 306, 16-25.
[http://dx.doi.org/10.1016/S0006-291X(03)00908-2] [PMID: 12788060]

Nardecchia, S, Sánchez-Moreno, P, Vicente, J, Marchal, JA, Boulaiz, H & Boulaiz, H (2019) Clinical trials of thermosensitive nanomaterials: an overview. *Nanomaterials (Basel),* 9, 191.
[http://dx.doi.org/10.3390/nano9020191] [PMID: 30717386]

Asl, MN & Hosseinzadeh, H (2008) Review of pharmacological effects of Glycyrrhiza sp. and its bioactive compounds. *Phytother Res,* 22, 709-24.
[http://dx.doi.org/10.1002/ptr.2362] [PMID: 18446848]

Neil, PD, Chunlin, T, Andrew, Y, Leslie, L, Tianli, Z, Zhiwen, Y, Patrik, S-S & Shlomo, M (2000) Methods and compositions useful for administration of chemotherapeutic agents US5916596A

Nikam, RR & Gore, KR (2018) Journey of siRNA: clinical developments and targeted delivery. *Nucleic Acid Ther,* 28, 209-24.
[http://dx.doi.org/10.1089/nat.2017.0715] [PMID: 29584585]

Numata, K (2015) Advances in ultrasound systems for hepatic lesions in Japan. Springer.
[http://dx.doi.org/10.1007/s10396-015-0630-8]

Numata, K, Luo, W, Morimoto, M, Kondo, M, Kunishi, Y, Sasaki, T, Nozaki, A & Tanaka, K (2010) Contrast enhanced ultrasound of hepatocellular carcinoma. *World J Radiol,* 2, 68-82.
[http://dx.doi.org/10.4329/wjr.v2.i2.68] [PMID: 21160920]

Okusaka, T, Okada, S, Ueno, H, Ikeda, M, Iwata, R, Furukawa, H, Takayasu, K, Moriyama, N, Sato, T & Sato, K (2002) Transcatheter arterial embolization with zinostatin stimalamer for hepatocellular carcinoma. *Oncology,* 62, 228-33.
[http://dx.doi.org/10.1159/000059570] [PMID: 12065870]

O'Shaughnessy, JA, Fisherman, JS & Cowan, KH (1994) Combination paclitaxel (Taxol) and doxorubicin therapy for metastatic breast cancer. *Semin Oncol,* 21 (Suppl. 8), 19-23.https://europepmc.org/article/med/7939757
[PMID: 7939757]

Park, JW (2002) Liposome-based drug delivery in breast cancer treatment. *Breast Cancer Res,* 4, 95-9.
[http://dx.doi.org/10.1186/bcr432] [PMID: 12052251]

Pattni, BS, Chupin, VV & Torchilin, VP (2015) New developments in liposomal drug delivery. *Chem Rev,* 115, 10938-66.
[http://dx.doi.org/10.1021/acs.chemrev.5b00046] [PMID: 26010257]

Phillips, M M, Sheaff, M T & Szlosarek, P W (2013) Targeting arginine-dependent cancers with arginine-degrading enzymes: opportunities and challenges, *Cancer research and treatment: official journal of Korean Cancer Association,* 45, 251.

Pohl, VG, Galvan, G, Maier, F & Balke, C (1974) Erfahrungen mit dem "Effective-Thyroxin-Ratio"-(E-R)-Test. *Acta Med Austriaca,* 1, 122-7.https://pubmed.ncbi.nlm.nih.gov/4219254/
[PMID: 4219254]

Pottier, A, Levy, L & Meyre, ME (2014) NANOBIOTIX, (2014) *Nanoparticles comprising metallic and hafnium oxide materials, preparation and uses thereof*. WO2013087920A1

Qu, Z (2019) Natural nano-vesicle and preparation method and applications thereof CN110420221A

Reed, RA & Daishui, SU (2019) Thermosensitive nanoparticle formulations and method of making the same US10251901B2

Sackstein, R (2011) The biology of CD44 and HCELL in hematopoiesis: the 'step 2-bypass pathway' and other emerging perspectives. *Curr Opin Hematol,* 18, 239-48.
[http://dx.doi.org/10.1097/MOH.0b013e3283476140] [PMID: 21546828]

Saetrom, P Mina Therapeutics Ltd (2019) C/EBPα short activating RNA compositions and methods of use, US10633659B2

Salonen, J, Kaukonen, AM, Hirvonen, J & Lehto, V-P (2008) Mesoporous silicon in drug delivery applications *Journal of Pharmaceutical Sciences* John Wiley and Sons Inc. 632-53.
[http://dx.doi.org/10.1002/jps.20999]

Kudo, M, Gianstefani, A, Negrini, G, Allegretti, G, Galassi, M, Piscaglia, F, Joo, I, Lee, JM, Lin, C-C & Cheng, Y-T (2016) Defect reperfusion imaging with Sonazoid®: a breakthrough in hepatocellular carcinoma. *Liver Cancer,* 5, 1-7.
[PMID: 26989655]

Sarker, D, Plummer, ER, Basu, B, Meyer, T, Huang, K-W, Evans, TJ, Spalding, D, Ma, YT, Palmer, DH & Chee, CE (2018) Preliminary results of a first-in-human, first-in-class phase I study of MTL-CEBPA, a small activating RNA (saRNA) targeting the transcription factor C/EBP-α in patients with advanced liver cancer American Society of Clinical Oncology.
[http://dx.doi.org/10.1200/JCO.2018.36.15_suppl.2509]

Sarker, D, Plummer, R, Meyer, T, Sodergren, M, Basu, B, Chee, C E, Huang, K-W, Palmer, D H, Ma, Y T & Evans, T J (2020) Preliminary results of a first-in-human, first-in-class phase I study of MTL-CEBPA, a small activating RNA (saRNA) targeting the transcription factor C/EBP-α in patients with advanced liver cancer, American Society of Clinical Oncology.

Scarabel, L, Perrone, F, Garziera, M, Farra, R, Grassi, M, Musiani, F, Russo Spena, C, Salis, B, De Stefano, L, Toffoli, G, Rizzolio, F, Tonon, F, Abrami, M, Chiarappa, G, Pozzato, G, Forte, G, Grassi, G & Dapas, B (2017) Strategies to optimize siRNA delivery to hepatocellular carcinoma cells. *Expert Opin Drug Deliv,* 14, 797-810.
[http://dx.doi.org/10.1080/17425247.2017.1292247] [PMID: 28266887]

Semple, SC, Judge, AD, Robbins, M, Klimuk, S, Eisenhardt, M, Crosley, E, Leung, A, Kwok, R, Ambegia, E & Mcclintock, K (2011) Preclinical characterization of TKM-080301, a lipid nanoparticle formulation of a small interfering RNA directed against polo-like kinase 1. AACR.

Senanayake, TH, Warren, G & Vinogradov, SV (2011) Novel anticancer polymeric conjugates of activated nucleoside analogues. *Bioconjug Chem,* 22, 1983-93.
[http://dx.doi.org/10.1021/bc200173e] [PMID: 21863885]

Seo, D Y, Lee, SR, Heo, JW, No, MH, Rhee, BD, Ko, KS, Kwak, HB & Han, J (2018) Ursolic acid in health and disease *Korean Journal of Physiology and Pharmacology,*, 235-48. Korean Physiological Soc. and Korean Soc. of Pharmacology
[http://dx.doi.org/10.4196/kjpp.2018.22.3.235]

Setten, RL, Lightfoot, HL, Habib, NA & Rossi, JJ (2018) Development of MTL-CEBPA: small activating RNA drug for hepatocellular carcinoma. *Curr Pharm Biotechnol,* 19, 611-21.
[http://dx.doi.org/10.2174/1389201019666180611093428] [PMID: 29886828]

Shafizadeh, N, Ferrell, LD & Kakar, S (2008) Utility and limitations of glypican-3 expression for the diagnosis of hepatocellular carcinoma at both ends of the differentiation spectrum. *Mod Pathol,* 21, 1011-8.
[http://dx.doi.org/10.1038/modpathol.2008.85] [PMID: 18536657]

Shilpi, S (2018) 'Drug targeting strategies for liver cancer and other liver diseases', *MOJ Drug Design Development & Therapy. MedCrave Group, LLC,* 2
[http://dx.doi.org/10.15406/mojddt.2018.02.00044]

Sobot, D, Mura, S & Couvreur, P (2016) How can nanomedicines overcome cellular-based anticancer drug resistance? *J Mater Chem B Mater Biol Med,* 4, 5078-100.
[http://dx.doi.org/10.1039/C6TB00900J] [PMID: 32263505]

Stylianopoulos, T (2013) EPR-effect: utilizing size-dependent nanoparticle delivery to solid tumors. *Ther Deliv,* 4, 421-3.
[http://dx.doi.org/10.4155/tde.13.8] [PMID: 23557281]

Sung, YK, Hwang, SY, Park, MK, Farooq, M, Han, IS, Bae, HI, Kim, JC & Kim, M (2003) Glypican-3 is overexpressed in human hepatocellular carcinoma. *Cancer Sci,* 94, 259-62.
[http://dx.doi.org/10.1111/j.1349-7006.2003.tb01430.x] [PMID: 12824919]

Svenson, S (2012) Clinical translation of nanomedicines. *Curr Opin Solid State Mater Sci,* 16, 287-94.
[http://dx.doi.org/10.1016/j.cossms.2012.10.001]

Synakiewicz, A, Stachowicz-Stencel, T & Adamkiewicz-Drozynska, E (2014) The role of arginine and the modified arginine deiminase enzyme ADI-PEG 20 in cancer therapy with special emphasis on Phase I/II clinical trials. *Expert Opin Investig Drugs,* 23, 1517-29.
[http://dx.doi.org/10.1517/13543784.2014.934808] [PMID: 24965808]

Tangkijvanich, P, Chanmee, T, Komtong, S, Mahachai, V, Wisedopas, N, Pothacharoen, P & Kongtawelert, P (2010) Diagnostic role of serum glypican-3 in differentiating hepatocellular carcinoma from non-malignant chronic liver disease and other liver cancers. *J Gastroenterol Hepatol,* 25, 129-37.
[http://dx.doi.org/10.1111/j.1440-1746.2009.05988.x] [PMID: 19793164]

Tomasz, M (1995) 'Mitomycin C: small, fast and deadly (but very selective)', *Chemistry and Biology* Chem Biol 575-9.
[http://dx.doi.org/10.1016/1074-5521(95)90120-5]

Tuerk, C & Gold, L (1990) Systematic evolution of ligands by exponential enrichment: RNA ligands to bacteriophage T4 DNA polymerase. *Science,* 249, 505-10.
[http://dx.doi.org/10.1126/science.2200121] [PMID: 2200121]

Wan, C, Allen, TM & Cullis, PR (2014) Lipid nanoparticle delivery systems for siRNA-based therapeutics. *Drug Deliv Transl Res,* 4, 74-83.
[http://dx.doi.org/10.1007/s13346-013-0161-z] [PMID: 25786618]

Wang, G, Wang, Y, Xue, J & Yang, Q (2015) AFP antibody modification PLGA load DCN nanoparticle targeting anticancer medicine CN104840947A.

Wiradharma, N, Tong, YW & Yang, Y-Y (2009) Self-assembled oligopeptide nanostructures for co-delivery of drug and gene with synergistic therapeutic effect. *Biomaterials,* 30, 3100-9.
[http://dx.doi.org/10.1016/j.biomaterials.2009.03.006] [PMID: 19342093]

Wong, N & Yeo, W (2011) Methods for treating hepatocellular carcinoma US9370494B2.

Wong, RJ, Cheung, R & Ahmed, A (2014) Nonalcoholic steatohepatitis is the most rapidly growing indication for liver transplantation in patients with hepatocellular carcinoma in the U.S. *Hepatology,* 59, 2188-95.
[http://dx.doi.org/10.1002/hep.26986] [PMID: 24375711]

Yazdani, A, Alirezaire, Z, Motamedi, MJ & Amani, J (2018) 'Gene Therapy: A New Approach in Modern Medicine', *International Journal of Medical Reviews. Armenian Green Publishing Co,* 5, 106-17.
[http://dx.doi.org/10.29252/IJMR-050304]

Yi, Yimu (2002) Ursolic acid bean phospholipid nano particle freeze drying powder for ampoule agent and its preparation method CN1243538C

Zhang, G (2018) Preparation method of biosynthesis silver nanoparticles CN109276559A

Zhang, L, Liao, Y & Tang, L (2019) MicroRNA-34 family: a potential tumor suppressor and therapeutic candidate in cancer. *J Exp Clin Cancer Res,* 38, 53.
[http://dx.doi.org/10.1186/s13046-019-1059-5] [PMID: 30717802]

CHAPTER 12

Future Direction of Nanotherapy in the Management of Hepatocellular Carcinoma

Biswajit Mukherjee[1,*], Laboni Das[2], Sanchari Bhattacharya[3], Apala Chakraborty[1], Shreyasi Chakraborty[1], Ashique Al Hoque[1] and **Debasmita Dutta[1,4]**

[1] *Department of Pharmaceutical Technology, Jadavpur University, Kolkata 700032, WB, India*

[2] *School of Pharmacy, Techno India University, EM-4, Sector-V, Salt Lake, Kolkata, WB, India*

[3] *Guru Nanak Institute of Pharmaceutical Science and Technology, 157 f, Nilgunj Rd, Sahid Colony, Panihati, Kolkata, West Bengal 700114, India*

[4] *Department of Molecular and Human Genetics, Baylor College of Medicine,Houston, Texas 77030, United States*

Abstract: Worldwide, hepatocellular carcinoma (HCC) is one of the leading causes of cancer-related deaths among humans. Several conventional therapies, including surgical and non-surgical methods such as liver transplantation, radiation, and chemotherapy, have been explored to combat this disease and improve the patients' quality of life. However, due to poor diagnosis of the disease, drug toxicity issues, and difficulties related to liver transplantation, scientists search for novel techniques to treat HCC that ensure targeted drug delivery and help in diagnosing the disease. Nanotherapeutics are a new trend in drug discovery and medicine which deals with nano-sized formulations loaded with various types of materials such as drugs, antibodies, aptamers, genes, viruses, *etc*., and targeted delivery. Moreover, controlled release of the materials can be achieved through modifying their external and internal structures as per requirement. Drug delivery through nano theranostics has taken a new turn as the diagnostic tools tagged with the nano-architectures ensure diagnosis and treatment simultaneously. Nanotheranostics have significant application in the identification of cancer progression through continuous monitoring and treatment of cancer. In this review, we will discuss different beneficial effects and applications of nanotherapeutics against HCC. Along with that, different upcoming strategies, such as personalized medicine, layer-by-layer technologies, implant theory, 3D printing technology, nanorobots, nanocrystals, nano-chips, *etc*., will be discussed here, which may pave the path towards successful diagnosis and treatment of HCC to improve the health of the patients.

[*] **Corresponding author Biswajit Mukherjee:** Department of Pharmaceutical Technology, Jadavpur University, Kolkata 700032, India, Tel/Fax: +913324146677; Mobile: +91-84208248897; E-mails: biswajit.mukherjee@jadavpuruniversity.in, biswajit55@yahoo.com

Keywords: Diagnosis, Future therapy, Hepatocellular carcinoma, Nanoparticles, Nanotherapeutics, Technology.

INTRODUCTION

Hepatocellular carcinoma (HCC) is a primary malignancy that starts in the liver and differs from the other "secondary" liver cancers which spread from other organs to the liver. Early diagnosis can cure HCC with the help of transplant or surgery, but in more advanced cases, the cure is quite tricky where better treatment and proper support can increase the life span of the patients (https://www.webmd.com/cancer/hepatocellular-carcinoma#1). Important risk factors that may lead to developing HCC include hepatitis B virus (HBV) and hepatitis C virus (HCV) infection, liver cirrhosis, alcohol consumption in excessive level, non-alcoholic steatohepatitis (NASH), and also by ingestion of aflatoxin B1 (Pimenta *et al.,* 2010, Gomes *et al.,* 2013, Tunissiolli *et al.,* 2017). The asymptomatic nature of this cancer causes the patients to be undiagnosed at early stages. When detected at the terminal stages, the patients suffer from the severe fatality of liver dysfunction. Therefore, the lack of a sophisticated and efficient tool for HCC diagnosis and late diagnosis at the advanced non-curable stage that excludes the patients from definitive surgical resection (Daher *et al.,* 2018) leaves the option to treat the patients with HCC with palliative care only. Thus the fatal HCC case rate increases worldwide (Stewart 2014, Baig *et al.,* 2019).

Further, the unavailability of competent diagnostic tools for early detection and suitable curable treatment options are the primary reasons that increase cancer-related deaths in HCC patients. Researchers have explored new cases of HCC and its high mortality rate. The investigation aims to improve the existing therapy in patients. In the future, more unique treatments that combat the current lacuna in treating HCC may be developed (Tao *et al.,* 2020).

Choice of treatment for HCC depends on the stage of the disease of the individual. The interdisciplinary evaluation that can guide individual treatment profile of HCC patient includes the tumor stage, liver functioning, performance status, comorbidities if any, and center expertise (Wege *et al.,* 2019).

Management of HCC therapy includes loco-regional therapy such as arterial chemoembolization, radiofrequency ablation, yttrium-90 intra-arterial delivery as microspheres, intra-tumor ethanol injection, microwave coagulation, and last but not least, surgical treatment, which includes surgical resection and liver transplantation (Alnajjar and Elsiesy 2015). Currently, in the late stage HCC therapy, sorafenib has also been considered as first-line therapy, although the incidence of drug resistance for sorafenib is becoming increasingly common (Tang *et al.,* 2020, Daher *et al.,* 2018).

In current research in the therapeutic management of HCC, the commonly associated complications of conventional therapies are being given attention by scientists worldwide. For the last two decades, they have been involved in finding innovative approaches to understand the development of HCC better and tackle it. Nanotechnology is a novel approach that has established its importance in different areas, including medicine, as confirmed by the interdisciplinary field's speedy growth. It offers unique opportunities for improved therapy for cancer and other diseases through different nanoformulations for improved and targeted drugs with reduced systemic toxicity (Gharpure *et al.,* 2015). Advancement in nanotechnology has drawn attention through the targeted delivery of bioactive anticancer molecules (Baig *et al.,* 2019). Though the application is not limited to treating cancer, it also has an improved profile in cancer diagnostics and imaging (Baetke *et al.,* 2015, Baig *et al.,* 2019). In the field of therapeutic approaches to HCC, nanomedicine has emerged as a great promise for management. Anticancer drug-loaded nanoparticles improve the pattern of biodistribution of the loaded drug, thus reducing the cytotoxic effect of the encapsulated potent anticancer drug and ultimately can overcome the problems associated with HCC management successfully (Malla *et al.,* 2020). Researchers are involved in developing nanomedicines with high biocompatibility, stability, degradability, and lower level of immunogenicity and toxicity,which have been recognized as an emerging field of biomedical research. Targeting of HCC cells with nanotherapeutics may be an obvious path for the treatment of HCC because, in comparison to other hepatic cells, HCC cells undergo genetic and phenotypic changes (Sun *et al.,* 2019).

Various nanomaterials include polymeric nanoparticles, metallic nanoparticles, liposomes, quantum dots, dendrimers, micelles, carbon nanotubes, and nanoshells (Elsabahy *et al.,* 2012, Mohamed *et al.,* 2017). By modifying chemistries of the building blocks and for functional optimization, nanoparticles should be designed to improve permeability through biological barriers, cellular uptake, and protection to the loaded drug from degradation and optimization (Mohamed *et al.,* 2017). Researchers have designed different types of drug delivery and targeting strategies for nanoparticles, nanoliposomes, nano micelles, *etc*., for effective targeting to HCC cells through both passive and active targeting (Sun *et al.,* 2019). A tumor can be targeted through nanomedicines in passive mode through leaky vasculature of the tumors by involving enhanced permeability and retention (EPR) effect (Sun *et al.,* 2019). In contrast, the nanoparticles' surface can be modified by incorporating conjugating surface legends with specificity to cancer cell surface receptors (Ghosh *et al.,* 2012, Baig *et al.,* 2019).

Nanoparticles can be designed to target the altered cell properties in a tumor, including malformed morphological changes, quick rate of cell proliferation, overexpression of various antigens that express on the cancer cell surface, and immature vasculature (Iyer *et al.,* 2012; Praetorius and Mandal, 2007).

Different nanotherapeutics and nanodiagnostics that have shown their potential in treatment and diagnosis of HCC are being commercialized, or they have been in preclinical and clinical trials in recent years (Mizrahy *et al.,* 2012, Sun *et al.,* 2019), which can bring a newer hope to the treatment of liver cancer.

In this chapter, we will discuss different nanoformulations currently in the pipeline for the management of HCC. We will also summarize various diagnostic approaches that can help overcome the challenges of HCC diagnosis. We will discuss different patented formulations, along with different nanotherapeutics in clinical development and preclinical settings. We will also highlight future possibilities of appraisal that can be a more recent nanotechnology aspect for combating HCC in revolutionizing chemotherapeutic modalities' status.

Nanotherapeutics and Their Primary Objectives

The difficulties in offering tailored, effective treatment to the desired tissue are some of the most significant modern medicine obstacles. Selective treatment of diseased cells can significantly decrease side effects or dosage complications while saving healthier ones, but lately, new approaches have appeared to achieve these effects. Nanotechnology to treat or diagnose diseases by nanocarriers using the delivery of drugs is generally known as Nanotherapy (https://onlinelibrary.wiley.com/doi/toc/10.1002/(ISSN)2192-2659). As a field of medicine, monotherapies have a wide variety of diagnostic research and advancement. The drugs bind to the nanoparticles that trigger it to function more effectively and reliably with fewer or no side effects than the conventional treatment methods. Nanotherapeutics propose new possibilities to boost the mode of protection and efficiency compared to the existing treatment (Prasad *et al.,* 2018). The health care system is also working to improve sustainability, greater access, and better treatment efficiency at lower prices. The problems associated with chronic diseases such as cancer, diabetes, HIV/AIDS, hepatitis C, hepatitis B, and infectious diseases, which contribute to the development of side effects and multiple drug resistance in traditional antimicrobial medicines, are pre-existing. The specificity of drug delivery to the target organs could be one of the keys to therapeutic success in such cases. Drug targeting using nanoparticles has proven to be successful as a vehicle for the site-specific delivery of drugs. Nanoformulations improve the bioavailability, pharmacokinetic properties, and drug targeting capability for various drugs. In the field, nanomedicine provides possible help in diagnosis, therapy, the discovery of medicines, and gene transmission through molecular knowledge of the human system and the prevention and treatment of diseases (Prasad *et al.,* 2018).

In general, the creation of modern nanotherapy has some sequential envisions. Nanotherapeutics must show sufficient stability, biodegradability, non/less toxicity, biocompatibility, and provide wide functionality, and be capable of encapsulating or combining their drug payload. They need specific means of targeting the targeted cells or receptors, thereby focusing on their desired site in the body. Once they are gathered to their target sites, the delivery system should release drugs or diagnostic molecules in a regulated manner. Then, once their payloads have been safely delivered to the desired areas, the system should have a way out of the body to prevent long-term toxicity issues (https://onlinelibrary.wiley.com/doi/toc/10.1002/(ISSN)2192-2659).

Beneficial Effects of Nanotherapeutics

Nanotechnology is believed to have a significant influence on public health in drug delivery and therapy. Nanotherapeutics are nano-size range devices used to detect, prevent, and manage diseases. They are used in diverse applications, such as drug distribution, *in vivo* imaging, *in vitro* diagnostic, active implants, *etc*. In the past two decades, significant developments in the area of nanomedicine have come up, resulting in a wide range of devices, including medicinal and imagery products, allowing care and diagnostic approaches that are more effective and less harmful (Murthy *et al.,* 2007). Nanotherapeutics' ability to provide a target drug delivery, increase the solubility of a drug, prolong drug half-life, enhance the medicinal therapeutic index, and reduce the immunogenicity of a drug has grown to revolutionize therapy for many diseases (Hafner *et al.,* 2014).

Prospective of Nanotherapeutic Devices For Therapeutic Management of Cancers Includes HCC

Recent times have successfully explained many drug delivery technologies, but there are still obstacles in successfully addressing cutting-edge technology to distribute medications to its target locations. However, nano-sized drug delivery systems have shown enormous prospects to facilitate site-specific delivery of drugs. In this context, we will discuss the opportunities of some potential nanoscale carriers.

Nanoparticles

Nanoparticles are solid particles ranging in size from 10 to 1000 nm. The drug is dissolved, entrapped, loaded, or bound to a matrix of nanoparticles. Nanoparticles, nanocapsules, and nanospheres can be obtained depending on the preparation process. Nanocapsule is a structure in which a drug substance remains in the polymer membrane's cavity. A nanosphere is a matrix system in which the drug is chemically and evenly distributed (Mohanraj and Chen 2006).

Many forms of drug delivery systems with nanoparticles probably have been most widely studied among the different nanoformulations at different levels. These particles were made from many materials with unique structures to treat a specific disease as a potential pharmaceutical vehicle. Most recent research focuses mainly on nanoparticles' use to treat many chronic diseases such as cancer, HIV, diabetes, *etc.*, as drug carriers. At present, traditional care may be felt as insufficient for these diseases, resulting in high mortality in most cases. Nanoparticles can be a useful device for battling these diseases to deliver medicines safely to the infected sites. Anticancer medications need to resolve the drug resistance on the organs, tissue, and/or cells. For this, it is of utmost importance to precisely deliver anticancer therapeutic agents to cancer cells.

In some cases, conventional chemotherapy does not work, as anticancer medications appear to spread to the whole body, killing both cancer and normal human cells. A promising tactical strategy that can face these obstacles is targeting cancer cells with nanoparticles filled with anticancer drugs (Yih and Al-fandi 2006, Brigger *et al.,* 2002). Several biodegradable nanoparticles can carry various therapeutic agents, including DNA, proteins, peptides, and low molecular weight compounds. Polymeric nanoparticles can be utilized as a possible potential drug carrier for a wide range of pharmacological therapies for different types of tumors, diabetes, bone healing, and vaccination (Yih and Al-fandi 2006).

Nanoliposomes

Liposomes are nano dimension lipid vesicles under intensive study as drug carriers to improve therapeutic agents' delivery and have enormous potential to deliver drugs across the physiological barriers. They are usually made of a comparatively biocompatible and biodegradable substance, and it comprises an aqueous volume entrapped by one or multiple bilayers of natural and/or synthetic lipids. A liposome encapsulates the aqueous solution inside a hydrophobic membrane, which cannot effectively move through lipids and contains dissolved hydrophilic solutes. The distribution of hydrophobic chemicals into the membrane will cause the liposome to be filled with hydrophobic and hydrophilic molecules. The lipid bilayer can fuse with some other bilayers, such as the cell membrane, and liposome content is endocytosed in the cells to carry drug molecules to operation locations in the cells (Satapathy *et al.,* 2016).

Due to their subcellular size, nanoliposomes allow comparatively higher intracellular absorption than other particle systems. They have been well investigated in treating the central nervous system's disorders such as infections in the brain, brain ischemia, brain tumors, and neurodegenerative conditions such as Parkinson's and Alzheimer's. Several studies have indicated improved transport of entrapped drugs by the blood-brain barrier (BBB) through intra-cerebral and intravenous delivery (Conti *et al.*, 2017, Agrawal *et al.*, 2017, Garcia-Garcia *et al.*, 2005). Many anti-HIV therapies cannot sufficiently cross BBB. Nanoliposomal formulation may be a good solution for taking these treatments to the brain to efficiently treat HIV infection (Dutta *et al.*, 2018). Antibiotics-loaded liposomal formulations have also been tried to be used for active targeting purposes. Pinheiro *et al.*, 2011 reported rifampicin-loaded liposomes containing ligands administered through an aerosol formulation and they were used for direct targeting of the infected alveolar macrophages (Pinheiro *et al.*, 2011). Nanoliposomes are significantly involved in the management of diabetes (Amjadi *et al.*, 2019) and active targeting of various cancers such as liver cancer (Ye *et al.*, 2020), lung cancer (Zare Kazemabadi *et al.*, 2019), colon cancer (Adiseshaiah *et al.*, 2013), pancreatic cancer (Glassman *et al.*, 2018), prostate cancer (Singh *et al.*, 2018), *etc*. Soon, nanoliposome may be extensively used for drug targeting and site-specific drug delivery across the physiological barriers.

Nanoemulsions

Nanoemulsions are kinetically stable, liquid in liquid dispersion with an average droplet size of 100 nm. Small dimensions of the droplets in the nanoemulsions contribute to beneficial characteristics such as high surface area per unit volume, good stability, a translucent visual appearance and tuning rheology, *etc*. Nanoemulsions are used in various fields, such as drug delivery, food, medicine, cosmetics, and material production. They also act as models for understanding colloidal nanoscale dispersions. Nanoemulsions are prepared using many processes, including high-pressure homogenization, phase inversion temperature, ultrasonication, emulsion inversion point, and newly established techniques such as the bubble bursting technique (Gupta *et al.*, 2016).

In the field of drug delivery, nanoemulsions provide some crucial advantages over other treatments that include increasing the rate of absorption, eliminating variability in absorption, providing an aqueous dosage form for water-insoluble drugs, increasing the bioavailability of active drugs, rapid and efficient penetration of the drug moiety, liquid dosage form which increases patient compliance, *etc*. (Sharma *et al.*, 2013). Clark *et al*. 2001 reported in a study about the use of nanoemulsions in the intranasal drug delivery system, which has achieved important brain targeting effects in the treatment of central nervous system-related diseases (Clark *et al.*, 2001). Many experiments have shown that nanoemulsion formulations have enhanced *in vitro* and *in vivo* transdermal and dermal drug distribution properties. Over traditional topical formulations such as emulsions and gels, nanoemulsions have increased transdermal permeation for many drug molecules (Lovelyn *et al.*, 2011). Apart from these beneficial effects, nanoemulsions are also widely used in cancer targeting, vaccine delivery, pulmonary drug delivery, and many more (Lovelyn *et al.*, 2011).

Nanocrystals

Nanocrystals are excellent drug particles within a size of 1000 nm. These are 100% drugs without any carrier molecule bound to them and are typically stabilized by using polymeric steric stabilizers or surfactant substances. The nanocrystals have unique characteristics such as increased saturation solubility, enlarged dissolution velocity,and increased adhesion to surface/cell membranes that allow them to overcome various difficulties (Patra *et al.*, 2018). A significant benefit of nanocrystal drugs is that they can be administered by various administration routes, such as oral, parenteral, ocular, pulmonary delivery, and have demonstrated considerable superiority to the equivalent conventional formulation products by each route of administration. Furthermore, drug nanocrystals can also be converted into different dose types compared to traditional formulation methods, such as tablets, capsules, injections, aerosols, and more (Gao *et al.*, 2008). Hence, nanocrystals have tremendous future potential in nanomedicine.

Quantum Dots

Quantum dots (QDs) are effective as fluorescent probes for long-term, multiplexed, and quantitative imaging and detection methods. Various engineered quantum dots with optimized targeting, visualization, and therapeutic capabilities have made them excellent drug delivery study materials to cells and small animals (Qi and Gao, 2008). More specifically, QDs have arisen from their particular photophysical and solid surface chemistry as one of the potential and promising classes of nanoparticles for biomedical imaging, medicinal products distribution, and sensing. Inorganic QD cores' biofunctionalization enables the association of nanoparticles with biological structures and allows for active intervention in the various biological processes. Consequently, quantum dot probes have been used widely in *in vivo* drug distribution, tracing, live-cell imaging, and *in vitro* molecular pathology. With every usage, QDs have opened up new horizons for quantitative multiplex detection, insightful high-resolution fluorescence imaging, and real-time monitoring of probe dynamics for a longer time (Zrazhevskiy *et al.*, 2010).

Applications of Nanotherapeutics in HCC

HCC is usually diagnosed at the late stage, and chemotherapy usually becomes a single option for treating HCC at this stage. It is essential to reduce the dose-related toxicity of the drug, and nano therapy could be an incredible option to tackle such challenges by using passive and active targeting. Some predominant modes of application of nanotherapeutics have been described below.

Drug Delivery

Nanotherapeutics play a major role in drug delivery because of the various limitations of active pharmaceutical agents. Many important drugs such as docetaxel, doxorubicin, paclitaxel, curcumin, diltiazem cannot be administered directly because of their low water solubility or extremely high water solubility (Tran and Tran 2019). These drugs can be delivered well to increase bioavailability/sustain drug release for an extended period when formulated in nanoformulations. First-generation nanotherapeutics have several advantages: enhancement of solubility, increased half-life, prolonged release, and reduced toxicity (Shi *et al.*, 2010). United States Food and Drug Administration (USFDA) approved some nanotherapeutics that are listed in Table **1**.

Table 1. US-FDA approved nanotherapeutics.

Name of Nanotherapeutic	Carrier and Drug Used	Indication	References
AmBisome®	Liposomes of Amphotericin B	Systemic fungal infection	(Hiemenz and Walsh 1996)
Marqibo®	Sphingomyelin-cholesterol liposome of vincristine sulfate	Acute lymphoid leukemia	(Weissig *et al.*,2014)
Opaxio®	Solid nanoparticles of paclitaxel	Glioblastoma	(Weissig *et al.*,2014)
Eligard	Leuprolide acetate and polymer	Prostate cancer	(Ventola 2017)
Avinza	Nanocrystals of morphine sulfate	Psychostimulant	(Ventola 2017)

The development of nanotherapeutics containing protein and peptide drugs is another emerging field in drug delivery. Protein and peptide drugs are called biopharmaceuticals, which have been found to be beneficial in treating various human ailments such as neurological disorders, metabolic disorders, microbial diseases, cancer, and diabetes. Significant disadvantages of protein and peptide drugs include sizeable molecular size, hydrophilic nature, and low stability, which result in low bioavailability (Srinivas *et al.,* 2019). Another problem associated with protein and peptide drugs is the oral delivery restriction, as these drugs undergo degradation in gastrointestinal pH. Better clinical efficacies of the protein/peptide-loaded nanocarriers have been exploited to enable new therapeutics and the development of innovative drug delivery (Table **2**).

Table 2. Some reported protein and peptide drugs loaded nanotherapeutics

Nanoformulation	Application	References
Liposomal formulation of Cetuximab-oxaliplatin	Targeted chemotherapy of colorectal cancer	(Zalba *et al.*, 2015)
Mesoporous silica nanoparticle-containing bone-forming peptide	Promote osteo-differentiation in bone tissue engineering	(Luo *et al.*,2015)
Iron oxide-tannic acid-containing trypsin	*In vitro* enzyme stability	(Atacan and Ozacar 2015)
Chitosan-polyethylene glycol monomethyl ether nano complex containing insulin	Enhanced hypoglycemic activity in oral delivery	(Liu C *et al.*, 2019)
Insulin-loaded alginate-dextran sulfate nanoparticle, coated with chitosan and albumin	Higher permeability and better oral delivery was achieved in type 1 diabetes	(Lopes *et al.*, 2016)

Targeted Delivery and Personalized Medicine

Surface modifications of nanotherapeutics can achieve active targeted therapy to reduce systemic side-effects and enhance the therapeutic potential of the drug. Ligand conjugated nanoparticles can reach specific cells and exert drug action. Ligand conjugated nanotherapeutics were evidenced to improve the uptake and retention of drugs within cancerous cells. The most important criterion in this regard is choosing the ligand to recognize the overexpressed receptor on the target cells (Weissig *et al.*, 2014). Antibody-conjugated nanoparticles augment the delivery of a chemotherapeutic agent to the specific tissue and increase drug payload into that particular tissue/site of action. These drug conjugates are used to deliver cytotoxic drugs to minimize systemic cytotoxicity. One such antibody conjugated nanotherapeutic is Kadcyla®, approved by US-FDA and used to treat HER2+ breast cancer. Kadcyla® is composed of a maytansine derivative, covalently conjugated to trastuzumab through the lysine residues of the antibody. Targeted delivery is also a vital technique to combat multidrug resistance (Yetisgin *et al.*, 2020). Personalized nanotherapy is a healthcare strategy where specific treatment is given to individual patient. Customized medicines have some advantages: targeting particular organs, offering individual treatment patterns to each patient (dose and frequency), versatility, and reducing the dose of drugs (Fornaguera and García-Celma 2017). It can open a new avenue in the management of chemotherapy of various cancers, including HCC.

Controlled Release

Tissue regeneration and growth require localization and control delivery of biological factors, which are remarkably achieved by nanotherapeutics. For example, for maintaining a continuous blood supply in HCC-developing tissue, controlled delivery of angiogenic factors is essential. In such cases, nanotherapeutics may be highly recommended (Weiss 2009). Some nanocarriers can deliver multiple drugs to a target site or trigger drug release in response to environmental changes such as pH, temperature, or mechanical stress (Shi *et al.*, 2010).

Delivery of siRNA and Gene Therapy

Small interfering RNA (siRNA) is a potential therapeutic agent for cancer, infectious diseases, immunological diseases where there is overexpression of multiple genes. In recent days 'Silencing of gene' has been the area of interest for most scientists. However, the delivery of siRNA has a few challenges. It requires the protection of siRNA in the circulation to successfully deliver the siRNA to the target site, enabling cellular uptake and excretion. Nanotherapeutics of siRNA opened a new paradigm in the future treatment of many critical diseases, including HCC (Schroeder *et al.*, 2010).

Co Delivery

Poor specificity of drug and complications of the hepatic tumor are challenging in the treatment by chemotherapy. In overcoming multidrug resistance, a combination of chemotherapeutic agents with nucleic acid is a promising strategy. Zhou *et al.* developed two combination nanotherapeutics. HPMA (hydroxypropyl methacrylate) copolymer-cyclopamine conjugate worked on stem cell signaling hedgehog pathway, and the HPMA copolymer-docetaxel conjugate was involved in cell differentiation (Zhou *et al.*, 2013). This study showed a better survival rate. Feng *et al.* showed the synergistic inhibitory activity of a combination of VEGF (vascular endothelial growth factor) siRNA and paclitaxel *via* vapreotide-modified core/shell nanoparticles in breast cancer (Pelaz *et al.*, 2017).

Photodynamic Therapy

Treatment with photosensitizing drugs requires a proper delivery system. Nanotherapeutics containing photosensitizing drugs are often used for the treatment of cancer, acne, skin diseases. Nanotherapeutics are applied in the skin near the target site or to the bloodstream through the vein (Prasad *et al.*, 2018). These nanotherapeutics are further categorized as passive nanotherapeutics and active nanotherapeutic (Naidoo *et al.*, 2018). Passive nanotherapeutics contain encapsulated photosensitizing agents as carriers of the drug, whereas in active nanotherapeutics, nanoparticles act as photo-sensitizer on their own. Passive nanoparticles become activated in exposure to light, and the exciting nanoparticles produce free oxygen radicals. These molecules are absorbed by the target cells, which in turn destroy the cancerous cells. This strategy became popular because it is a non-invasive method than surgery and has no side effects in the long term (Smith *et al.,* 2012). Such an approach is potentially practical for HCC therapy. Some nanotherapeutics containing photosensitizing agents are listed in Table **3**.

Table 3. Nanotherapeutics containing photosensitizing agent for the treatment of HCC.

Serial No:	Composition of Nanotherapeutic	Application in HCC	References
1.	Nanotherapeutics containing doxorubicin-loaded nanoparticles modified with hematoporphyrin	Markedly improved *in vivo* anticancer efficacy in mice bearing HepG2 tumor	(Chang *et al.*, 2014)
2.	Nanotherapeutics containing copper-cysteamine nanoparticles	Induced apoptosis, reduced HepG2cell activity *in vitro*, and inhibited tumor growth *in vivo*	(Huang *et al.*, 2019)
3.	Hollow silica nanoparticle-containing photos	Better efficacy in terms of tumor cell apoptosis was found for nanoparticle-containing photosan compared to free photo san in HCC	(Liu Z *et al.*, 2014)
4	Poly(dopamine) nanoparticle conjugated with chlorin e6	Produced higher efficacy of photothermal/photodynamic therapy compared to free chlorin e6 in HCC	(Zhang *et al.*, 2015)
5	An organic framework of folic acid-nanoscale gadolinium-porphyrin metal	After laser irradiation, HCC tumor cells were eliminated	(Chen *et al.*, 2018)

Diagnostics for HCC

Nano-ranged sensors have been developed for the detection of various pathological conditions, foreign particles, or antigens. Nanoparticles are used as an imaging agent for ultrasound, MRI (magnetic resonance imaging), or PET (positron emission tomography). Nano-sized diagnostics provide better contrast and controlled biodistribution. For example, a high X-ray attenuation coefficient of gold has been utilized to develop gold nanoparticles, a contrasting agent for X-ray and CT (computed tomography) scans. AuroVist™ is a search-use only gold nanoparticle which is also commercially available (Matthew *et al.,* 2018). Radiolabeled nanoparticles are often used for molecular imaging purposes. The most commonly used isotopes for radiolabeling of nanoparticles are ^{99m}technetium and radioiodine (^{131}I) in single-photon emission computed tomography (SPECT), where gamma emission is detected (Hong *et al.,* 2009). Though many types of nanoparticles are available, quantum dots are ideal as an imaging agent. These agents' major drawback is that they cannot be applied to renal problems due to renal toxicity. A gold nanoparticle is a diagnostic tool for prostate cancer. Infectious diseases caused by *Mycobacterium tuberculosis* complex (MTB), *Salmonella typhimurium*, or *S. aureus* can be diagnosed by using fluorescent silica nanoparticles within 4 h. A study has been reported by Valizadeh A, 2016, where quantum dots-based nanosensors are used for the detection of HIV1 and HIV2 viruses. Nanoparticles are also used for renal problems like ischemia or acute renal failure (El-Sayed and Kamel 2020). It is believed that late detection of HCC is the primary cause of mortality for HCC patients. However, efforts should be focused on developing such nanodiagnostic imaging agents/diagnostics to detect HCC at an early stage, bringing a new strategy for therapeutic management of HCC.

Projected Areas of Nanotherapeutics in HCC

Recent Updates on HCC Targeted Nanotherapeutics Based on Clinical and Preclinical Studies

Until recently, the life expectancy of HCC patients could only be improved by invasive methods such as radiofrequency ablation, liver transplantation, transcatheter arterial chemoembolization, or surgical resection process before the approval of the drug sorafenib, a multiple kinase inhibitor, as a first anti-HCC drug approved by USFDA on 2007 (Bruix *et al.,* 2015). The poor bioavailability (around 8%), aqueous insolubility, rapid systemic clearance, and various side effects such as chances of high blood pressure, nausea, fatigue, and diarrhea reduce the efficacy of sorafenib for the treatment of HCC (Thapa *et al.,* 2015). Hence, the nano-drug delivery system has come to the forefront as an approach to overcome the solubility problem and the side effects of the drug. Moreover, the development and application of biopolymers, proteins, and peptides in drug delivery have also accelerated the discovery of advanced nanotechnological approaches to target cancer therapy (Ferrari 2015, Yu *et al.,* 2013). In the recent past, nano-drug delivery systems such as liposomes, solid lipid nanoparticles, and polymeric metallic nanoparticles have been approached by various investigators to increase bioavailability and to reduce the side effects of sorafenib. However, to achieve the HCC cell-targeting, various approaches are now under rigorous trial for a more satisfactory therapeutic outcome. Along with the increased bioavailability of the drug inside the drug carrier system, the ultimate focus of the nanotechnological application to treat HCC is to enhance the response of HCC cells toward drug therapy by enhancing their cellular binding, internalization, drug retention, toxicity, and efficacy (Sun *et al.,* 2019). For instance, pH-responsive HCC targeting of sorafenib can increase the tumor selectivity and the half-life of the drug by almost 4 folds (Li and Zhao, 2019). Li *et al.*, 2019, depict that the weak acidic microenvironment of the tumor helps break the micelles at the amide bond and carboxy dimethyl maleic bond followed by the rapid release and intracellular uptake of the drug, preferably in the HCC cells. Combination of sorafenib and small interfering RNA (siRNA) in pH-triggered liposomes using carboxymethyl chitosan is another approach to suppress HCC cells' progression (Liu F *et al.*, 2014). The pH-responsive nanoliposome has protected sorafenib and protects siRNA from degradation in serum in the presence of RNase enzymes. Another novel approach for HCC treatment is to induce ferroptosis inside the tumor cells by reducing glutathione (GSH), which can be achieved by incorporating sorafenib in mesoporous silica nanoparticles. The thiol-containing tripeptide GSH that is abundantly found in tumor cells can be targeted by disulfide linkage of poly (acrylic acid)-D-α-tocopherol succinate polymer or manganese-oxidation bond of mesoporous silica nanoparticles. Both the vehicles have been used for the delivery of sorafenib in high GSH overexpressed HCC cells (Tang *et al.*, 2019, Sang *et al.*, 2019). In another approach, the interruption of tumor microvasculature has been achieved by forming bubble cavitation using ultrasound-based nano delivery. This delivery system has shown an increase in the drug release and its uptake into the tumor cells. The same has been applied for sorafenib's successful delivery combined with doxorubicin in HCC cells (Yang *et al.*, 2019). The dual drug-loaded nanodroplets formed a strong cavity that can disrupt microvessels in tumors and increase the penetrability of drugs, followed by a reduced level of tumor-angiogenesis and growth inhibition of tumor cells in HCC patients (Yang *et al.*, 2019). A multi-responsive nano-delivery system is also a novel approach for the delivery of sorafenib in HCC cells. The investigation of Liu *et al.* depicts the idea of co-delivery of the Fe^{3+} and tannic acid along with sorafenib by forming a ferrous-supply-regeneration nanoengineering system for its delivery in the tumor cells. Along with sorafenib's delivery, the system further initiates an iron-redox system followed by lipid peroxidation and ferroptosis, which can inhibit tumor cell proliferation (Liu *et al.*, 2018). Along with cancer therapy, nano-drug delivery research is now greatly applied in imaging studies. The liposomal formulation containing sorafenib and gadolinium is applied as a contrast agent in MRI study and its therapeutic activities towards HCC (Xiao *et al.*, 2016). Superparamagnetic iron oxide nanoparticle is another contrast agent in MRI imaging, which has been co-loaded with sorafenib in a solid-lipid nanoparticle or folate-modified PEG-PCL polymeric micelles for inhibiting cell proliferation and inducing apoptosis specifically to the HCC cells for dual application (Agarwal *et al.*, 2008, Zhang *et al.*, 2013). Combination of sorafenib with other chemotherapeutic agents, immunomodulatory agents, or photo-therapeutic agents can help reduce the drug resistance and induce the chances of cancer cell deaths (Wang *et al.*, 2013). For instance, a combination of doxorubicin, a topoisomerase II inhibitor in DNA replication, with sorafenib has shown synergistic antitumor properties in HCC patients. This combination has shown improvement in phase II clinical trials on advanced HCC patients (Lencioni *et al.*, 2016). For further improvement in this combination, Xiong and his colleague applied a reduction-responsive nano delivery system. As per their investigation, a prodrug of doxorubicin (modified by disulfide) and sorafenib have been incorporated in the PEG-b-cyclodextrin amphiphiles polymeric nanoparticle which in the presence of dithiothreitol shows cytotoxicity in the HepG2 cells in-vitro (Xiong *et al.*, 2018). In another experiment, sorafenib and doxorubicin accumulated in the core-shell lipid nanosystem and have been shown to improve the cytotoxic stress and found to be effective up to 92% on HCC cells (Malarvizhi *et al.*, 2014). Co-loading of paclitaxel, tubulin targeting anticancer drug, and sorafenib in hyaluronic acid-modified multifunctional liposome has also been synergistically effective on cell apoptosis and inhibition of proliferation of cancer cells (Zhu and Chen 2019). The hyaluronic acid modification helps target the CD44 receptor overexpressed cancer cells and allows a high drug accumulation in the tumor microenvironment by endo-lysosomal escape (Lei *et al.*, 2019). The overexpressed asialoglycoprotein receptor in HepG2 cells has also been targeted by galactose modified solid lipid nanoparticles of sorafenib. This modification shows an increase in cellular uptake and enhanced cytotoxicity in the asialoglycoprotein overexpressed HepG2 cells. As mentioned above, the pharmacokinetic data of the formulation has also shown an improved bioavailability compared to the free drug (Tunki *et al.*, 2019). In this context, it may be mentioned that co-delivery of drugs with other chemotherapeutic agents is beneficial over a single dose. It reduces the dosing of a single drug and its associated toxicity. The application of targeted nanoparticles to deliver the combination of drugs to target HCC can further enhance the treatment's efficacy. The application of immune-modulating agents in cancer therapy is already an well-established thought in the recent trend of cancer research. Multikinase-inhibitor sorafenib has been shown to promote immunosuppression by enhancing the programmed death-ligand 1 (PD-L1) expression in cancer cells (Lu *et al.*, 2019). Co-delivery of sorafenib with immunomodulating agents may improve the antitumor immune response and inhibit tumor progression. This strategy has been applied for the co-delivery of AMD31, C-X-C receptor type 4 (CXCR4) antagonist, and sorafenib. Targeting CXCR4 helps regulate PD-L1-mediated immunosuppression, which can further help in the reduction of tumor-associated macrophage infiltration. The combination of AMD31 with sorafenib reduces angiogenesis and tumor progression (Gao *et al.*, 2015). Combination therapy of sorafenib and selumetinib to target CXCR4 overexpressed HCC cells has been found to prevent the

RAF/ERK pathway. PD-L1 expression increases the CD8+ T cells infiltration, followed by suppression of fibrosis of liver tissues (Chen *et al.*, 2014, Chen *et al.*, 2017). A combination of sorafenib and anti- PD-1 nivolumab for metastatic liver cancer treatment is under phase II clinical trial (Kelley RK, 2018). Co-delivery of PI3Kγ inhibitor TG100-115 and sorafenib in a nano micelle responsive to the HCC microenvironment has been found to enhance the antitumor effect in the HCC-induced mice model (Li and Zhao 2019). Photodynamic therapy is a newer approach in cancer therapies, which applies the redox mechanism, promotes oxidative stress to the cancer cells, and reduces tumor growth (Zhao *et al.*, 2018). As sorafenib also enhances reactive oxygen species generation, a combination of a phototherapeutic agent with sorafenib can act synergistically (Lin *et al.*, 2016). Chemo-thermal combination of IR780 iodide and sorafenib targeted glypican-3 (GPC3) overexpressed HCC cells and improved sorafenib's efficacy. Mu *et al.* has observed that near-infra-red light IR780 produces a cytotoxic heat and enhances sorafenib's affinity toward HCC cells (Mu *et al.*, 2019). Recently, US-FDA has approved another multiple kinase inhibitor, lenvatinib, as a first-line treatment for unresectable HCC. It is more efficacious than sorafenib (Kudo *et al.*, 2018). Lenvatinib can target vascular endothelial growth factor (VEGF) A and C, VEGF receptor 3, tyrosine-protein kinase, fibroblast growth factors (1-4), fibroblast gr-owth factors and reduce the angiogenesis of tumor cells (Yamamoto *et al.*, 2014). In the last few years, some more anticancer drugs have been approved clinically as potent anti-HCC molecules. Though the delivery of those drugs is in a very nascent development stage, future HCC therapy research will tend to those drug substances (Table **4**). In preparation for cancer-targeting drug delivery, clinical trials' failure generally comes from the lack of information on tumor progression's molecular mechanism. Further, the involvement of critical techniques, the requirement of advanced facilities in the laboratory, storage and shelf-life of the biological products, their stability, non-selective biodistribution, and undesirable toxicity are also critical for the successful development of a nano formulated drug delivery in cancer targeting.

Nanocrystals for HCC Targeted Drug Delivery

The nanocrystals, a beneficial tool for drug delivery, are 10-1000 nm sized particles of the drugs prepared with 100% drugs and no polymer or lipids (Muller *et al.*, 2011). This type of drug delivery provides better solubility, larger surface area followed by better bioavailability (Zhou *et al.*, 2016). Various studies are in progress regarding nanocrystal application in cancer therapy to increase the anticancer drug's bioavailability after oral administration (Jain *et al.*, 2016). The intravenous delivery of nanocrystals may also enhance the drug's permeability and retention time compared to the other delivery devices and improve the tumor-targeting as ligand-attachment is possible with this nanocarrier. Along with the therapeutic application, nanocrystal can be used for diagnostic purposes as a tool for bioimaging. Thus, this delivery vehicle can appear in tumor theranostics, *i.e.*, concurrent application of tumor recognition and evaluation and its therapy (Tan and Wu 2016, Li *et al.*, 2016). For example, paclitaxel and two bioimaging-specific fluorophores, near-infrared FPR-648 and bioactivatable MMPSense 750 FAST, have been delivered by a hybrid nanocrystal for the theranostic application in a murine xenograft model for breast cancer. The finding suggests that along with paclitaxel's anticancer activity, the hybrid nanocrystals release MMPSense molecules after getting activated by matrix metalloproteinase *in vivo* and help in monitoring cancer progression (Hollis *et al.*, 2014). Liquid crystalline nanoparticles (LCN) (prepared with an assembly of layer-by-layer (LbL) monoolein-based polymer) delivery system of sorafenib helped in the pH-responsive drug release in the HCC tumor microenvironment. They increased the bioavailability of the drug (Thapa *et al.*, 2015). So far, there are minimal applications of nanocrystals in HCC theranostics, and further exploration is needed. This method can be useful for monitoring and targeting tumor biomarkers.

Table 4. US-FDA approved drugs in last five years used in the treatment of HCC.

Drug	Approved On	Treatment Time	Mechanism of Action	Limitations	References
Sorafenib	Year of approval: 2007 Company name: Bayer AG, Leverkusen, Germany	1st line of treatment	Inhibit multiple kinases, platelet-derived growth factor -α, β; Vascular endothelial growth factor receptor -1-3, c-kit, Ras, C- Rapidly accelerated fibrosarcoma, B- Rapidly accelerated fibrosarcoma, extracellular-signal-regulated kinase, mitogen-activated protein kinase, *etc.* Ameliorate the abnormality of glycosylation in HCC cells.	Drug resistance Poor bioavailability	(Zhai and Sun, 2013)
Regorafenib	Year of approval: 2017 Company name: Bayer AG, Leverkusen, Germany	Second-line therapy for Sorafenib-refractory patients	inhibitor of STAT3 signaling. Induce src homology 2 domain -phosphatase 1 (SHP1). Inhibits V600-mutated BRAF and Tie2 like oncogenic factors.	Toxicities, complications like hypertension, proteinuria, gastrointestinal perforation, Thromboembolic events, hemorrhage, *etc.*	(Bruix *et al.*, 2017)

(Table 4) cont.....

Drug	Approved On	Treatment Time	Mechanism of Action	Limitations	References
Nivolumab	Year of approval: 2017 Company name: Bristol-Myers Squibb, NY, US	The second line of treatment	A human anti-programmed cell death protein 1 (PD1) helps in the prevention of immune tolerance. Inhibit the conjugation of PD1 with its ligands and promote a T-cell response in HCC cells	Serious side effects like fatigue, abdominal pain, rash, decreased appetite, cough	(El-Khoueiry *et al.*, 2017)
Lenvatinib	Year of approval: 2018 Company name: Eisai Inc, Tokyo, Japan	The first line of treatment	targets vascular endothelial growth factor (VEGF) A, C; VEGFR 3, tyrosine-protein kinase, fibroblast growth factors (1-4); fibroblast growth factors and stem cell factor (SCF) followed by a reduction in angiogenesis	Drug resistance	(Yamamoto *et al.*, 2014)
Cabozantinib	Year of approval: 2019 Company name: ExelixisInc California, USA	The second line of treatment	multikinase inhibitor superior over sorafenib in terms of the overall survival rate	Fatigue, diarrhea, palmar-plantar erythrodysesthesia	(Schoffski *et al.*, 2017)
Pembrolizumab	Year of approval: 2018 Company name: Merck &Co., Inc. New Jersey, US	The second line of treatment	recombinant humanized IgG4 monoclonal antibody against PD1	An adverse effect like fatigue, and an increase in the level of aspartate aminotransferase (AST) and alanine aminotransferase (ALT), hypothyroidism.	(Zhu *et al.*, 2018)

Implant Therapy

Interstitial radiotherapy with or without external beam radiotherapy has application in cancer research. Radioactive implantation of brachytherapy inside the tumor can deliver a high dose of radiation (Minniti *et al.*, 2012). The most commonly used isotopes are iridium-192 or iodine-125. Iodine seeds with a half-life of 60 days can be implanted temporarily or as a permanent implant. The knowledge about hepatocellular tumors' radiosensitivity has provided new insight into the development of HCC specific brachytherapy or implantation therapy. In this therapeutic process, a radioisotope of Iodine (^{125}I) is implanted inside HCC patients' tumors. Implantation of ^{125}I brachytherapy has shown almost 70% efficacy in inducing substantial tumor response, and the survival rate has enhanced up to 75% for 1 year, 46% for 2, and 27% for 3 years, respectively, for the patient of HCC who had failed transcatheter arterial chemoembolization (Lv *et al.*, 2009).

The Layer-by-Layer (LBL) Nanotechnology

The layer-by-layer (LBL) nanotechnology was first established by Moehwald, Lvov, and Decherin in the early 90s (Decher *et al.*, 1992, Decher *et al.*, 1997). The multilayered nanoparticles or films can be engineered using alternative adsorption of polyelectrolyte components to build up a self-assembled system (Lvov *et al.*, 1993). Several technological advancements of LBL nanoparticles have been introduced for drug delivery and tissue imaging, therapeutic and diagnostic requirements, respectively, after its invention. Multifunctional LBL assemblies showed promising results in targeted drug delivery, diagnosis, and theranostic potential for different cancer types. This technology has a versatile range of targeting categories such as the low pH, hypoxic region of the tumor microenvironment, and siRNA, miRNA, and DNA. Although several drugs are available for the treatment of HCC, their poor water solubility, off-target toxicity, and fast clearance make them difficult for clinical use (Günthert *et al.*, 1991). In the first step of the self-assembled system, a hydrophobic drug can be encapsulated at the polymer's nonpolar shell.

Furthermore, additional layering with polyelectrolyte materials forms an outer nanoshell for making it a stimuli-responsive system. USFDA approved polymers such as PLGA, protein molecules such as albumin, or some synthetic polymers to encapsulate the drug molecule, which generates a negative surface charge for the core nanoparticles. Thus, positively charged polymers, poly-L-lysine (PLL), or poly-arginine coating can form the first layer due to electrostatic attraction with the negatively charged core drug-loaded nanoparticle. The negatively charged hyaluronic acid is considered for the compatible second layering component on the PLL layer for most of the cases for its negative charge and its targeting efficiency to cancer tissue. There are several receptors overexpressed on cancer cells. They include folate receptors, integrins, EpCAM (Epithelial cell adhesion molecules) receptors, and so on (Okamoto *et al.*, 1999). One of such widely expressed receptors in many cancers, including liver cancer, is CD44, which plays a pivotal role in cancer migration, tumorigenicity in cancer stem cells, and spreading metastasis. The outermost layer of an LBL formulation coated with hyaluronic acid (HA) can target the CD44 receptor. The low pKa value of hyaluronic acid facilitates maintaining its secondary structure in blood pH and electrostatic adhesion on the positively charged PLL in the bloodstream. Once the formulation reaches the hypoxic region, *i.e.*, tumor microenvironment and the HA layer starts to be swollen in its neutral structure (Knudson *et al.*, 2002).

Eventually, a burst drug release can be possible at the hypoxic region. The multiple layering with polyelectrolytes inside nanoparticles can make a pH-responsive formulation for stimuli-responsive drug delivery. Thapa *et al.*, 2015 designed layer-by-layer nano assemble for a USFDA-approved drug, sorafenib, to treat HCC. They layered sorafenib with poly-L-lysine (PLL) and poly(ethylene glycol)- poly (aspartic acid) (PEG-b-PAsp). They observed a significant increase in cell death induction toward HepG2 cells than free drugs (Thapa *et al.*, 2015). Additionally, off-target cytotoxicity was found to reduce in the case of LBL particles. Multifunctional nanoengineered LBL formulation can maneuver multidirectional challenges in cancer treatment.

Quantum Dot

The treatment of HCC is one of the most challenging stages of liver cancer, with some viable options such as surgical resection or liver transplantation. However, it is tough to diagnose patients developing primary liver cancers. Thus, an early-stage liver cancer diagnosis is of utmost importance to prevent the deadly disease's progression. One type of the most promising imaging agent used for cancer tissue detection is Quantum dots (QDs). QDs are fluorescent semiconductors with unique photoluminescence properties, which enables them to be used as optical probes. Near-infrared, NRI (650–900 nm NIR-I and 1000–1450 nm NIR-II) QDs are considered the most efficient luminescence probe for bioimaging purposes, with the capability to penetrate in depth tissue regions with a nominal tissue absorbance (Michalet *et al.,* 2005).

Additionally, QDs can also be used for therapeutic purposes along with their diagnostic function. The dual advantage, diagnosis as well as therapeutic use are called the theranostic applications of QDs. Several types of coating with biocompatible polymers and surface modifications with antibodies, aptamers for targeting the desired organ of interest are extremely helpful to make QDs a multidimensional nanosystem (Li *et al.*, 2013, Park *et al.,* 2017). Al-Jamal *et al.* developed liposome-encapsulated NRI-QDs for liver cancer diagnosis. They found significant QD fluorescence signaling, *i.e*., accumulation of QDs in the mice tumor tissue (Al-Jamal *et al.,* 2009). Shao *et al.* also reported QDs coated with the liposomal carrier for liver cancer diagnosis of suicide gene therapy (Shao *et al.,* 2015). Olerile *et al.* demonstrated that NLC nanoengineered lipid carrier encapsulated QD sufficiently detected liver tumors (Olerile *et al.*, 2017). Das and Mohapatra reported QDs incorporated in the bioimaging system as a suitable targeted imaging tool for detecting liver cancer cells (Das and Mohapatra*et al.*, 2017). Thus, the outstanding optical features of QDs, including broad absorption spectrum, narrow light emission, high quantum yield, and resistance to photobleaching, introduce new opportunities in imaging and theranostic application of QD nanoformulations for the diagnostic and therapeutic management of HCC.

Personalized Treatment

Several molecular signaling pathways are involved in the progression of liver cirrhosis, followed by HCC. The most widely mutated signaling cascades include P53, Wnt/β-catenin, Akt/mTOR, endothelial growth factor receptor (EGFR)/RAS/MAPK, and vascular endothelial growth factor receptor (VEGFR) mediated signaling cascade. A comprehensive genomic description of HCC tumor tissue and normal tissue by exosome sequencing can determine the lethal mutation inherited or acquired by the patient. The particular mutational change in the genome alters the regulation of a signaling pathway. Based on the mutational status, personalized treatment options can be considered for the early detected HCC patients. Moreover, the potential therapeutic strategies such as liver resection, radiofrequency or microwave ablation, liver transplantation, and chemotherapeutic doses depend on overall liver functioning, extra-hepatic disease, and other co-morbidity condition of a patient. Thus, personalized treatment may be a future goal for effective therapeutic management of HCC patients.

Future Nanotherapeutics Services to Combat HCC

When we talk about future directions in nanotechnology driven future drug delivery devices to combat HCC, we should remember that this is an upcoming field of medicine where the diagnosis of the disease as well as targeted drug delivery and release of drug will be monitored externally with the help of computer according to the patient's requirement. Nanotherapeutics are going to lead us to a world of personalized medicine and an individualistic approach to treating a specific disease. Here, we will discuss three significant divisions of recent nanotherapeutics for the detection and treatment of HCC.

Nanotheranostics

The application of nano theranostics involves the simultaneous treatment and diagnosis (*via* imaging) of the disease in an individual patient (Tutar 2020). In cancer treatment, conventional chemotherapies affect both the cancer tissue as well as normal tissues, which lead to moderate to severe adverse drug reactions in patients. Treatment of HCC involves surgical and non-surgical approaches, but in both cases, normal hepatic architecture gets affected and worsens the patient's quality of life (Bhattacharya *et al., 2018*). The use of nanotheranostics, where an imaging technique is paired with nanosize drug delivery systems, may help reach the particular tumor site. Real-time monitoring and visualization of the tumor site may be achieved to understand the tumor growth and treatment effect in that individual.

The successful conversions of light and sound into heat *via* nano-radiation (photothermal therapy and photoacoustic imaging) are the two most promising applications of nano theranostics in the field of cancer-related research (Liu *et al.*, 2019). Another study revealed that poly-amidoamine dendrimers (generation-5) (PAMAM-G5) are used as a delivery system of a particular adenovirus that is replication-deficient (5/hNIS). These dendrimers ensured targeted delivery of the adenovirus in the HCC xenograft mouse model. They showed a significant reduction in transgenes' expression in the cancer site, which is monitored *via* the I^{-123} scintigraphy technique (Muthu *et al.*, 2014). Not only in primary liver cancer (HCC) but also in cancer metastasis (development of secondary malignant growth in other organs) and in the case of multidrug resistance (MDR), nano theranostics may play a crucial role by improving the prognosis as well as detecting the tumor growth with the help of the diagnostic mechanism involved. Thus, therapy and simultaneously monitoring the modulation of the progress of cancers, including HCC, could soon make a tremendous change in cancer therapy.

Nanosized 3D Printing/Bio-Printing

In today's world, 3D bio-printing is another emerging area of drug delivery technology whereby using layer-by-layer techniques, functional three-dimensional biomaterials (such as living cells, biochemicals, nanomedicines, *etc.*) are grafted in the desired tissue/organ to improve the biological stability of the tissue. One of the most promising advantages of 3D bioprinting is to replace damaged tissue with functional tissues in a living host. The liver is a highly vascularized organ. In acute liver failure or end-stage liver diseases (such as HCC), liver resection and liver transplantation, as already mentioned, are the only choice of treatments left but may lead to donor rejection or reduced quality of life. Thus, hepatic tissue engineering and artificial liver transplantation may serve as better surgical methods for patients with terminal liver diseases (Kryou *et al.*, 2019, Murphy *et al.*, 2014, Munaz *et al.*, 2016, Derakhshanfar *et al.*, 2018). Besides, 3D bio-imaging plays a vital role in cancer detection. Using this technology, minor tumors may also be detectable in hepatic tissue, which are not visible by conventional methods (Wang *et al.*,2018). Moreover, research findings suggest that 3D bio-printing may play a role in detoxification systems inside the liver *via* a nanocomposite (hydrogel) based biomimetic device, which serves as an innovative medical device useful in detecting and treating liver diseases. Another study revealed that in hepatoblastoma cells and human HCC cells (Hep-G2), a 3D printed biosensor electrochemically detects tumor biomarker CD133 with specific recombinant protein (Gou *et al.*, 2014, Damiati *et al.*, 2017, Oldani *et al.*, 2016).

In clinical practice, during a complicated surgery, the 2D imaging of the liver is generally done by ultrasonography (USG)/Computed Tomography Angiography (CTA)/Magnetic Resonance Imaging (MRI), which gives an indirect viewing of the organ. On the other hand, 3D bio-printing ensures a three-dimensional view of the tissue and elaborates the exact location of hepatic vasculature in a real-time manner, and gives an accurate diagnosis of the disease HCC (Xiang *et al.*, 2015). The paradigm shift from 2D to 3D imaging also involves the use of nanotechnology in various drug delivery systems targeted to specific hepatocellular carcinoma cells without affecting the normal hepatocytes. In the surgical treatment of HCC, 3D bioprinting is used extensively for a better understanding of the disease and to lower the surgical risks. They may also be paired with nano-architecture-based drug delivery systems, which ensure the medicine's availability in the cancer tissue for the desired time frame.

Nanorobots for Diagnosis and Therapy of HCC

Nanorobots (also known as nanobots) are hypothetical nano-sized medical devices prepared so that they can navigate through the bloodstream and attach to specific tumor sites using bio-sensing technologies (Mukherjee *et al.*, 2020). After attachment to the cancer cells, they can be monitored externally by a computer and used to detect and treat cancer. The tiny size (0.1 to 10 μm) of nanorobots often makes them suitable for bypassing the body's natural immune system and ensures target-specific drug delivery. With the help of computer-based technologies, nanorobots may also replicate themselves if required (Venkatesan *et al.*, 2010, Tripathi *et al.*, 2018). Theoretically, the nanorobots' navigation should be smooth through the vascular system (bloodstream and lymphatic system) and should possess minimal destructive effects on normal cells. Nanorobots may also have tentacles, which only get activated by detecting cancer cells and are able to capture them precisely. Different types of nano-architectures such as nano-cantilevers, nanopores, nanotubes, quantum dots, liposomes, dendrimers, nanoparticles, nanoshells, and micelles, *etc.*, may be useful in designing nanorobots for diagnosis and drug delivery related to the cancer tissue (Venkatesan *et al.*,2018).

Projected Utilization Area of Nanotherapeutics in HCC in Near Future

Various newer nanotherapeutics are currently under extensive investigation, that ensures target-specific delivery of the medicines and helps ease cancer and external monitoring of the cancer sites. Exploiting particular proteins that are over-expressed in HCC, these medical devices locate the proliferating cells, identify them, reach them and treat them with specific technologies. These methods also open a new window of individual drug delivery strategies for patients with distinct abnormalities in particular genes. The shift of paradigm from conventional therapies toward digital nanotherapeutics is already in progress. In the recent future, a person suffering from a life-threatening disease such as HCC may receive a definite diagnosis and treatment according to the genetic configuration of that person.

CONCLUSION

Nanotherapy is continuously upgrading to a new level of advancement in every aspect of HCC. The engineered nanoscale systems, upon functionalizing with various ligands (small molecules, peptides, antibody, aptamer, DNA, *etc.*), increase the chances of targeted tumor therapy and reduce the toxicities of anticancer drugs and their related side effects to the cancer patients. Moreover, co-delivery of diagnostic biomolecules and the therapeutic application may help develop the theranostic approaches for HCC. However, there are certain limitations of nanosystems yet to be overcome to apply nanotherapy in HCC clinically. They include (i) the preparation and characterization of nanoformulations that need a sophisticated facility and critical techniques, which often make it difficult for the production of them on a large scale, (ii) the nonspecific biodistribution and toxic by-products of delivery vehicles may produce undesirable side effects, although these side effects are relatively less compared to the conventional cancer therapy and thus the efficacy for their tissue-specific delivery has to be enhanced for a better outcome, and (iii) systematic investigations of preclinical and clinical trials are essential to achieve a reproducible and effective therapy. Apart from the treatment, the application of nanotechnology is considerably associated with detection, more particularly imaging of the HCC tumor cells. Lastly, transferring the nanotechnological research to clinical practice also involves ethical and social perceptions. We expect that human society will be benefited from this application of nanotherapy in various types of cancers, including HCC.

CONSENT FOR PUBLICATION

Not applicable.

CONFLICT OF INTEREST

The authors declare no conflict of interest, financial or otherwise.

ACKNOWLEDGEMENTS

Declared none.

REFERENCES

Adiseshaiah, PP, Clogston, JD, McLeland, CB, Rodriguez, J, Potter, TM, Neun, BW, Skoczen, SL, Shanmugavelandy, SS, Kester, M, Stern, ST & McNeil, SE (2013) Synergistic combination therapy with nanoliposomal C6-ceramide and vinblastine is associated with autophagy dysfunction in hepatocarcinoma and colorectal cancer models. *Cancer Lett,* 337, 254-65. [http://dx.doi.org/10.1016/j.canlet.2013.04.034] [PMID: 23664889]

Advanced healthcare materials. *Wiley online library.*https://onlinelibrary.wiley.com/doi/toc/10.1002/(ISSN)2192-2659.Nanotherapeutics

Agarwal, A, Saraf, S, Asthana, A, Gupta, U, Gajbhiye, V & Jain, NK (2008) Ligand based dendritic systems for tumor targeting. *Int J Pharm,* 350, 3-13. [http://dx.doi.org/10.1016/j.ijpharm.2007.09.024] [PMID: 18162345]

Agrawal, M, Ajazuddin, Tripathi, DK, Saraf, S, Saraf, S, Antimisiaris, SG, Mourtas, S, Hammarlund-Udenaes, M & Alexander, A (2017) Recent advancements in liposomes targeting strategies to cross blood-brain barrier (BBB) for the treatment of Alzheimer's disease. *Journal of controlled release : official journal of the Controlled Release Society,* 260, 61-77. [http://dx.doi.org/10.1016/j.jconrel.2017.05.019]

Al-Jamal, WT, Al-Jamal, KT, Cakebread, A, Halket, JM & Kostarelos, K (2009) Blood circulation and tissue biodistribution of lipid--quantum dot (L-QD) hybrid vesicles intravenously administered in mice. *Bioconjug Chem,* 20, 1696-702. [http://dx.doi.org/10.1021/bc900047n] [PMID: 19655725]

Alnajjar, AM & Elsiesy, HA (2015) Natural products and hepatocellular carcinoma: a review. *Hepatoma Res,* 1, 119-24. [http://dx.doi.org/10.4103/2394-5079.167379]

Amjadi, S (2019) Enhancement of therapeutic efficacy of betanin for diabetes treatment by liposomal nanocarriers. *J Funct Foods,* 59, 119-28. [http://dx.doi.org/10.1016/j.jff.2019.05.015]

Atacan, K & Özacar, M (2015) Characterization and immobilization of trypsin on tannic acid modified Fe3O4 nanoparticles. *Colloids Surf B Biointerfaces,* 128, 227-36. [http://dx.doi.org/10.1016/j.colsurfb.2015.01.038] [PMID: 25686792]

Baetke, SC, Lammers, T & Kiessling, F (2015) Applications of nanoparticles for diagnosis and therapy of cancer. *Br J Radiol,* 88, 20150207. [http://dx.doi.org/10.1259/bjr.20150207] [PMID: 25969868]

Baig, B, Halim, SA, Farrukh, A, Greish, Y & Amin, A (2019) Current status of nanomaterial-based treatment for hepatocellular carcinoma. *Biomedicine & pharmacotherapy Biomedecine & pharmacotherapie,* 116, 108852. [http://dx.doi.org/10.1016/j.biopha.2019.108852]

Bhattacharya, S, Mondal, L, Mukherjee, B, Dutta, L, Ehsan, I, Debnath, MC, Gaonkar, RH, Pal, MM & Majumdar, S (2018) Apigenin loaded nanoparticle delayed development of hepatocellular carcinoma in rats. *Nanomedicine,* 14, 1905-17. [http://dx.doi.org/10.1016/j.nano.2018.05.011] [PMID: 29802937]

Brigger, I, Dubernet, C & Couvreur, P (2002) Nanoparticles in cancer therapy and diagnosis. *Adv Drug Deliv Rev,* 54, 631-51. [http://dx.doi.org/10.1016/S0169-409X(02)00044-3] [PMID: 12204596]

Bruix, J, Takayama, T, Mazzaferro, V, Chau, GY, Yang, J, Kudo, M, Cai, J, Poon, RT, Han, KH, Tak, WY, Lee, HC, Song, T, Roayaie, S, Bolondi, L, Lee, KS, Makuuchi, M, Souza, F, Berre, MA, Meinhardt, G & Llovet, JM (2015) Adjuvant sorafenib for hepatocellular carcinoma after resection or ablation (STORM): a phase 3, randomised, double-blind, placebo-controlled trial. *Lancet Oncol,* 16, 1344-54. [http://dx.doi.org/10.1016/S1470-2045(15)00198-9] [PMID: 26361969]

Calderaro, J, Couchy, G, Imbeaud, S, Amaddeo, G, Letouzé, E, Blanc, JF, Laurent, C, Hajji, Y, Azoulay, D, Bioulac-Sage, P, Nault, JC & Zucman-Rossi, J (2017) Histological subtypes of hepatocellular carcinoma are related to gene mutations and molecular tumour classification. *J Hepatol,* 67, 727-38. [http://dx.doi.org/10.1016/j.jhep.2017.05.014] [PMID: 28532995]

Chakraborty, S, Dlie, ZY, Chakraborty, S, Roy, S, Mukherjee, B, Besra, SE, Dewanjee, S, Mukherjee, A, Ojha, PK, Kumar, V & Sen, R (2020) Aptamer-functionalized drug nanocarrier improves hepatocellular carcinoma toward normal by targeting neoplastic hepatocytes. *Mol Ther Nucleic Acids,* 20, 34-49. [http://dx.doi.org/10.1016/j.omtn.2020.01.034] [PMID: 32146417]

Chakraborty, S, Ehsan, I, Mukherjee, B, Mondal, L, Roy, S, Saha, KD, Paul, B, Debnath, MC & Bera, T (2019) Therapeutic potential of andrographolide-loaded nanoparticles on a murine asthma model. *Nanomedicine,* 20, 102006. [http://dx.doi.org/10.1016/j.nano.2019.04.009] [PMID: 31059793]

Chang, JE, Yoon, IS, Sun, PL, Yi, E, Jheon, S & Shim, CK (2014) Anticancer efficacy of photodynamic therapy with hematoporphyrin-modified, doxorubicin-loaded nanoparticles in liver cancer. *J Photochem Photobiol B,* 140, 49-56. [http://dx.doi.org/10.1016/j.jphotobiol.2014.07.005] [PMID: 25090224]

Chen, Y, Liu, W, Shang, Y, Cao, P, Cui, J, Li, Z, Yin, X & Li, Y (2018) Folic acid-nanoscale gadolinium-porphyrin metal-organic frameworks: fluorescence and magnetic resonance dual-modality imaging and photodynamic therapy in hepatocellular carcinoma. *Int J Nanomedicine,* 14, 57-74. [http://dx.doi.org/10.2147/IJN.S177880] [PMID: 30587985]

Chen, Y, Liu, YC, Sung, YC, Ramjiawan, RR, Lin, TT, Chang, CC, Jeng, KS, Chang, CF, Liu, CH, Gao, DY, Hsu, FF, Duyverman, AM, Kitahara, S, Huang, P, Dima, S, Popescu, I, Flaherty, KT, Zhu, AX, Bardeesy, N, Jain, RK, Benes, CH & Duda, DG (2017) Overcoming sorafenib evasion in hepatocellular carcinoma using CXCR4-targeted nanoparticles to co-deliver MEK-inhibitors. *Sci Rep,* 7, 44123. [http://dx.doi.org/10.1038/srep44123] [PMID: 28276530]

Clark, MA, Jepson, MA & Hirst, BH (2001) Exploiting M cells for drug and vaccine delivery. *Adv Drug Deliv Rev,* 50, 81-106. [http://dx.doi.org/10.1016/S0169-409X(01)00149-1] [PMID: 11489335]

Conti, E, Gregori, M, Radice, I, Da Re, F, Grana, D, Re, F, Salvati, E, Masserini, M, Ferrarese, C, Zoia, CP & Tremolizzo, L (2017) Multifunctional liposomes interact with Abeta in human biological fluids: Therapeutic implications for Alzheimer's disease. *Neurochem Int,* 108, 60-5. [http://dx.doi.org/10.1016/j.neuint.2017.02.012] [PMID: 28238790]

Daher, S, Massarwa, M, Benson, AA & Khoury, T (2018) Current and future treatment of hepatocellular carcinoma: an updated comprehensive review. *J Clin Transl Hepatol,* 6, 69-78. [http://dx.doi.org/10.14218/JCTH.2017.00031] [PMID: 29607307]

Damiati, S, Küpcü, S, Peacock, M, Eilenberger, C, Zamzami, M, Qadri, I, Choudhry, H, Sleytr, UB & Schuster, B (2017) Acoustic and hybrid 3D-printed electrochemical biosensors for the real-time immunodetection of liver cancer cells (HepG2). *Biosens Bioelectron,* 94, 500-6. [http://dx.doi.org/10.1016/j.bios.2017.03.045] [PMID: 28343102]

Das, RK & Mohapatra, S (2017) Highly luminescent, heteroatom-doped carbon quantum dots for ultrasensitive sensing of glucosamine and targeted imaging of liver cancer cells. *J Mater Chem B Mater Biol Med,* 5, 2190-7. [http://dx.doi.org/10.1039/C6TB03141B] [PMID: 32263692]

Decher, G (1997) Fuzzy nanoassemblies: toward layered polymeric multicomposites. *Science,* 277, 1232-7. [http://dx.doi.org/10.1126/science.277.5330.1232]

Decher, G, Hong, JD & Schmitt, J (1992) Buildup of ultrathin multilayer films by a self-assembly process: III. Consecutively alternating adsorption of anionic and cationic polyelectrolytes on charged surfaces. *Thin Solid Films,* 210 211, 831-5.

[http://dx.doi.org/10.1016/0040-6090(92)90417-A]

Derakhshanfar, S, Mbeleck, R, Xu, K, Zhang, X, Zhong, W & Xing, M (2018) 3D bioprinting for biomedical devices and tissue engineering: A review of recent trends and advances. *Bioact Mater,* 3, 144-56. [http://dx.doi.org/10.1016/j.bioactmat.2017.11.008] [PMID: 29744452]

Dutta, L, Mukherjee, B, Chakraborty, T, Das, MK, Mondal, L, Bhattacharya, S, Gaonkar, RH & Debnath, MC (2018) Lipid-based nanocarrier efficiently delivers highly water soluble drug across the blood-brain barrier into brain. *Drug Deliv,* 25, 504-16. [http://dx.doi.org/10.1080/10717544.2018.1435749] [PMID: 29426257]

El-Khoueiry, AB, Sangro, B, Yau, T, Crocenzi, TS, Kudo, M, Hsu, C, Kim, TY, Choo, SP, Trojan, J, Welling, TH, Meyer, T, Kang, YK, Yeo, W, Chopra, A, Anderson, J, Dela Cruz, C, Lang, L, Neely, J, Tang, H, Dastani, HB & Melero, I (2017) Nivolumab in patients with advanced hepatocellular carcinoma (CheckMate 040): an open-label, non-comparative, phase 1/2 dose escalation and expansion trial. *Lancet,* 389, 2492-502. [http://dx.doi.org/10.1016/S0140-6736(17)31046-2] [PMID: 28434648]

Elsabahy, M & Wooley, KL (2012) Design of polymeric nanoparticles for biomedical delivery applications. *Chem Soc Rev,* 41, 2545-61. [http://dx.doi.org/10.1039/c2cs15327k] [PMID: 22334259]

El-Sayed, A & Kamel, M (2020) Advances in nanomedical applications: diagnostic, therapeutic, immunization, and vaccine production. *Environ Sci Pollut Res Int,* 27, 19200-13. [http://dx.doi.org/10.1007/s11356-019-06459-2] [PMID: 31529348]

Ferrari, M (2005) Cancer nanotechnology: opportunities and challenges. *Nat Rev Cancer,* 5, 161-71. [http://dx.doi.org/10.1038/nrc1566] [PMID: 15738981]

Fornaguera, C & García-Celma, MJ (2017) Personalized nanomedicine: a revolution at the nanoscale. *J Pers Med,* 7, 12. [http://dx.doi.org/10.3390/jpm7040012] [PMID: 29023366]

Gao, DY, Lin, TsT, Sung, YC, Liu, YC, Chiang, WH, Chang, CC, Liu, JY & Chen, Y (2015) CXCR4-targeted lipid-coated PLGA nanoparticles deliver sorafenib and overcome acquired drug resistance in liver cancer. *Biomaterials,* 67, 194-203. [http://dx.doi.org/10.1016/j.biomaterials.2015.07.035] [PMID: 26218745]

Gao, L, Zhang, D & Chen, M (2008) Drug nanocrystals for the formulation of poorly soluble drugs and its application as a potential drug delivery system. *J Nanopart Res,* 10, 845-62. [http://dx.doi.org/10.1007/s11051-008-9357-4]

Garcia-Garcia, E, Andrieux, K, Gil, S & Couvreur, P (2005) Colloidal carriers and blood-brain barrier (BBB) translocation: a way to deliver drugs to the brain? *Int J Pharm,* 298, 274-92. [http://dx.doi.org/10.1016/j.ijpharm.2005.03.031] [PMID: 15896933]

Gharpure, KM, Wu, SY, Li, C, Lopez-Berestein, G & Sood, AK (2015) Nanotechnology: future of oncotherapy. *Clin Cancer Res,* 21, 3121-30. [http://dx.doi.org/10.1158/1078-0432.CCR-14-1189] [PMID: 26180057]

Ghosh, D, Choudhury, ST, Ghosh, S, Mandal, AK, Sarkar, S, Ghosh, A, Saha, KD & Das, N (2012) Nanocapsulated curcumin: oral chemopreventive formulation against diethylnitrosamine induced hepatocellular carcinoma in rat. *Chem Biol Interact,* 195, 206-14. [http://dx.doi.org/10.1016/j.cbi.2011.12.004] [PMID: 22197969]

Glassman, DC, Palmaira, RL, Covington, CM, Desai, AM, Ku, GY, Li, J, Harding, JJ, Varghese, AM, O'Reilly, EM & Yu, KH (2018) Nanoliposomal irinotecan with fluorouracil for the treatment of advanced pancreatic cancer, a single institution experience. *BMC Cancer,* 18, 693. [http://dx.doi.org/10.1186/s12885-018-4605-1] [PMID: 29945562]

Gomes, MA, Priolli, DG, Tralhão, JG & Botelho, MF (2013) Hepatocellular carcinoma: epidemiology, biology, diagnosis, and therapies. *Revista da Associacao Medica Brasileira (1992),* 59, 514-24. [http://dx.doi.org/10.1016/j.ramb.2013.03.005]

Gou, M, Qu, X, Zhu, W, Xiang, M, Yang, J, Zhang, K, Wei, Y & Chen, S (2014) Bio-inspired detoxification using 3D-printed hydrogel nanocomposites. *Nat Commun,* 5, 3774. [http://dx.doi.org/10.1038/ncomms4774] [PMID: 24805923]

Günthert, U, Hofmann, M, Rudy, W, Reber, S, Zöller, M, Haussmann, I, Matzku, S, Wenzel, A, Ponta, H & Herrlich, P (1991) A new variant of glycoprotein CD44 confers metastatic potential to rat carcinoma cells. *Cell,* 65, 13-24. [http://dx.doi.org/10.1016/0092-8674(91)90403-L] [PMID: 1707342]

Gupta, A, Eral, HB, Hatton, TA & Doyle, PS (2016) Nanoemulsions: formation, properties and applications. *Soft Matter,* 12, 2826-41. [http://dx.doi.org/10.1039/C5SM02958A] [PMID: 26924445]

Hafner, A, Lovrić, J, Lakoš, GP & Pepić, I (2014) Nanotherapeutics in the EU: an overview on current state and future directions. *Int J Nanomedicine,* 9, 1005-23. [http://dx.doi.org/10.2147/IJN.S55359] [PMID: 24600222]

Hiemenz, JW & Walsh, TJ (1996) Lipid formulations of amphotericin B: recent progress and future directions. *Clin Infect Dis,* 22 (Suppl. 2), S133-44. [http://dx.doi.org/10.1093/clinids/22.Supplement_2.S133] [PMID: 8722841]

Hollis, CP, Weiss, HL, Evers, BM, Gemeinhart, RA & Li, T (2014) *In vivo* investigation of hybrid Paclitaxel nanocrystals with dual fluorescent probes for cancer theranostics. *Pharm Res,* 31, 1450-9. [http://dx.doi.org/10.1007/s11095-013-1048-x] [PMID: 23619595]

Hong, H, Zhang, Y, Sun, J & Cai, W (2009) Molecular imaging and therapy of cancer with radiolabeled nanoparticles. *Nano Today,* 4, 399-413. [http://dx.doi.org/10.1016/j.nantod.2009.07.001] [PMID: 20161038]

Huang, X, Wan, F, Ma, L, Phan, JB, Lim, RX, Li, C, Chen, J, Deng, J, Li, Y, Chen, W & He, M (2019) Investigation of copper-cysteamine nanoparticles as a new photosensitizer for anti-hepatocellular carcinoma. *Cancer Biol Ther,* 20, 812-25. [http://dx.doi.org/10.1080/15384047.2018.1564568] [PMID: 30727796]

Iyer, AK, He, J & Amiji, MM (2012) Image-guided nanosystems for targeted delivery in cancer therapy. *Curr Med Chem,* 19, 3230-40. [http://dx.doi.org/10.2174/092986712800784685] [PMID: 22612697]

Jain, S, Reddy, VA, Arora, S & Patel, K (2016) Development of surface stabilized candesartan cilexetil nanocrystals with enhanced dissolution rate, permeation rate across CaCo-2, and oral bioavailability. *Drug Deliv Transl Res,* 6, 498-510. [http://dx.doi.org/10.1007/s13346-016-0297-8] [PMID: 27129488]

Kelley, RK (2018) Sorafenib and nivolumab in treating participants with unresectable, locally advanced or metastatic liver cancer. *NCT03439891.*https://clinicaltrials.gov/ct2/show/NCT03439891

Knudson, W, Chow, G & Knudson, C B (2002) CD44-mediated uptake and degradation of hyaluronan. *Matrix biology: journal of the International Society for Matrix Biology,* 21, 15-23. [http://dx.doi.org/10.1016/S0945-053X(01)00186-X]

Kryou, C, Leva, V, Chatzipetrou, M & Zergioti, I (2019) Bioprinting for liver transplantation. *Bioengineering (Basel),* 6, 95. [http://dx.doi.org/10.3390/bioengineering6040095] [PMID: 31658719]

Kudo, M, Finn, RS, Qin, S, Han, KH, Ikeda, K, Piscaglia, F, Baron, A, Park, JW, Han, G, Jassem, J, Blanc, JF, Vogel, A, Komov, D, Evans, TRJ, Lopez, C, Dutcus, C, Guo, M, Saito, K, Kraljevic, S, Tamai, T, Ren, M & Cheng, AL (2018) Lenvatinib *versus* sorafenib in first-line treatment of patients with unresectable hepatocellular carcinoma: a randomised phase 3 non-inferiority trial. *Lancet,* 391, 1163-73.
[http://dx.doi.org/10.1016/S0140-6736(18)30207-1] [PMID: 29433850]

Langer, R (2009) A conversation with Robert Langer: pioneering biomedical scientist and engineer. Interview by Paul S. Weiss. *ACS Nano,* 3, 756-61.
[http://dx.doi.org/10.1021/nn900350p] [PMID: 19397341]

Lei, M, Ma, G, Sha, S, Wang, X, Feng, H, Zhu, Y & Du, X (2019) Dual-functionalized liposome by co-delivery of paclitaxel with sorafenib for synergistic antitumor efficacy and reversion of multidrug resistance. *Drug Deliv,* 26, 262-72.
[http://dx.doi.org/10.1080/10717544.2019.1580797] [PMID: 30856352]

Lencioni, R, Llovet, JM, Han, G, Tak, WY, Yang, J, Guglielmi, A, Paik, SW, Reig, M, Kim, DY, Chau, GY, Luca, A, Del Arbol, LR, Leberre, MA, Niu, W, Nicholson, K, Meinhardt, G & Bruix, J (2016) Sorafenib or placebo plus TACE with doxorubicin-eluting beads for intermediate stage HCC: The SPACE trial. *J Hepatol,* 64, 1090-8.
[http://dx.doi.org/10.1016/j.jhep.2016.01.012] [PMID: 26809111]

Li, G & Zhao, L (2019) Sorafenib-loaded hydroxyethyl starch-TG100-115 micelles for the treatment of liver cancer based on synergistic treatment. *Drug Deliv,* 26, 756-64.
[http://dx.doi.org/10.1080/10717544.2019.1642418] [PMID: 31357893]

Li, J & Zhu, JJ (2013) Quantum dots for fluorescent biosensing and bio-imaging applications. *Analyst (Lond),* 138, 2506-15.
[http://dx.doi.org/10.1039/c3an36705c] [PMID: 23518695]

Li, SY, Cheng, H, Xie, BR, Qiu, WX, Song, LL, Zhuo, RX & Zhang, XZ (2016) A ratiometric theranostic probe for tumor targeting therapy and self-therapeutic monitoring. *Biomaterials,* 104, 297-309.
[http://dx.doi.org/10.1016/j.biomaterials.2016.07.024] [PMID: 27475726]

Lin, T, Gao, D Y, Liu, Y C, Sung, Y C, Wan, D, Liu, J Y, Chiang, T, Wang, L & Chen, Y (2016) Development and characterization of sorafenib-loaded PLGA nanoparticles for the systemic treatment of liver fibrosis. *Journal of controlled release: official journal of the Controlled Release Society,* 221, 62-70.
[http://dx.doi.org/10.1016/j.jconrel.2015.11.003]

Liu, C, Kou, Y, Zhang, X, Dong, W, Cheng, H & Mao, S (2019) Enhanced oral insulin delivery *via* surface hydrophilic modification of chitosan copolymer based self-assembly polyelectrolyte nanocomplex. *Int J Pharm,* 554, 36-47.
[http://dx.doi.org/10.1016/j.ijpharm.2018.10.068] [PMID: 30385377]

Liu, F, Li, M, Liu, C, Liu, Y & Zhang, N (2014) PH-sensitive self-assembled carboxymethyl chitosan-modified DNA/polyethylenimine complexes for efficient gene delivery. *J Biomed Nanotechnol,* 10, 3397-406.
[http://dx.doi.org/10.1166/jbn.2014.1901] [PMID: 26000398]

Liu, T, Liu, W, Zhang, M, Yu, W, Gao, F, Li, C, Wang, SB, Feng, J & Zhang, XZ (2018) Ferrous-supply-regeneration nanoengineering for cancer-cell-specific ferroptosis in combination with imaging-guided photodynamic therapy. *ACS Nano,* 12, 12181-92.
[http://dx.doi.org/10.1021/acsnano.8b05860] [PMID: 30458111]

Liu, Y, Bhattarai, P, Dai, Z & Chen, X (2019) Photothermal therapy and photoacoustic imaging *via* nanotheranostics in fighting cancer. *Chem Soc Rev,* 48, 2053-108.
[http://dx.doi.org/10.1039/C8CS00618K] [PMID: 30259015]

Liu, ZT, Xiong, L, Liu, ZP, Miao, XY, Lin, LW & Wen, Y (2014) *In vivo* and *in vitro* evaluation of the cytotoxic effects of Photosan-loaded hollow silica nanoparticles on liver cancer. *Nanoscale Res Lett,* 9, 319.
[http://dx.doi.org/10.1186/1556-276X-9-319] [PMID: 25024681]

Lopes, M, Shrestha, N, Correia, A, Shahbazi, MA, Sarmento, B, Hirvonen, J, Veiga, F, Seiça, R, Ribeiro, A

& Santos, H A (2016) Dual chitosan/albumin-coated alginate/dextran sulfate nanoparticles for enhanced oral delivery of insulin. *Journal of controlled release : official journal of the Controlled Release Society,* 323, 29-41.
[http://dx.doi.org/10.1016/j.jconrel.2016.04.012]

Lovelyn, C & Attama, AA (2011) Current state of nanoemulsions in drug delivery. *J Biomater Nanobiotechnol,* 2, 626-39.
[http://dx.doi.org/10.4236/jbnb.2011.225075]

Lu, LC, Lee, YH, Chang, CJ, Shun, CT, Fang, CY, Shao, YY, Liu, TH, Cheng, AL & Hsu, CH (2019) Increased expression of programmed death-ligand 1 in infiltrating immune cells in hepatocellular carcinoma tissues after sorafenib treatment. *Liver Cancer,* 8, 110-20.
[http://dx.doi.org/10.1159/000489021] [PMID: 31019901]

Luo, Z, Deng, Y, Zhang, R, Wang, M, Bai, Y, Zhao, Q, Lyu, Y, Wei, J & Wei, S (2015) Peptide-laden mesoporous silica nanoparticles with promoted bioactivity and osteo-differentiation ability for bone tissue engineering. *Colloids Surf B Biointerfaces,* 131, 73-82.
[http://dx.doi.org/10.1016/j.colsurfb.2015.04.043] [PMID: 25969416]

Lv, J, Cao, XF & Zhu, B (2009) ^{125}I Radioactive Seeds Implantation Therapy for Hepatocellular Carcinoma. *Gastroenterol Res,* 2, 141-7.
[http://dx.doi.org/10.4021/gr2009.05.1289] [PMID: 27933123]

Lvov, Y, Decher, G & Moehwald, H (1993) Assembly, structural characterization and thermal behavior of layer-by-layer deposited ultrathin films of poly- (vinylsulfate) and poly (allylamine. *Langmuir,* 9, 481-6.
[http://dx.doi.org/10.1021/la00026a020]

Mahan, MM & Doiron, AL (2018) Gold nanoparticles as X-Ray, CT, and multimodal imaging contrast agents: formulation, targeting, and methodology. *J Nanomater,* 2018, 1-15.
[http://dx.doi.org/10.1155/2018/5837276]

Malarvizhi, GL, Retnakumari, AP, Nair, S & Koyakutty, M (2014) Transferrin targeted core-shell nanomedicine for combinatorial delivery of doxorubicin and sorafenib against hepatocellular carcinoma. *Nanomedicine,* 10, 1649-59.
[http://dx.doi.org/10.1016/j.nano.2014.05.011] [PMID: 24905399]

Malla, RR, Kumari, S, Kgk, D, Momin, S & Nagaraju, GP (2020) Nanotheranostics: their role in hepatocellular carcinoma. *Crit Rev Oncol Hematol,* 151, 102968.
[http://dx.doi.org/10.1016/j.critrevonc.2020.102968] [PMID: 32416345]

Michalet, X, Pinaud, FF, Bentolila, LA, Tsay, JM, Doose, S, Li, JJ, Sundaresan, G, Wu, AM, Gambhir, SS & Weiss, S (2005) Quantum dots for live cells, *in vivo* imaging, and diagnostics. *Science,* 307, 538-44.
[http://dx.doi.org/10.1126/science.1104274] [PMID: 15681376]

Minniti, G, Goldsmith, C, Brada, M & Dick F., Swaab (2012) Radiotherapy In: Michael J., Aminoff, François, Boller, Dick F., Swaab, (Eds.), *Handbook of Clinical Neurology* Elsevier 215-28.

Mizrahy, S & Peer, D (2012) Polysaccharides as building blocks for nanotherapeutics. *Chem Soc Rev,* 41, 2623-40.
[http://dx.doi.org/10.1039/C1CS15239D] [PMID: 22085917]

Mohamed, NK, Hamad, MA, Hafez, MZ, Wooley, KL & Elsabahy, M (2017) Nanomedicine in management of hepatocellular carcinoma: Challenges and opportunities. *Int J Cancer,* 140, 1475-84.
[http://dx.doi.org/10.1002/ijc.30517] [PMID: 27861850]

Mohanraj, VJ & Chen, Y (2006) Nanoparticles - A review. *Trop J Pharm Res,* 5, 561-73.

Mondal, L, Mukherjee, B, Das, K, Bhattacharya, S, Dutta, D, Chakraborty, S, Pal, MM, Gaonkar, RH & Debnath, MC (2019) CD-340 functionalized doxorubicin-loaded nanoparticle induces apoptosis and reduces tumor volume along with drug-related cardiotoxicity in mice. *Int J Nanomedicine,* 14, 8073-94.
[http://dx.doi.org/10.2147/IJN.S220740] [PMID: 31632019]

Mu, W, Jiang, D, Mu, S, Liang, S, Liu, Y & Zhang, N (2019) Promoting early diagnosis and precise therapy

of hepatocellular carcinoma by glypican-3-targeted synergistic chemo-photothermal theranostics. *ACS Appl Mater Interfaces,* 11, 23591-604.
[http://dx.doi.org/10.1021/acsami.9b05526] [PMID: 31179679]

Mukherjee, B, Engblom, J, Ho, PC & Karunaratne, V (2020) Editorial: Advances in Drug Formulation. *Front Pharmacol,* 11, 608771.
[http://dx.doi.org/10.3389/fphar.2020.608771] [PMID: 33390997]

Müller, R H, Gohla, S & Keck, C M (2011) State of the art of nanocrystals--special features, production, nanotoxicology aspects and intracellular delivery. *European journal of pharmaceutics and biopharmaceutics : official journal of Arbeitsgemeinschaft fur PharmazeutischeVerfahrenstechnike,* 78, 1-9.
[http://dx.doi.org/10.1016/j.ejpb.2011.01.007]

Murphy, SV & Atala, A (2014) 3D bioprinting of tissues and organs. *Nat Biotechnol,* 32, 773-85.
[http://dx.doi.org/10.1038/nbt.2958] [PMID: 25093879]

Murthy, SK (2007) Nanoparticles in modern medicine: state of the art and future challenges. *Int J Nanomedicine,* 2, 129-41.
[PMID: 17722542]

Muthu, MS, Leong, DT, Mei, L & Feng, SS (2014) Nanotheranostics - application and further development of nanomedicine strategies for advanced theranostics. *Theranostics,* 4, 660-77.
[http://dx.doi.org/10.7150/thno.8698] [PMID: 24723986]

Naidoo, C, Kruger, CA & Abrahamse, H (2018) Photodynamic therapy for metastatic melanoma treatment: a review. *Technol Cancer Res Treat,* 17, 1533033818791795.
[http://dx.doi.org/10.1177/1533033818791795] [PMID: 30099929]

Okamoto, I, Kawano, Y, Tsuiki, H, Sasaki, J, Nakao, M, Matsumoto, M, Suga, M, Ando, M, Nakajima, M & Saya, H (1999) CD44 cleavage induced by a membrane-associated metalloprotease plays a critical role in tumor cell migration. *Oncogene,* 18, 1435-46.
[http://dx.doi.org/10.1038/sj.onc.1202447] [PMID: 10050880]

Oldani, G, Lacotte, S, Orci, LA, Delaune, V, Slits, F, Gex, Q, Morel, P, Rubbia-Brandt, L & Toso, C (2016) Efficient nonarterialized mouse liver transplantation using 3-dimensional-printed instruments. *Liver Transpl,* 22, 1688-96.
[http://dx.doi.org/10.1002/lt.24637] [PMID: 27616447]

Olerile, LD, Liu, Y, Zhang, B, Wang, T, Mu, S, Zhang, J, Selotlegeng, L & Zhang, N (2017) Near-infrared mediated quantum dots and paclitaxel co-loaded nanostructured lipid carriers for cancer theragnostic. *Colloids Surf B Biointerfaces,* 150, 121-30.
[http://dx.doi.org/10.1016/j.colsurfb.2016.11.032] [PMID: 27907859]

Park, Y, Jeong, S & Kim, S (2017) Medically translatable quantum dots for biosensing and imaging. *J Photochem Photobiol Photochem Rev,* 30, 51-70.
[http://dx.doi.org/10.1016/j.jphotochemrev.2017.01.002]

Patra, JK, Das, G, Fraceto, LF, Campos, EVR, Rodriguez-Torres, MDP, Acosta-Torres, LS, Diaz-Torres, LA, Grillo, R, Swamy, MK, Sharma, S, Habtemariam, S & Shin, HS (2018) Nano based drug delivery systems: recent developments and future prospects. *J Nanobiotechnology,* 16, 71.
[http://dx.doi.org/10.1186/s12951-018-0392-8] [PMID: 30231877]

Pelaz, B, Alexiou, C, Alvarez-Puebla, RA, Alves, F, Andrews, AM, Ashraf, S, Balogh, LP, Ballerini, L, Bestetti, A, Brendel, C, Bosi, S, Carril, M, Chan, WC, Chen, C, Chen, X, Chen, X, Cheng, Z, Cui, D, Du, J, Dullin, C, Escudero, A, Feliu, N, Gao, M, George, M, Gogotsi, Y, Grünweller, A, Gu, Z, Halas, NJ, Hampp, N, Hartmann, RK, Hersam, MC, Hunziker, P, Jian, J, Jiang, X, Jungebluth, P, Kadhiresan, P, Kataoka, K, Khademhosseini, A, Kopeček, J, Kotov, NA, Krug, HF, Lee, DS, Lehr, CM, Leong, KW, Liang, XJ, Ling Lim, M, Liz-Marzán, LM, Ma, X, Macchiarini, P, Meng, H, Möhwald, H, Mulvaney, P, Nel, AE, Nie, S, Nordlander, P, Okano, T, Oliveira, J, Park, TH, Penner, RM, Prato, M, Puntes, V, Rotello, VM, Samarakoon, A, Schaak, RE, Shen, Y, Sjöqvist, S, Skirtach, AG, Soliman, MG, Stevens, MM, Sung, HW, Tang, BZ, Tietze, R, Udugama, BN, VanEpps, JS, Weil, T, Weiss, PS, Willner, I, Wu, Y, Yang, L, Yue, Z, Zhang, Q,

Zhang, Q, Zhang, XE, Zhao, Y, Zhou, X & Parak, WJ (2017) Diverse applications of nanomedicine. *ACS Nano,* 11, 2313-81.
[http://dx.doi.org/10.1021/acsnano.6b06040] [PMID: 28290206]

Pimenta, JR & Massabki, OS (2010) Hepatocellular carcinoma: a clinical outlook. *Rev Bras Clin Med,* 8, 59-67.

Pinheiro, M, Lúcio, M, Lima, JL & Reis, S (2011) Liposomes as drug delivery systems for the treatment of TB. *Nanomedicine (Lond),* 6, 1413-28.
[http://dx.doi.org/10.2217/nnm.11.122] [PMID: 22026379]

Praetorius, NP & Mandal, TK (2007) Engineered nanoparticles in cancer therapy. *Recent Pat Drug Deliv Formul,* 1, 37-51.
[http://dx.doi.org/10.2174/187221107779814104] [PMID: 19075873]

Prasad, M, Lambe, U P, Brar, B, Shah, I, J, M, Ranjan, K, Rao, R, Kumar, S, Mahant, S, Khurana, S K, Iqbal, H, Dhama, K, Misri, J & Prasad, G (2018) Nanotherapeutics: An insight into healthcare and multi-dimensional applications in medical sector of the modern world. *Biomedicine & pharmacotherapy = Biomedecine & pharmacotherapie,* 97, 1521-37.
[http://dx.doi.org/10.1016/j.biopha.2017.11.026]

Qi, L & Gao, X (2008) Emerging application of quantum dots for drug delivery and therapy. *Expert Opin Drug Deliv,* 5, 263-7.
[http://dx.doi.org/10.1517/17425247.5.3.263] [PMID: 18318649]

Sang, M, Luo, R, Bai, Y, Dou, J, Zhang, Z, Liu, F, Feng, F, Xu, J & Liu, W (2019) Mitochondrial membrane anchored photosensitive nano-device for lipid hydroperoxides burst and inducing ferroptosis to surmount therapy-resistant cancer. *Theranostics,* 9, 6209-23.
[http://dx.doi.org/10.7150/thno.36283] [PMID: 31534546]

Satapathy, BS, Mukherjee, B, Baishya, R, Debnath, MC, Dey, NS & Maji, R (2016) Lipid nanocarrier-based transport of docetaxel across the blood brain barrier. *RSC Advances,* 6, 85261-74.
[http://dx.doi.org/10.1039/C6RA16426A]

Schöffski, P, Gordon, M, Smith, DC, Kurzrock, R, Daud, A, Vogelzang, NJ, Lee, Y, Scheffold, C & Shapiro, GI (2017) Phase II randomised discontinuation trial of cabozantinib in patients with advanced solid tumours. *European journal of cancer (Oxford, England : 1990),* 86, 296-304.
[http://dx.doi.org/10.1016/j.ejca.2017.09.011]

Schroeder, A, Levins, CG, Cortez, C, Langer, R & Anderson, DG (2010) Lipid-based nanotherapeutics for siRNA delivery. *J Intern Med,* 267, 9-21.
[http://dx.doi.org/10.1111/j.1365-2796.2009.02189.x] [PMID: 20059641]

Shao, D, Li, J, Pan, Y, Zhang, X, Zheng, X, Wang, Z, Zhang, M, Zhang, H & Chen, L (2015) Noninvasive theranostic imaging of HSV-TK/GCV suicide gene therapy in liver cancer by folate-targeted quantum dot-based liposomes. *Biomater Sci,* 3, 833-41.
[http://dx.doi.org/10.1039/C5BM00077G] [PMID: 26221843]

Sharma, N, Mishra, S, Sharma, S, Deshpande, RD & Sharma, RK (2013) Preparation and optimization of nanoemulsions for targeting drug delivery. *Int J Drug Dev & Res,* 5, 37-48.

Shi, J, Votruba, AR, Farokhzad, OC & Langer, R (2010) Nanotechnology in drug delivery and tissue engineering: from discovery to applications. *Nano Lett,* 10, 3223-30.
[http://dx.doi.org/10.1021/nl102184c] [PMID: 20726522]

Singh, S, Asal, R & Bhagat, S (2018) Multifunctional antioxidant nanoliposome-mediated delivery of PTEN plasmids restore the expression of tumor suppressor protein and induce apoptosis in prostate cancer cells. *J Biomed Mater Res A,* 106, 3152-64.
[http://dx.doi.org/10.1002/jbm.a.36510] [PMID: 30194716]

Smith, L, Kuncic, Z, Ostrikov, K & Kumar, S (2012) Nanoparticles in cancer imaging and therapy. *J Nanomater,* 2012, 1-7.
[http://dx.doi.org/10.1155/2012/891318]

Srinivas, L, Manikanta, V & Jaswitha, M (2019) Protein and peptide drug delivery-A brief review. *Research Journal of Pharmacy and Technology,* 12, 1369.

Stewart, B (2014). *World Cancer Report 2014.* IARC Press, Lyon.

Sun, Y, Ma, W, Yang, Y, He, M, Li, A, Bai, L, Yu, B & Yu, Z (2019) Cancer nanotechnology: Enhancing tumor cell response to chemotherapy for hepatocellular carcinoma therapy. *Asian journal of pharmaceutical sciences,* 14, 581-94.
[http://dx.doi.org/10.1016/j.ajps.2019.04.005]

Tan, M & Wu, A (2016) Nanomaterials for tumor targeting theranostics: a proactive clinical perspective. World Scientific. *publishing company,* 73, 626-7.

Tang, H, Chen, D, Li, C, Zheng, C, Wu, X, Zhang, Y, Song, Q & Fei, W (2019) Dual GSH-exhausting sorafenib loaded manganese-silica nanodrugs for inducing the ferroptosis of hepatocellular carcinoma cells. *Int J Pharm,* 572, 118782.
[http://dx.doi.org/10.1016/j.ijpharm.2019.118782] [PMID: 31678528]

Tang, W, Chen, Z, Zhang, W, Cheng, Y, Zhang, B, Wu, F, Wang, Q, Wang, S, Rong, D, Reiter, FP, De Toni, EN & Wang, X (2020) The mechanisms of sorafenib resistance in hepatocellular carcinoma: theoretical basis and therapeutic aspects. *Signal Transduct Target Ther,* 5, 87.
[http://dx.doi.org/10.1038/s41392-020-0187-x] [PMID: 32532960]

Tao, Y, Wang, J & Xu, X (2020) Emerging and innovative theranostic approaches for mesoporous silica nanoparticles in hepatocellular carcinoma: current status and advances. *Front Bioeng Biotechnol,* 8, 184.
[http://dx.doi.org/10.3389/fbioe.2020.00184] [PMID: 32211399]

Tasnim, N, De la Vega, L, Anil Kumar, S, Abelseth, L, Alonzo, M, Amereh, M, Joddar, B & Willerth, SM (2018) 3D bioprinting stem cell derived tissues. *Cell Mol Bioeng,* 11, 219-40.
[http://dx.doi.org/10.1007/s12195-018-0530-2] [PMID: 31719887]

Thapa, RK, Choi, JY, Poudel, BK, Hiep, TT, Pathak, S, Gupta, B, Choi, HG, Yong, CS & Kim, JO (2015) Multilayer-coated liquid crystalline nanoparticles for effective sorafenib delivery to hepatocellular carcinoma. *ACS Appl Mater Interfaces,* 7, 20360-8.
[http://dx.doi.org/10.1021/acsami.5b06203] [PMID: 26315487]

Tran, TTD & Tran, PHL (2019) Nanoconjugation and encapsulation strategies for improving drug delivery and therapeutic efficacy of poorly water-soluble drugs. *Pharmaceutics,* 11, 325.
[http://dx.doi.org/10.3390/pharmaceutics11070325] [PMID: 31295947]

Tripathi, R & Kumar, A (2018) Application of nanorobotics for cancer treatment. *Mater Today Proc,* 5, 9114-7.
[http://dx.doi.org/10.1016/j.matpr.2017.10.029]

Tunissiolli, NM, Castanhole-Nunes, MMU, Biselli-Chicote, PM, Pavarino, EC, da Silva, RF, da Silva, RC & Goloni-Bertollo, EM (2017) Hepatocellular carcinoma: a comprehensive review of biomarkers, clinical aspects, and therapy. *APJCP,* 18, 863-72.
[PMID: 28545181]

Tunki, L, Kulhari, H, Vadithe, L N, Kuncha, M, Bhargava, S, Pooja, D & Sistla, R (2019)). Modulating the site-specific oral delivery of sorafenib using sugar-grafted nanoparticles for hepatocellular carcinoma treatment. *European journal of pharmaceutical sciences : official journal of the European Federation for Pharmaceutical Sciences,* 137, 104978.
[http://dx.doi.org/10.1016/j.ejps.2019.104978]

Tutar, Y (2020). *Advances in cancer nanotheranostics for experimental and personalized medicine.*Bentham Science Publishers.
[http://dx.doi.org/10.2174/97898114569161200101]

Valizadeh, A (2016) Nanomaterials and optical diagnosis of HIV. *Artif Cells Nanomed Biotechnol,* 44, 1383-90.
[http://dx.doi.org/10.3109/21691401.2015.1052469] [PMID: 26099718]

Venkatesan, M & Jolad, B (2010) Nanorobots in cancer treatment.*INTERACT-2010*.IEEE.
[http://dx.doi.org/10.1109/INTERACT.2010.5706154]

Ventola, C L (2017) Progress in nanomedicine: approved and investigational nanodrugs. *P & T : a peer-reviewed journal for formulary management,* 42, 742-55.

Wang, JL, Xi, Y, Liu, YL, Wang, ZH & Zhang, Q (2013) Combination of targeted PDT and anti-VEGF therapy for rat CNV by RGD-modified liposomal photocyanine and sorafenib. *Invest Ophthalmol Vis Sci,* 54, 7983-9.
[http://dx.doi.org/10.1167/iovs.13-13068] [PMID: 24204046]

Wang, JZ, Xiong, NY, Zhao, LZ, Hu, JT, Kong, DC & Yuan, JY (2018) Review fantastic medical implications of 3D-printing in liver surgeries, liver regeneration, liver transplantation and drug hepatotoxicity testing: A review. *Int J Surg,* 56, 1-6.
[http://dx.doi.org/10.1016/j.ijsu.2018.06.004] [PMID: 29886280]

Wege, H, Li, J & Ittrich, H (2019) Treatment lines in hepatocellular carcinoma. *Visc Med,* 35, 266-72.
[http://dx.doi.org/10.1159/000501749] [PMID: 31602390]

Weissig, V, Pettinger, TK & Murdock, N (2014) Nanopharmaceuticals (part 1): products on the market. *Int J Nanomedicine,* 9, 4357-73.
[http://dx.doi.org/10.2147/IJN.S46900] [PMID: 25258527]

Xiang, N, Fang, C, Fan, Y, Yang, J, Zeng, N, Liu, J & Zhu, W (2015) Application of liver three-dimensional printing in hepatectomy for complex massive hepatocarcinoma with rare variations of portal vein: preliminary experience. *Int J Clin Exp Med,* 8, 18873-8.
[PMID: 26770510]

Xiao, Y, Liu, Y, Yang, S, Zhang, B, Wang, T, Jiang, D, Zhang, J, Yu, D & Zhang, N (2016) Sorafenib and gadolinium co-loaded liposomes for drug delivery and MRI-guided HCC treatment. *Colloids Surf B Biointerfaces,* 141, 83-92.
[http://dx.doi.org/10.1016/j.colsurfb.2016.01.016] [PMID: 26844644]

Xiong, Q, Cui, M, Yu, G, Wang, J & Song, T (2018) Facile fabrication of reduction-responsive supramolecular nanoassemblies for co-delivery of doxorubicin and sorafenib toward hepatoma cells. *Front Pharmacol,* 9, 61.
[http://dx.doi.org/10.3389/fphar.2018.00061] [PMID: 29487523]

Yamamoto, Y, Matsui, J, Matsushima, T, Obaishi, H, Miyazaki, K, Nakamura, K, Tohyama, O, Semba, T, Yamaguchi, A, Hoshi, SS, Mimura, F, Haneda, T, Fukuda, Y, Kamata, JI, Takahashi, K, Matsukura, M, Wakabayashi, T, Asada, M, Nomoto, KI, Watanabe, T, Dezso, Z, Yoshimatsu, K, Funahashi, Y & Tsuruoka, A (2014) Lenvatinib, an angiogenesis inhibitor targeting VEGFR/FGFR, shows broad antitumor activity in human tumor xenograft models associated with microvessel density and pericyte coverage. *Vasc Cell,* 6, 18.
[http://dx.doi.org/10.1186/2045-824X-6-18] [PMID: 25197551]

Yang, T, Ming, X, Jie, L, Wei, W, Guangliang, H, Manxia, L, Huanling, G, Xiangzi, S, Chunyang, Z, Bai, L, Dan, W, Zhong, C & Xiaoyan, X (2019) Ultrasound-triggered nanodroplets for targeted co-delivery of sorafenib/doxorubicin for hepatocellular carcinoma therapy. *J Biomed Nanotechnol,* 15, 1881-96.
[http://dx.doi.org/10.1166/jbn.2019.2823] [PMID: 31387676]

Ye, H, Zhou, L, Jin, H, Chen, Y, Cheng, D & Jiang, Y (2020) Sorafenib-loaded long-circulating nanoliposomes for liver cancer therapy. *BioMed Res Int,* 2020, 1351046.
[http://dx.doi.org/10.1155/2020/1351046] [PMID: 32461962]

Yetisgin, AA, Cetinel, S, Zuvin, M, Kosar, A & Kutlu, O (2020) Therapeutic nanoparticles and their targeted delivery applications. *Molecules,* 25, 2193.
[http://dx.doi.org/10.3390/molecules25092193] [PMID: 32397080]

Yih, TC & Al-Fandi, M (2006) Engineered nanoparticles as precise drug delivery systems. *J Cell Biochem,* 97, 1184-90.
[http://dx.doi.org/10.1002/jcb.20796] [PMID: 16440317]

Yu, Z, Schmaltz, RM, Bozeman, TC, Paul, R, Rishel, MJ, Tsosie, KS & Hecht, SM (2013) Selective tumor cell targeting by the disaccharide moiety of bleomycin. *J Am Chem Soc,* 135, 2883-6.
[http://dx.doi.org/10.1021/ja311090e] [PMID: 23379863]

Zalba, S, Contreras, AM, Haeri, A, Ten Hagen, TL, Navarro, I, Koning, G & Garrido, MJ (2015) Cetuximab-oxaliplatin-liposomes for epidermal growth factor receptor targeted chemotherapy of colorectal cancer. *Journal of controlled release : official journal of the Controlled Release Society,* 210, 26-38.
[http://dx.doi.org/10.1016/j.jconrel.2015.05.271]

Zare Kazemabadi, F, Heydarinasab, A, Akbarzadeh, A & Ardjmand, M (2019) Preparation, characterization and *in vitro* evaluation of PEGylated nanoliposomal containing etoposide on lung cancer. *Artif Cells Nanomed Biotechnol,* 47, 3222-30.
[http://dx.doi.org/10.1080/21691401.2019.1646265] [PMID: 31373225]

Zhai, B & Sun, XY (2013) Mechanisms of resistance to sorafenib and the corresponding strategies in hepatocellular carcinoma. *World J Hepatol,* 5, 345-52.
[http://dx.doi.org/10.4254/wjh.v5.i7.345] [PMID: 23898367]

Zhang, L, Gong, F, Zhang, F, Ma, J, Zhang, P & Shen, J (2013) Targeted therapy for human hepatic carcinoma cells using folate-functionalized polymeric micelles loaded with superparamagnetic iron oxide and sorafenib *in vitro. Int J Nanomedicine,* 8, 1517-24.
[http://dx.doi.org/10.2147/IJN.S43263] [PMID: 23620667]

Zhang, D, Wu, M, Zeng, Y, Wu, L, Wang, Q, Han, X, Liu, X & Liu, J (2015) Chlorin e6 Conjugated Poly(dopamine) Nanospheres as PDT/PTT Dual-Modal Therapeutic Agents for Enhanced Cancer Therapy. *ACS Appl Mater Interfaces,* 7, 8176-87.
[http://dx.doi.org/10.1021/acsami.5b01027] [PMID: 25837008]

Zhao, C, Tong, Y, Li, X, Shao, L, Chen, L, Lu, J, Deng, X, Wang, X & Wu, Y (2018) Photosensitive Nanoparticles Combining Vascular-Independent Intratumor Distribution and On-Demand Oxygen-Depot Delivery for Enhanced Cancer Photodynamic Therapy. *Small (Weinheim an der Bergstrasse, Germany),* 14, e1703045.
[http://dx.doi.org/10.1002/smll.201703045]

Zhou, Y, Du, J, Wang, L & Wang, Y (2017) Nanocrystals Technology for Improving Bioavailability of Poorly Soluble Drugs: A Mini-Review. *J Nanosci Nanotechnol,* 17, 18-28.
[http://dx.doi.org/10.1166/jnn.2017.13108] [PMID: 29616786]

Zhou, Y, Yang, J, Rhim, J S & Kopeček, J (2013) HPMA copolymer-based combination therapy toxic to both prostate cancer stem/progenitor cells and differentiated cells induces durable anti-tumor effects. Journal of controlled release *official journal of the Controlled Release Society,* 172, 946-53.
[http://dx.doi.org/10.1016/j.jconrel.2013.09.005]

Zhu, AX, Finn, RS, Edeline, J, Cattan, S, Ogasawara, S, Palmer, D, Verslype, C, Zagonel, V, Fartoux, L, Vogel, A, Sarker, D, Verset, G, Chan, SL, Knox, J, Daniele, B, Webber, AL, Ebbinghaus, SW, Ma, J, Siegel, AB, Cheng, AL & Kudo, M (2018) Pembrolizumab in patients with advanced hepatocellular carcinoma previously treated with sorafenib (KEYNOTE-224): a non-randomised, open-label phase 2 trial. *Lancet Oncol,* 19, 940-52.
[http://dx.doi.org/10.1016/S1470-2045(18)30351-6] [PMID: 29875066]

Zhu, L & Chen, L (2019) Progress in research on paclitaxel and tumor immunotherapy. *Cell Mol Biol Lett,* 24, 40.
[http://dx.doi.org/10.1186/s11658-019-0164-y] [PMID: 31223315]

Zrazhevskiy, P, Sena, M & Gao, X (2010) Designing multifunctional quantum dots for bioimaging, detection, and drug delivery. *Chem Soc Rev,* 39, 4326-54.
[http://dx.doi.org/10.1039/b915139g] [PMID: 20697629]

SUBJECT INDEX

A

B

C

D

E

F

G

H

I

K

L

M

N

O

P

R

S

U

V

W

Z

Made in the USA
Las Vegas, NV
03 November 2026

57424412R00331